The 5-Minute Infectious Diseases Consult

ASSOCIATE EDITORS

ELEFTHERIOS MYLONAKIS, M.D.
HOWARD HUGHES PHYSICIAN
POSTDOCTORAL FELLOW IN MEDICINE
MASSACHUSETTS GENERAL HOSPITAL
HARVARD UNIVERSITY
BOSTON, MASSACHUSETTS

DAVID R. STONE, M.D.
ASSISTANT PROFESSOR OF MEDICINE
TUFTS UNIVERSITY SCHOOL OF MEDICINE
PHYSICIAN
GEOGRAPHIC MEDICINE AND INFECTIOUS DISEASE
NEW ENGLAND MEDICAL CENTER AND LEMUEL SHATTUCK HOSPITAL
BOSTON, MASSACHUSETTS

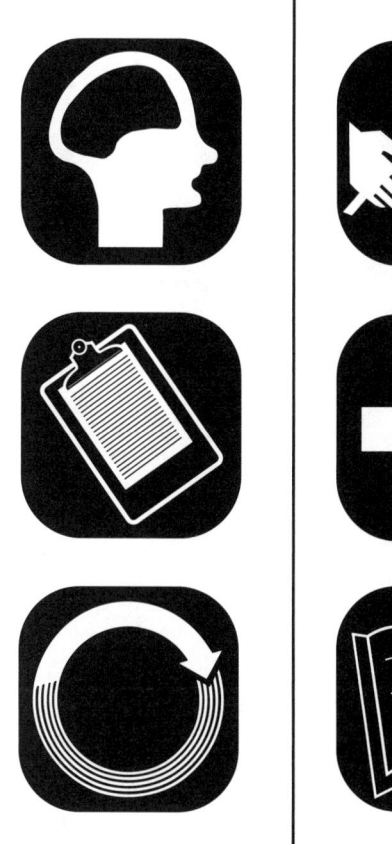

The 5-Minute Infectious Diseases Consult

EDITORS

SHERWOOD L. GORBACH, M.D.

PROFESSOR OF COMMUNITY HEALTH AND MEDICINE

TUFTS UNIVERSITY SCHOOL OF MEDICINE

BOSTON, MASSACHUSETTS

MATTHEW FALAGAS, M.D., MSc

ADJUNCT ASSISTANT PROFESSOR OF MEDICINE

TUFTS UNIVERSITY SCHOOL OF MEDICINE

BOSTON, MASSACHUSETTS

INFECTIOUS DISEASES CONSULTANT

HYGEIA HOSPITAL

ATHENS, GREECE

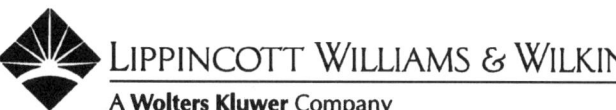

A **Wolters Kluwer** Company

Philadelphia • Baltimore • New York • London
Buenos Aires • Hong Kong • Sydney • Tokyo

Acquisitions Editor: Jonathan W. Pine, Jr.
Developing Editor: Joyce A. Murphy
Supervising Editor: Steven P. Martin
Manufacturing Manager: Benjamin Rivera
Production Service: Colophon
Cover Designer: Christine Jenny
Compositor: TechBooks
Printer: R. R. Donnelly Willard

The 5 Minute Logo is a registered trademark of Lippincott Williams & Wilkins. This mark may not be used without written permission from the publisher.

© 2001 by LIPPINCOTT WILLIAMS & WILKINS. This book is protected by copyright. No part of this book may be reproduced in any form or by any means, including photocopying, or utilized by any information storage and retrieval system without written permission from the copyright owner, except for brief quotations embodied in critical articles and reviews. Materials appearing in this book prepared by individuals as part of their official duties as U.S. government employees are not covered by the above-mentioned copyright.

Printed in the USA

Library of Congress Cataloging-in-Publication Data

The 5 minute infectious diseases consult / editors, Sherwood L. Gorbach, Matthew
   Falagas ; associate editors, Eleftherios Mylonakis, David R. Stone.
       p. ; cm.
    Includes bibliographical references and index.
    ISBN 0-683-30736-3 (alk. paper)
       1. Communicable diseases—Handbooks, manuals, etc.   I. title: Five minute infectious
    diseases consult.   II. Gorbach, Sherwood L., 1934–
       [DNLM: 1. Communicable diseases—Handbooks.   WC 39 Z999 2001]
    RC122 .A15 2001
    616.9—dc21   2001029911

Care has been taken to confirm the accuracy of the information presented and to describe generally accepted practices. However, the authors, editors, and publisher are not responsible for errors or omissions or for any consequences from application of the information in this book and make no warranty, express or implied, with respect to the currency, completeness, or accuracy of the contents of the publication. Application of this information in a particular situation remains the professional responsibility of the practitioner.

The authors, editors, and publisher have exerted every effort to ensure that drug selection and dosage set forth in this text are in accordance with current recommendations and practice at the time of publication. However, in view of ongoing research, changes in government regulations, and the constant flow of information relating to drug therapy and drug reactions, the reader is urged to check the package insert for each drug for any change in indications and dosage and for added warnings and precautions. This is particularly important when the recommended agent is a new or infrequently employed drug.

Some drugs and medical devices presented in this publication have Food and Drug Administration (FDA) clearance for limited use in restricted research settings. It is the responsibility of the health care provider to ascertain the FDA status of each drug or device planned for use in their clinical practice.

10 9 8 7 6 5 4 3 2 1

To my wife, Judy, who has supported me in this work, and to my students and colleagues, who provided the inspiration for our efforts

    Sherwood L. Gorbach

To my wife, Vana

    Matthew Falagas

To my family, parents, and teachers

    Eleftherios Mylonakis

To my wife Marguerite and my children Alex, Sam, and Sophia

    David R. Stone

Preface

Managing infectious diseases is practicing "Medicine of the Possible." Most of the common infections are treatable by anti-infective drugs or have a self-limited course that can be ameliorated by symptomatic therapy. Upon making a diagnosis and instituting treatment, both the patient and the physician are generally assured a favorable outcome. While this homily is widely accepted, the "devil is in the details." The correct diagnosis must be established, usually on clinical grounds by a careful history and physical exam. If indicated, the proper laboratory tests must be obtained. And last, but certainly not least from the patient's perspective, effective treatment must be applied. What this book provides is a quick and ready reference for most of the infections seen in medical practice, with expert guidance on these critical issues—clinical diagnosis, laboratory tests, and appropriate therapy. While key articles are provided for more detailed study, the main need that is served by this book is for a brief, easily-digested source of critical information that can be applied instantly in managing infection.

Current trends in the United States indicate that infectious diseases account for about 20% of visits to a doctor's office or an emergency room, a minimum of 150 million visits each year. In the past 20 years the death rate from infectious diseases has increased along with an increase in the proportion of hospitalizations for these illnesses. These figures do not take into account the added burden of patients with human immunodeficiency virus (HIV) infection, which has risen in recent years. Despite advances in antimicrobial agents, vaccines, and preventive medicine, infection continues to exact significant morbidity and mortality on all stratum of our population, with its greatest impact on the young, the old, and the infirm.

"Medicine of the Possible" means that physicians and healthcare workers can make a substantial difference in improving the outcome of a patient with an infectious disease by applying the correct principles of good diagnosis and judicious treatment. Many illnesses in medicine are chronic and unrelenting conditions which can be improved but not necessarily cured by treatment. On the other hand, most infections are transient interruptions in the course of life which, if managed properly, can pass without significant damage to the fabric of one's existence. The authors of this book have tried to provide guidance to manage infectious diseases, thereby relieving the patient's misery and giving physicians the satisfaction of performing their sacred calling of curing disease and relieving suffering.

Sherwood L. Gorbach, M.D.
Matthew Falagas, M.D.
Eleftherios Mylonakis, M.D.
David R. Stone, M.D.

Contents

Preface / vii

SECTION I: CHIEF COMPLAINTS

Abdominal Pain and Fever / 2–5
Animal/Human Bite Infections, Including Clenched-Fist Injuries / 6–7
Atypical Lymphocytosis / 8–9
Back Pain and Fever / 10–11
Cough and Fever / 12–13
Diarrhea and Fever / 14–15
Dysuria / 16–17
Ear Pain / 18–19
Fever of Unknown Origin / 20–21
Genital Lesions / 22–23
Hepatosplenomegaly and Fever / 24–25
Insect Bites and Stings / 26–27
Jaundice and Fever / 28–29
Joint Pain and Fever / 30–31
Lymph Node Enlargement and Fever / 32–33
Neurologic Symptoms/Signs and Fever / 34–35
Pancytopenia and Fever / 36–37
Pleural Effusion and Fever / 38–39
Pleuritic and Chest Pain and Fever / 40–41
Postoperative Fever / 42–43
Rash and Fever / 44–45
Red Eye / 46–47
Rhinorrhea / 48–49
Sepsis Syndrome / 50–51
Sexual Assault / 52–53
Sore Throat / 54–55
Trauma-related Infections / 56–57
Urethritis and Urethral Discharge / 58–59
Vaginal Discharge/Vaginitis / 60–61

SECTION II: SPECIFIC INFECTIONS AND DISEASES

Acne Vulgaris / 64–65
Actinomycosis / 66–67
Adenovirus Infections / 68–69
Amebiasis / 70–71
Anaerobic Infections / 72–73
Anorectal Infections / 74–75
Anthrax / 76–77
Antibiotic- and *Clostridium difficile*-associated Diarrhea and Colitis / 78–79
Appendicitis / 80–81
Aspergillosis / 82–83
Atypical Mycobacteria / 84–85
Babesiosis / 86–87
Bacillary Angiomatosis/Peliosis Hepatica / 88–89
Bacterial Vaginosis / 90–91
Balanitis / 92–93
Bartonellosis (Oroya Fever and Verruga Peruana) / 94–95
Bell's Palsy / 96–97
Blastomycosis / 98–99
Blepharitis and Chalazion / 100–101
Botulism / 102–103
Brain Abscess / 104–105
Bronchiolitis / 106–107
Bronchitis / 108–109
Brucellosis / 110–111
Bursitis / 112–113
Campylobacter Infections / 114–115
Candida Vaginitis / 116–117
Candidiasis / 118–119
Cat-Scratch Disease / 120–121
Cervicitis/Mucopurulent Cervicitis (MCP) / 122–123
Chancroid / 124–125
Chickenpox / 126–127
Cholecystitis/Cholangitis / 128–129
Cholera / 130–131
Chorioretinitis (Uveitis and Retinitis) / 132–133
Chronic Fatigue Syndrome / 134–135
Coccidioidomycosis / 136–137
Common Cold / 138–139
Conjunctivitis / 140–141
Creutzfeldt-Jakob Disease / 142–143
Cryptococcal Infections / 144–145
Cryptosporidiosis / 146–147
Cysticercosis / 148–149
Cystitis / 150–151
Cytomegalovirus Infections / 152–153
Dengue / 154–155
Diphtheria / 156–157
Diverticulitis / 158–159
Echinococcosis / 160–161
Ehrlichiosis / 162–163
Encephalitis / 164–165
Endocarditis, Native Valves / 166–167

Endocarditis, Prosthetic Valves / 168–169
Endophthalmitis / 170–171
Epidemic Pleurodynia (Bornholm Disease) / 172–173
Epididymitis / 174–175
Epidural Abscess / 176–177
Epiglottitis / 178–179
Escherichia coli Infections / 180–181
Esophagitis, Infective / 182–183
Exanthem Subitum / 184–185
Filariasis / 186–187
Food-borne Diseases / 188–189
Fungal Infections of the Hair, Nails, and Skin / 190–191
Gas Gangrene / 192–193
Genital Herpes / 194–195
Giardiasis / 196–197
Gingivitis / 198–199
Granuloma Inguinale (Donovanosis) / 200–201
Hantavirus Pulmonary Syndrome / 202–203
Helicobacter pylori Infection / 204–205
Hemolytic-Uremic Syndrome and Enterohemorrhagic Escherichia coli Infection / 206–207
Hepatitis / 208–209
Herpes Simplex Virus Infections / 210–211
Herpes Zoster / 212–213
Histoplasmosis / 214–217
HIV Infection and AIDS / 218–221
Infectious Mononucleosis / 222–223
Influenza / 224–225
Intraabdominal Abscesses / 226–227
Kaposi's Sarcoma / 228–229
Kawasaki Syndrome / 230–231
Keratitis / 232–233
Larva Migrans Syndromes / 234–235
Laryngitis/Laryngotracheobronchitis (Croup) / 236–237
Legionnaires' Disease / 238–239
Leishmaniasis / 240–241
Leprosy / 242–243
Leptospirosis / 244–245
Lice / 246–247
Listeriosis / 248–249
Lung Abscess / 250–251
Lyme Disease / 252–253
Lymphangitis / 254–255
Lymphogranuloma Venereum / 256–257
Malaria / 258–259
Mastitis / 260–261
Mastoiditis / 262–263
Measles / 264–265
Mediastinitis / 266–267
Meningitis, Acute / 268–269
Meningitis, Chronic / 270–271

Mesenteric Adenitis / 272–273
Mites/Chiggers / 274–275
Mucormycosis / 276–277
Mumps / 278–279
Mycotic Aneurysms / 280–281
Myelitis / 282–283
Myocarditis / 284–285
Myositis / 286–287
Necrotizing Skin and Soft-Tissue Infections / 288–289
Neuritis / 290–291
Nocardiosis / 292–295
Nontyphoidal *Salmonella* Infections / 296–297
Odontogenic Infections / 298–299
Orchitis / 300–301
Osteomyelitis / 302–303
Otitis Externa / 304–305
Otitis Media / 306–307
Parvovirus Infections / 308–309
Pelvic Inflammatory Disease / 310–311
Pericarditis / 312–313
Peritonitis / 314–315
Pertussis / 316–317
Pharyngitis/Tonsillitis / 318–321
Pilonidal Abscess / 322–323
Plague / 324–325
Pneumocystis carinii Infection / 326–327
Pneumonia / 328–329
Poliomyelitis / 330–331
Progressive Multifocal Leukoencephalopathy / 332–333
Prostatitis / 334–335
Pseudomonas Infections/Melioidosis/Glanders / 336–337
Psittacosis / 338–339
Pyelonephritis / 340–341
Q Fever / 342–343
Rabies / 344–345
Relapsing Fever / 346–347
Respiratory Syncytial Virus Infection / 348–349
Rheumatic Fever / 350–351
Rocky Mountain Spotted Fever / 352–353
Roundworms, Intestinal / 354–355
Rubella (German Measles) / 356–357
Scabies / 358–359
Scarlet Fever / 360–361
Schistosomiasis / 362–363
Septic Arthritis / 364–365
Shigellosis / 366–367
Sinusitis / 368–371
Sporotrichosis / 372–373
Stomatitis / 374–375
Strongyloidiasis / 376–377
Superficial Skin and Soft-Tissue Infections / 378–379

Surgical Site Infections (Surgical Wound Infections) / 380–381
Syphilis / 382–383
Tetanus / 384–385
Thrombophlebitis, Suppurative / 386–387
Thyroiditis, Infectious / 388–389
Toxic Shock Syndrome / 390–391
Toxoplasmosis / 392–393
Trachoma and Inclusion Conjunctivitis / 394–395
Traveler's Diarrhea / 396–397
Trichinosis / 398–399
Trichomoniasis / 400–401
Trypanosomiasis / 402–403
Tuberculosis / 404–405
Tularemia / 406–407
Typhoid Fever / 408–409
Typhus / 410–411
Uveitis. See Chorioretinitis
Warts / 412–413
Yellow Fever / 414–415
Yersinia enterocolitica Infections / 416–417

SECTION III: MICROORGANISMS

Absidia corymbifera / 420
Acanthamoeba Species / 420
Acinetobacter Species / 420
Acremonium Species / 421
Actinobacillus Species / 421
Actinomadura Species / 421
Actinomyces Species / 421
Aeromonas Species / 421
Afipia Species / 422
Agrobacterium radiobacter / 422
Alcaligenes Species / 422
Alphavirus / 422
Alternaria Species / 423
Anaerobiospirillum / 423
Ancylostoma / 423
Angiostrongylus Species / 424
Anisakis Species / 424
Apophysomyces elegans / 424
Arcanobacterium Species / 424
Arenaviral Hemorrhagic Fevers in South America / 425
Ascaris lumbricoides / 425
Aspergillus Species / 425
Aureobasidium pullulans / 425
Babesia Species / 425
Bacillus Species / 426
Bacteroides Species / 426

Balantidium coli / 427
Bartonella bacilliformis / 427
Bartonella (Rochalimaea) henselae / 427
Bartonella (Rochalimaea) quintana / 427
Basidiobolus ranarum / 427
Baylisascaris procyonis / 428
Bilophila wadsworthia / 428
Bipolaris Species / 428
Blastocystis hominis / 428
Blastomyces dermatitidis / 428
Blastoschizomyces capitatus / 429
Bordetella bronchiseptica / 429
Bordetella Species / 429
Borrelia burgdorferi / 429
Borrelia Species / 429
Brucella Species / 429
Brugia Species / 430
Burkholderia (Pseudomonas) mallei / 430
Burkholderia (Pseudomonas) pseudomallei / 430
Burkholderia (Pseudomonas) Species / 430
Caliciviruses and Calici-like Viruses / 431
Calymmatobacterium granulomatis / 431
Campylobacter Species / 431
Candida Species / 431
Capillaria Species / 431
Capnocytophaga Species / 431
Chlamydia Species / 432
Chromobacterium violaceum / 432
Chromomycosis Agents / 432
Chryseomonas luteola / 432
Chrysosporium parvum / 433
Citrobacter Species / 433
Clonorchis sinensis (Opisthorchis sinensis) / 433
Clostridium botulinum / 433
Clostridium difficile / 433
Clostridium Species / 433
Clostridium tetani / 434
Coccidioides immitis / 434
Colorado Tick Fever Virus / 434
Comamonas Species / 434
Conidiobolus Species / 434
Coronavirus / 435
Corynebacterium diphtheriae / 435
Corynebacterium jeikeium / 435
Corynebacterium minutissimum / 435
Corynebacterium pseudotuberculosis / 435
Corynebacterium Species / 436
Corynebacterium urealyticum / 436
Coxiella burnetii / 436
Coxsackievirus / 436
Crimean-Congo Hemorrhagic Fever Virus / 436

Cryptococcus neoformans / 436
Cryptosporidium parvum / 436
Cunninghamella bertholetiae / 437
Curvularia Species / 437
Cyclospora cayatanensis / 437
Cytomegalovirus / 437
Dengue Virus / 438
Dermatobia hominis / 438
Dicrocoelium dendriticum / 438
Dientamoeba fragilis / 438
Diphyllobothrium Species / 438
Dipylidium caninum / 439
Dirofilaria Species / 439
Dracunculus medinensis / 439
Ebola-Marburg Viral Diseases / 439
Echinococcus Species / 439
Echinostoma ilocanum / 440
Echovirus / 440
Edwardsiella tarda / 440
Ehrlichia Species / 440
Eikenella corrodens / 440
Emmonsia parva / 441
Encephalitis Viruses of the Flaviviridae Family / 441
Endolimax nana / 441
Entamoeba histolytica / 441
Entamoeba Species / 441
Enterobacter Species / 442
Enterobius vermicularis / 442
Enterococcus Species / 442
Enterocytozoon bieneusi / 442
Enterovirus / 443
Epidermophyton floccosum / 443
Epstein-Barr Virus / 443
Erysipelothrix rhusiopathiae / 443
Escherichia coli / 443
Eubacterium Species / 443
Ewingella americana / 444
Exophiala Species / 444
Fasciola Species / 444
Fasciolopsis buski / 444
Flavimonas oryzihabitans / 445
Flavobacterium / 445
Fonsecaea Species / 445
Francisella tularensis / 445
Fusarium Species / 445
Fusobacterium Species / 445
Gardnerella vaginalis / 446
Gemella Species / 446
Geotrichum candidum / 446
Giardia lamblia / 446
Gnathostoma spinigerum / 446

Haemophilus ducreyi / 447
Haemophilus influenzae / 447
Haemophilus Species / 447
Hafnia alvei / 447
Hansenula Species / 448
Hantaan Virus / 448
Helicobacter Species / 448
Hendersonula toruloidea / 448
Hepatitis Viruses / 448
Herpes Simplex Virus Type 1 and 2 / 448
Human Herpesvirus Type 6 / 448
Human Herpesvirus Type 8 / 449
Herpes Zoster Virus / 449
Heterophyes heterophyes / 449
Hymenolepsis Species / 449
Hypoderma Species / 449
Influenza A, B, and C Virus / 449
Isospora belli / 449
Junin Virus (Argentine Hemorrhagic Fever) / 449
Kingella Species / 450
Klebsiella Species / 450
Kluyvera Species / 450
Kurthia Species / 450
Kyasanur Forest Disease Virus / 451
Lactobacillus Species / 451
Lassa Virus / 451
Leclercia adecarbxylata / 451
Legionella Species / 451
Leishmania Species Complex / 451
Leptomyxid Species / 452
Leptospira Species / 452
Leuconostoc Species / 452
Linguatula serrata / 452
Listeria monocytogenes / 452
Loa loa / 452
Lymphocytic Choriomeningitis Virus / 453
Lymphotropic T-Cell Human Virus / 453
Machupo Virus (Bolivian Hemorrhagic Fever) / 454
Madurella Species / 454
Malassezia Species / 454
Mansonella Species / 454
Marburg Virus / 454
Measles Virus / 454
Metagonimus yokogawai / 455
Methylobacterium Species / 455
Microsporidia / 455
Microsporum Species / 455
Mobiluncus Species / 456
Molluscum contagiosum Virus / 456
Moraxella (Branhamella) Species / 456
Morganella morganii / 456

Mucor Species / 456
Muerto Canyon Virus / 456
Multiceps multiceps / 457
Mumps Virus / 457
Myiasis Agents / 457
Mycobacterium, Atypical / 457
Mycobacterium bovis / 457
Mycobacterium leprae / 457
Mycobacterium tuberculosis / 457
Mycoplasma Species / 457
Myiasis Agents / 458
Naegleria fowleri / 458
Nanophyetus salmincola / 458
Necator americanus / 458
Neisseria gonorrhoeae / 458
Neisseria meningitidis / 458
Neisseria Species / 459
Nocardia Species / 459
Norwalk Virus / 459
Nosema Species / 459
Ochrobactrum anthropi / 459
Oerskovia Species / 459
Oligella Species / 460
Omsk Virus (Hemorrhagic Fever) / 460
Onchocerca volvulus / 460
Opisthorchis Species / 460
ORF Virus / 460
Paecilomyces Species / 461
Pantoea agglomerans / 461
Papillomavirus / 461
Paracoccidioides brasiliensis / 461
Paragonimus Species / 462
Parainfluenza Virus / 462
Parvovirus B-19 / 462
Pasteurella Species / 463
Pediculus and *Phthirus* Species (Lice) / 463
Pediococcus Species / 464
Penicillium Species / 464
Peptococcus niger / 464
Peptostreptococcus Species / 465
Phialophora Species / 465
Phthirus pubis / 465
Piedraia hortae / 465
Plasmodium Species / 465
Pleistophora Species / 465
Plesiomonas shigelloides / 466
Pneumocystis carinii / 466
Poliomyelitis Virus / 466
Polyomaviruses / 466
Porphyromonas Species / 466
Prevotella Species / 466

Prions / 467
Propionibacterium propionicus / 467
Propionibacterium Species / 467
Proteus Species / 467
Protomonas Species / 467
Prototheca Species / 467
Providencia Species / 468
Pseudallescheria boydii / 468
Pseudomonas aeruginosa / 468
Psychrobacter immobilis / 468
Rabies Virus / 469
Respiratory Syncytial Virus / 469
Rhinocladiella aquaspersa / 469
Rhinosporidium seeberi / 469
Rhinovirus / 469
Rhizomucor Species / 469
Rhizopus Species / 469
Rhodococcus Species / 470
Rhodotorula Species / 470
Rickettsia Species / 470
Rotavirus, Human / 471
Rothia dentocariosa / 471
Rubella Virus / 471
Saccharomyces cerevisiae / 472
Saksenaea vasiformis / 472
Salmonella Species / 472
Sarcocystis Species / 472
Sarcoptes scabiei / 472
Scedosporium prolificans / 472
Schistosoma Species / 472
Scopulariopsis Species / 473
Septata intestinalis / 473
Serratia Species / 473
Shigella Species / 473
Smallpox Virus / 474
Sphingobacterium Species / 474
Spirillum minus (minor) / 474
Spirometra Species / 474
Sporobolomyces Species / 474
Sporothrix schenckii / 474
Staphylococcus Species / 475
Stenotrophomonas Species / 475
Stomatococcus mucilaginosus / 475
Streptobacillus moniliformis / 476
Streptococcus agalactiae (Group B) / 476
Streptococcus pneumoniae / 476
Streptococcus pyogenes (Group A β-Hemolytic Streptococcus) / 476
Strongyloides Species / 476
Taenia saginata / 476
Taenia solium / 476

Toxocara Species / 477
Toxoplasma gondii / 477
Treponema carateum / 477
Treponema pallidum / 477
Trichinella spiralis / 477
Trichomonas vaginalis / 477
Trichophyton Species / 477
Trichosporon beigelii / 478
Trichostrongylus Species / 478
Trichuris trichiura / 478
Tropheryma whippelii / 478
Trypanosoma Species / 478
Tunga penetrans / 479
Ureaplasma urealyticum / 479
Varicella Zoster Virus / 479
Veillonella parvula / 479
Vibrio cholerae / 479
Vibrio Species / 480
Weeksella Species / 480
Wohlfahrtia magnifica / 480
Wuchereia bancrofti / 480
Yellow Fever Virus / 480
Yersinia pestis / 480
Yersinia Species / 480

SECTION IV: DRUGS AND VACCINES

Table 1a. Adverse Reactions to Antimicrobial Agents / 482–483

Table 1b. Reported Percentage Frequency of Selected Adverse Effects after Oral Administration of Antibacterial Drugs in Different Studies / 484–485
Table 1c. Selected Drug-Drug Interactions Involving an Oral Antibacterial Agent / 486
Table 2a. Antimicrobial Dosing Regimens in Renal Failure / 487–488
Table 2b. Drug Therapy Dosing Guidelines / 489–493
Table 3. Antimicrobial Dosing Regimens in Severe Liver Disease / 494
Table 4. Guidelines for Adult Immunizations / 495–497
Table 5. Guidelines for Childhood Immunizations / 498–499
Table 6. Vaccines Available in the United States by Type and Recommended Routes of Administration / 500–501
Table 7a. Vaccines in the Immunocompromised Host / 502
Table 7b. Summary of Recommendations on Nonroutine Immunization of Immunocompromised Persons / 503
Table 8a. Characteristics, Activity, and Adverse Effects of Immunoglobulins / 504
Table 8b. Use of Vaccines and Immunoglobulins / 505–508
Table 9a. Prophylaxis of Endocarditis / 509–510
Table 9b. Prophylactic Regimens for Dental, Respiratory Tract, or Esophageal Procedures / 511
Table 9c. Prophylactic Regimens for Genitourinary and Gastrointestinal (Excluding Esophageal) Procedures / 512
Table 10. Trade Names of Antimicrobial Agents / 513–514
Table 11. Prevention of Travel-related Illness / 515–521

Index / 523

SECTION I
Chief Complaints

Abdominal Pain and Fever

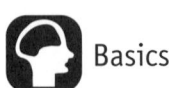 Basics

DEFINITION
This chapter examines the causes of temperature elevation that are accompanied by abdominal pain.

APPROACH TO THE PATIENT
- In evaluating patients with abdominal pain and fever, the first decision concerns whether the patient requires immediate surgical treatment.
- Patients with catastrophic abdominal infections can present with low or no fever and limited abdominal pain. This is more common among neonates, the elderly, immunocompromised patients, patients with overwhelming sepsis, and patients with renal failure.
- The physician needs to clarify quickly the severity, onset, and characteristics of the symptoms; check the vital signs; and perform a thorough physical examination.
- The physical examination should include, in addition to the meticulous abdominal examination, evaluation of the characteristics of the fever and pulse and evaluation of skin, eyes, oral cavity, oropharynx, lymph nodes, and chest.
- Rectal examination should be performed, unless the patient is severely neutropenic (in which case, clinicians should perform careful inspection and further testing as needed).

ETIOLOGY

Infectious Causes of Abdominal Pain
The most common infectious causes of abdominal pain are the following:

- Right upper quadrant pain: acute cholecystitis, hepatitis, pyelonephritis, pneumonia, liver abscess, and perforation of the gallbladder with bile ascites
- Left upper quadrant pain: pyelonephritis, pneumonia, and splenic abscess
- Epigastric pain: diverticulitis, appendicitis (early phase), peritonitis (primary, secondary, tuberculous), acute gastroenteritis, pancreatic abscess, Crohn's disease, ulcerative colitis, and colitis due to *Clostridium difficile*
- Right lower quadrant pain: appendicitis, salpingitis, psoas abscess, mesenteric adenitis, pelvic inflammatory disease, and bowel perforation
- Left lower quadrant pain: diverticulitis, salpingitis, abscess involving the psoas muscle, mesenteric adenitis, pelvic infection, and bowel perforation

Noninfectious Causes of Abdominal Pain
The most common noninfectious causes of abdominal pain are the following:

- Acute porphyria
- Addisonian crisis
- Collagen and granulomatous diseases (polyarteritis nodosa or other vasculitis, sarcoidosis, Crohn's disease, Still's disease, granulomatous hepatitis, etc.)
- Diabetic ketoacidosis
- Esophageal disease
- Lead intoxication
- Malignancy (intraabdominal or hematologic)
- Mediastinal tumors
- Mesenteric artery embolus
- Mesenteric vessel thrombus
- Myocardial infarction (usually inferior)
- Pancreatitis
- Pneumothorax complicating pneumonia (e.g., due to *Pneumocystis carinii*)
- Pulmonary embolism
- Ruptured ovarian follicle
- Sickle cell anemia crisis

Fever
- Enteric fever is characterized by sustained fever, headache, abdominal pain, splenomegaly, bacteremia, and, occasionally, skin rash.
- Typhoid fever (caused by *Salmonella typhi*) is the prototype of enteric fever, but several bacteria can cause enteric fever, and a range of systemic bacterial, rickettsial, viral, fungal, and parasitic infections can cause enteric fever-like syndrome (e.g., *Yersinia enterocolitica*, *Yersinia pestis*, *Leptospira*, *Mycobacterium tuberculosis*, *Chlamydia*, hepatitis viruses, Epstein-Barr virus, etc.).
- Mesenteric adenitis, a syndrome that may mimic acute appendicitis, most frequently is due to a viral infection or *Y. enterocolitica*.
- Eosinophilia associated with abdominal cramps or diarrhea is often accompanied by fever and may be caused by parasites (usually helminths), several diseases of unknown cause, and intestinal lymphoma (see also chapter, "Diarrhea and Fever").
- Patients infected with enterohemorrhagic *Escherichia coli* can present with abdominal cramps before developing bloody diarrhea. However, patients with *E. coli* 0157:H7 infection usually are afebrile.

EPIDEMIOLOGY
- Patients with *Salmonella*-induced fever are frequently less than 30 years of age, whereas the vast majority of patients with non-*Salmonella* enteric fever-like syndromes are over 40 years of age.
- Most of the cases of typhoid fever in the United States are acquired abroad, usually in Mexico, India, and Pakistan.
- Travel to tropical areas may suggest malaria. Travel to areas where louse-borne relapsing fever is endemic (Ethiopia, South America, the Far East) raises the possibility of *Borrelia recurrentis* infection.
- Ingestion of unpasteurized milk and milk products, malnutrition, and HIV infection are associated with intestinal tuberculosis.
- Animal contact may suggest leptospirosis, toxoplasmosis, brucellosis, or Q fever.

Abdominal Pain and Fever

- Vector exposure may suggest dengue fever (mosquito), typhus (flea, mite, louse), and psittacosis (parrots and related birds).
- Patients with sickle cell disease or splenectomy are more prone to salmonellosis.
- Melena or guaiac-positive stools and weight loss make solid tumors and lymphomas a possible diagnosis.

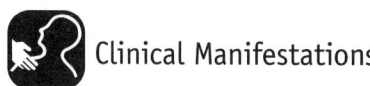

Clinical Manifestations

See the table, Most Common Causes of Enteric Fever and Conditions That May Mimic Enteric Fever: Data from the History and the Physical Examination.

HISTORY

The location of pain, mode of onset, rate of change in intensity, relation to eating, presence of diarrhea (see relevant chapter) or constipation, recent travel, and exposure to animals, are all pertinent information.

PHYSICAL EXAMINATION

- The physical examination should include the location and degree of muscle spasm and rebound tenderness (if any), changes in the breathing pattern, the location of tenderness to percussion, and the existence of changes in cutaneous sensitivity.
- Relative bradycardia suggests enteric fever. Conjunctivitis, pharyngitis, or abnormal lung examination may also be present in enteric fever.
- Acute diarrhea and non-suppurative arthritis are often prominent features of infection with *Y. enterocolitica*.
- Because of increased frequency of chronic liver disease in patients with enteric fever-like syndromes, physical examination is more likely to reveal stigmata of chronic liver disease, such as spider angiomata, gynecomastia, and ascites.
- Pain and rebound tenderness localized in the lower right quadrant, mimicking acute appendicitis, is typically associated with mesenteric adenitis.

Diagnosis

- Blood, stool, and urine specimens should be obtained for cultures from every patient with a syndrome compatible with enteric fever or enteric fever-like syndrome before initiating antimicrobial therapy.
- If typhoid fever is suspected, bone marrow cultures could be considered, because they have a higher yield than blood cultures.
- Widal's reaction (a serology test) is not helpful in the diagnosis of enteric fever caused by organisms other than *S. typhi*.
- Additional laboratory tests that may be of value include WBC count and differential, liver function tests, urinalysis, and chest radiograph.
- Leukopenia is common in typhoid fever.
- When mesenteric adenitis is suspected, studies of the small bowel may help in the diagnosis, particularly if ileitis is associated with mesenteric adenitis. Blood cultures are rarely positive in this

Most Common Causes of Enteric Fever and Conditions That May Mimic Enteric Fever: Data from History and Physical Examination

Etiologic Agent	Travel History	Animal Exposure	Vector Exposure	Diet	Clinical Clues
S. typhi	India	—	—	—	Relative bradycardia, splenomegaly, rose spots, conjunctivitis
S. choleraesius	Mexico				
S. paratyphi A,B					
Y. enterocolitis	—	Pets	—	—	Signs of chronic liver disease
Y. pseudotuberculosis					
C. fetus	—	Farm animals	—	—	Signs of chronic liver disease
Brucella	—	Goats, sheep, cattle	—	Unpasteurized cheese	
Y. pestis	+	Rodent	Fleas	—	Prostration
Bacillus anthracis	+	—	—	Undercooked meat	
Leptospira	—	Cattle, dogs	—	—	Relative bradycardia, conjunctival suffusion
Borrelia species	Southeast and Far East Asia, Ethiopia	—	Louse, tick	—	Relapsing fever pattern, conjunctival suffusion, splenomegaly, skin rash
Legionella species	—	—	—	—	Compromized host, Pneumonia, CNS symptoms
M. Tuberculosis	+	—	—	Unpasteurized milk and milk products	Signs of TB or HIV.
M. avium Tuberculosis					
Actinomyces	—	—	—	—	Abdominal mass or fistula
Chlamydiae	—	Parrots	—	—	Cough, headache, nausea, vomiting
Rickettsia species	+	Rats	Flea, mouse, mites	—	Headache, myalgia, skin rash (except Q fever)
Malaria	+	—	Mosquito	—	Splenomegaly, fever pattern
Toxoplasma gondii	—	Cats	—	Undercooked pork	Lymphadenopathy

Abdominal Pain and Fever

- syndrome, whereas methylene blue examination of feces may reveal polymorphonuclear leukocytes.
- When eosinophilia is present, laboratory tests can include examination of stool and, if necessary, small bowel contents for ova and parasites, and radiologic studies or bowel tissue biopsy.
- Flat and upright abdominal radiographs can provide some clues for the diagnosis of abdominal pain (free air, loss of psoas muscle shadow, radiopaque stones, etc.). Further testing with the use of ultrasound or computed tomography is often necessary.
- Ultrasound remains the initial investigation of choice in patients with suspected intraabdominal abscess because of its rapid availability and simplicity and reported superiority in liver lesions. However, studies highlight its limitations, particularly in the postoperative patient, and if results are equivocal or inconsistent with clinical findings, the patient should be further investigated with radiolabelled white cell scanning or CT scanning.
- Transcutaneous ultrasonography is generally used for the initial evaluation of patients presenting with symptoms consistent with choledocholithiasis.
- Diagnostic accuracy of endoscopic ultrasonography for biliary tract stone disease is greater than 95%.
- Magnetic resonance cholangiography is a noninvasive, but still under study, method of imaging the biliary tract.
- Acute acalculous cholecystitis, inflammation of the gall bladder without evidence of calculi, accounts for 2% to 15% of all cases of acute cholecystitis. Hydroxyindole diaminoacetic acid (HIDA) scanning is costly and rarely used as a first-line study to evaluate biliary tract disease, but it is very useful in evaluating acalculous cholecystitis.
- Bile leaks occur in 30% of patients following cholecystectomy and are best detected by Tc-99m scanning rather than ultrasonography.
- Helical CT cholangiography (HCT cholangiography), first described in 1993, has been found to be suitable for biliary tree visualisation and useful for detection of bile duct stones.
- Endoscopic retrograde cholangiography, percutaneous transhepatic cholangiography, and intraoperative cholangiography are considered the best diagnostic methods for common bile duct stones; however, these procedures are invasive.

Abdominal Pain and Fever

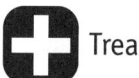 Treatment

- For many patients with the enteric fever syndrome, antimicrobial therapy must be initiated before the diagnosis is documented by culture.
- A third-generation cephalosporin or a fluoroquinolone is used in most areas for the treatment of enteric fever.
- The patient's travel history should be considered before initial empiric antimicrobial therapy.
- Mesenteric adenitis is a self-limited illness in the vast majority of cases. Specific antimicrobial therapy often is not required. Therapeutic agents to be considered include trimethoprim—sulfamethoxazole, a third-generation cephalosporin, or a fluoroquinolone.

COMPLICATIONS

N/A

 Follow-Up

When the fever persists or recurs, intraabdominal abscesses should be strongly suspected.

PREVENTION

N/A

 Selected Readings

Samuels J, Aksentijevich I, Torosyan Y, et al. Familial Mediterranean fever at the millennium. Clinical spectrum, ancient mutations, and a survey of 100 American referrals to the National Institutes of Health. *Medicine* 1998;77:268–297.

Wagner JM, McKinney, Carpenter JL. Does this patient have appendicitis? *JAMA* 1996;276:1589–1594.

Weldon MJ, Joseph AE, French A., et al. Comparison of 99m technetium hexamethylpropylene-amine oxime labelled leucocyte with 111-indium tropolonate labeled granulocyte scanning and ultrasound in the diagnosis of intra-abdominal abscess. *Gut* 1995;37:557–564.

Zidi SH, Prat F, Le Guen O, et al. Use of magnetic resonance cholangiography in the diagnosis of choledocholithiasis: Prospective comparison with a reference imaging method. *Gut* 1999;44:118–122.

Animal/Human Bite Infections, Including Clenched-Fist Injuries

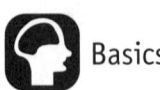 Basics

DEFINITION

Human bites are categorized as occlusional injuries, which are inflicted by actual biting, and clenched-fist injuries, which are sustained when the fist of one individual strikes the teeth of another, causing traumatic laceration of the hand.

APPROACH TO THE PATIENT

- Physicians must focus initially on diagnosing and treating any potentially life-threatening injuries.
- All wounds require careful exploration, because even trivial injuries may involve lacerated tendons, vessels, or nerves; extend into body cavities; or penetrate joint spaces.
- Copious irrigation at high pressure markedly decreases the concentration of bacteria in contaminated wounds. Debridement of devitalized tissue further decreases the likelihood of infection.
- Physicians must then decide whether to close cutaneous wounds, weighing the cosmetic benefits against the increased risk of infection. Usually, such wounds should be treated and left open initially if they
  —Are punctures rather than lacerations
  —Are not potentially disfiguring
  —Are inflicted by humans
  —Involve the legs and arms (particularly the hands), as opposed to the face
  —Occurred more than 6 to 12 hours earlier (or 12 to 24 hours in the case of bites to the face)
- Suspicious human bite wounds should provoke careful questioning regarding domestic or child abuse.
- Details on antibiotic allergies, immunosuppression, splenectomy, liver disease, mastectomy, and immunization history should be obtained.
- The type of wound (puncture, laceration, or scratch), the depth of penetration, and the possible involvement of joints, tendons, nerves, and bone should be evaluated.
- In cases of hand bites, physicians should consider consulting a hand surgeon.

ETIOLOGY

- *Pasteurella canis* is the most common pathogen in infections from dog bites, and *Pasteurella multocida* is the most common isolate of cat bites.
- Other pathogens include the following:
  —*Capnocytophaga* spp
  —*Bartonella henselae*
  —*Francisella tularensis*
  —*Leptospira* spp
  —*Streptobacillus moniliformis*
  —*Spirillum minus* (which causes rat-bite fever)
- Less common aerobes include *Streptococci* spp, *Staphylococci* spp, *Moraxella* spp, and *Neisseria* spp. Anaerobes are usually involved in polymicrobial infections and include *Fusobacterium* spp, *Bacteroides* spp, *Porphyromonas* spp, and *Prevotella* spp.
- Bite wounds from aquatic animals such as alligators or piranhas may contain *Aeromonas hydrophila*.
- Small rodents, including rats, mice, and gerbils, as well as animals that prey on rodents, may transmit *S. moniliformis* or *S. minor* (which, as mentioned, causes a clinical illness known as rat-bite fever).
- In human bites, common aerobic isolates include *Streptococcus* spp, *Staphylococcus aureus*, *Eikenella corrodens*, and *Haemophilus influenzae*. Anaerobic species include *Fusobacterium nucleatum*, *Prevotella* spp, *Porphyromonas* spp, *Peptococcus* spp, and *Peptostreptococcus* spp.

EPIDEMIOLOGY

Incidence

- Each year in the United States, between one and two million animal bite wounds are sustained, resulting in approximately 300,000 visits to emergency departments and 10,000 hospitalizations. Ninety percent of these bites are from dogs and cats.
- Incidence of infection after animal studies varies from 2% to 45%, or even higher in different studies.
- Human bites more frequently become infected than do bites inflicted by other animals.
- Most wounds involve the arms, especially the hands.

Risk Factors

- Infections have been attributed to bites from many animal species, often as a consequence of occupational exposure (farmers, laboratory workers, veterinarians) or recreational exposure (hunters, campers, owners of exotic pets).
- Systemic infections after animal or human bites are particularly likely in hosts with edema or compromised lymphatic drainage in the involved extremity and in patients who are immunocompromised by medication or disease.
- When fever occurs in immunosuppressed patients after a dog bite, the possibility of an infection with *Capnocytophaga canimorsus*, an invasive organism, should be considered.

INCUBATION

- *Pasteurella* infections from animals and mixed infectious human bites tend to advance rapidly, often within hours, causing severe inflammation and spreading cellulitis accompanied by purulent drainage.
- In rat-bite, fever symptoms start after an incubation period of 3 to 10 days.

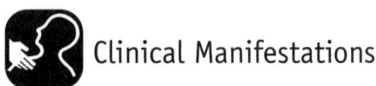 Clinical Manifestations

SYMPTOMS

- The most common symptoms of infection after a bite wound include the following:
  —Fever
  —Wound-associated erythema
  —Spreading cellulitis
  —Induration or swelling at the wound site
  —Purulent drainage
- In rat-bite fever, fever, chills, myalgias, headache, and arthralgias are usually followed by a maculopapular rash, which characteristically involves the palms and soles and may become confluent or purpuric.

SIGNS

- The most common signs include the following:
  —Local erythema and swelling
  —Fever
  —Abscess
  —Lymphangitis

Animal/Human Bite Infections, Including Clenched-Fist Injuries

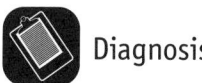 Diagnosis

LABORATORY

- Culture and Gram staining of all infected wounds can be helpful, but cultures obtained at the time of injury are of limited value because they cannot predict whether infection will develop or identify the causative pathogens.
- Anaerobic cultures should be undertaken if abscesses or foul-smelling exudate is present.
- A white blood cell count should be determined and blood cultured if systemic infection is suspected.

IMAGING

Radiographs should be obtained when the bone might have been penetrated or a tooth fragment might be present.

DIAGNOSTIC/TESTING PROCEDURES

C. canimorsus is a thin gram-negative rod that is difficult to culture on most solid media, but it grows in a variety of liquid media.

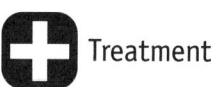 Treatment

MAIN TREATMENT

- Whether antibiotics prevent infection after bites remains controversial. Currently, antibiotics are not given routinely for superficial animal bites, but they are recommended for the following:
  —High-risk wounds, particularly those associated with human bites
  —Deep punctures
  —Those that require surgical repair
  —Those involving the hands or the face
- Cat/dog bite: amoxicillin/clavulanic acid (500/125 mg orally tid); or ampicillin/sulbactam (1.5–3.0 g i.v. q6h)
- Human bite: amoxicillin/clavulanic acid or ampicillin/sulbactam (dosing as for dog bite; if signs of infection, intravenous therapy is indicated)
- Human clenched-fist injury: ampicillin/sulbactam (dosing as for dog bite)
- Monkey bite: as for human bite; also, acyclovir for prevention or treatment of *Herpesvirus simiae*
- Snake bite: ampicillin/sulbactam (as for dog bite). Use antivenin for possible venomous snake bite.
- Rodent bite: penicillin VK (500 mg orally bid)
- Duration of therapy depends on the characteristics of each wound. At least 7 to 14 days of antibiotic therapy is indicated.

ALTERNATIVE TREATMENT

- Cat/dog bite: clindamycin (150–300 mg orally qid) plus either ciprofloxacin (500 mg orally bid) or, for children, trimethoprim–sulfamethoxazole (1 double-strength tablet bid)
- Human bite: clindamycin plus either trimethoprim–sulfamethoxazole or a fluoroquinolone (as in dog bites above)
- Human clenched-fist injury: imipenem (500 mg intravenously q6h) or cefoxitin (1.5 g intravenously q6h)
- Snake bite: clindamycin plus either trimethoprim–sulfamethoxazole or a fluoroquinolone (as for dog bite)
- Rodent bite: doxycycline (100 mg orally bid)

SURGICAL TREATMENT

- Primary closure is recommended for bites involving the face or when a poor cosmetic result is expected.
- Debridement of necrotic material may be needed.
- If abscess develops, drainage is indicated.
- For bites involving the hand, elevation is recommended.

COMPLICATIONS

- Occasionally, severe infections (e.g., sepsis, endocarditis, septic arthritis, and meningitis) develop after bites as a result of either hematogenous spread or undetected penetration of deeper structures.
- Infection with *C. canimorsus* following dog bite wounds may result in fulminant sepsis, disseminated intravascular coagulation, and renal failure, particularly in hosts who have impaired hepatic function, who have undergone splenectomy, or who are immunosuppressed.
- Cat bites are more likely than dog bites to cause septic arthritis and osteomyelitis.
- Human bites arouse special concern because they can transmit organisms such as HIV, hepatitis B virus, and even syphilis.

 Follow-Up

After 72 hours, physicians may choose to reevaluate wounds that were initially left open to determine whether delayed primary closure would be appropriate.

PREVENTION

- Tetanus immune globulin and tetanus toxoid should be administered to patients who have had two or fewer primary immunizations. Tetanus toxoid alone can be given to those who have completed a primary immunization series but who have not received a booster for more than 5 years.
- Please see Section II, "Rabies," for details on prevention of this infection.
- Physicians may provide prophylactic therapy for persons who are bitten by those at high risk for infection with HIV or hepatitis B virus.

 Selected Readings

Fleisher GR. The management of bite wounds. *N Engl J Med* 1999;340:138.

Talan DA, Citron DM, Abrahamian FM, et al. Bacteriologic analysis of infected dog and cat bites. *N Engl J Med* 1999;340:85–92.

Atypical Lymphocytosis

 Basics

DEFINITION

- Lymphocytosis is defined as any lymphocyte count in excess of 5×10^9 per liter.
- Atypical lymphocytosis is present when atypical lymphocytes account for more than 20% of the total peripheral blood lymphocyte population.
- The atypical lymphocytes are usually CD8+ cells and have cytoplasmic vacuoles and cell membrane indentations.

APPROACH TO THE PATIENT

- The evaluation of the patient with atypical lymphocytosis should be guided by the age of the patient, results of previous complete blood counts, history of previous viral infections or exposures, and presence of accompanying symptoms.
- The first step in the evaluation of a patient with lymphocytosis is to differentiate between infectious and noninfectious causes (usually a hematologic malignancy).
- A peripheral blood smear should be carefully evaluated by an experienced physician, and, in case of diagnostic difficulties, by a hematologist.

ETIOLOGY

Differential Diagnosis

- The most common infectious causes of lymphocytosis are the following:
  —Infectious mononucleosis
  —Cytomegalovirus (CMV)
  —Acute infectious lymphocytosis
- Less common infectious causes of lymphocytosis are the following:
  —Adenovirus
  —Babesiosis
  —Brucellosis
  —Coxsackievirus
  —Dengue
  —Human herpesvirus 6
  —HIV (especially during acute seroconversion)
  —Infectious hepatitis
  —Malaria
  —Measles
  —Mumps
  —Pertussis
  —Rubella
  —Secondary or congenital syphilis
  —Toxoplasmosis
  —Tuberculosis
  —Tularemia
  —Typhoid fever
  —Varicella
- Infectious mononucleosis, acute infectious lymphocytosis, pertussis, and rubella may cause significant lymphocytosis ($>10 \times 10^9$ lymphocytes per liter of blood)
- Acute infectious lymphocytosis is a benign, moderately contagious disease with an incubation period of 12 to 21 days. It is more common among children and young adults. Patients are asymptomatic or could present with the following:
  —Diarrhea
  —Nausea or vomiting
  —Abdominal pain
  —Symptoms from the respiratory tract
  —Symptoms from the central nervous system
  —Skin rash
- The most common noninfectious causes of lymphocytosis are the following:
  —Acute lymphocytic leukemia
  —Chronic lymphocytic leukemia
  —Hairy-cell leukemia
  —Drug hypersensitivity reactions
  —Graves' disease
  —Lymphomas
  —Serum sickness
  —Solid tumors
  —Stress lymphocytosis
     —Cardiovascular collapse
     —Major surgery
     —Sickle cell anemia crisis
     —Trauma
     —Status epilepticus
- Chronic lymphocytosis is usually due to noninfectious diseases causes, such as the following:
  —Autoimmune disorders
  —Cancer
  —Cigarette smoking
  —Chronic inflammation
  —Sarcoidosis
  —Thymoma

EPIDEMIOLOGY

- CMV usually affects older patients (average age, 29 years) than does Epstein-Barr virus (EBV).
- Syndromes caused by CMV in the immunocompromised host often begin with prolonged fever, malaise, anorexia, night sweats, arthralgias, or myalgias.
- Atypical lymphocytes are found more commonly during the acute than the chronic phase of viral hepatitis.
- Patients with chronic lymphocytic leukemia can be asymptomatic.

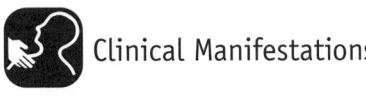 Clinical Manifestations

- Clinical manifestations of infectious mononucleosis include the following:
  —Fever
  —Pharyngitis
  —Lymphadenopathy
  —Generalized weakness
  —Anorexia or nausea
  —Hepatomegaly
  —Splenomegaly
  —Petechiae
  —Rash

PHYSICAL EXAMINATION

- In CMV mononucleosis, exudative pharyngitis, splenomegaly, and cervical lymphadenopathy are rare.
- Maculopapular eruption is present in both infectious mononucleosis and in mononucleosis-like syndrome due to CMV, especially if the patient was exposed to ampicillin or amoxicillin.
- Toxoplasmosis usually causes lymphadenopathy, especially involving posterior auricular lymph nodes; however, it does not cause pharyngitis and hepatosplenomegaly as often as EBV or CMV infection.
- Lymphadenopathy and splenomegaly are usually absent in cases of acute infectious lymphocytosis.
- Clinicians should evaluate the patients for the presence of jaundice or for other signs of hepatitis. However, these findings are not diagnostic of infectious hepatitis; they can be present in a variety of infections, including infectious mononucleosis and CMV infection.
- Drug-induced hypersensitivity reactions can lead to erythema, urticaria, fever, arthralgias, high eosinophil count, and abnormal liver function tests.

Atypical Lymphocytosis

 ## Diagnosis

- In most of the diseases that cause atypical lymphocytosis, the total lymphocyte count can be low, normal, or significantly elevated.
- The heterophile antibody test (an IgM antibody) is used for the diagnosis of infectious mononucleosis. A titer of 1:40 or greater is diagnostic of acute EBV infection in a patient with compatible clinical symptoms and atypical lymphocytosis. Tests for heterophile antibodies are positive in about one-half of the patients during the first week of illness and in more than 80% during the third week.
- CMV is the most common cause of heterophile antibody-negative mononucleosis-like syndrome; it causes about half of such cases.
- Acute bacterial infections rarely cause lymphocytosis; however, pertussis can lead to high lymphocyte count (even greater than 30×10^9 per liter of blood).
- In acute infectious lymphocytosis, lymphocytosis persists for 3 to 7 weeks and consists mostly of normal mature lymphocytes.
- Low-grade neutropenia and thrombocytopenia are common during the first month of infectious mononucleosis. Liver function tests are abnormal in more than 90% of patients.
- EBV can also cause aseptic meningitis. In this case, atypical lymphocytes can be found in the cerebrospinal fluid.
- Lymphocyte markers can provide evidence for or against dominance of one lymphocytic type, and flow cytometry and cytogenetics should be performed in cases in which the morphology suggests that the dysplastic cells are due to a hematologic or lymphoid neoplastic disorder.
- Patients with atypical lymphocytosis due to HIV might be at the "window period" (HIV antibody-negative cases). In such patients, the diagnosis of HIV requires clinical follow-up and evaluation of the plasma viral load.

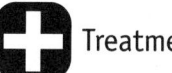 ## Treatment

- Treatment of the patient with atypical lymphocytosis should be based on the specific etiology.
- Infectious mononucleosis (the most common cause of atypical lymphocytosis) does not usually require a specific treatment, except for rare cases with complications such as the following:
  —Hemolytic anemia
  —Thrombocytopenia
  —Aplastic anemia
  —Respiratory obstruction
  —Splenic rupture
  —Jaundice
  —Guillain-Barré syndrome
  —Encephalitis
  —Myelitis
  —Renal failure
  —Pneumonitis
  —Myocarditis
- CMV infection (the second most common cause of atypical lymphocytosis) does not usually require specific treatment in the immunocompetent host. CMV infection should be treated in neonates and in immunocompromised hosts and in patients with complications such as the following:
  —Guillain-Barré syndrome
  —Hemolytic anemia
  —Thrombocytopenia
  —Jaundice
  —Encephalitis
  —Myelitis
  —Pneumonitis

COMPLICATIONS

N/A

 ## Follow-Up

- Failure to recognize heterophile antibody-negative causes of atypical lymphocytosis can result in unnecessary lymph node or liver biopsies, bone marrow aspiration, or other unnecessary testing.
- Most authorities suggest bone marrow aspiration and biopsy when lymphocytosis coexists with leukoerythroblastosis or peripheral lymphoblasts and if atypical lymphocytosis persists without evidence of infection.
- Patients with atypical lymphocytosis due to possible HIV infection need close observation and further testing. Early HIV infection is one of the indications for early antiretroviral therapy with highly active antiretroviral treatment.
- Patients with atypical lymphocytosis due to unclear etiology require clinical and laboratory follow-up.

PREVENTION

N/A

 ## Selected Readings

Steeper TA, Horwitz CA, Hanson M, et al. Heterophil-negative mononucleosis-like illnesses with atypical lymphocytosis in patients undergoing seroconversions to the human immunodeficiency virus. *Am J Clin Pathol* 1988;90:169–174.

Teggatz JR, Parkin J, Peterson L. Transient atypical lymphocytosis in patients with emergency medical conditions. *Arch Pathol Lab Med* 1987;111:712–714.

Back Pain and Fever

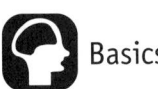 ## Basics

DEFINITION

The term *back pain* is usually used to describe acute or chronic spinal or paraspinal pain.

APPROACH TO THE PATIENT

- Patients who present with back pain and fever should have a thorough evaluation to detect possible sources of nonmechanical pain.
- Clinicians should obtain a careful history and inquire for symptoms of weight loss, recumbency pain, morning stiffness, and acute severe or colicky pain.
- Repeated spinal and neurologic examinations are essential, and when there is spinal pain or tenderness, full investigation is warranted.
- Back pain exacerbated by motion and unrelieved by rest, spine tenderness over the involved spine segment, and an elevated erythrocyte sedimentation rate are the most common findings in vertebral osteomyelitis.
- Pain due to neoplastic infiltration of nerves is typically continuous, progressive in severity, and unrelieved by rest at night. In contrast, mechanical low back pain is usually improved with rest.
- Patients will generally require a plain roentgenographic examination with subsequent scintigraphy, magnetic resonance imaging (MRI), computed tomography (CT), laboratory work, and biopsy as indicated by any positive findings during the diagnostic work-up.

ETIOLOGY

- Infectious causes of back pain and fever:
  - Biliary tract infection
  - Chronic prostatitis
  - Herpes zoster
  - Pyelonephritis
  - Retroperitoneal abscess
    - Spinal epidural abscess
    - Vertebral osteomyelitis
- Noninfectious causes of back pain and fever:
  - Colonic neoplasms
  - Diseases of the pancreas
  - Histiocytosis X
  - Metastatic carcinoma (breast, lung, prostate, thyroid, kidney, gastrointestinal tract)
  - Multiple myeloma
  - Neoplastic invasion of pelvic nerves
  - Lymphoma
  - Pregnancy
  - Vertebral fracture
  - Renal artery or vein thrombosis
  - Renal stones
  - Retroperitoneal hemorrhage and tumors
  - Tumor of the posterior wall of the stomach or duodenum
- *Staphylococcus aureus* is the most commonly recognized causative organism of spinal epidural abscess and accounts for 57% to 73% of reported abscesses. Other pathogens include the following:
  - *Actinomyces israelii*
  - *Aspergillus* spp
  - *Blastomyces* spp
  - *Brucella* spp
  - *Cryptococcus* spp
  - *Haemophilus parainfluenzae*
  - *Mycobacterium tuberculosis*
  - *Streptococcus milleri*
- Vertebral osteomyelitis is usually caused by staphylococci, but other bacteria or *M. tuberculosis* (Pott's disease) may be the responsible organisms. However, this is variable. In a retrospective multicentre study conducted in the south of Spain, 48% of patients had vertebral osteomyelitis due to *Brucella* spp, 33% had pyogenic vertebral osteomyelitis, and 19% had tuberculous vertebral osteomyelitis.

EPIDEMIOLOGY

Incidence

- Spinal epidural abscess is an uncommon condition, with an estimated incidence of 0.2 to 2.0 per 10,000 hospital admissions, and a peak incidence in the sixth and seventh decades of life.
- Spinal epidural abscess may result as a complication of pyogenic vertebral osteomyelitis in as many as 33% of presenting cases.
- Annual incidence of vertebral osteomyelitis is estimated up to seven per one million individuals.
- In adults, brucellosis produces vertebral osteomyelitis in 6% to 12% of cases.
- Thoracic involvement is more frequent in tuberculous vertebral osteomyelitis.

Risk Factors

- Conditions commonly associated with vertebral osteomyelitis and spinal epidural abscess include the following:
  - Diabetes mellitus (in up to 25% to 33% of cases)
  - Injecting drug use
  - Chronic renal failure
  - Ethanol abuse
  - Focal infections and bacteremia
  - Malignancy
- Most spinal epidural abscesses are thought to result from the hematogenous spread of bacteria, usually from a cutaneous or mucosal source. The direct spread of infection into the epidural space from a source adjacent to the spine is also well described. Postoperative abscesses account for 16% of all spinal epidural abscesses, and epidural catheter insertion is another recognized predisposing factor.
- Blunt trauma is reported to precede the symptoms of spinal epidural abscess in 15% to 35% of cases, and it is postulated that trauma may result in the formation of an epidural hematoma that subsequently becomes infected.

 ## Clinical Manifestations

- The typical features of spinal epidural abscess include fever, spinal pain and tenderness, and radiating root pain followed by limb weakness. Pain is the most consistent symptom and occurs in virtually all patients at some time during their illness. However, spinal pain and fever can be the only features before a precipitous neurologic deterioration occurs.
- When septicemia dominates the clinical picture, the neurologic symptoms may go unnoticed. This also may be the case in patients confined to bed.
- Fever can be absent in up to 30% of patients with pyogenic vertebral osteomyelitis. The absence of fever is more frequent in the group of tuberculous vertebral osteomyelitis.

 ## Diagnosis

DIFFERENTIAL DIAGNOSIS

- Reports of new-onset backache after epidural anesthesia vary from 2% to 31%. The most common causes of back pain after regional anesthesia are thought to include ligamentous trauma, reflex paraspinous muscle spasm, or ligamentous strain during patient positioning secondary to skeletal muscle relaxation. Back pain after regional anesthesia that occurs concomitantly with neurologic dysfunction is rare and should immediately alert the physician to search for other potential causes.

Back Pain and Fever

- Vertebral osteomyelitis should be considered in the differential diagnosis of pleural effusion of uncertain cause, especially if there is associated back pain.

LABORATORY

- The usual hematologic and biochemical parameters are of little value in the diagnosis of vertebral osteomyelitis. However, when leucocytosis, neutrophilia, and very high values of erythrocyte sedimentation rate (ESR) and C-reactive protein are present, they suggest pyogenic vertebral osteomyelitis.
- CT and MRI have significantly improved the sensitivity and specificity of simple radiography in the diagnosis of vertebral osteomyelitis.
- Blood culture is the most useful routine test, resulting in the isolation of the responsible microorganism in about half the cases of vertebral osteomyelitis due to pyogenic and *Brucella* spp.
- Bone biopsy is necessary to establish the diagnosis in 50% of pyogenic vertebral osteomyelitis and in almost 75% of tuberculous vertebral osteomyelitis.

IMAGING

- Plain x-ray films of the spine may be normal early in vertebral osteomyelitis.
- The extent and location of a spinal epidural abscess is best visualized using MRI.
- MRI or CT-myelography are the studies of choice in the setting of suspected spinal metastasis.

DIAGNOSTIC/TESTING PROCEDURES

- CT-guided needle biopsy is a reliable procedure for diagnosing carcinoma but not lymphoma. The reliability of needle biopsy for the diagnosis of lymphoma has improved with the advent of CT guidance, the addition of immunophenotyping, and the use of larger bore needles, but the failure rate is still high.
- Etiologic diagnosis of vertebral osteomyelitis is frequently difficult, requiring in 30% to 70% of cases the performance of percutaneous or surgical vertebral bone biopsies.

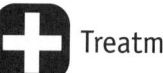 Treatment

- Empirical medical treatment should only be started once.
- Empirical antimicrobial treatment of spinal epidural abscess should be bactericidal and start early, but after blood cultures and, if possible, bone biopsy have been obtained.
- If a methicillin-sensitive *S. aureus* is isolated, successful treatment is possible with a first-generation cephalosporin, a penicillinase-resistant penicillin, combination vancomycin plus aminoglycoside, or trimethoprim-sulfamethoxazole.
- Parenteral treatment should be continued for at least 4 weeks, and may be prolonged for 8 weeks or longer if vertebral osteomyelitis is suspected.
- Surgical treatment of spinal epidural abscess entails emergency evacuation of the pus with decompression of the spinal cord and nerve roots.

COMPLICATIONS

Although the mortality rate from spinal epidural abscess has improved from that described in the early reports, it has remained surprisingly consistent over the past several decades, at about 14%.

 Follow-Up

- Among patients with pleural effusion of unknown cause, the possibility of vertebral osteomyelitis should be considered, and possibly more so in diabetics.
- Patients with vertebral osteomyelitis and spinal epidural abscess should be followed up for several months—even after completion of antibiotic therapy—because of the spinal instability that may result from the infection or the necessary surgical intervention.

PREVENTION

Some authors suggest that epidural anesthesia should be avoided among patients that are at risk for bacteremia.

 Selected Readings

Anonymous. Case records of the Massachusetts General Hospital. Weekly clinicopathological exercises. Case 21-1996. A 52-year-old man with back pain, fever, and abnormal imaging studies. *N Engl J Med* 1996;335:115–122.

Bass SN, Ailani RK, Shekar R, Gerblich AA. Pyogenic vertebral osteomyelitis presenting as exudative pleural effusion: A series of five cases. *Chest* 1998;114:642–647.

Colmenero JD, Jimenez-Mejias ME, Sanchez-Lora FJ, et al. Pyogenic, tuberculous, and brucellar vertebral osteomyelitis: A descriptive and comparative study of 219 cases. *Ann Rheum Dis* 1997;56:709–715.

Engstrom JW, Bradford DS. Back and neck pain. In: Fauci AS, Braunwald E, Isselbacher KJ, et al., eds. *Harrison's principles of medicine*, 14th ed. New York: McGraw-Hill, 1998:73–84.

Mackenzie AR, Laing RB, Smith CC, et al. Spinal epidural abscess: The importance of early diagnosis and treatment. *J Neurol Neurosurg Psychiatry* 1998;65:209–212.

McCowin PR, Borenstein D, Wiesel SW. The current approach to the medical diagnosis of low back pain. *Orthop Clin North Am* 1991;22:315–325.

Pinczower GR, Gyorke A. Vertebral osteomyelitis as a cause of back pain after epidural anesthesia. *Anesthesiology* 1996;84:215–217.

Cough and Fever

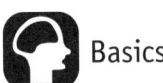 Basics

DEFINITION
- *Cough* is an explosive expiration that provides a protective mechanism for clearing the tracheobronchial tree of secretions and foreign material.
- *Chronic cough* is generally defined as cough persisting for 3 weeks or longer.

APPROACH TO THE PATIENT
- Some patients who complain of persistent coughing may in fact be experiencing frequent throat clearing, "hawking," or symptoms of the upper respiratory tract other than cough. When the clinician is unsure whether the patient is truly describing cough, having the patient reproduce the "cough" in the office is helpful.
- Acute and self-limited episodes of cough commonly stem from viral infections of the respiratory tract and usually do not pose a diagnostic problem.
- A detailed history frequently provides the most valuable clues for etiology of the cough.
- Clinicians should question patients about whether the cough is acute or chronic and whether it is associated with the following:
  —Hemoptysis
  —Production of phlegm
  —Symptoms suggestive of a respiratory infection
  —Symptoms suggestive of postnasal drip (nasal discharge, frequent throat clearing) or gastroesophageal reflux (heartburn or sensation of regurgitation)
- A thorough travel history and investigation for the presence of signs or history of immunodeficiency can be useful.
- Examination of the patient, with special attention to the lungs, ears, nose, and mouth, may yield useful clues.
- A chest roentgenogram may be helpful in narrowing the differential diagnosis.
- The use of empiric broad-spectrum antibiotics or bronchoscopy with BAL, protected specimen brush, or biopsy depends on the clinical situation.
- Sinus imaging and otolaryngologic consultation may be considered in difficult cases. vfill

- A search for extrapulmonary spread (especially brain abscess) is imperative in all patients with pulmonary infection who have neurologic or other extrapulmonary symptoms.

ETIOLOGY
- As a protective mechanism against foreign or noxious material, cough can be initiated by a variety of airway irritants, which enter the tracheobronchial tree by inhalation (smoke, dust, fumes) or by aspiration (upper airway secretions, gastric contents, foreign bodies).
- The clinical syndrome of cough and fever is often associated with a viral nasopharyngitis. The causes of such infection are usually influenza virus, parainfluenza virus, respiratory syncytial virus, rhinovirus, coronavirus, and adenovirus. Other infectious causes of cough and fever include the following:
  —Actinomycosis
  —Aspergillosis
  —*Bordetella pertussis*
  —Bronchiectasis
  —*Chlamydia pneumoniae*
  —Coccidioidomycosis
  —*Cryptococcus neoformans* pneumonia
  —Cytomegalovirus pneumonia
  —Endocarditis
  —Histoplasmosis
  —Legionellosis
  —Lung abscess
  —Mycobacterial infections, particularly *Mycobacterium tuberculosis* and *Mycobacterium avium* complex (MAC)
  —*Mycoplasma pneumoniae*
  —Nocardiosis
  —*Pneumocystis carinii* pneumonia
  —Pulmonary toxoplasmosis
  —Viral bronchitis.
- Other inflammatory and noninfectious causes of cough and fever include the following:
  —Endobronchial sarcoidosis
  —Kaposi's sarcoma
  —Lymphoma
  —Neoplasms infiltrating the airway wall, such as bronchogenic carcinoma or a carcinoid tumor
  —Pulmonary embolism
  —Treatment with antihypertensives (ACE inhibitors).

- Inflammatory pseudotumor of the lung generally represents an organizing pneumonia that fails to decrease in size over time. Inflammatory pseudotumors have been associated with a variety of infections, such as bacteroides, *Corynebacterium equi*, *Coxiella burnetii*, intracellular mycobacteria, *M. pneumoniae* infections, and so on.

EPIDEMIOLOGY
- Cough is the fifth most common symptom encountered by physicians who treat outpatients.
- Up to 5% of patients with AIDS in the United States have active tuberculosis.
- The reason for the increased incidence of pertussis over the past years is unclear, but a combination of factors is likely involved. Adolescents and adults are currently considered the major reservoir for *B. pertussis*, playing a predominant role in the transmission of pertussis to young children, in whom the disease is most severe.

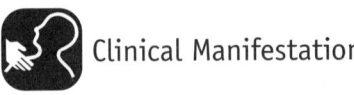 Clinical Manifestations

- Pertussis is an acute respiratory tract infection characterized by severe coughing spasms that may end with an inspiratory whoop. The Chinese name for this illness, "the 100-day cough," attests to its prolonged course.
- Because pertussis is generally milder in older people, the diagnosis tends to be overlooked. Persistent cough may be the sole manifestation, and the characteristic whoop occurs in only a few of those infected. Fever and lower respiratory tract signs are usually absent.
- Patients with Kaposi's sarcoma involvement of their lungs may progress in the extent and the severity of their pulmonary disease at a time that skin lesions remain quiescent or even regress. Dyspnea and dry cough are characteristic symptoms, and hypoxemia is common. There is an association of pulmonary Kaposi's sarcoma with fever in about 50% of the patients.

Cough and Fever

 ## Diagnosis

DIFFERENTIAL DIAGNOSIS

- Tuberculosis tends to be one of the early opportunistic infections occurring in AIDS patients, often an AIDS-defining illness, whereas MAC infection tends to occur in the late stage of HIV infection when the CD4 count is usually 50 to 75 cells per milliliter or less.
- Pertussis should be considered in anyone who has a pure or predominant complaint of cough, especially if there is a history of paroxysmal coughing, inspiratory whoop, posttussive vomiting, cough resulting in sleep disturbance, or close contact with others who have similar symptoms.

LABORATORY

- Blood cultures and a sputum Gram stain and culture are appropriate investigations in a febrile immunocompromised patient with cough and fever.
- Purulent sputum suggests chronic bronchitis, bronchiectasis, pneumonia, or lung abscess. Blood in the sputum may be seen in the same disorders, but its presence also raises the question of an endobronchial tumor.

IMAGING

- Chest radiography may be particularly helpful in suggesting or confirming the cause of the cough. Important potential findings include the presence of an intrathoracic mass lesion, a localized pulmonary parenchymal infiltrate, or diffuse interstitial or alveolar disease.
- In lower respiratory tract infection, diffuse pulmonary involvement is common in patients with *P. carinii*, herpesvirus, *Legionella* spp, or *M. pneumoniae* infection. A nodular or cavitary pattern may be detected in patients who have an infection with *Nocardia* spp, actinomycosis, atypical mycobacteria, cryptococcosis, or aspergillosis, or who have a bacterial lung abscess. Focal infiltrates are common with bacteria (including *Nocardia* spp), mycobacteria, *Cryptococcus* spp, or *Aspergillus* spp.
- High-resolution computed tomography (HRCT) is the procedure of choice for demonstrating dilated airways and confirming the diagnosis of bronchiectasis.

DIAGNOSTIC/TESTING PROCEDURES

Fiberoptic bronchoscopy is the procedure of choice for visualizing an endobronchial tumor and collecting cytologic and histologic specimens. Inspection of the airway mucosa by bronchoscopy can also demonstrate the characteristic appearance of endobronchial Kaposi's sarcoma in patients with AIDS.

 ## Treatment

- Definitive treatment of cough depends on determining the underlying cause and then initiating specific therapy.
- Although usually resected, inflammatory pseudotumors have been treated successfully with antibiotics, radiation, and corticosteroids, and may regress spontaneously.
- An irritative, nonproductive cough may be suppressed by an antitussive agent, which increases the latency or threshold of the cough. Such agents include codeine (15 mg qid) or nonnarcotics such as dextromethorphan (15 mg qid).
- Cough productive of significant quantities of sputum should usually not be suppressed, because retention of sputum in the tracheobronchial tree may interfere with the distribution of ventilation, alveolar aeration, and the ability of the lung to resist infection.
- Other agents (such as ipratropium bromide 24 puffs qid and inhaled glucocorticoids) have also been used to control cough, but objective information assessing their benefit is meager.

COMPLICATIONS

- Paroxysms of coughing may precipitate syncope.
- Patients with tuberculosis and cough are considered infectious and can spread the infection.

 ## Follow-Up

- The term *postinfectious cough* has been used to refer to cough that persists after respiratory tract infections. In some patients, transient bronchial hyperreactivity may be demonstrated. This type of cough generally fades over a period of a few months.
- Although cough fractures of the ribs may occur in otherwise normal patients, their occurrence should at least raise the possibility of pathologic fractures, which are seen with multiple myeloma, osteoporosis, and osteolytic metastases.

PREVENTION

- Chest physiotherapy can be useful to enhance clearance of secretions in patients with bronchiectasis.
- Routine use of whole-cell pertussis vaccines was suspended in some countries in the late 1970s and early 1980s, leading to a resurgence of whooping cough. Acellular pertussis vaccines containing purified or recombinant *B. pertussis* antigens were developed in the hope that they would be as effective but less toxic than the whole-cell vaccines.

 ## Selected Readings

Anonymous. Case records of the Massachusetts General Hospital. Weekly clinicopathological exercises. Case 201993. A 5-year-old girl with recurrent cough and fever and an enlarging pulmonary mass. *N Engl J Med* 1994;330:1439–1446.

Anonymous. Fever, cough, and dyspnea in a 38-year-old man with acquired immunodeficiency syndrome. *Am J Med* 1995;98:85–94.

Evans G, Radisch N, McReynolds M, Shepherd A. Pertussis. *Can Med Assoc J* 1996;155:1439–1440.

Tam TW, Bentsi-Enchill A. The return of the 100-day cough: Resurgence of pertussis in the 1990s. *Can Med Assoc J* 1998;159:695–696.

Weinberger SE, Braunwald E. Cough and hemoptysis. In: Fauci AS, Braunwald E, Isselbacher KJ, et al., eds. *Harrison's principles of medicine*, 14th ed. New York: McGraw-Hill, 1998:194–198.

Windgassen EB, Gillespie DJ. 39-year-old man with fever, cough, and chest pain. *Mayo Clinic Proc* 1995;70:1191–1194.

Yu ML, Ryu JH. Assessment of the patient with chronic cough. *Mayo Clin Proc* 1997;72:957–959.

Diarrhea and Fever

 ## Basics

DEFINITION

- Diarrhea is increased frequency and liquidity of fecal discharge. It is formally defined as an increase in daily stool weight above 200 g. A working definition is any bowel movement that assumes the shape of the container.
- A noninflammatory diarrheal syndrome is characterized by watery stools that may be of large volume (>1 L/d), without blood, pus, severe abdominal pain, or fever.
- An inflammatory diarrheal syndrome is characterized by frequent, small-volume, mucoid or bloody stools (or both), and may be accompanied by tenesmus, fever, or severe abdominal pain. The hallmark of inflammatory diarrheas is the presence of leukocytes in the stool.
- Diarrhea is considered acute when lasting less than 7 to 14 days, and chronic when lasting longer than 23 weeks.

APPROACH TO THE PATIENT

- An adequate medical history and a physical examination are essential in determining the possible diagnoses, degree of severity, and complications and to suggest further investigations. The presence of volume depletion should be observed as manifested by postural hypotension, tachycardia, decreased skin turgor, and so forth.
- High fever, systemic toxicity, bloody diarrhea, dehydration, a known outbreak of food poisoning, recent overseas travel, immunosuppression, male homosexuality, or recent antibiotic use are reasons for diagnostic testing.
- Examination of a stool sample is important. Grossly bloody or mucoid stool suggests an inflammatory process; all stools should be examined for fecal leukocytes.
- The cornerstone of diagnosis in patients with severe diarrhea, especially bloody diarrhea, is bacterial culture and microscopic examination of the stool for ova and parasites.

ETIOLOGY

- The most common causes of inflammatory diarrhea include the following:
  —*Salmonella* spp
  —*Shigella* spp
  —*Campylobacter jejuni*
  —Enterohemorrhagic and enteroinvasive *Escherichia coli*
  —*Clostridium difficile*
  —*Vibrio parahaemolyticus*
  —*Entamoeba histolytica*
  —*Yersinia enterocolitica*
- Patients with atypical microorganisms (such as *Cryptosporidium*, *Microsporidium*, *Isospora belli*, cytomegalovirus, and *Mycobacterium avium-intracellulare*) along with fever are usually associated with the following:
  —IgA deficiency
  —AIDS
  —Impaired intestinal motility (due to opiates or antimotility drugs, diabetes mellitus, etc.)
  —Immunosuppressive therapy (for chemotherapy, etc.)
  —Achlorhydria, gastric surgery, or receiving medications (such as antacids, H_2 blockers, etc.) that neutralize gastric acid
  —Use of corticosteroids
- The acute inflammatory diarrheal syndrome can also be of noninfectious etiology, such as ulcerative colitis, Crohn's disease, radiation or ischemic colitis, or diverticulitis.
- Fever and diarrhea also may result from infection outside the gastrointestinal tract, as in malaria.

EPIDEMIOLOGY

Incidence

- In developing countries, more than half of the deaths of children are directly attributable to acute diarrheal illnesses, and they account for more than 58 million deaths each year in children under 5 years of age.
- In the United States, acute infectious diarrhea accounts for 250,000 hospital admissions and nearly eight million office visits to physicians each year.

Risk Factors

- Antibiotic-associated diarrhea caused by *C. difficile* infection is the most common cause of acute diarrhea in hospitalized patients (please see relevant chapter).
- Organisms with higher attack rates among children than among adults include enterotoxigenic and enteropathogenic *E. coli*, *C. jejuni*, and *Giardia lamblia*.
- Among children, the incidence of *Salmonella* infections is highest among infants under 1 year of age, while the attack rate for *Shigella* infections is greatest among children aged 6 months to 4 years.

 ## Clinical Manifestations

SYMPTOMS

- Inflammatory diarrhea usually presents with abdominal pain and, often, a high fever. Abdominal pain may be the main symptom.
- Food poisoning due to *Clostridium perfringens* rarely causes fever. It presents with moderately severe abdominal cramps and diarrhea and has a slightly longer incubation period (8–14 h).
- Fever is uncommon in bacterial disease caused by an enterotoxin elaborated outside the host, such as that due to *Staphylococcus aureus* or *Bacillus cereus*. Such cases usually present with diarrhea, nausea, vomiting, abdominal cramping, and short incubation period (1–6 h).
- *Yersinia* and *Salmonella* often infect the terminal ileum and cecum and present with right lower quadrant pain and tenderness suggestive of acute appendicitis.
- Extraintestinal manifestations such as arthritis, skin lesions, or ocular symptoms suggest idiopathic inflammatory bowel disease, but they may be associated with pathogens causing inflammatory diarrhea, e.g., *Shigella*, *Salmonella*, *Yersinia*, and *C. difficile*.

 ## Diagnosis

LABORATORY

- All patients with fever and evidence of inflammatory disease should have stool cultured for *Salmonella*, *Shigella*, and *Campylobacter*. Isolation of *C. jejuni* requires inoculation of fresh stool onto selective growth medium and incubation at 42°C in a microaerophilic atmosphere.
- In most microbiology laboratories, stool sent for culture of enteric pathogens will be processed for *Shigella*, *Salmonella*, and *Campylobacter*. Other enteric pathogens, such as *Yersinia*, *Vibrio*, and *E. coli* O157: H7, are not routinely sought. Therefore, if the clinical suspicion for these organisms is high, the microbiology department needs to be notified.
- If the medical history suggests risk factors for *C. difficile*, such as recent antibiotic exposure, recent hospitalization, day-care exposure, or recent chemotherapy, stool should be tested for *C. difficile* toxin.

Diarrhea and Fever

- In patients with AIDS and chronic diarrhea, multiple stool specimens for culture and examination for ova and parasites should be obtained.

IMAGING

- Barium radiographs are best deferred until the initial course of illness has been observed and appropriate stool specimens obtained.
- In rare instances, a CT scan with oral contrast is a useful technique.

DIAGNOSTIC/TESTING PROCEDURES

- Further evaluation usually involves upper gastrointestinal endoscopy or colonoscopy with diagnostic biopsies.
- While colonoscopic and radiographic findings may be indistinguishable in infectious colitis and inflammatory bowel disease, histologic findings may be diagnostic.
- Small-intestine biopsy is generally diagnostic in diseases characterized by diffuse involvement of the small intestine, such as Whipple's disease and *M. avium* complex infection, but may be falsely negative in diseases with a patchy distribution, such as lymphoma, eosinophilic gastroenteritis, or amyloidosis.
- Certain organisms, such as *Giardia* and *Strongyloides*, as well as *Cryptosporidium* and *I. belli*, may be difficult to detect in stool and are better diagnosed by duodenal aspiration or intestinal biopsy.
- In patients with bloody diarrhea, sigmoidoscopy and occasionally colonoscopy are generally reserved for those with symptoms lasting longer than 10 days.

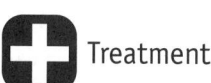

Treatment

- Therapy should be directed at preventing dehydration and restoring fluid losses. Although this is often done intravenously, it can also be accomplished with oral fluid–electrolyte therapy.
- In many patients with acute inflammatory diarrhea, a specific pathogen can be diagnosed, and the patient may benefit from antibiotic therapy.
- Patients should avoid milk and other lactose-containing products, because viral or bacterial enteropathogens often result in transient lactase deficiency, leading to lactose malabsorption.
- Pharmacotherapy with antidiarrheal agents for acute infectious diarrhea can reduce the number of bowel movements and diminish the magnitude of fluid and electrolyte loss. The most commonly used agents include opiates and opiate derivatives (loperamide and diphenoxylate), bismuth subsalicylate, and kaolin-containing agents. Also, bismuth subsalicylate (Pepto-Bismol) is safe and efficacious in the treatment of infectious bacterial diarrhea. There is concern that agents that decrease intestinal transit time are contraindicated in invasive infectious diarrhea, but the use of these medications in such patients is generally safe.
- Antibiotic therapy for *C. jejuni* is ciprofloxacin 500 mg PO bid for 5 days or azithromycin 500 mg PO once daily for 3 days.
- Antibiotic therapy for *V. parahaemolyticus* does not shorten the course of the infection (fluoroquinolones and doxycycline effective *in vitro*).
- See respective chapters for antibiotic treatment of other inflammatory causes of diarrhea.

COMPLICATIONS

- Both shigellosis and infection with enterohemorrhagic *E. coli* may be accompanied by the hemolytic–uremic syndrome, particularly in persons who are very young or very old.
- *Yersinia* infection and occasionally other enteric bacterial infections may be accompanied by Reiter's syndrome (arthritis, urethritis, and conjunctivitis), thyroiditis, pericarditis, or glomerulonephritis.

Follow-Up

Many isolates of *C. jejuni*, *Shigella*, and *Salmonella* are resistant to many antibiotics, and patients should be monitored for treatment failure.

PREVENTION

Improvements in hygiene to limit fecal–oral spread of enteric pathogens will be necessary if the prevalence of diarrheal diseases is to be significantly reduced in developing countries.

Selected Readings

Aranda-Michel J, Giannella RA. Acute diarrhea: A practical review. *Am J Med* 1999;106:670–676.

Butterton JR, Calderwood SB. Acute infectious diarrheal diseases and bacterial food poisoning. In: Fauci AS, Braunwald E, Isselbacher KJ, et al., eds. *Harrison's principles of medicine*, 14th ed. New York: McGraw-Hill, 1998:796–801.

Friedman LS, Isselbacher KJ. Diarrhea and constipation. In: Fauci AS, Braunwald E, Isselbacher KJ, et al., eds. *Harrison's principles of medicine*, 14th ed. New York: McGraw-Hill, 1998:236–244.

Gorbach SL. Treating diarrhoea. *BMJ* 1997;314:1776–1777.

Lopez AP, Gorbach SL. Diarrhea in AIDS. *Infect Dis Clin North Am* 1988;2:705–718.

Dysuria

 ## Basics

DEFINITION
- The term *dysuria* is used to characterize painful or difficult urination.
- Some authors use the term *acute urethral syndrome* to describe symptoms of dysuria, urgency, and frequency unaccompanied by significant bacteriuria.

APPROACH TO THE PATIENT
- Many physicians equate dysuria with urinary tract infection and treat with antibiotics. This therapeutic trial represents undertreatment for many patients and inappropriate treatment for others.
- A careful history and examination (including rectal and pelvic examination) can lead to a diagnosis and minimize laboratory testing.
- If dysuria is accompanied by fever, consider an infectious etiology (pyelonephritis, cystitis, acute prostatitis, and genital herpes).
- If dysuria is accompanied by hematuria, consider cystitis, interstitial cystitis, schistosomiasis, tuberculous cystitis, and bladder carcinoma.
- If dysuria is accompanied by urethral or vaginal discharge, consider urethral syndrome and gonorrhea (women) or gonorrhea, prostatitis, nonspecific urethritis, and Reiter's syndrome (men).
- If dysuria is accompanied by severe pain with urination, consider urethritis, acute cystitis, interstitial cystitis, a renal stone, and prostatitis.
- Urinalysis, urine culture, and urinal and vaginal smears are the initial diagnostic tests.

ETIOLOGY
- In addition to the causes noted above, dysuria can be due to the following:
  — Atrophic vaginitis (caused by urine contact with the inflamed atrophic tissues themselves or because of the increased incidence of urinary tract infections in these women)
  — Bladder irritation from a distal urethral stone
  — Chemical exposure (irritant or topical allergic responses to soaps, douches, vaginal lubricants, spermicidal jellies, contraceptive foams and sponges, soaps, toilet paper, tampons, and sanitary napkins)
  — Compression from an adnexal mass
  — Radiation
  — Vaginal and urethral trauma, including sexual abuse and the insertion of a foreign body
- Among women presenting with acute dysuria and frequency, 60% to 70% have significant bacteriuria, but most of those without significant bacteriuria also have infections of the kidneys, bladder, or urethra.
- Atrophic vaginitis increases the risk for urinary tract infections.
- Pathogens causing dysuria vary with the underlying cause.
- *Ureaplasma urealyticum* has frequently been isolated from the urethra and urine of patients with dysuria, but it is also found in specimens from patients without urinary symptoms.
- *U. urealyticum* and *Mycoplasma hominis* have been isolated from prostatic and renal tissues of patients with dysuria.
- Adenoviruses cause acute hemorrhagic cystitis in children and in some young adults, often in epidemics. Although many other viruses can be isolated from urine, they are thought not to cause urinary infection.

EPIDEMIOLOGY
- Up to 25% of women in the United States have dysuria each year.
- Eighty percent of patients with primary symptomatic genital herpes will have dysuria; however, dysuria is usually not present if the infection recurs.
- Sexual intercourse is associated with many causes of dysuria. Women with postcoital cystitis typically develop symptoms within a few days of intercourse, as women with urethritis develop symptoms 1 to 2 weeks later, and women with vaginitis develop symptoms weeks to months later.
- Acute urinary tract infections account for more than six million office visits annually in the United States. These infections occur in 1% to 3% of schoolgirls and then increase markedly in incidence with the onset of sexual activity in adolescence.
- Ten percent to 15% of women over 60 years of age have frequent urinary tract infections.
- Atrophic vaginitis is a common disorder, affecting 20% to 30% of postmenopausal women.
- Acute symptomatic urinary infections are unusual in men under the age of 50.

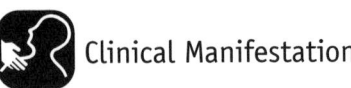 ## Clinical Manifestations

- Atrophic vaginitis is associated with decreased vaginal discharge, vaginal tenderness, bloody vaginal spotting (especially after intercourse), and dyspareunia.
- Dysuria, frequency, urgency, and suprapubic tenderness are common symptoms of bladder and urethral inflammation.
- Prostatitis leads to frequency, dysuria, and urgency, and the prostate may be boggy and tender on rectal examination.
- Symptoms of acute pyelonephritis generally develop rapidly over a few hours or a day and include a temperature of 39.4°C (103°F), shaking chills, nausea, vomiting, and diarrhea. Symptoms of cystitis may or may not develop. In addition to fever, tachycardia, and generalized muscle tenderness, physical examination reveals marked tenderness on deep pressure in one or both costovertebral angles or on deep abdominal palpation.
- Flank pain, chills, fever, nausea and vomiting, hypotension from sepsis, and leukocyte casts all suggest true renal parenchymal infection (i.e., pyelonephritis); their absence, however, does not exclude pyelonephritis.

Dysuria

Diagnosis

- The most sensitive laboratory indicator for urinary tract infections is pyuria. A positive leukocyte esterase dipstick test is 75% to 95% sensitive in detecting pyuria secondary to infection.
- Bacterial colony counts of 10^5 organisms per milliliter or greater in urine generally indicate urinary tract colonization and infection. Levels above 10^2 colonies per milliliter are sufficient to indicate infection in symptomatic patients and in urine samples obtained by suprapubic aspiration or bladder catheter.
- Most of the subtypes of the known bacterial pathogens (with the exception of *Staphylococcus saprophyticus* and *Enterococcus* spp) can convert urinary nitrate to nitrite. Positive nitrite is over 90% specific for urinary tract infections, but sensitivity is only about 30%.
- Rapid methods of detection of bacteriuria have been developed as alternatives to standard culture methods. These methods detect bacterial growth by photometry, bioluminescence, or other means and provide results rapidly, usually in 1 to 2 hours. Compared with urine cultures, these techniques generally exhibit a sensitivity of 95% to 98% and a negative predictive value of >99% when bacteriuria is defined as 10^5 colony-forming units per milliliter. However, the sensitivity of these tests falls to 60% to 80% when 10^2 to 10^4 colony-forming units per milliliter is the standard of comparison.
- Pyuria in the absence of bacteriuria (sterile pyuria) may indicate infection with unusual bacterial agents, such as *C. trachomatis*, *U. urealyticum*, and *Mycobacterium tuberculosis*, or with fungi. Sterile pyuria may also indicate prostatitis and noninfectious urologic conditions such as calculi, anatomic abnormality, nephrocalcinosis, vesicoureteral reflux, interstitial nephritis, or polycystic disease.
- Potassium hydroxide and normal saline vaginal smears may reveal mycelia and motile trichomonads in patients with suspected vaginitis. Most women with urethritis are found to have greater than five white blood cells per high-power field on urethral smear.

Treatment

- The choice of treatment for women with acute urethritis depends on the etiologic agent involved and is discussed in the chapters. Section I, "Urethritis and Urethral Discharge" and Section II, "Prostatitis" and "Vaginal Discharge/Vaginitis."
- If dysuria is caused by chemical exposure, avoidance of the irritative agent generally leads to the resolution of symptoms.
- Women with acute dysuria and frequency, negative urine cultures, and no pyuria usually do not respond to antimicrobial agents.

COMPLICATIONS

- Complicated urinary tract infections are defined as those occurring in patients with anatomically or functionally abnormal urinary tracts, or in patients who are immunocompromised or have iatrogenic infections. Clinical recognition of complicated urinary tract infections is important because these patients are more likely to harbor resistant organisms. Therapy consists of broader spectrum agents such as the fluoroquinolones. Cystitis should be treated for 1 week. Upper urinary tract infections should be treated for 2 weeks. A urine culture should be obtained to confirm sensitivity.
- Cystitis may result in upper tract infection.

Follow-Up

- Of the more than 30% of women who will experience at least one episode of cystitis in their lifetime, 20% will have recurrent cystitis.
- Recurrent urinary tract infections are usually reinfections separated by an asymptomatic interval of at least 1 month's duration. They are usually caused by vaginal and rectal colonization with uropathogens. Anatomic abnormalities in young women with recurrent cystitis are rare.

PREVENTION

Topical estriol vaginal cream is an effective treatment in postmenopausal women with recurrent infections.

Selected Readings

Collins RD. Dysuria. In: Collins RD, ed. *Algorithmic diagnosis of symptoms and signs: Cost-effective approach.* New York: Igaku-Shoin Medical Publishers, 1995:165–166.

Kurowski K. The women with dysuria. *Am Fam Physician* 1998;57:2155–2164, 2169–2170.

Richardson DA. Dysuria and urinary tract infections. *Obstet Gynecol Clin North Am* 1990;17:881–888.

Stamm WE. Urinary tract infections and pyelonephritis. In: Fauci AS, Braunwald E, Isselbacher KJ, et al., eds. *Harrison's principles of medicine*, 14th ed. New York: McGraw-Hill, 1998:131, 817–824.

Wathne B, Hovelius B, Mardh PA. Causes of frequency and dysuria in women. *Scand J Infect Dis* 1987;19:223–229.

Ear Pain

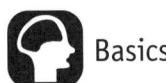 ## Basics

DEFINITIONS
The terms *otalgia* and *earache* are used to describe pain involving the ear.

APPROACH TO THE PATIENT
- The age of the patient and the presence of sore throat, fever, or other symptoms, as well as the duration of these symptoms, should be investigated.
- Examining the ear itself is the most critical assessment in the evaluation of ear pain. The auricle and external auditory meatus should be examined first, because the presence or absence of signs of infection can aid in the differential diagnosis.
- During the otoscopic examination, adequate visualization of the external canal and tympanic membrane is essential. For this, removal of cerumen should be undertaken first.
- If there is an exudate, a culture and sensitivity should be obtained.
- Physical examination may also reveal lymphadenopathy, posterior nasal or pharyngeal inflammation, and discharge.

ETIOLOGY
- Otalgia is often related to pathology in areas of the head and neck apart from the ear. This is due to the rich innervation of the ear via the fifth, seventh, ninth, and tenth cranial nerves and the cervical plexus.
- Severe pain in the ear and its vicinity can be caused by the following:
  —Disease of the teeth (abscess, impacted teeth, etc.)
  —Laryngeal foreign body
  —Inflammatory and neoplastic disease of the larynx and nasopharynx
  —Temporomandibular joint disorders
  —Tonsillitis
  —Tumors
  —Diseases of the cervical spine
  —Tumor of the acoustic nerve
  —Gastroesophageal reflux (in infants and children)
  —Medications (such as mesalazine and sulfasalazine)
  —Acute bacterial thyroiditis
  —Inflammation and thrombosis of the lateral sinus
  —Inflammation of the posterior fossa
- Otalgia due primarily to ear processes also has a broad differential diagnosis that includes the following:
  —Acute otitis media
  —Furunculosis of the ear canal
  —Traumatic rupture of the tympanum
  —Fracture of the anterior wall of the body canal
  —Osteomyelitis of the mastoid bone
- Ear pain is also associated with vascular headaches, atypical facial pain, and herpes simplex of the fifth and seventh cranial nerves and the glossopharyngeal nerve.
- Herpes zoster in the external canal is often accompanied by ipsilateral facial paralysis (Ramsay Hunt syndrome) due to the involvement of the geniculate ganglion of cranial nerve VII.
- Bell's palsy may be caused by herpes zoster and Lyme disease.
- The infratemporal fossa is a relatively protected region that may be the site of malignant neoplasms causing otalgia.
- The most common pathogens of acute otitis externa are *Pseudomonas aeruginosa*, *Staphylococcus aureus*, and streptococci, and the disease is seen most commonly in diabetics.
- *P. aeruginosa* is often found in the external auditory canal, particularly under moist conditions and in the presence of inflammation or maceration (as in "swimmer's ear").

EPIDEMIOLOGY
- It is estimated that 50% of ear pain is referred from nonotologic sites.
- Acute otitis externa (or "swimmer's ear") occurs mostly in the summer.
- Annual health care costs for treatment of otitis media in children younger than age 6 years are estimated at $5 billion.
- About 20% of children have multiple, recurrent episodes of acute otitis media.
- Most head and neck cancers occur after age 50, although these cancers can appear in younger patients, including those without known risk factors.
- In auricular cellulitis, there may be a history of minor trauma to the ear.
- Perichondritis (infection of the perichondrium of the ear) usually follows burns or significant trauma to the ear. *P. aeruginosa* and *S. aureus* are the most common pathogens.
- Chronic otitis externa is often due to irritation from either repeated minor trauma to the canal (e.g., scratching or use of cotton swabs) or drainage of a chronic middle ear infection.

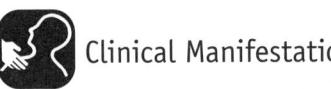 ## Clinical Manifestations

- Auricular cellulitis usually presents as a swollen, erythematous, hot, mildly tender ear. The lobule usually is especially swollen and red.
- Perichondritis is often accompanied by infection of the underlying cartilage of the pinna (chondritis). Patients present with a swollen, hot, red, and exquisitely tender pinna, usually with sparing of the lobule.
- Chronic otitis externa causes pruritus rather than ear pain.
- In acute otitis externa, the ear is pruritic and painful, and the canal appears swollen and red.
- Cancer of the nasopharynx typically does not cause early symptoms. However, on occasion, it may cause unilateral serous otitis media due to obstruction of the eustachian tube, unilateral or bilateral nasal obstruction, or epistaxis.
- Advanced nasopharyngeal carcinoma can cause neuropathies of the cranial nerves.
- Patients with malignant external otitis usually have diabetes and present with otalgia and otorrhea. Facial nerve paralysis tends to occur early, while other cranial nerve palsies appear later. There may be a

Ear Pain

loss of hearing, the pinna of the ear is typically tender, and trismus indicates temporomandibular involvement. Constitutional symptoms such as fever and weight loss are relatively uncommon. Physical examination almost always reveals abnormalities of the external auditory canal, including swelling, erythema, purulent discharge, debris, and granulation tissue in the canal wall.
- Temporomandibular joint dysfunction may be diagnosed by finding tenderness of the joint or masticatory muscles in at least two separate sites.
- A vesicular rash of the drum and external auditory canal may indicate herpes zoster.
- Hearing loss with an abdominal drum suggests serous or bacterial otitis media or cholesteatoma.
- Polyposis, severe deviation of the nasal septum, or a nasopharyngeal tumor may be associated with otitis media.

 Diagnosis

DIFFERENTIAL DIAGNOSIS

- Pain on moving the ear suggests otitis externa, foreign body, and impacted wax.
- A trial of carbamazepine or phenytoin may be useful in diagnosing glossopharyngeal neuralgia.
- Perichondritis must be distinguished from relapsing polychondritis, a rheumatologic condition.

LABORATORY

Peripheral leukocytosis is relatively infrequent in malignant external otitis, while the erythrocyte sedimentation rate usually is markedly elevated. Cerebrospinal fluid occasionally exhibits pleocytosis and an elevation in the protein level.

IMAGING

- Dental disease can be excluded by radiographic examination.
- In malignant external otitis, computed tomography (CT) of the mastoid or temporal bone typically reveals bony erosions and new bone formation, while the floor of the skull may have soft-tissue densities associated with areas of cellulitis. Magnetic resonance imaging (MRI) may delineate soft-tissue involvement with greater sensitivity and accuracy.

 Treatment

- Treatment of acute otitis externa consists of cleansing of the ear with alcohol–acetic acid mixtures and the administration of topical antibiotic ear drops, such as polymyxin–neomycin (4 drops four times daily for 5 days).
- Malignant otitis externa is tested with ciprofloxacin 500 mg bid PO or i.v., if indicated. Treatment should be extended for 3 to 4 weeks, and even longer if bone is involved.
- Treatment of auricular cellulitis consists of warm compresses and i.v. administration of antibiotics active against *S. aureus* and streptococci.
- Severe perichondritis should be treated with antibiotics, such as i.v. ticarcillin/clavulanic acid (3.1 g i.v. q4h) or i.v. nafcillin (2 g i.v. every 4–6 hours) plus oral ciprofloxacin (750 mg PO bid), for at least 4 weeks. Incision and drainage may be helpful for culture and for resolution of infection, which is often slow.
- Although the antiviral agent acyclovir (acyclovir 400 mg PO five times orally for 10 days, with or without prednisone 30 mg PO bid for 5 days, and then taper) is currently used for the treatment of Ramsay Hunt syndrome, its effects on facial nerve and hearing recovery remain controversial. A retrospective analysis among 80 patients with Ramsay Hunt syndrome, early administration of acyclovir–prednisone was proved to reduce nerve degeneration by nerve excitability testing. Hearing recovery also tended to be better in patients with early treatment. There was no significant difference in facial nerve outcome between i.v. and oral acyclovir treatment.

COMPLICATIONS

- Complications of otitis media and mastoiditis include epidural abscess, dural venous thrombophlebitis (usually sigmoid sinus), meningitis, and brain abscess.
- Osteomyelitis of the mastoid bone can affect the periosteum and lead to epidural abscess.
- The cavernous sinus can become involved in malignant external otitis, as can the contralateral petrous apex; meningitis and brain abscess are relatively rare complications.

 Follow-Up

If otalgia does not resolve in a short period, further work-up and probably referral to an otorhinolaryngologist are indicated. To simply continue monitoring may lead to losing the chance of early diagnosis of a malignancy.

PREVENTION

Ear pain is not uncommon in children traveling by commercial aircraft. The predeparture use of pseudoephedrine does not decrease the risk for in-flight ear pain in children but is associated with drowsiness.

 Selected Readings

Collins RD. Earache. In: Collins RD, ed. *Algorithmic diagnosis of symptoms and signs: Cost-effective approach*. Collins RD, ed. Igaku-Shoin Medical Publishers, 1995:167–168.

Durand M, Joseph M, Baker AS. Infections of the upper respiratory tract. In: Fauci AS, Braunwald E, Isselbacher KJ, et al., eds. *Harrison's principles of medicine*, 14th ed. New York: McGraw-Hill,. 1998:179–184.

Gates GA. Otitis media—The pharyngeal connection. *JAMA* 1999;282:987–989.

Murakami S, Hato N, Horiuchi J, et al. Treatment of Ramsay Hunt syndrome with acyclovir-prednisone: Significance of early diagnosis and treatment. *Ann Neurol* 1997;41:353–357.

Fever of Unknown Origin

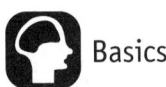 ## Basics

DEFINITION
The term *fever of unknown origin* (FUO) is used to describe fever that does not resolve spontaneously in the period expected for self-limited infection and whose cause cannot be ascertained despite considerable diagnostic effort.

APPROACH TO THE PATIENT
- Initially, FUO was defined as the following:
  — Illness of more than 3 weeks' duration
  — Temperatures higher than 38.3°C on several occasions
  — Diagnosis uncertain after 1 week of stay in hospital
- Because thorough diagnostic testing can now be done in an outpatient setting, the definition was modified to remove the requirement of hospitalization for the week of evaluation.
- More recently, a new system has been proposed for classification of FUO:
  — Classic FUO
  — Nosocomial FUO
  — Neutropenic FUO
  — FUO associated with human immunodeficiency virus infection
  — Based on this approach, neutropenic patients, hospitalized individuals that were afebrile prior to their admission, and those with advanced HIV infection can be considered as having FUO only after 3 to 5 days of evaluation in the hospital.
- In order to qualify for the diagnosis of FUO, a minimum diagnostic evaluation should include the following:
  — Detailed history
  — Repeat physical examination
  — Complete blood count with differential and platelet count
  — Routine blood chemistry, including liver enzymes, LDH, and bilirubin
  — Urinalysis (including microscopy)
  — Chest radiograph
  — Erythrocyte sedimentation rate
  — Antinuclear antibodies
  — Rheumatoid factor
  — Three sets of routine blood cultures (while not on antibiotics)
  — Tuberculin skin test
  — Computerized tomography of abdomen
  — Evaluation for viral causes (HIV antibodies or viral load, cytomegalovirus antibodies, heterophile antibody, etc.) based on the clinical scenario

ETIOLOGY
Differential Diagnosis
- The most common infectious causes of FUO include the following:
  — Intravascular infections
  — Endocarditis
  — Bacterial aortitis
  — Intravenous catheter infection
    — Septic jugular phlebitis
    — Vascular graft infection
  — Systemic bacterial infections: bartonellosis, brucellosis, *Campylobacter* infection, cat-scratch disease/bacillary angiomatosis, ehrlichiosis, gonococcemia, legionellosis, leptospirosis, listeriosis, Lyme disease, meningococcemia, rat-bite fever, relapsing fever (*Borrelia recurrentis*), salmonellosis (including typhoid fever), syphilis, tularemia, and yersiniosis
  — Chlamydial infections: psittacosis, lymphogranuloma venereum, *C. pneumoniae* infection, etc.
  — Fungal infections: candidemia, cryptococcosis, histoplasmosis, coccidioidomycosis, blastomycosis, sporotrichosis, aspergillosis, mucormycosis, *Pneumocystis carinii*, *Malassezia furfur*
  — Parasitic infections: amebiasis, babesiosis, Chagas' disease, leishmaniasis, malaria, strongyloidiasis, toxoplasmosis, trichinosis, infected hydatid cyst, trypanosomiasis, and so forth
  — Tuberculosis and infections caused by atypical mycobacteria
  — Viral infections: cytomegalovirus, Epstein-Barr virus, viral hepatitis, HIV infection, parvovirus B19 infection, and so forth
- Also, FUO can be caused by localized infections such as appendicitis, cholangitis and cholecystitis, dental abscess, diverticulitis, intraabdominal abscess (such as subphrenic, liver, splenic, pancreatic, perinephric, placental, etc.), intracranial abscess, lung abscess, mastoiditis, mesenteric lymphadenitis, osteomyelitis or infected joint prosthesis, otitis media, pelvic inflammatory disease, perinephric abscess, prostatic abscess, prostatitis, pyometra, sinusitis, tracheobronchitis, and wound infection.
- The most common noninfectious causes of FUO are the following:
  — Neoplasms
    — Malignant (colon cancer, hepatoma, Hodgkin's lymphoma, leukemia, malignant histiocytosis, nephroma, non-Hodgkin's lymphoma, pancreatic cancer, sarcoma, etc.)
    — Benign (atrial myxoma, etc.)
  — Collagen and granulomatous diseases: adult Still's disease, ankylotic spondylitis, Behçet's syndrome, Crohn's disease, cryoglobulinemia, erythema multiforme, erythema nodosum, giant-cell arthritis, hypersensitivity vasculitis, polyarteritis nodosa, polymyalgia rheumatica, Reiter's syndrome, rheumatic fever, rheumatoid arthritis, sarcoidosis, Sjögren's syndrome, systemic lupus erythematosus, Takayasu's aortitis, and urticaria vasculitis
  — Miscellaneous conditions: hematoma, recurrent pulmonary embolism, aortic dissection, after myocardial infarction, subacute thyroiditis, hyperthyroidism, drug fever, gout, pseudogout, hypersensitivity pneumonitis, encephalitis, cerebrovascular accident, familial Mediterranean fever, pheochromocytoma, etc.
  — Factitious fever
  — Exaggerated circadian rhythm

EPIDEMIOLOGY
- Infections count for about one-third of cases of FUO, followed by neoplasms and collagen vascular diseases.

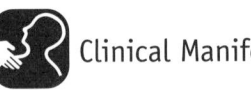 ## Clinical Manifestations

The diagnostic approach in FUO includes a thorough history, careful physical examination, laboratory tests, and radiographic studies.

HISTORY
- A thorough history is important, and this should include information about alcohol intake, medications, occupational exposures, pets, travel, familial diseases, and previous illnesses.
- Specific fever patterns have been described for many infectious and noninfectious causes of FUO. However, entities that usually have a distinctive fever pattern (e.g., malaria) are rare, and fever patterns thought to be distinctive for other diseases, such as Pel-Ebstein fever in lymphoma, are uncommon.

Fever of Unknown Origin

PHYSICAL EXAMINATION

- The specific findings that have led to a diagnosis in FUO are diverse, and a thorough clinical assessment is the cornerstone for diagnosis. This should include evaluation of the following:
  — Oropharynx (dental abscess)
  — Thyroid (thyroiditis)
  — Temporal area (temporal arteritis)
  — Heart murmurs (atrial myxoma)
  — Skin (Whipple's disease)
- Relative bradycardia may be useful, but it is associated with a substantial differential diagnosis, including brucellosis, drug fever, factitious fever, hepatitis A, legionnaire's disease, leptospirosis, neoplasms, psittacosis, subacute necrotising lymphadenitis, and typhoid fever.
- Fever due to solid tumors and many collagen diseases usually subsides promptly with the use of nonsteroidal antiinflammatories, while fever due to other causes may persist.
- Other features, such as sweats, chills, or weight loss, have not discriminated among causes of FUO.

Diagnosis

- Noninvasive laboratory tests have provided a diagnosis in perhaps one-fourth of FUO cases. These include serologic tests for microbial pathogens or rheumatologic diseases.
- Imaging has been used primarily to localize abnormalities for subsequent evaluation. Abdominal computed tomography (CT), in particular, has increased the rate of positive results when subsequent invasive diagnostic procedures are done.
- False-negative CT results have occasionally been reported, even with abscesses in solid organs.
- MRI is preferred if a spinal or paraspinal lesion is suspected.
- When infection or malignancy is the cause of FUO, scanning with gallium-67- or indium-111-labeled autologous leucocytes has been helpful, and the overall yield may be higher than that with CT or ultrasound. Limitations include false-negative gallium results with secondary infected lesions (e.g., hematomas or pseudocysts), difficulty detecting splenic abscesses due to a high level of background uptake in the spleen, and a low positive predictive value with indium.
- If imaging and serologic studies are unrevealing, invasive studies (including liver and bone marrow biopsy) should be considered.
- Diagnosis in fewer than half the cases of FUO has resulted from excisional or needle biopsy or laparotomy.
- The yield from open or under-CT-guidance biopsies is greater than that of bedside biopsy procedures.
- The only biopsy that may often be rewarding in the absence of prior localizing information is the temporal artery biopsy in elderly patients with a very high erythrocyte sedimentation rate.
- Disseminated tuberculosis probably is the most treatable cause of death in patients with FUO and warrants vigorous diagnostic efforts when the disease is suspected. A tuberculin skin test may be negative in up to one-half of patients, and sputum smears may be positive for acid-fast bacilli in only one-fourth to one-half of cases.
- Lymph node biopsy may be helpful if nodes are enlarged. Inguinal nodes are often palpable but are seldom diagnostically useful.
- Hospitalized patients should be evaluated for sinus infection (common in intubated patients) or for other nosocomial complications, such as acalculous cholecystitis, *Clostridium difficile* colitis, and drug reactions.
- Infection with *Brucella canis* may be missed with standard antibody tests for *Brucella*.
- *Salmonella* infection elevates antibody titers to the H and O antigens. High titers of antibody to the H antigen persist for years and may reflect previous infection or immunization.
- The measurement of specific antirickettsial titers should be requested for the diagnosis of Rocky Mountain spotted fever and Q fever.

Treatment

- Therapy varies based on the underlying condition.
- The emphasis in patients with classic FUO is on continuing the observation and examination, with avoidance of empirical therapy.
- If the PPD skin test is positive or if granulomatous disease (with possible anergy) is present, then a therapeutic trial for tuberculosis should be undertaken, with treatment continued for up to 6 weeks. Failure of the fever to respond over this period suggests an alternative diagnosis.
- Glucocorticoids and nonsteroidal antiinflammatories could mask fever, while permitting the spread of infection, so their use should be avoided unless infection has been largely excluded.
- Details on the management of nosocomial, neutropenic, and HIV-associated fever are discussed elsewhere in this book.

COMPLICATIONS

N/A

Follow-Up

- In half of cases of FUO, the abnormalities are detected only by repeat examinations.
- As the duration of fever increases, the likelihood of an infectious cause decreases.
- FUO patients who remain undiagnosed after extensive evaluation generally have a favorable outcome.
- Physicians should do the following:
  — Discontinue as many medicines as possible.
  — Repeatedly interview and examine the patient.
  — Review laboratory test results and imaging studies.

PREVENTION

N/A

Selected Readings

Arnow PM, Flaherty JP. Fever of unknown origin. *Lancet* 1997;350:575–580.

Gelfand JA, Dinarello CA. Fever of unknown origin. In: Fauci AS, Braunwald E, Isselbacher KJ, et al., eds. *Harrison's principles of internal medicine,* 14th ed. New York: McGraw-Hill, 1998:780–785.

Genital Lesions

Basics

DEFINITION
- Lesions involving the reproductive organs

APPROACH TO THE PATIENT
- Several infectious and noninfectious diseases cause genital lesions. The relative frequency of these diseases in a population is determined by many factors, including age, sexual behavior, residence, and travel.
- Physicians should clarify when the genital lesions first appeared, identify any possible accompanying symptoms, and investigate any underlying immunodeficiency, previous sexually transmitted diseases, or history of similar genital lesions.
- Obtaining a detailed sexual history and a careful travel history is necessary.
- On physical examination, the physician should identify the type and the extent of the lesions; investigate whether these are confined to the genitalia or have spread to other skin areas; evaluate for associated tenderness, inguinal or generalized lymphadenopathy, or any vaginal or urethral discharge; and perform a careful examination of the buccal mucosa and the perianal area.
- Pelvic examination or evaluation of the prostate is often indicated.
- Clinicians are not always able to establish the diagnosis of genital lesions based on morphology alone.
- When the diagnosis is unclear or the lesion could be due to skin cancer, a consultation by an experienced dermatologist and biopsies by a gynecologist or a urologist should be obtained.

ETIOLOGY

Differential Diagnosis
- Genital ulcers are the most common type of genital lesion caused by sexually transmitted diseases.
- Infectious: genital herpes, syphilis (*Treponema pallidum*), chancroid (*Haemophilus ducreyi*), lymphogranuloma venereum (*Chlamydia trachomatis* serovars L$_1$, L$_2$, or L$_3$), donovanosis or granuloma inguinale (*Calymmatobacterium granulomatis*), tuberculosis, and tularemia
  —Less common causes: candidiasis, histoplasmosis, amebiasis, gonorrhea, trichomoniasis
- Noninfectious: trauma, fixed drug eruption, malignancy (skin cancer, leukemia, etc.), and systemic lupus erythematosus
- Unclear etiology: Behçet's disease

- Less common genital lesions
  —Papules: candidiasis, molluscum contagiosum, scabies (*Sarcoptes scabiei*), syphilis, veneral warts or condylomata acumulata (human papillomavirus; types 6 and 11 most common, types 16, 18, 31, 33, and 35 associated with cervical dysplasia)
  —Vesicles and bullae: herpes genitalis, impetigo, scabies
  —Diffuse erythema: candidiasis, erysipelas (usually associated with trauma or surgery), contact dermatitis, drug eruption, psoriasis, trauma
  —Benign cysts
  —Nodules: hidradenitis, furunculosis
  —Crusts: herpes genitalis, scabies

EPIDEMIOLOGY
N/A

Clinical Manifestations

HISTORY
- *Candida albicans* and herpes simplex virus are common causes among neonates.
- In North America and Europe, sexually transmitted diseases most likely to cause genital ulcers are, in decreasing order of frequency, genital herpes, syphilis, and chancroid.
- Chancroid is more prevalent in Africa, Asia, and Latin America.
- Lymphogranuloma venereum and donovanosis occur mainly in certain tropical areas.
- Up to 10% of patients with genital ulcers have more than one pathogen.
- Genital lesions that develop within hours of sexual exposure suggest trauma, chemical irritation, or hypersensitivity.
- Usual incubation period:
  —Chancroid: 5 to 7 days (can be from 1 day to 3 weeks)
  —Donovanosis: 2 to 3 weeks
  —Genital warts: 4 to 12 weeks (occasionally longer)
  —Herpes genitalis: 2 to 7 days (can be up to 4 weeks)
  —Molluscum contagiosum: up to 8 months
  —Pubic lice and scabies: 4 to 6 weeks
  —Syphilis: 1 to 3 weeks (can be up to 3 months)
- Pruritus is almost always present among patients with herpes genitalis (especially during incubation), scabies, and pubic lice. Severe pruritus is uncommon among patients with secondary syphilis, but mild itching can be present.

PHYSICAL EXAMINATION
- Behçet's disease can present with recurrent, multiple genital ulcerations (>80%) that usually involve the scrotum or vulva. It is also characterized by recurrent oral ulcerations (>97%) and lesions that involve other areas of the skin (75%) or the eyes (50%).
- Linear tracks suggest scabies, while reddish flecks can be due to crab louse excreta.
- Primary syphilis usually causes a single lesion, while chancroid usually presents as multiple ulcerations of variable size.
- The classic initial lesion of genital herpes is grouped vesicles on an erythematous base. Umbilications are sometimes observed. The lesion is extremely painful, and the vesicles have often ruptured by the time the patient seeks medical attention.
- Tenderness on palpation characterizes herpes genitalis, chancroid, and tularemia.
- Ulcerated lesions of donovanosis are nontender.
- Ulcer base
  —Behçet's disease: yellow and necrotic
  —Chancroid: necrotic
  —Donovanosis: beefy red with hypertrophy
  —Syphilitic and herpetic ulcers: clean
- Ulcer edge
  —Chancroid: nonindurated ("soft chancre"), erythematous, irregular
  —Donovanosis: white
  —Herpetic ulcers: erythematous
  —Syphilitic: indurated
- Urethral discharge suggests gonorrhea or Reiter's syndrome.
- The genital ulcer caused by lymphogranuloma venereum can go unnoticed by the patient. The ulcer spontaneously heals, and 24 weeks later, painful inguinal lymphadenopathy develops, often associated with signs of systemic infection (headache, arthralgia, leukocytosis, and hypergammaglobulinemia).
- Inguinal lymphadenopathy is not always associated with acute or local disease. However, the presence of inguinal lymphadenopathy in an adult with a genital lesion suggests the following:
  —Chancroid
  —Lymphogranuloma venereum
  —Syphilis
  —Genital herpes
  —Lymphoma
  —Tuberculosis
- Inguinal lymphadenopathy is usually unilateral in chancroid and lymphogranuloma venereum, and bilateral in genital herpes.

Genital Lesions

- Molluscum contagiosum is mildly infectious. Lesions are usually umbilicated and vary in size up to 1 cm. Patients with advanced HIV infection can have generalized molluscum contagiosum.
- Lymphogranuloma venereum can lead to elephantiasis and marked distortion of the genitalia.
- Tuberculous lesions usually manifest as chronic, minimally painful "sores" that are red, moderately firm, and nodular.
- For details on the diagnosis and treatment of syphilis, please see the chapter, "Syphilis" (Section II). Gonorrhea is discussed in the Section I chapter, "Urethritis and Urethral Discharge."

Diagnosis

- The differential diagnosis of genital lesions is challenging. History and physical examination alone often lead to an inaccurate diagnosis.
- Evaluation should include laboratory tests to investigate all three main possibilities: genital herpes, syphilis, and chancroid. However, this approach is often impractical because some tests are not readily available.
- Every patient with genital ulcer(s) should have at least the following:
  —A serologic test for syphilis
  —An HIV test, if HIV status is unknown, particularly in suspected cases of syphilis or chancroid
- Other tests of specimens obtained from genital lesions are based on availability and clinical or epidemiologic suspicion:
  —Dark-field microscopic examination or direct immunofluorescence test for *T. pallidum*
  —Culture or antigen test for herpes simplex virus
  —Culture for *H. ducreyi*
- Proper specimen collection technique is necessary. Lesions should be gently abraded with a sterile gauze pad to provoke oozing but not gross bleeding. Exudate from the lesion is increased if the lesion is squeezed between gloved thumb and forefinger. Direct application of exudate onto a microscope slide is used for dark-field and direct immunofluorescence tests.
- Donovanosis is usually diagnosed based on morphology. When indicated, confirmation can be obtained by demonstrating intracellular "Donovan bodies," using Giemsa or Wright stain, from lesion scrapings or biopsies. (Biopsy is preferred when malignancy is also a possibility.)
- Chancroid is usually diagnosed based on clinical data and morphologic demonstration of typical organisms in the lesion or culture. Culture is the preferred method (>80% sensitive), but selective culture media are not readily available.
- Diagnosis of lymphogranuloma venereum is based on serology or by isolating *C. trachomatis* and confirming the isotype (definitive diagnosis). Biopsy of lesions and lymph nodes should be performed in selected cases, due to low yield and the possibility of fistula formation.
- Diagnosis of molluscum contagiosum can be confirmed by histology and electron microscopy.

Treatment

MAIN

- Chancroid
  —Azithromycin (1 g orally) or
  —Ceftriaxone (250 mg intramuscular injection) given once
- Condylomata acumulata
  —No optimal treatment established.
  —Imiquimod 5% cream three times per week for 16 weeks or
  —Podophyllotoxin (podofilox 0.5% solution or gel) twice daily for 3 days, followed by 1 day off; repeat four times
- Donovanosis
  —Trimethoprim–sulfamethoxazole (one double-strength tablet orally bid) for >3 weeks
  —Tetracycline (500 mg orally qid) or
  —Doxycycline (100 mg orally bid) for >3 weeks
- Herpes simplex virus infection
  —Acyclovir (400 mg orally tid or 200 mg five times a day) for 7 to 10 days
  —Famciclovir (250 mg orally tid) for 7 to 10 days
  —Valacyclovir (1 g orally bid) for 7 to 10 days
  —See also Section II chapter, "Herpes Simplex Virus Infections."
- Tuberculous lesions: systemic antituberculosis treatment
- Lymphogranuloma venereum: doxycycline (100 mg bid orally) for 21 days
- Molluscum contagiosum: desiccation, freezing, or curettage of lesions

ALTERNATIVE

- Chancroid
  —Erythromycin (500 mg orally qid) for 7 days or
  —Ciprofloxacin (500 mg orally bid) for 3 days
- Condylomata acuminata: cryosurgery, excision, electrosurgical destruction, and laser evaporation
- Donovanosis: ciprofloxacin (750 mg orally bid) for >3 weeks, erythromycin, chloramphenicol
- Lymphogranuloma venereum: erythromycin (500 mg qid orally) for 21 days

COMPLICATIONS

N/A

Follow-Up

- The presence of sexually transmitted lesions in a child should prompt evaluation for sexual abuse.
- Women with human papilloma virus infection need to be counseled regarding the need for regular cytologic screening.
- Consider Pap smears for all patients evaluated for sexually transmitted diseases that did not have a documented Pap smear within the preceding 12 months.
- Patients on empiric treatment for chancroid should be reexamined 3 to 7 days after initiation of therapy. Ulcers should improve symptomatically within 3 days and objectively after 7 days.

PREVENTION

N/A

Selected Readings

Centers for Disease Control and Prevention. 1998 Guidelines for treatment of sexually transmitted diseases. Centers for Disease Control and Prevention. *Morbid Mortal Wkly Rep* 1998;47(RR1):1–111.

Rein MF. Genital skin and mucous membrane lesions. In: Mandell GL, Bennett JE, Dolin R, eds. *Principles and practice of infectious diseases,* 4th ed. New York: Churchill Livingstone, 1995:1055–1063.

Hepatosplenomegaly and Fever

Basics

DEFINITION

- Liver span (midclavicular line) equal to or higher than 15.5 cm suggests hepatomegaly.
- Any spleen greater than 250 g or that is palpable is deemed enlarged. The ultrasound criterion of enlargement is a cephalocaudad diameter of 13 cm or more.

APPROACH TO THE PATIENT

Evaluation for Hepatosplenomegaly

- Palpate to locate the lower liver border in the midclavicular line in situations of low probability of liver disease. If the liver is not palpable, one can defensibly forgo any further examination in patients without reason to suspect liver disease. With a palpable lower edge, the midclavicular line span can be ascertained by light percussion of the upper border. A span <12 to 13 cm on physical examination reduces the probability of hepatomegaly.
- A nonpalpable liver does reduce the probability of hepatomegaly, even though a palpable organ has less than a 50% chance of being enlarged.
- The bedside examination of the spleen should start with percussion. If percussion is not dull, there is no need to palpate, because the results of palpation will not effectively rule in or rule out splenic enlargement. If the possibility of missing splenic enlargement remains an important clinical concern, ultrasonography or scintigraphy is indicated. In the presence of percussion dullness, palpation should follow. If both tests are positive, the diagnosis of splenomegaly is established (provided that the clinical suspicion of splenomegaly was at least 10% before examination). If palpation is negative, diagnostic imaging is required to confidently rule in or rule out splenomegaly.

Approach to Patient with Liver and/or Spleen Enlargement and Fever

- History of travel, immigration, and immunodeficiency
- Evaluate for the following:
  —The presence of jaundice
  —The duration and characteristics of fever
  —The presence of lymphadenopathy
  —Consistency, nodularity, and tenderness of a palpable liver edge
  —The presence of enlarged gallbladder or another abdominal mass
  —The size and the consistency of the spleen
- Diagnostic tests include general laboratory evaluation, Monospot test, hepatitis profile, imaging studies, and, in certain cases, bone marrow examination, endoscopy, and/or liver biopsy.

ETIOLOGY

Hepatomegaly and Fever

- Infectious causes
  —Abscess
  —Ascending cholangitis
  —Chronic granulomatous disease of childhood
  —Chronic Q fever
  —Ehrlichiosis
  —Histoplasmosis
  —Infectious hepatitis
  —Infectious mononucleosis
  —Leptospirosis
  —Miliary tuberculosis
  —Parasitosis
  —Syphilis
- Noninfectious causes
  —Angiosarcoma
  —Diffuse hepatic carcinoma
  —Diffuse metastases
  —Familial Mediterranean fever
  —Lymphoma
- Other
  —Sarcoidosis

Splenomegaly and Fever

- Infectious causes
  —Brucellosis
  —Ehrlichiosis
  —Endocarditis
  —Infectious hepatitis
  —Infectious mononucleosis
  —Leptospirosis
  —Miliary tuberculosis
  —Parasitosis
  —Salmonellosis
  —Sepsis
- Noninfectious causes
  —Acute leukemia
  —Lymphoma
  —Systemic lupus erythematosus

- Numerous parasitic diseases can lead to liver and spleen enlargement. The causes vary based on epidemiologic data and include the following:
  —Schistosomiasis
  —Hydatidosis
  —Leishmaniasis
  —Toxocariasis
  —Toxoplasmosis
  —Fascioliasis (*Fasciola hepatica*)
- Fever is found in nearly 50% of cases with either *Toxoplasma* or *Toxocara* infections.

EPIDEMIOLOGY

- One study has reported data on a palpable liver among one thousand military personnel. In 57% of subjects, the liver either was not palpable in the right upper quadrant or was felt just at the costal margin. An additional 28% descended only 1 to 2 cm below the costal margin. Findings were similar for both sexes.
- In two other studies, about 3% of otherwise healthy students entering a U.S. college had unexplained palpable spleens, and 12% of otherwise normal postpartum women at a Canadian hospital had palpable spleens.
- In splenomegaly, percussion is somewhat more sensitive than palpation.

Clinical Manifestations

- In the tropics, a finding of splenomegaly can be due to tropical splenomegaly syndrome (also known as hyperreactive malarial splenomegaly). This syndrome is characterized by fever, anemia, weight loss, abdominal discomfort, and lassitude. Laboratory hallmarks include abnormal results of liver function tests, elevated IgM levels, and hepatic sinusoidal lymphocytosis.
- A constellation of fever, abdominal pain (whether or not localized in the right upper abdomen), vomiting or anorexia, hepatomegaly, elevated white blood cell count and sedimentation rate, and an unexplained anemia should prompt the clinician to include occult liver abscess in the differential diagnosis.

Hepatosplenomegaly and Fever

Diagnosis

DIFFERENTIAL DIAGNOSIS

- Differential diagnosis of jaundice and hepatomegaly in a person with AIDS:
  - Bacillary peliosis hepatis
  - Cholangitis
  - Chronic Q fever
  - Coccidioidomycosis
  - *Cryptococcus* spp
  - *Cryptosporidium* spp
  - Cytomegalovirus
  - Drug-induced
  - Histoplasmosis
  - Kaposi's sarcoma
  - Lymphoma
  - Microsporidiosis
  - *Mycobacterium avium-intracellulare*
  - *Mycobacterium tuberculosis*
  - *Pneumocystis carinii*
  - Viral hepatitis
- Cirrhosis or infiltrative disorders increase the firmness of the liver edge and the likelihood of its being felt independent of effect on organ size.
- A pulsatile liver edge is noted in tricuspid valvular disease. Pulsatile hepatomegaly is also found in constrictive pericarditis.

LABORATORY

- An elevated WBC with a shift to the left is suggestive of a bacterial infection.
- Eosinophilia can be found in cases of liver or spleen enlargement caused by parasitic diseases.

DIAGNOSTIC/TESTING PROCEDURES

- In HIV-seropositive patients who undergo percutaneous liver biopsy, the most common infectious causes are the following:
  - Chronic active viral hepatitis
  - *Mycobacterium avium* complex
  - *M. tuberculosis*
  - Other opportunistic hepatic infections
- For splenomegaly of unknown origin, the invasive procedure of choice for patients with hematologic associations is bone marrow biopsy; for those with hepatic association, a liver biopsy; and for those with infectious disease associations, a blood culture and lymph node biopsy.

Treatment

- Treatment of the infection with appropriate drugs
- Percutaneous aspiration of the liver abscess is preferred over surgery.
- Praziquantel is an effective and well-tolerated drug for treatment of *Schistosoma mansoni* infection in patients with advanced hepatosplenic schistosomiasis, and it is the drug of choice for patients with coexisting *Schistosoma haematobium* infection.
- Fascioliasis is usually managed with bithionol, at a dose of 40 mg/kg every other day in three divided doses for 30 days, or triclabendazole. The efficacy of praziquantel is controversial.

COMPLICATIONS

In the United States, nearly all cases of spontaneous splenic rupture are associated with infectious mononucleosis. Splenic rupture is a rare complication that is estimated to occur in 0.1% to 0.5% of the patients with infectious mononucleosis. However, this complication is the most frequent cause of death associated with infectious mononucleosis.

Follow-Up

Patients with splenomegaly should be monitored for the development of signs and symptoms suggestive of spontaneous splenic rupture. Severe upper abdominal pain is the presenting complaint in virtually all patients with spontaneous splenic rupture. The pain usually begins in the left upper quadrant and spreads throughout the abdomen, frequently radiating to the left shoulder. Patients may have tachycardia as well as signs that are suggestive of infectious mononucleosis, including pharyngitis, scleral jaundice, and lymphadenopathy.

PREVENTION

N/A

Selected Readings

Arjona R, Riancho JA, Aguado JM, et al. Fascioliasis in developed countries: A review of classic and aberrant forms of the disease. *Medicine* 1995;74:13–23.

Grover SA, Barkun AN, Sackett DL. Does this patient have splenomegaly? *JAMA* 1993;270:2218–2221.

Naylor CD. Physical examination of the liver. *JAMA* 1994;271:1859–1865.

O'Reilly RA. Splenomegaly in 2,505 patients at a large university medical center from 1913 to 1995. 1963 to 1995: 449 patients. *West J Med* 1998;169:88–97.

Poles MA, Dieterich DT, Schwarz ED, et al. Liver biopsy findings in 501 patients infected with human immunodeficiency virus (HIV). *J Acquir Immune Defic Syndr Hum Retrovirol* 1996;11:170–177.

Schuler JG, Filtzer H. Spontaneous splenic rupture. The role of nonoperative management. *Arch Surg* 1995;130:662–665.

Vinetz JM, Li J, McCutchan TF, Kaslow DC. *Plasmodium malariae* infection in an asymptomatic 74-year-old Greek woman with splenomegaly. *N Engl J Med* 1998;338:367–371.

Insect Bites and Stings

Basics

DEFINITION

- The vector is an animal, bird, or insect that transfers a pathogen from one host to another.
- Zoonosis is a disease of animals that may be transmitted to humans.

APPROACH TO THE PATIENT

- Insect bites and stings can cause an array of illnesses that can present with protean manifestations. Awareness of both their geographic distribution and their clinical presentations is critical in determining the probable cause of these illnesses.
- A history of mosquito bite has little diagnostic importance, while a history of tick bite has greater significance.
- A thorough travel history can be useful.
- Laboratory diagnosis of a transmitted agent often is elusive, particularly during the acute stage of illness. Specific diagnostic laboratory tests should be used, not for screening but to confirm the clinical diagnosis of insect-borne illness.
- Coinfection with another pathogen should be considered. For example, *Borrelia burgdorferi*, *Ehrlichia* spp, and *Babesia microti* are transmitted to humans by *Ixodes scapularis*, and patients can have infection with more than one of these pathogens.
- Because of the substantial morbidity and mortality associated with a delay in diagnosing and treating these infections, empiric administration of appropriate antimicrobial therapy is often justified. For example, empiric treatment with doxycycline can be life-saving in Rocky Mountain spotted fever and ehrlichiosis.

ETIOLOGY

- The most compelling vector-borne diseases that can be encountered by physicians in the United States are the following:
  —Lyme disease
    —Dengue
    —Eastern equine and other viral causes of encephalitis
    —Human granulocytic ehrlichiosis
    —Human monocytic ehrlichiosis
    —Rocky Mountain spotted fever
    —Bartonelloses of immunocompetent and immunocompromised persons, particularly those with AIDS
    —Yellow fever and malaria (usually among travelers returning from endemic areas)
    —A novel cat flea–associated, typhus-group rickettsiosis due to *Rickettsia felis*
    —A Southern erythema migrans–like illness
- Most of these infections are discussed in more detail in the Section I chapter, "Encephalitis," and in separate topics in this book.
- One unexplained phenomenon in the southeastern and south central states is the report of erythema migrans rash and constitutional symptoms. The probable vector of the agent causing this "Lyme disease-like" illness is *Amblyomma americanum*, the Lone Star tick.
- In the United States, most cases of tick paralysis in humans have occurred in the Pacific Northwest and Rocky Mountain states, usually in spring and summer. Most cases are in girls, but among adults, men are more likely than women to be affected.
- During 1999, West Nile virus infection associated with encephalitis was reported in the state of New York and is now recognized elsewhere.
- *R. felis* is transovarially (vertical from generation to generation through the egg) maintained in cat fleas (*Ctenocephalides felis*) and has been demonstrated infecting the tissues of opossums. Wild infected cat fleas have been detected in California, Texas, Louisiana, and New York. Human cases apparently similar to murine typhus by routine clinical and laboratory evaluation have occurred in Texas and California. The etiologic rickettsia is quite distinct genetically but shares substantial antigens with *Rickettsia typhi*.

EPIDEMIOLOGY

- In the United States in 1995, the reported incidence of Lyme disease was 4.4 cases per 100,000 population.
- From 1981 to 1992, the incidence of Rocky Mountain spotted fever was 0.6 to 1.5 cases per 100,000 in the United States. Approximately 5% to 12% of high-risk populations have evidence of antibodies.
- The incidence of ehrlichioses in the United States is low (1 per 100,000 per year) but may be as high as 14 to 16 cases per 100,000 in endemic areas.
- Eastern equine encephalitis is a life-threatening, mosquito-borne arboviral infection found principally along the East and Gulf coasts of the United States. Cases have occurred sporadically and in small epidemics: 223 cases were reported to the Centers for Disease Control and Prevention (CDC) between 1955 and 1993.
- Several hundred cases of Colorado tick fever are reported annually in the United States. The infection is acquired between March and November through the bite of an infected *Dermacentor andersoni* tick in mountainous western regions at altitudes of 1,200 to 3,000 m. Ground squirrels are the main vertebrate reservoirs for Colorado tick fever, but other rodents and mammals, such as rabbits and deer, may be infected.

Clinical Manifestations

- See other chapters for specific diseases.
- Patients with Colorado tick fever, after an incubation period of 3 to 6 days, develop the primary phase of illness that typically begins with the abrupt onset of fever, chills, severe headache, photophobia, and myalgias. These symptoms persist for 5 to 8 days, then, after resolution, recur within 3 days in approximately 50% of patients. This secondary phase of illness usually lasts 2 to 4 days. A transient petechial or macular rash may develop.
- Symptoms of tick paralysis begin 2 to 7 days after the tick begins feeding. Symmetric weakness of the lower extremities progresses to an ascending

Insect Bites and Stings

flaccid paralysis over several hours or days. Sensory function is usually spared, and the sensorium is clear. Alternatively, the disease can present as acute ataxia without muscle weakness. The blood and cerebrospinal fluid are normal. Nerve conduction velocity and compound muscle action potentials are decreased.

Diagnosis

DIFFERENTIAL DIAGNOSIS

- The occurrence of Rocky Mountain spotted fever, human monocytotropic ehrlichiosis, tularemia, tick-borne relapsing fever, and a southern erythema migrans–like illness (Lyme/Lymelike disease) is determined by the geographic distribution and seasonal activity of the particular vector tick(s).
- The flulike signs and symptoms early in the course of spotted fever rickettsiosis, ehrlichiosis, tularemia, and relapsing fever are nonspecific and do not readily suggest a particular diagnosis.
- Among patients with eastern equine encephalitis, the characteristic early involvement of the basal ganglia and thalami distinguishes this illness from herpes simplex encephalitis.

LABORATORY

- See other chapters.
- Colorado tick fever can be diagnosed by isolation of the virus from blood or cerebrospinal fluid inoculated into suckling mice. The clinical laboratory detects leukopenia and thrombocytopenia.

IMAGING

Among patients with eastern equine encephalitis, MRI is a sensitive technique to identify the characteristic early radiographic manifestations of this viral encephalitis.

DIAGNOSTIC/TESTING PROCEDURES

Confirmation of eastern equine encephalitis requires either specific serologic findings or the demonstration of the virus in cerebrospinal fluid or brain tissue.

Treatment

- See other chapters.
- The diagnosis of tick paralysis is made by finding an embedded tick, usually on the scalp. After the removal of the tick, symptoms generally resolve within several hours or days, although, in one case, weakness persisted for several months. If untreated, tick paralysis can be fatal, with reported mortality rates of 10% to 12%.
- No specific treatment exists for Colorado tick fever; therapy is limited to supportive care.

COMPLICATIONS

- The mortality rate in eastern equine encephalitis is 35%, and 35% of the survivors are moderately or severely disabled.
- Epistaxis and scattered petechiae are often noted in uncomplicated dengue, and preexisting gastrointestinal lesions may bleed during the acute illness.
- Rare complications, such as encephalitis, aseptic meningitis, hemorrhage, pericarditis, orchitis, atypical pneumonitis, and hepatitis, have been described among patients with Colorado tick fever.

Follow-Up

Serologic evidence of exposure to the human granulocytic *Ehrlichia* among Lyme disease patients approaches 30%.

PREVENTION

- In regions where tick exposure is likely, preventive measures are recommended and should include the wearing of long-sleeved shirts, long pants, and closed-toed shoes. To remove an embedded tick, one should use tweezers to grasp the tick as close as possible to the skin, then pull with slow, steady pressure in a direction perpendicular to the skin.
- *N,N*-diethyl-3-methylbenzamide (DEET) is the most effective, and best studied, insect repellent currently on the market. When DEET-based repellents are applied in combination with permethrin-treated clothing, protection against bites of nearly 100% can be achieved. However, toxic reactions can occur (usually when the product is misused). Plant-based repellents are generally less effective than DEET-based products. Ultrasonic devices, outdoor bug "zappers," and bat houses are not effective against mosquitoes.
- Information can be obtained from the CDC, Atlanta, GA 30333, or on the World Wide Web at http://www.cdc.gov.

Selected Readings

Billings AN, Rawlings JA, Walker DH. Tick-borne diseases in Texas: A 10-year retrospective examination of cases. *Tex Med* 1998;94:66–76.

Deresiewicz RL, Thaler SJ, Hsu L, Zamani AA. Clinical and neuroradiographic manifestations of eastern equine encephalitis. *N Engl J Med* 1997;336:1867–1874.

Fradin MS. Mosquitoes and mosquito repellents: A clinician's guide. *Ann Intern Med* 1998;128:931–940.

Peters CJ. Infections caused by arthropod and rodent-borne viruses. In: Fauci AS, Braunwald E, Isselbacher KJ, et al., eds. *Harrison's principles of medicine*, 14th ed. New York: McGraw-Hill, 1998:1132–1146.

Spach DH, Liles WC, Campbell GL, et al. Tick-borne diseases in the United States. *N Engl J Med* 1993;329:936–947.

Walker DH, Barbour AG, Oliver JH, et al. Emerging bacterial zoonotic and vector-borne diseases. Ecological and epidemiological factors. *JAMA* 1996;275:463–449.

Jaundice and Fever

Basics

DEFINITIONS
- Jaundice (or icterus) is characterized by hyperbilirubinemia and deposition of bile pigment in the skin, mucous membranes, and the sclera.
- For further discussion on this topic, please see also the Section I chapters, "Abdominal Pain and Fever" and "Hepatosplenomegaly and Fever," and the Section II chapters, "Cholecystitis/Cholangitis" and "Hepatitis."

APPROACH TO THE PATIENT
- Historic evaluation should include the following:
  - Determination of the length of symptoms
  - Duration of fever
  - History of blood product transfusions or injecting drug use
  - History of medication (including over-the-counter drugs)
  - History of travel to developing countries
  - Presence and character of abdominal pain
  - Presence of pruritus, myalgias, constitutional symptoms, and changes in appetite, weight, and bowel habits
- Once jaundice is recognized clinically or chemically, it is important to clarify whether hyperbilirubinemia is predominantly unconjugated or conjugated. Absence of bilirubin in the urine suggests unconjugated hyperbilirubinemia.
- The presence of alcoholic and heme-positive stools suggests a tumor of the distal biliary tract.

ETIOLOGY
- The most common causes of *unconjugated* hyperbilirubinemia and fever include the following:
  - Sepsis that can cause decreased hepatic uptake and bilirubin conjugation
  - Hepatitis that can cause hepatocellular disease. Acute viral infection is the most common cause. Other viral diseases, such as infectious mononucleosis; those due to cytomegalovirus, herpes simplex, and coxsackieviruses; and toxoplasmosis, may share certain clinical features with viral hepatitis and cause jaundice and elevation in serum aminotransferases. Infections with *Leptospira*, *Candida*, *Brucella*, *Mycobacteria*, *Babesia* spp, and *Pneumocystis* and right ventricular failure with passive hepatic congestion or hypoperfusion syndromes can cause hepatic injury that can be confused with viral hepatitis.
- The most common causes of *conjugated* hyperbilirubinemia and fever include the following:
  - Sepsis that can impair hepatic excretion
  - Extrahepatic biliary obstruction due to malignancy, inflammation (pancreatitis, etc.), infection (*Ascaris*, *Clonorchis*, etc.), and gallstones (that may lead to cholecystitis/cholangitis)

EPIDEMIOLOGY
N/A

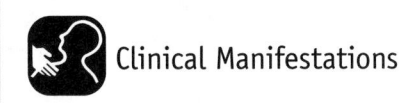

Clinical Manifestations

SYMPTOMS
- Jaundice is usually visible in the sclera or skin when the serum bilirubin value exceeds 43 mol/L (2.5 mg/dL).
- The diagnosis of anicteric hepatitis is difficult and requires a high index of suspicion, and it is based on clinical features and on aminotransferase elevations.

SIGNS
- Epigastric or right upper quadrant tenderness is frequently associated with choledocholithiasis and cholangitis or cholecystitis.
- An enlarged, tender liver suggests acute hepatic inflammation or a rapidly enlarging hepatic tumor, while a palpable gallbladder suggests distal biliary obstruction from a malignant tumor.
- The presence of splenomegaly may provide a clue to the presence of portal hypertension, from chronic active hepatitis, severe alcoholic or acute viral hepatitis, or cirrhosis.

Summary of Serologic Testing in Acute and Chronic Hepatitis

	Anti-HAV IgM	Anti-HAV IgG	HBsAg	Anti-HBs	Anti-HBc IgG	Anti-HBc IgM	HBeAg	Anti-HDV
Acute HAV	+	−	−	−	−	−	−	−
Previous HAV	−	+	−	−	−	−	−	−
Acute HBV	−	−	+ early	+ late	−	+	± If (+), infectivity is high	− If (+), coinfection with HDV
Chronic HBV	−	−	+	−	+	−	± If (+), infectivity is high	− If (+), superinfection with HDV
Previous HBV (recovery)	−	−	−	+	+	−	±	−
Immunization against HBV	−	−	−	+	−	−	−	−

Jaundice and Fever

Diagnosis

- Chronic hepatitis can present with a history of unexplained episodes of acute hepatitis.
- Malignancies metastatic to the liver can mimic acute or even fulminant viral hepatitis.

LABORATORY

- Tests such as the differential heterophile and serologic tests for these agents may be helpful in the differential diagnosis.
- In the appropriate clinical setting, serologic studies are extremely helpful for establishing or excluding the diagnosis of hepatitis A; acute and chronic hepatitis B; hepatitis C, D, and E; and hepatitis from cytomegalovirus (CMV) or Epstein-Barr virus.
- When acute viral hepatitis is considered, the patient should undergo four serologic tests:
  —HBsAg
  —IgM anti-HAV
  —IgM anti-HBc
  —Anti-HCV
- See also the table, Summary of Serologic Testing in Acute and Chronic Hepatitis, for a review.

IMAGING

- For patients whose clinical evaluation and liver chemistries suggest cholestasis or extrahepatic biliary obstruction, biliary imaging is an important early diagnostic tool to differentiate intrahepatic causes from extrahepatic obstruction. Both ultrasonography and computed tomography detect dilated extrahepatic biliary ducts with great sensitivity.
- Further definition and relief of extrahepatic biliary obstruction can frequently be accomplished by percutaneous or endoscopic cholangiography.

DIAGNOSTIC/TESTING PROCEDURES

- Endoscopic retrograde cholangiopancreatography (ERCP) is frequently the preferred technique for diagnosing and treating distal biliary obstructions.
- In some cases, identification of focal lesions by computed tomography, transabdominal ultrasonography, or magnetic resonance imaging can increase the diagnostic accuracy of liver biopsy.
- The results of percutaneous, transjugular, or laparoscopic biopsy may also provide important information for optimal therapy.

Treatment

See the Section II chapter, "Hepatitis."

COMPLICATIONS

N/A

Follow-Up

N/A

PREVENTION

N/A

Selected Readings

Anonymous. Case records of the Massachusetts General Hospital. Weekly clinicopathological exercises. Case 29-1998. A 57-year-old man with fever and jaundice after intravesical instillation of bacille Calmette-Guerin for bladder cancer. *N Engl J Med* 1998;339:831–837.

Dienstag JL, Isselbacher KJ. Acute viral hepatitis. In: Fauci AS, Braunwald E, Isselbacher KJ, et al., eds. *Harrison's principles of medicine*, 14th ed. New York: McGraw-Hill, 1998:1677–1692.

Kaplan LM, Isselbacher KJ. Jaundice. In: Fauci AS, Braunwald E, Isselbacher KJ, et al., eds. *Harrison's principles of medicine*, 14th ed. New York: McGraw-Hill, 1998:249–255.

McNair AN, Tibbs CJ, Williams R. Hepatology. *BMJ* 1995;311:1351–1355.

Joint Pain and Fever

Basics

DEFINITIONS

- Joint disorders are classified as monarticular (one joint involved), oligoarticular (two to three joints involved), or polyarticular (more than three joints involved).
- *Arthritis* describes inflammatory process that involves the joint(s).
- *Arthralgia* describes pain that involves the joint(s).

APPROACH TO THE PATIENT

- Musculoskeletal disorders are generally classified as inflammatory (infectious, crystal-induced, immune-related, reactive, idiopathic) or noninflammatory, and are called *acute* if they last less than 6 weeks and *chronic* if they last longer. Acute arthropathies tend to be infectious, crystal-induced, or reactive.
- Noninflammatory disorders may be related to trauma, osteoarthritis, synovitis, or fibromyalgia and usually are not associated with fever.
- The term *arthritis* is not specific enough to be regarded as a diagnosis. Many patients believe any joint pain is due to "arthritis," but their understanding of the term can be vague. Clinicians must discriminate the anatomic site(s) of origin of the patient's complaint. Aspects of the patient profile, including age, sex, race, and family history, can provide important information. The chronology of the complaint (onset, evolution, and duration) is an important diagnostic feature. The onset of certain disorders, such as septic arthritis and gout, tends to be abrupt.
- The goal of the physical examination is to ascertain the structures involved, the nature of the underlying pathology, the extent and functional consequences of the process, and the presence of systemic or extraarticular manifestations.
- Examination of involved and uninvolved joints determines whether warmth, erythema, or swelling is present.
- Aspiration and analysis of synovial fluid is always indicated in acute monarthritis or when an infectious or crystal-induced arthropathy is suspected.
- If examination and cultures of the synovial fluid are nondiagnostic, the likelihood of viral arthritis, reactive arthritis, or systemic rheumatic illness increases. Serologic studies should be obtained, particularly assays for antinuclear and antistreptococcal antibodies and for antibodies to *Borrelia burgdorferi* in the case of patients who live in or have visited areas where Lyme disease is endemic.

ETIOLOGY

- Fever and arthritis often accompanies septic arthritis, but has been reported in a number of other local and systemic infections, including the following:
  —Acute HIV conversion
  —Chronic meningococcaemia caused by *Neisseria meningitidis*
  —Dengue
  —Ebola hemorrhagic fever
  —Endocarditis
  —Epstein-Barr virus
  —Lyme disease
  —Necrotizing lymphadenitis (Kikuchi's disease)
  —Parvovirus B19 infection
  —Rickettsial diseases
  —Rubella
  —Secondary syphilis
  —Viral hepatitis
  —Whipple's disease
- The systemic form of juvenile rheumatoid arthritis (Still's disease) is characterized by high fever and polyarthritis. It may appear in young adults, and occasionally in older adults, either as a new illness or as a recrudescence of a dormant childhood disease.
- Fever and polyarthritis can be early features of systemic lupus erythematosus and vasculitis.
- Acute sarcoid arthritis, usually associated with erythema nodosum and hilar adenopathy, is frequently accompanied by low-grade or moderate fever.
- Fever is frequent in polyarticular gout. In pseudogout, high fever has been reported, even with monoarthritis.
- Lymphoma and other neoplasias can rarely present with arthritis and fever.

EPIDEMIOLOGY

- In bacterial arthritis, only 10% to 20% of adults have polyarticular involvement, with simultaneous onset in several large joints or serial onset over 1 or 2 days.
- *Staphylococcus aureus* is the most common cause of both monoarticular and polyarticular sepsis.
- Musculoskeletal symptoms are frequent in endocarditis, occurring in 45% of patients in one large series.
- A large-joint oligoarthritis occurs in 10% to 20% of patients with inflammatory bowel disease, usually during periods of active disease. In these patients, it can be a reflection of the intraabdominal process.
- Familial Mediterranean fever appears during childhood, with brief episodes of fever, arthritis, and abdominal and pleuritic pain.
- The post–Q-fever fatigue syndrome (inappropriate fatigue, myalgia and arthralgia, night sweats, changes in mood and sleep patterns) has been reported in up to 20% of laboratory-proven, acute primary Q-fever cases.

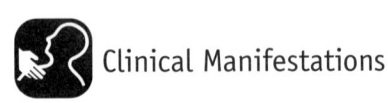

Clinical Manifestations

- An asymmetric, additive polyarthritis predominantly involving large joints in a lower extremity may be a sequel to enteritis (usually caused by *Salmonella*, *Shigella*, *Campylobacter*, or *Yersinia*) or urogenital infection with certain organisms (principally *Chlamydia trachomatis*).
- The clinical manifestations of Whipple's disease are many and diverse. Almost all organ systems can be involved. In approximately two-thirds of patients, the disease begins insidiously with either arthralgia or a migratory, nonerosive, nondeforming seronegative arthritis. This may precede any other features by up to 24 years.
- Dissemination of *B. burgdorferi*, the causative agent of Lyme disease in the United States, is often accompanied by fever and migratory arthralgia, with little

Joint Pain and Fever

or no joint swelling, but frank arthritis may appear weeks or months later (mean interval, 6 months).
- *Neisseria* arthritis may present as a migratory arthritis with chills, fever, and tenosynovitis, especially in the wrist and ankle extensor-tendon sheaths.
- In secondary syphilis, symmetrical polyarthritis and fever are the predominant presenting features in rare cases, but most patients also have a maculopapular rash that is most likely to appear on the palms and soles.
- In mycobacterial and fungal arthritis, an indolent monoarthritis is the rule, but occasionally two or three large joints may be involved. Because fever is either absent or mild, an infectious process may not be considered.
- Systemic candidiasis may present with polyarthritis, particularly in immunosuppressed patients and intravenous drug users.
- Among patients with hepatitis B virus infection, the arthritis precedes the symptoms of hepatitis and resolves when jaundice appears.
- In children with rheumatic fever, cardiac involvement is a dominant feature, but adults generally present with abrupt onset of polyarthritis and fever.

Diagnosis

DIFFERENTIAL DIAGNOSIS

- The diagnosis of septic arthritis in young children requires a high index of suspicion, and the disease cannot be excluded on the basis of lack of fever or normal results of laboratory tests.
- Among children, fever, rash, and arthritis can be due to several different diseases, including the following:
  —Rheumatic fever
  —Systemic juvenile rheumatoid arthritis
  —Recent streptococcal infection with osteomyelitis or septic arthritis
  —Lyme disease

- Whipple's disease may resemble inflammatory bowel disease in its clinical presentation, and arthritis may be an early complication, although the patient is usually afebrile.

DIAGNOSTIC/TESTING PROCEDURES

- Examination of the synovial fluid may identify bacterial and crystal-induced arthritis and is often helpful in reducing the number of conditions warranting continued consideration.
- Synovial fluid leukocyte counts over 50,000/mL suggest a bacterial infection but are occasionally seen in rheumatoid, crystal-induced, and reactive arthritis.
- Infectious synovial fluid is turbid and opaque, with a predominance of polymorphonuclear leukocytes (>75%) and low viscosity. Whenever infection is suspected, synovial fluid should be Gram stained and cultured appropriately.
- Transiently positive rheumatoid factors have been reported early in the course of Lyme disease.

IMAGING

- Plain x-rays are most appropriate when there is a history of trauma, suspected chronic infection, progressive disability, or monarticular involvement; when therapeutic alterations are considered; or when a baseline assessment is desired for what appears to be a chronic process.
- Computed tomography and, especially, magnetic resonance imaging have significantly advanced the ability to image musculoskeletal structures.

Treatment

For patients with septic arthritis, therapy should be initiated promptly after the samples for cultures have been obtained (see Section II chapter, "Septic Arthritis").

COMPLICATIONS

- For septic arthritis, spread to bone or frank bacteremia
- Before the introduction of antibiotic regimens, diagnosed Whipple's disease was universally fatal. A variety of antibiotic regimens are suggested, and none is universally successful. Patients often relapse, even after prolonged courses of antibiotics, and the relapses often involve the central nervous system and may be progressive.

Follow-Up

In Lyme arthritis, recurrent episodes of arthritis can persist over periods of 1 week to 8 years.

PREVENTION

- For Lyme arthritis, protection against tick bites

Selected Readings

Cush JJ, Lipsky PE. Approach to articular and musculoskeletal disorders. In: Fauci AS, Braunwald E, Isselbacher KJ, et al., eds. *Harrison's principles of medicine*, 14th ed. New York: McGraw-Hill, 1998:1928–1935.

Gerber MA, Zemel LS, Shapiro ED. Lyme arthritis in children: Clinical epidemiology and long-term outcomes. *Pediatrics* 1998;102:905–908.

Knight SM, Symmons DP. A man with intermittent fever and arthralgia. *Ann Rheum Dis* 1998;57:711–714.

Pinals RS. Polyarthritis and fever. *N Engl J Med* 1994;330:769–774.

Vecchio P. Is it arthritis? Beware the mimics. *Aust Fam Physician* 1998;27:17–20.

Lymph Node Enlargement and Fever

Basics

DEFINITION
- Lymphadenitis is inflammation of one or more lymph nodes, usually caused by a primary focus of infection elsewhere in the body.
- Mesenteric lymphadenitis is a condition clinically resembling acute appendicitis and is caused by inflammation of the mesenteric lymph nodes.
- Lymph nodes greater than 1 cm in diameter are significantly enlarged. Epitrochlear nodes more than 0.5 cm, and inguinal nodes more than 1.5 to 2.0 cm should be regarded as abnormal.
- *Generalized lymphadenopathy* has been defined as involvement of three or more noncontiguous lymph node areas.

APPROACH TO THE PATIENT
- Almost all causes of lymph node enlargement can also cause fever. Infection is the leading cause.
- Lymphadenopathy may be an incidental finding in patients being examined for various reasons, or it may be a presenting sign or symptom of an illness. The physician must eventually decide whether the lymphadenopathy is a normal finding or one that requires further study, up to and including biopsy.
- A detailed history should focus both on diagnostic clues and on features suggestive of more sinister pathology.
- Duration of lymphadenopathy may be helpful. Most infectious causes produce a short (<2 weeks) history. Long-standing lymphadenopathy may be caused by a variety of diseases, including infections (HIV, Epstein-Barr virus, tuberculosis), malignancy, inflammation, and autoimmune disease.
- Attention should be paid to associated rashes (exanthemata), travel, and exposure to pets (particularly cats).
- Associated symptoms should be sought: weight loss, fever and night sweats, sore throat, cough, pruritus, fatigue, pain in the nodes, and myalgia/arthralgia.
- Full examination of all nodal sites should be undertaken to determine whether it is localized or generalized. The distinction between localized or generalized lymphadenopathy is important, as a specific pathologic cause is more likely to be found in patients with generalized lymphadenopathy.
- Abdominal examination should determine the presence of liver or splenic enlargement.
- Anemia, petechiae, or bleeding points to infiltrative disease of the bone marrow, such as leukemia.
- Long-standing lymphadenopathy may suggest tuberculosis, and a history of contact should be sought.
- Many infectious agents cause fever and lymphadenopathy, but only a few, including *Francisella tularensis, Bartonella henselae*, and various mycobacteria, commonly result in a single prominent lymph node with fever.

ETIOLOGY
- Infectious diseases
  - Viral (infectious mononucleosis syndromes due to Epstein-Barr virus or cytomegalovirus, hepatitis, herpes simplex, herpesvirus 6, varicella-zoster virus, dengue fever, rubella, measles, adenovirus, HIV, epidemic keratoconjunctivitis, etc.)
  - Bacterial (streptococci, staphylococci, cat-scratch disease, brucellosis, Calmette-Guerin bacillus infection, tularemia, plague, chancroid, melioidosis, glanders, tuberculosis, listeriosis, leptospirosis, atypical mycobacterial infection, syphilis, diphtheria, leprosy)
  - Fungal (histoplasmosis, coccidioidomycosis, paracoccidioidomycosis, cryptococcosis)
  - Chlamydial (lymphogranuloma venereum, trachoma)
  - Parasitic (toxoplasmosis, leishmaniasis, trypanosomiasis, filariasis)
  - Rickettsial
  - Helminthic (filariasis, loiasis, oncocerciasis)
- Immunologic diseases, such as angioimmunoblastic lymphadenopathy, dermatomyositis, graft-versus-host disease, juvenile rheumatoid arthritis, mixed connective-tissue disease, primary biliary cirrhosis, rheumatoid arthritis, serum sickness, Sjögren's syndrome, systemic lupus erythematosus, and vasculitis syndromes
- Malignant diseases (hematologic)
  - Hodgkin's disease, non-Hodgkin's lymphomas, acute or chronic lymphocytic leukemia, hairy-cell leukemia, Sézary syndrome, histiocytosis amyloidosis
- Malignant diseases (nonhematologic)
  - Sarcomas, metastasis, etc.
- Lipid storage diseases
  - Gaucher's, Niemann-Pick, Fabry, Tangier
- Endocrine disease
  - Hyperthyroidism
- Other disorders, such as Castleman's disease (giant lymph node hyperplasia), dermatopathic lymphadenitis, drugs (particularly phenytoin and carbamazepine), familial Mediterranean fever, histiocytic necrotizing lymphadenitis (Kikuchi's disease), histiocytosis X, inflammatory pseudotumor of lymph node, Kawasaki disease (usually presents with a combination of fever, rash, changes to the peripheral extremities, mucosal changes, conjunctival injection, and cervical lymphadenopathy), lymphomatoid granulomatosis, Rosai-Dorfman disease (sinus histiocytosis with massive lymphadenopathy), sarcoidosis, severe hypertriglyceridemia, and vascular transformation of sinuses
- Acute mesenteric lymphadenitis: It has been recognized that some of these patients have infection with *Y. pseudotuberculosis* or *Y. enterocolitica*, in which case the diagnosis can be established by culture of the mesenteric nodes or by serologic titers.
- Lymphadenopathy is a common finding in patients with HIV infection, ranging from the generalized follicular hyperplasia seen early in disease to involvement secondary to opportunistic infections and neoplasms. In this population, Kaposi's sarcoma, lymphoma and mycobacterial infection, toxoplasmosis, systemic fungal infection, and bacillary angiomatosis are common causes of lymphadenopathy.

EPIDEMIOLOGY
- Acute mesenteric lymphadenitis is more common among children.
- In developed countries, lymphadenopathy due to mycobacteria is likely to be nontuberculous.
- Children and young adults usually have benign (i.e., nonmalignant) disorders, such as viral or bacterial infections, and, in some countries, tuberculosis. After age 50, the incidence of malignant disorders increases.

Lymph Node Enlargement and Fever

Clinical Manifestations

- Nodes involved by lymphoma tend to be large, discrete, symmetric, rubbery, firm, mobile, and nontender.
- Some malignant diseases, such as acute leukemia, produce rapid enlargement and pain in the nodes.
- In some patients, the portal of entry for *F. tularensis* is the conjunctiva, causing purulent conjunctivitis with regional lymphadenopathy (preauricular, submandibular, or cervical).
- Oral inoculation of *F. tularensis* may result in acute, exudative, or membranous pharyngitis associated with cervical lymphadenopathy.

Diagnosis

DIFFERENTIAL DIAGNOSIS

- The most frequent site of regional adenopathy is the neck, and most common infectious causes include upper respiratory infections, oral and dental lesions, infectious mononucleosis, and other viral illnesses.
- Occipital adenopathy often reflects an infection of the scalp, and preauricular adenopathy accompanies conjunctival infections and cat-scratch disease. Painful preauricular lymphadenopathy is unique to tularemia and distinguishes it from cat-scratch disease, tuberculosis, sporotrichosis, and syphilis.
- Enlargement of supraclavicular and scalene nodes is always abnormal. Tuberculosis, sarcoidosis, and toxoplasmosis are nonmalignant causes of supraclavicular adenopathy.
- Axillary adenopathy is usually due to injuries or localized infections of the ipsilateral upper extremity.
- In the young, mediastinal adenopathy is associated with infectious mononucleosis and sarcoidosis. In endemic regions, tuberculosis and histoplasmosis can cause unilateral paratracheal lymph node involvement that mimics lymphoma. In older patients, the differential diagnosis includes primary lung cancer (especially among smokers), lymphomas, metastatic carcinoma (usually lung), tuberculosis, fungal infection, and sarcoidosis.
- Enlarged intraabdominal or retroperitoneal nodes are usually malignant. Although tuberculosis may present as mesenteric lymphadenitis, these masses usually contain lymphomas or, in young men, germ-cell tumors.

LABORATORY

- Erythrocyte sedimentation rate (ESR) is a nonspecific test and is of limited benefit, as it is commonly raised in a wide range of inflammatory, reactive, and malignant conditions. Similarly, a normal ESR does not necessarily exclude significant pathology.
- Lymph node fine-needle aspiration has an important roll in diagnosis, but interpretation of samples requires a higher degree of expertise.

IMAGING

Computed tomography can be very useful in assessing the extent of lymphadenopathy and aid in the diagnosis of localized infections, such as psoas and iliacus muscle collections.

DIAGNOSTIC/TESTING PROCEDURES

The diagnostic test of choice in nontuberculous lymphadenopathy is excision, with the specimen being sent for both mycobacterial culture and routine histology.

Treatment

- Treatment of lymphadenitis depends on etiology.
- In cervical pyogenic lymphadenitis due to pharyngeal or periodontal process, consider antibiotics active against streptococci and oral anaerobes (e.g., penicillin 4 μ q4h i.v. and metronidazole 500 mg tid i.v. or cefoxitin 2 g q8h i.v. or ampicillin/sulbactam).
- For the management of pyogenic lymphadenitis complicating skin infections, a penicillinase-resistant penicillin is usually the drug of choice (e.g., dicloxacillin 250–500 mg PO qid or nafcillin 2 g i.v. q4–6h).
- For the therapy of cat-scratch disease and bubonic plague, see the relevant chapters in Section II.

COMPLICATIONS

- Acute axillary lymphadenitis (usually due to *Streptococcus pyogenes*) can lead to ipsilateral pleural effusion (caused by blockage of the lymphatic vessels) and thrombosis of the axillary and subclavian veins.
- Scrofula (tuberculous cervical lymphadenitis) can lead to drainage of caseous material onto the skin surface.

Follow-Up

Based on the clinical situation, among children in whom the diagnosis is not immediately obvious and other clinical signs are absent, a period of observation could be undertaken.

PREVENTION

- Incision and drainage or needle biopsy in nontuberculous lymphadenopathy can produce sinus formation and scarring.
- Appropriate treatment should be instituted immediately while awaiting results of cultures (from blood and bubo aspirates) if bubonic plague is suspected.

Selected Readings

Anonymous. Case records of the Massachusetts General Hospital. Weekly clinicopathological exercises. Case 14-1999. A nine-year-old girl with fever and cervical lymphadenopathy. *N Engl J Med* 1999;340:1491–1497.

Henry PH, Longo DL. Enlargement of lymph nodes and spleen. In: Fauci AS, Braunwald E, Isselbacher KJ, et al., eds. *Harrison's principles of medicine*, 14th ed. New York: McGraw-Hill, 1998:345–351.

Morland B. Lymphadenopathy. *Arch Dis Child* 1995;73:476–479.

Swartz MN. Lymphadenitis and lymphangitis. In: Mandell GL, Bennett JE, Dolin R, eds. *Principles and practice of infectious diseases*, 4th ed. New York: Churchill Livingstone, 1995:936–944.

Neurologic Symptoms/Signs and Fever

Basics

DEFINITION
- *Drowsiness* is a disorder that simulates light sleep, from which the patient can be easily aroused by touch or noise and can maintain alertness for some time.
- *Stupor* defines a state in which the patient can be awakened only by vigorous stimuli, and an effort to avoid uncomfortable or aggravating stimulation is displayed.
- *Coma* indicates a state from which the patient cannot be aroused by stimulation, and no purposeful attempt is made to avoid painful stimuli.
- *Confusion* is clouding of consciousness.
- When there is, in addition to confusion, an element of drowsiness, the patient is said to have an encephalopathy.
- *Chronic meningitis* is defined as signs and symptoms of meningitis persisting for more than 4 weeks, with abnormal findings in the cerebrospinal fluid.

APPROACH TO THE PATIENT
- Patients with fever and neurologic symptoms should be evaluated for localized or systemic infections and for noninfectious pathology.
- Details of preceding neurologic symptoms; the use of medications, illicit drugs, or alcohol; and a history of other medical disease are elicited.
- Physical examination specifically for meningitis includes assessing neck stiffness, testing for Kernig and Brudzinski signs, and assessing jolt accentuation of headache.
- A complete neurologic examination follows, including examination of the cranial nerves, the motor and sensory systems, and reflexes, and testing for the Babinski reflex. A general examination follows, with an emphasis on the ears, sinuses, and respiratory system.
- The funduscopic examination is used to detect subarachnoid hemorrhage, hypertensive encephalopathy, and increased intracranial pressure.

ETIOLOGY
- Among patients with neurologic signs, fever suggests systemic infection, bacterial meningitis, encephalitis, or a brain lesion that has disturbed the temperature-regulating centers.
- High body temperature (42°C–44°C) that is associated with dry skin should arouse the suspicion of heat stroke or anticholinergic drug intoxication.
- Lymphomas and paraneoplastic neurologic disorders should be considered.
- Granulomas involving the central nervous system (CNS) can be due to syphilis, cysticercosis, and tuberculoma. Although more frequently associated with chronic meningitis, *Cryptococcus neoformans* infections can cause solitary granulomas.
- *Listeria* rhombencephalitis is associated with signs of cranial nerve or brainstem involvement and abnormalities on MRI scan.
- Among the respiratory infectious agents associated with cerebellitis, *Mycoplasma pneumoniae*, influenza virus, and Q fever are the more common.
- Cerebellar encephalitis has occurred in patients with measles, varicella, Lyme disease, rabies, and legionellosis.
- *Echinococcus granulosus* is a major cause of cerebral infection worldwide.
- Schistosomiasis generally affects the spinal canal, producing myelopathy. In rare cases, it causes intracranial lesions.
- Amebiasis (*Entamoeba histolytica*) can be complicated by meningoencephalitis and suppurative brain abscesses in a small percentage of patients, but they usually have hepatic abscesses and are acutely ill.
- Paragonimiasis is a frequent cause of solitary brain masses in the Far East.
- Viruses are most often implicated in aseptic meningitis in the enterovirus group (coxsackievirus, echoviruses, and poliovirus). Also, recent HIV seroconversion and Epstein-Barr virus infection have caused cerebellitis.
- The most common type of fungal meningitis is cryptococcal. Coccidioidomycosis and histoplasmosis can disseminate to the nervous system. Blastomycosis generally infects the brain and meninges late in the course of advanced disease. *Aspergillus* spp, mucor, and *Pseudallescheria boydii* cause widespread disease in immunocompromised persons.
- Acute disseminated encephalomyelitis typically follows a viral exanthem, respiratory infection, or vaccination. In the United States today, the disease most commonly follows respiratory infections. Demyelination typically involves the cerebral hemispheres but may be restricted to the spinal cord, as in acute transverse myelitis, or to the cerebellum, as in acute cerebellitis.
- Acute hemorrhagic leukoencephalitis typically develops 3 to 14 days after a respiratory tract infection but occasionally as long as 3 weeks after the infection. Because of the time lag, the fever from the initial infection has often resolved.

EPIDEMIOLOGY
- Herpes simplex virus type 1 accounts for approximately 10% of all cases of encephalitis and 20% to 75% of all cases of necrotizing encephalitis.
- In India, tuberculomas account for 20% to 30% of intracranial masses.
- The annual incidence of bacterial meningitis ranges from approximately 3 per 100,000 population in the United States, to 45.8 per 100,000 in Brazil, to 500 per 100,000 in the "meningitis belt" of Africa.
- In one county in Minnesota, there was an incidence rate of viral meningitis of 10.9 per 100,000 person-years from 1950 to 1981, with most cases occurring in the summer months.

Neurologic Symptoms/Signs and Fever

Clinical Manifestation

- Absence of neck stiffness and altered mental status effectively eliminates meningitis. However, individual items of the clinical history have low accuracy for the diagnosis of meningitis in adults (for headache, 50%; and for nausea/vomiting, 30%).
- The most generalized form of postinfectious disease of the nervous system is postinfectious encephalomyelitis, which is characterized by multifocal or disseminated demyelination of the brain and spinal cord. Ataxia develops within days after the onset of the infection, and sometimes before it. The cerebellar signs can be mild; the presence of nystagmus and dysarthria varies.
- In tuberculosis of the CNS, fever occurs at some time during the course of the illness in more than 80% of patients.
- *Brucella* can cause a chronic granulomatous meningitis, but it is typically associated with fever, constitutional symptoms, and a history of exposure to infected animal tissues or products.

Diagnosis

DIFFERENTIAL DIAGNOSIS

- Tuberculosis should be considered not only in patients who have emigrated from areas in which the disease is endemic, but also in those who live in medically underserved areas, such as inner cities, where tuberculosis is still endemic.
- Neoplastic meningitis must be seriously considered in a patient presenting with headache, cranial nerve palsies, and dural enhancement or imaging. Lymphoma and leukemia, as well as adenocarcinoma and melanoma, can involve the meninges diffusely.

LABORATORY

Laboratory tests used most frequently in the evaluation of patients with fever and neurologic symptoms are chemical-toxicologic analysis of blood and urine, CT or MRI, electroencephalogram, and cerebrospinal fluid examination.

IMAGING

In most cases, infectious meningitis presents as leptomeningeal enhancement, and carcinomatous meningitis presents as dural enhancement.

CEREBROSPINAL FLUID

In both acute hemorrhagic leukoencephalitis and acute disseminated encephalomyelitis, the protein level is elevated and the glucose level is normal. In acute disseminated encephalomyelitis, the pleocytosis is predominantly lymphocytic, with counts ranging from a few cells to several hundred, whereas in acute hemorrhagic leukoencephalitis, the pleocytosis is more frequently polymorphonuclear. Also, massive edema associated with acute hemorrhagic leukoencephalitis usually raises the cerebrospinal fluid opening pressure.

Treatment

- The immediate goal in acute coma is the prevention of further nervous system damage.
- Therapy with acyclovir should be instituted without delay once the diagnosis of herpes virus is suspected.

COMPLICATIONS

- Meningitis
- Increased intracranial pressure
- Survival is poor for HIV patients with intracerebral pathology other than CNS toxoplasmosis.
- Patients with herpes encephalitis have a poor prognosis if coma is present, especially in the elderly.

Follow-Up

Early clinical recognition of meningitis is imperative to allow clinicians to efficiently complete further tests and initiate appropriate therapy.

PREVENTION

Headache accompanied by fever and meningismus indicates an urgent need for examination of the cerebrospinal fluid to diagnose meningitis, and lumbar puncture should not be delayed while awaiting a CT scan.

Selected Readings

Anonymous. Case records of the Massachusetts General Hospital. Weekly clinicopathological exercises. Case 9-1999. A 74-year-old woman with hydrocephalus and pleocytosis. *N Engl J Med* 1999;340:945–953.

Anonymous. Case records of the Massachusetts General Hospital. Weekly clinicopathological exercises. Case 1-1999. A 53-year-old man with fever and rapid neurologic deterioration. *N Engl J Med* 1999;340:127–135.

Anonymous. Case records of the Massachusetts General Hospital. Weekly clinicopathological exercises. Case 2-1998. A 50-year-old woman with increasing headache and a left abducent-nerve palsy. *N Engl J Med* 1998;338:180–188.

Anonymous. Case records of the Massachusetts General Hospital. Weekly clinicopathological exercises. Case 39-1996. A 30-year-old man with a generalized tonic-clonic seizure and a left temporal-lobe mass. *N Engl J Med* 1996;335:1906–1914.

Attia J, Hatala R, Cook DJ, Wong JG. Does this adult patient have acute meningitis? *JAMA* 1999;282:175–181.

Ropper AH. Acute confusional states and coma. In: Braunwald E, Fauci AS, Kasper DL, Hauser SL, Longo DL, Jameson JL, eds. *Harrison's principles of internal medicine*, 15th ed. New York: McGraw-Hill, 2001:132–140.

Pancytopenia and Fever

Basics

DEFINITION

- Pancytopenia is deficiency of all cell elements of the blood. Leukopenia is usually defined as <5,000 leukocytes per milliliter. Anemia and thrombocytopenia are less well defined. Thrombocytopenia with 50,000 to 100,000 platelets per milliliter is usually considered mild.

APPROACH TO THE PATIENT

- Cytopenias can be due to systemic infections as well as to infectious and noninfectious processes involving the bone marrow.
- Fever involving neutropenic patients is a medical emergency. The first issue is to determine whether the patient is suffering from a febrile illness that is associated with cytopenias or whether the fever is caused by a secondary infection.
- A complete history, including a thorough medication list and review of travel history and previous exposure to tuberculosis and histoplasmosis, is necessary.
- Patients should be questioned about the presence of concurrent symptoms (such as weight loss, night sweats, etc.).
- Review of previous complete blood count results is helpful.
- In evaluating anemia without reticulocytosis, especially in the setting of pancytopenia, one must consider infiltrative diseases of the marrow.
- Patients with cytopenia(s) and fever should undergo blood cultures and serologic evaluation and be considered for an evaluation of the bone marrow that includes histology and cultures for bacteria, parasites, mycobacteria, and fungi.

ETIOLOGY

- The reactive hemophagocytic syndrome is a benign histiocytic disorder characterized by hemophagocytosis by stimulated histiocytes in the bone marrow and reticuloendothelial system, resulting in pancytopenia, liver dysfunction, and disseminated coagulopathy. Several diseases, including viral (particularly herpesviruses) or bacterial infection, lymphoma, and other malignancies, are known to be causative disorders for this syndrome. However, the underlying disease sometimes remains unclear.
- Bone marrow necrosis, defined morphologically as destruction of hematopoietic tissue, including the stroma, with preservation of the bone, is a rare condition. It is seen in sickle cell diseases, AIDS, leukemia, lymphoma, metastatic carcinoma, anemia, parvovirus infections, enterovirus infection, sepsis, Kaposi's sarcoma, mucormycosis, disseminated tuberculosis, and other systemic diseases. Bone marrow invasion is associated with leishmaniasis, malignancy, myelodysplastic syndromes, and tuberculosis.
- Thrombocytopenia, a shift to the left in the neutrophil count, and pancytopenia have been described in patients with tuberculosis. In a study of miliary tuberculosis, thrombocytopenia was recorded in 83% of the patients, leukopenia in 15%, lymphopenia in 87%, and pancytopenia in 5%; in three of the six patients with pancytopenia, it was reversed by antituberculosis treatment.
- Human ehrlichiosis should be considered in the differential diagnosis in patients with fever and cytopenia associated with hemophagocytosis. Pancytopenia associated with ehrlichiosis is usually transient; however, it may be severe when it is associated with destruction of normal blood elements.
- Familial erythrophagocytic lymphocytosis is a rare, nonmalignant class II histiocytosis characterized by fever, irritability, hepatosplenomegaly, pancytopenia, and hemophagocytosis.

- Infectious causes of aplastic anemia include Epstein-Barr virus, hepatitis viruses, and HIV.
- Acute infectious mononucleosis may lead to life-threatening thrombocytopenia.
- Systemic lupus erythematosus can present with lymphadenopathy, fever, anemia, and leukopenia.
- Leukopenia and thrombocytopenia are common abnormalities in patients with malaria.
- Kaposi's sarcoma and lymphoma can affect the bone marrow, among HIV-infected individuals.
- The infectious agent most often associated with a pure red-cell aplasia is parvovirus B19.
- Many of the AIDS-related opportunistic infections are associated with bone marrow suppression. With some of these infections, such as those due to *Mycobacterium tuberculosis*, histoplasmosis, and cryptococcosis, it occurs as a result of massive bone marrow infiltration in the setting of widely disseminated disease; the patients typically have fever, chills, sweats, and lymphadenopathy and/or hepatosplenomegaly. Disseminated *Mycobacterium avium* complex infection can cause pancytopenia as a result of massive bone marrow infiltration, but unlike other systemic infections, this disorder is often associated with a profound anemia disproportionate to the degree of leukopenia and thrombocytopenia.
- Of the disseminated viral opportunistic infections, cytomegalovirus infection is most commonly associated with bone marrow suppression in patients with AIDS, but the pancytopenia that results usually does not include a disproportionately pronounced anemia.

EPIDEMIOLOGY

Aplastic anemia is not a common disease. The most accurate prospective studies report an annual incidence of two new cases per one million population in Europe and Israel. However, the rate is much higher in the developing world, where aplastic anemia may rival acute myelogenous leukemia in frequency of diagnosis in hematology clinics. Studies in Thailand and China found the incidence to be about threefold higher than in the West.

Pancytopenia and Fever

Clinical Manifestations

- Patients with virus-associated hemophagocytic syndrome have high fever, skin rash, hepatosplenomegaly, pancytopenia, and coagulopathy. Morphologic examination of lymph node and bone marrow demonstrates prominent phagocytosis of erythrocytes and nucleated blood cells.
- Patients with hemophagocytic syndrome associated with Epstein-Barr virus generally have an abrupt onset of the disorder, are usually very ill, and have marked lymphadenopathy and hepatosplenomegaly.

Diagnosis

- Marrow microscopy can help in the diagnosis of disseminated lymphoma and infections such as toxoplasmosis, leishmaniasis, and disseminated fungal infections, including those caused by *Histoplasma capsulatum* and *Penicillium marneffei*.
- Bone marrow sampling has diagnostic utility in HIV-infected patients with pyrexia without localizing signs, in pancytopenia, and in the staging/investigation of lymphoma. However, this test has little value in the investigation of afebrile patients with isolated thrombocytopenia, anemia, or leukopenia.

Treatment

- Neutropenic fevers must be treated aggressively with parenteral, broad-spectrum antibiotics. Because aspergillosis is difficult to diagnose, antifungal therapy should be added when patients are persistently febrile.
- For the treatment of aplastic anemia, bone marrow or peripheral blood stem-cell transplantation from a histocompatible sibling usually cures the underlying bone marrow failure. Survival rates have been reported to be as high as 90% from a single experienced institution and 77% for registry data, which reflect the more general experience.
- Treatment of infectious mononucleosis-induced thrombocytopenia with steroids is variably successful. Intravenous immunoglobulin and, in selected cases, splenectomy are also used.
- Aggressive antiretroviral treatment may effectively diminish transfusion requirements among HIV-infected individuals with pure red blood cell aplasia resulting from parvovirus B19 infection.
- Anemia and thrombocytopenia can be corrected by transfusion.

COMPLICATIONS

The prognosis in aplastic anemia is directly related to the quantitative reduction in peripheral blood cell counts, particularly the neutrophil number. Prior to the introduction of practical blood transfusions, patients died of congestive heart failure caused by anemia or of hemorrhaging due to thrombocytopenia. Historically, mortality figures at 1 to 2 years were 80% to 90% in patients who were treated only with blood transfusions and antibiotics. Today, the most serious complication of aplastic anemia is the high risk of infection secondary to the absence of neutrophils; overwhelming bacterial sepsis and, especially, fungal infections are the most frequent causes of death. Patients who satisfy the criteria for severe disease, but who are refractory to treatment, have a less than 20% chance of long-term survival.

Follow-up

Limited numbers of blood transfusions probably do not affect the outcome of stem-cell transplantation; to avoid alloimmunization, family donors should not be used.

PREVENTION

Attention to the details of oral hygiene and hand-washing and avoidance of minor injuries or casual exposure to infectious agents can reduce the risk of serious complications among neutropenic patients.

Selected Readings

Anonymous. Case records of the Massachusetts General Hospital. Weekly clinicopathological exercises. Case 23-1995. A 44-year-old woman with pulmonary infiltrates, respiratory failure, and pancytopenia. *N Engl J Med* 1995;333:241–248.

Anonymous. Case records of the Massachusetts General Hospital. Weekly clinicopathological exercises. Case 36-1993. A 28-year-old man with AIDS, persistent pancytopenia, and lymphoma. *N Engl J Med* 1993;329:792–799.

Brook MG, Ayles H, Harrison C, et al. Diagnostic utility of bone marrow sampling in HIV positive patients. *Genitourin Med* 1997;73:117–121.

Greene WL, Craft J. A man with fever and petechiae. *Lancet* 1997;349:696.

Hiraoka N, Yoshioka K, Inoue K, et al. Chromobacterium violaceum sepsis accompanied by bacteria-associated hemophagocytic syndrome in a Japanese man. *Arch Intern Med* 1999;159:1623–1624.

Kumakura S, Ishikura H, Umegae N, et al. Autoimmune-associated hemophagocytic syndrome. *Am J Med* 1997;102:113–115.

Tsuda H. The use of cyclosporin-A in the treatment of virus-associated hemophagocytic syndrome in adults. *Leuk Lymphoma* 1997;28:73–82.

Young NS. Acquired aplastic anemia. *JAMA* 1999;282:271–278.

Pleural Effusion and Fever

Basics

DEFINITION

- A pleural effusion is defined by fluid in the pleural space.
- Light's criteria are usually used for separating transudates and exudates. Exudative pleural effusions meet at least one of the following criteria:
  —Pleural fluid protein/serum protein >0.5
  —Pleural fluid lactate dehydrogenase (LDH)/serum LDH >0.6
  —Pleural fluid LDH more than two-thirds normal upper limit for serum
- The term *parapneumonic effusion* is used when the pleural effusion is secondary to a bacterial process in the thoracic cavity.
- A patient has an uncomplicated parapneumonic effusion if the pleural fluid is not loculated, does not appear to be frank pus, and has one or more of the following:
  —Low pleural fluid pH (<7.00–7.20)
  —Low pleural fluid glucose level (<40–50 mg/dL)
  —Positive Gram stain
  —Positive culture
- A patient has a complex complicated parapneumonic effusion if the fluid meets the criteria for a simple parapneumonic effusion but, in addition, the pleural fluid is loculated.
- Empyema is pus in the pleural space. A patient has a simple empyema if the pleural fluid is frank pus and if the fluid is free-flowing or is in a single loculus. A patient has a complex empyema if the pleural fluid is frank pus and if the fluid is multiloculated.

APPROACH TO THE PATIENT

- When the patient is first evaluated, a careful history and physical examination should be obtained and a diagnostic thoracentesis should be performed. Initial laboratory studies include measurement of the levels of protein, glucose, amylase, and LDH and pleural fluid cytology. If the patient has an acute febrile illness or if the pleural fluid smells putrid or is turbid, the fluid should be analyzed for cell count, and Gram stain and aerobic and anaerobic cultures should be obtained. Also, consider evaluation of pH, acid-fast bacillus smear, tuberculosis culture, fungal smear, and fungal culture.
- The next procedure depends on the clinical situation. For example, if pleural tuberculosis or malignancy is strongly suspected, the procedure should be needle biopsy of the parietal pleura. Bronchoscopy is also recommended at this point.
- If indicated, the patient is subjected to thoracoscopy or open pleural biopsy.

ETIOLOGY

- Transudative pleural effusions are not often associated with fever, and the most common causes include the following:
  —Cirrhosis
  —Congestive heart failure
  —Myxedema
  —Nephrotic syndrome
  —Peritoneal dialysis
  —Pulmonary emboli
  —Superior vena cava obstruction
  —Urinothorax
- All leading causes of exudative pleural effusions can be accompanied by fever and include the following:
  —Infections (bacterial, fungal, mycobacterial, viral, or parasitic)
  —Malignancies (usually lung carcinoma, breast carcinoma, and lymphoma)
  —Collagen-vascular diseases (rheumatoid pleuritis, systemic lupus erythematosus, etc.)
  —Pulmonary embolism
- Other causes of exudative pleural effusions include the following:
  —Asbestos exposure
  —Chylothorax
  —Drug-induced pleural disease
  —Electrical burns
  —Gastrointestinal disease (esophageal perforation, pancreatitis, intraabdominal abscesses, etc.)
  —Hemothorax
  —Iatrogenic injury
  —Meigs' syndrome
  —Pericardial disease
  —Post–lung transplant
  —Post–cardiac injury syndrome
  —Radiation therapy
  —Sarcoidosis
  —Uremia
- Early in the process of a parapneumonic effusion, the effusion may appear transudative.
- Pleural fluid glucose concentration levels below 60 mg/dL suggest pleuritis due to bacterial infection, malignancy, or rheumatoid arthritis.
- Among hospitalized patients with AIDS, most causes of pleural effusion are noninfectious and include hypoalbuminemia, cardiac failure, atelectasis, Kaposi's sarcoma, uremic pleurisy, and adult respiratory distress syndrome. Most common infectious causes include bacterial pneumonia, *Pneumocystis carinii* pneumonia, *Mycobacterium tuberculosis*, septic embolism, *Nocardia asteroides*, *Cryptococcus neoformans*, and *Mycobacterium avium-intracellulare*.
- Tuberculous pleurisy usually occurs 3 to 7 months after infection. The fluid is straw colored and at times hemorrhagic; it is an exudate with a protein concentration greater than 50% of that in serum, a normal to low glucose concentration, a pH that is generally less than 7.2, and, usually, 500 to 2,500 white blood cells per milliliter. Neutrophils may predominate in the early stage, while mononuclear cells are the typical finding later.
- Vertebral osteomyelitis should be considered in the differential diagnosis of pleural effusion, especially if there is associated back pain.
- Hantavirus pulmonary syndrome often is associated with pleural effusion. The fluid is probably initially transudative but may take on characteristics of an exudate.
- Consider testing for antibodies to *Toxocara* larva in patients with eosinophilic pleurisy, particularly when associated with blood eosinophilia.
- Chagas' disease can cause a transudative effusion due to congestive heart failure.

Pleural Effusion and Fever

EPIDEMIOLOGY

- In many parts of the world, the most common cause of an exudative pleural effusion is tuberculosis, but this is relatively uncommon in the United States.
- In the medical intensive care unit, about 10% of the pleural effusions are parapneumonic.

Clinical Manifestations

- Patients with aerobic bacterial pneumonia and pleural effusion present with an acute febrile illness consisting of chest pain, sputum production, and leukocytosis. Patients with anaerobic infections present with a subacute illness, with weight loss, leukocytosis, mild anemia, and a history of some factor that predisposes them to aspiration.
- Patients with tuberculous pleuritis present with fever, weight loss, dyspnea, and/or pleuritic chest pain. However, pleural pain is absent in about one-fourth of the cases.

Diagnosis

- One-third of patients with tuberculous pleuritis can have a negative tuberculin skin test.
- In tuberculous pleuritis, pleural fluid culture results can be positive in less than 25% of cases, while a specimen from a single, closed pleural biopsy can show granulomas in about 60%, and three biopsies can demonstrate granulomas in about 80%. Mycobacterial culture of the biopsy specimen increases the diagnostic yield to about 90%. Thoracoscopic biopsy probably has an even higher yield. The use of polymerase chain reaction and levels of adenosine deaminase has not been found to be clinically useful.

IMAGING

- In tuberculous pleuritis, only about a third of the cases have parenchymal disease visible radiographically.
- In tuberculosis and other lung processes, computed tomography of the chest can reveal parenchymal disease that is not evident on simple radiographs.

Treatment

- Antibiotic therapy alone is adequate for the treatment of a typical parapneumonic effusion.
- The appropriate management of patients with complicated parapneumonic pleural effusion is tube thoracostomy (usually relatively small chest tubes inserted percutaneously).
- Patients with a complex complicated parapneumonic should be treated with tube thoracostomy. Streptokinase or urokinase administered through the chest tube can facilitate the drainage of loculated effusions. If drainage is still inadequate, thoracoscopy with the breakdown of adhesions and the optimal positioning of the chest tube or decortication is indicated.
- Patients with a simple empyema should be treated with a relatively large chest tube. If a sizable empyema cavity remains after 7 days of chest tube drainage, consideration should be given to performing more extensive drainage and a decortication.
- Patients with complex empyemas should initially be managed with large chest tubes and intrapleural thrombolytic therapy. However, most patients will require decortication.

COMPLICATIONS

- Even though the pleural reaction itself abates without treatment, active tuberculosis develops in approximately 65% of patients within 5 to 7 years. Treatment, therefore, is mandatory.
- Tuberculous empyema is usually the result of the rupture of a cavity and may result in severe pleural fibrosis and restrictive lung disease.

Follow-Up

In many series, no diagnosis is established for approximately 20% of exudative effusions, and these effusions often resolve spontaneously with no long-term residual.

PREVENTION

- The possibility of a parapneumonic effusion should be considered whenever a patient with a bacterial pneumonia is initially evaluated.
- A repeat diagnostic thoracentesis should be considered in a typical parapneumonic effusion if the effusion increases in size.

Selected Readings

Judson MA, Handy JR, Sahn SA. Pleural effusions following lung transplantation. Time course, characteristics, and clinical implications. *Chest* 1996;109:1190–1194.

Light RW. A new classification of parapneumonic effusions and empyema. *Chest* 1995;108:299–301.

Light RW. Disorders of the pleura, mediastinum, and diaphragm. In: Fauci AS, Braunwald E, Isselbacher KJ, et al., eds. *Harrison's principles of internal medicine*, 14th ed. New York: McGraw-Hill, 1998;1472–1476.

Marel M, Stastny B, Melinova L, et al. Diagnosis of pleural effusions. Experience with clinical studies, 1986 to 1990. *Chest* 1995;107:1598–1603.

Roth BJ. Evaluating pleural fluid. *Chest* 1996;110:7–8.

Pleuritic and Chest Pain and Fever

Basics

DEFINITION
- The term *pleuritic pain* is used to describe pain that is related to respiratory movements and is aggravated by cough and/or deep inspiration.
- Because the pleuritic component is not always apparent, chest pain in general is discussed.

APPROACH TO THE PATIENT
- Chest discomfort is one of the most frequent complaints for which patients seek medical attention.
- Failure to recognize a serious disorder, such as ischemic heart disease, may result in the dangerous delay of much-needed treatment, while an incorrect diagnosis of a potentially serious condition, such as angina pectoris, is likely to have harmful psychological and economic consequences and may lead to unnecessary cardiac catheterization.
- Clinicians should determine whether the syndrome represents new, acute, and often ongoing pain; recurrent, episodic pain; or pain that is persistent, perhaps for days.
- A complete history and a physical examination are needed to distinguish potentially life-threatening conditions, such as coronary artery disease, aortic dissection, or pulmonary embolism.
- Most infectious causes of chest pain present with pleuritic characteristics.
- Testing guided by data includes the following:
  - Electrocardiogram
  - Computed tomography (CT) of chest
  - Gastrointestinal evaluation
  - Spine, shoulder, or rib radiographs
  - Echocardiogram

ETIOLOGY
- *Infectious* causes of chest pain (often with pleuritic characteristics) include aspergillosis, biliary disease, Chagas' disease, coccidioidomycosis, echinococcosis of the lung, empyema, herpes zoster, infection with the *Mycobacterium avium* complex, mediastinitis, mucormycosis, pericarditis, pleurodynia (Bornholm disease), *Pneumocystis carinii* pneumonia, pneumonia (legionellosis, *Chlamydia* spp, *Mycoplasma* spp, *Streptococcus pneumoniae*), pneumonic plague, pulmonary actinomycosis, pulmonary tularemia, Q fever, tracheobronchitis, and tuberculosis.
- *Noninfectious* causes of chest pain include angina pectoris, aortic dissection, aortic stenosis, arthritis of the shoulder or spine, cholelithiasis, costochondritis, esophageal reflux, esophageal spasm, hypertropic cardiomyopathy, malignancy, myocardial infarction, pancreatitis, peptic ulcer disease, pericarditis, pneumothorax, primary pulmonary hypertension, pulmonary embolism, and sickle-cell crisis.
- The organisms detected in acute mediastinitis vary with the underlying cause. Mixed infections containing both aerobic and anaerobic organisms are commonly associated with acute mediastinitis, resulting from both esophageal perforation and spread from oropharyngeal sources.
- Although most cases of granulomatous or sclerosing mediastinitis have been ascribed to *Histoplasma capsulatum*, other recognized causes include tuberculosis, blastomycosis, actinomycosis, coccidioidomycosis, aspergillosis, and nocardiosis.

EPIDEMIOLOGY
- The most common cause of acute mediastinitis is iatrogenic esophageal perforation. The greatest risk for perforation is associated with stricture dilation or sclerotherapy.
- Acute mediastinitis complicates 1.3% of cardiothoracic surgical procedures (from 600 to 1,200 cases of mediastinitis annually in the United States). Reported mortality varies from 20% to 40%.
- Descending oropharyngeal infections such as Ludwig's angina give rise to descending necrotizing mediastinitis, the most aggressive type of acute mediastinitis.
- Factors predisposing to development of postsurgical mediastinitis include the following:
  - Duration of the surgical procedure
  - Previous sternotomy
  - Reoperation
  - Obesity
  - Presence of disease in other organ systems

- There are a number of causes of pericarditis, including infection, systemic illness, cardiac disease, trauma, and neoplasm. Iatrogenic causes include surgery, cardiac instrumentation, irradiation, and medications. In a study of 57 patients who underwent surgical treatment because of large pericardial effusions, pericardial fluid and tissue samples were studied cytologically, and cultures for aerobic and anaerobic bacteria, fungi, mycobacteria, *Mycoplasma*, and viruses were done. A diagnosis was made in 53 patients (93%). Malignant disease was the most common finding. Eight patients had an infectious cause, including *M. pneumoniae*, cytomegalovirus, herpes simplex virus, *Mycobacterium avium-intracellulare*, and *Mycobacterium chelonei*.

Clinical Manifestations

- Classically, acute mediastinitis manifests with the sudden onset of fever, chills, and prostration. Patients have severe, usually pleuritic, substernal chest pain, and examination reveals tachycardia, tachypnea, and signs of systemic toxicity.
- The clinical presentation of pericarditis varies, depending on the cause. Chest pain and dyspnea are characteristic complaints. Pericardial pain is sometimes brought on by swallowing, because the esophagus lies just behind the posterior portion of the heart, and is often altered by a change of body position, becoming sharper and more left-sided in the supine position and milder when the patient sits upright, leaning forward.
- Patients with pleurodynia present with an acute onset of fever and spasms of pleuritic chest or upper abdominal pain. Chest pain is more frequent in adults, and abdominal pain is more common in children. Paroxysms of severe, knifelike pain usually last 15 to 30 min and are associated with diaphoresis and tachypnea. Fever peaks within an hour after the onset of paroxysms and subsides when pain resolves. The involved muscles are tender to palpation, and a pleural rub may be detected.

Pleuritic and Chest Pain and Fever

- The triad of pleuritic chest pain, hemoptysis, and dyspnea occurs in less than 15% of patients with substantiated pulmonary embolism. The most frequent symptoms associated with pulmonary embolism are nonspecific (dyspnea and chest pain); cough, palpitations, syncope, and diaphoresis have also been reported.

Diagnosis

DIFFERENTIAL DIAGNOSIS

- Fever and pleuritic chest pain after a cardiac operation can be caused by postpericardiotomy syndrome or postmyocardial infarction syndrome (Dressler's syndrome). Postperfusion syndrome is another cause of fever in this population. It results from primary cytomegalovirus infection but is not associated with pleuritic chest pain.
- The radiographic finding of a widened mediastinum in the clinical setting of fever and pleuritic chest pain strongly suggests acute mediastinitis.
- A history of prior upper endoscopy should alert one to the possibility of an esophageal perforation.

LABORATORY

- Electrocardiographic abnormalities, including tachycardia, incomplete right bundle branch block, $S_1 Q_3 T_3$, right-axis deviation, and atrial arrhythmias, occur in 80% to 85% of patients with pulmonary embolism.
- Enzyme-linked immunosorbent assay measurement of D-dimers has a reported high sensitivity but is not specific for pulmonary embolism.

IMAGING

- For the diagnosis of mediastinitis, a Gastrografin swallow study (contrast esophagography) is the investigation of choice for visualization of the esophagus when an esophageal perforation is suspected. A CT scan of the chest is required at this stage to evaluate the mediastinum.
- The chest radiograph classically demonstrates a widened mediastinum, at times with air–fluid levels visible in the mediastinum on the lateral view. A CT scan of the chest typically shows abscesses and mediastinal emphysema and may reveal pleural or pericardial effusions.
- The chest roentgenographic findings may be normal in 20% to 30% of patients with pulmonary embolism. Frequently, however, an elevated hemidiaphragm, an infiltrate, or a pleural effusion is detected. Other possible radiologic findings include atelectasis, enlarged pulmonary arteries, or peripheral radiolucency indicative of decreased vascular filling (Westermark's sign). Hampton's hump is a pyramidal infiltrate peaked toward the hilum, indicating infarction.

DIAGNOSTIC/TESTING PROCEDURES

- Echocardiography is the most sensitive technique for detecting the presence of pericardial effusion.
- Thoracentesis with pleural fluid analysis should be performed in cases of suspected empyema, in conjunction with analysis of pH, protein, lactate dehydrogenase, and glucose, and Gram stain and culture. A bloody effusion would be supportive of the diagnosis of pulmonary embolism.

Treatment

For patients with acute severe mediastinitis, aggressive open surgical drainage and debridement are necessary to prevent serious morbidity and mortality. Percutaneous catheter drainage has been used in less urgent clinical settings, often as a temporizing measure, but open surgical drainage remains the standard of therapy.

COMPLICATIONS

- The mortality rate associated with acute mediastinitis from esophageal disruption is 5% to 30%, even with appropriate treatment.
- Common complications of mediastinitis result from extension of the infectious process into contiguous structures and spaces. Thus, abscess formation and empyema are relatively common complications of acute mediastinitis of any cause. Late complications of acute mediastinitis resulting from esophageal perforation include esophagocutaneous, esophagopleural, and esophagobronchial fistulas.

Follow-Up

- Any form of pericarditis may lead to the development of cardiac tamponade. Malignant effusion is probably the most common single cause.
- Progression of infection during the course of acute mediastinitis can result in mass effect and local tissue injury.

PREVENTION

Sternal osteomyelitis is a common complication of mediastinitis after a cardiothoracic operation. The incidences of pericardial effusion, abscess, and empyema formation all increase if treatment is delayed.

Selected Readings

Farraj RS, McCully RB, Oh JK, Smith TF. Mycoplasma-associated pericarditis. *Mayo Clinic Proc* 1997;72:33–36.

Goldman L. Chest discomfort and palpitation. In: Fauci AS, Braunwald E, Isselbacher KJ, et al., eds. *Harrison's principles of medicine*, 14th ed. New York: McGraw-Hill, 1998:59–65.

Prince SE, Cunha BA. Postpericardiotomy syndrome. *Heart Lung* 1997;26:165–168.

Sabers CJ, Levy NT, Bowen JM. 33-year-old man with chest pain and fever. *Mayo Clinic Proc* 1999;74:181–184.

Sternbach GL. Pericarditis. *Ann Emerg Med* 1988;17:214–220.

Windgassen EB, Gillespie DJ. 39-year-old man with fever, cough, and chest pain. *Mayo Clinic Proc* 1995;70:1191–1194.

Postoperative Fever

Basics

DEFINITION

Postoperative fever has been used to describe hyperthermia that occurs early (<48–96 hours) or late (>96 hours) after an invasive procedure.

APPROACH TO THE PATIENT

- Postoperative fever can be due to numerous infectious and noninfectious causes.
- The evaluation includes history, physical examination, and appropriate radiologic and laboratory tests, including cultures and Gram stains of body fluids.
- Fever in the early postoperative period is often noninfectious in origin, presuming that unusual breaks in sterile technique or pulmonary aspiration did not occur. However, once a patient is >96 hours postoperative, fever is likely to represent infection.
- Because bacterial etiology of fever is a major concern, clinical and laboratory findings can be used to predict patients at high risk for an infectious process.
- The patient could have aspirated during the postoperative period, or the patient might be incubating a community-acquired process prior to the operation.
- The degree of initial temperature elevation should not be used as a sole guide for initiating a search for a bacterial infection.
- New or persistent fever >4 days after surgery should raise a strong suspicion of persistent pathology or a new complication.
- It is mandatory to remove the surgical dressing to inspect the wound as well as all previous catheter sites.

ETIOLOGY

- Postoperative fever is a common occurrence.
- Urinary tract infection is common postoperatively because of the use of urinary drainage catheters. Also, respiratory tract infections, sinusitis, suppurative phlebitis, catheter-related infection, and *Clostridium difficile*–associated diarrhea are frequent causes of fever in the postoperative period.
- Wound infection is rare in the first 1 to 3 days after operation, except for group A streptococcal infections and clostridial infections, which can develop immediately after surgery.
- Many emergency abdominal operations are performed for control of an infection (e.g., peritonitis). Even under optimal circumstances, it may take 3 days or more for such patients to defervesce.
- If no infection is found, atelectasis, if present, may be blamed; however, attributing fever to atelectasis may lead to missing an infection or to inappropriate therapy.
- Other potentially serious causes of postoperative fever include deep venous thrombosis, pulmonary embolism, subarachnoid hemorrhage, gout, fat emboli, and transplant rejection.
- Crush injury syndrome and tetanus are two other rare complications of traumatic wounds that may cause fever.
- Among drug categories, fever is most often attributed to antimicrobials (especially beta-lactam drugs), antiepileptic drugs (especially phenytoin), antiarrhythmics (especially quinidine and procainamide), and antihypertensives (methyldopa).
- Drugs or their delivery systems (intravenous fluid, intravascular delivery devices, etc.) may also contain pyrogens or, rarely, microbial contaminants.
- Fever associated with transfusion of blood products, particularly red blood cells and platelets, occurs most frequently in patients who have received multiple transfusions.
- Certain inflammatory processes cause fever in the absence of infection, particularly pulmonary infarction and the fibroproliferative phase of adult respiratory distress syndrome (ARDS). Additionally, acute or chronic pancreatitis may be associated with fever as well as hemodynamic instability.
- Fever may be associated with acute myocardial infarction in the first few days. Higher temperature elevations have been associated with Dressler's syndrome in the later period after myocardial infarction or after cardiothoracic surgery involving incision of the pericardium—the so-called postpericardiotomy syndrome.
- Endocrine emergencies such as acute adrenal insufficiency and hyperthyroidism can be associated with fever.

EPIDEMIOLOGY

- The duration of catheterization is the most important risk factor for the development of nosocomial cystitis or pyelonephritis.
- Bacterial vaginosis is associated with increased vaginal concentrations of certain anaerobic and facultative bacteria. Bacterial vaginosis appears to be a risk factor for the development of postoperative infections in obstetrics and gynecology.
- Preoperative biliary stenting in proximal cholangiocarcinoma increases the incidence of contaminated bile and postoperative infectious complications.

Clinical Manifestations

- There is nothing characteristic about the fevers induced by drugs. Fevers do not invariably occur immediately after drug administration: It may be days after administration that fever occurs, and many more days before the fever abates.
- When erysipelas or myonecrosis is present, the diagnosis is often suspected by inspection alone, and such patients are usually toxic appearing.
- Malignant hyperthermia is more often identified in the operating room, but onset can be delayed for as long as 24 hours. It can be caused by succinylcholine and the inhalation anesthetics, of which halothane is the most frequently identified. This hyperthermic syndrome is believed to be a

Postoperative Fever

genetically determined response. It is caused by calcium dysregulation and intense muscle contraction, which generates fever and increasing creatinine phosphokinase concentrations.
- The neuroleptic malignant syndrome is rare but more often identified than malignant hyperthermia. It has been strongly associated with antipsychotic neuroleptic medications. Haloperidol is perhaps the most frequently reported drug. It manifests as muscle rigidity, generating fever as well as increasing creatinine phosphokinase concentrations. However, unlike malignant hyperthermia, the initiator of muscle contraction is central.
- Withdrawal of certain drugs may be associated with fever often with associated tachycardia, diaphoresis, and hyperreflexia. Alcohol, opiates (including methadone), barbiturates, and benzodiazepines have all been associated with this febrile syndrome. A history of use of these drugs may not be available when the patient is admitted. Withdrawal and related fever may therefore occur several hours or days after admission.

Diagnosis

LABORATORY

- A urinalysis and culture are not mandatory during the initial 72 hours postoperatively if fever is the only indication. Urinalysis and culture should be performed for those febrile patients who have indwelling bladder catheters for >72 hours.
- Eosinophilia is uncommon among patients with fevers induced by drugs.

IMAGING

- Clinicians should consider investigating (usually by duplex ultrasonography with color ODoppler flow studies) any new swelling of an extremity.
- A chest radiograph is not mandatory during the initial 72 hours postoperatively if fever is the only indication.

DIAGNOSTIC/TESTING PROCEDURES

Swabbing the wound for culture is rarely helpful if clinical assessment reveals no symptoms or signs suggesting infection.

Treatment

- Physicians should consider all the possible causes when they treat patients with postoperative fever and should avoid using antibiotics for noninfectious causes.
- Treatments for atelectasis include cough and deep breathing, incentive spirometry, percussion and postural drainage, beta-2 agonists, intermittent positive-pressure breathing, ultrasonic nebulizers, and even antibiotics.

COMPLICATIONS

Infections during the postoperative period can increase morbidity and mortality (lead to sepsis, affect the healing of the surgical wound, lead to respiratory failure, etc.).

Follow-Up

- The diagnosis of drug-induced fever is usually established by the temporal relationship of the fever to starting and stopping the drug. Patients can be rechallenged with the drug to confirm the diagnosis, but this is rarely done unless the drug in question is essential and alternatives are not available.
- Surgical wounds should be examined daily for infection. They do not need to be cultured if there is no symptom or sign suggesting infection.

PREVENTION

- A patient with fever in the early postoperative period should have aggressive pulmonary toilet, including incentive spirometry to reduce the likelihood or extent of atelectasis.
- A reduction in the number of invasive procedures, which partly depends on physicians' practice patterns, may decrease the incidence of postoperative fever.

Selected Readings

Arbo MJ, Fine MJ, Hanusa BH, et al. Lack of association between atelectasis and fever. *Chest* 1995;107:81–84.

Hochwald SN, Burke EC, Jarnagin WR, et al. Association of preoperative biliary stenting with increased postoperative infectious complications in proximal cholangiocarcinoma. *Arch Surg* 1999;134:261–266.

Klingler A, Henle KP, Beller S, et al. Laparoscopic appendectomy does not change the incidence of postoperative infectious complications. *Am J Surg* 1998;175:232–235.

O'Grady NP, Barie PS, Bartlett J, et al. Practice parameters for evaluating new fever in critically ill adult patients. Task Force of the American College of Critical Care Medicine of the Society of Critical Care Medicine in collaboration with the Infectious Disease Society of America. *Crit Care Med* 1998;26:392–408.

Soper DE. Bacterial vaginosis and postoperative infections. *Am J Obstet Gynecol* 1993;169:467–469.

Rash and Fever

Basics

DEFINITION

- The term *rash* describes temporary skin eruptions.
- Skin eruptions can accompany numerous infectious diseases and can be localized or generalized.
- Skin manifestations of infectious diseases are discussed throughout this book. In this chapter, the focus is on the differential diagnosis and early recognition of life-threatening, generalized skin eruptions.

APPROACH TO THE PATIENT

- A thorough history should elicit the following information:
  —Immune status
  —Complete medication list
  —Travel history
  —Immunization status
  —Exposure to domestic pets and other animals
  —History of animal or arthropod bites
  —Existence of cardiac abnormalities
  —Presence of prosthetic material
  —Recent exposure to ill individuals
  —Exposure to sexually transmitted diseases
- The history should also include the site of onset of the rash, whether it is pruritic or painful, and its direction and rate of spread.
- A thorough physical examination determines the type of lesions that make up the eruption, including their configuration (i.e., annular or target), the arrangement of their lesions, and their distribution (i.e., central or peripheral).

ETIOLOGY

The most common skin eruptions among adults include the following:

- Centrally distributed maculopapular eruptions
  —Adult-onset Still's disease
  —Allergic(drug)-induced eruptions
  —Dengue
  —Ehrlichiosis
  —Endemic (murine) typhus
  —Epidemic typhus
  —Erythema marginatum (rheumatic fever)
  —Infectious mononucleosis
  —Leptospirosis
  —Lyme disease
  —Primary HIV infection
  —Relapsing fever
  —Rubella (German measles)
  —Rubeola (measles)
  —Systemic lupus erythematosus
  —Typhoid fever
- Peripheral eruptions
  —Bacterial endocarditis
  —Chronic meningococcemia
  —Disseminated gonococcal infection
  —Erythema multiforme
  —Rocky Mountain spotted fever (RMSF)
  —Secondary syphilis
- Confluent desquamative erythemas
  —Graft-versus-host disease
  —Kawasaki disease
  —Scarlet fever
  —Staphylococcal and streptococcal toxic shock syndrome
- Vesiculobullous eruptions
  —Disseminated *Vibrio vulnificus* infection
  —Ecthyma gangrenosum
  —Rickettsial pox
- Urticarial vasculitis
- Nodular eruptions
  —Disseminated infections due to fungi and mycobacteria
  —Erythema nodosum
  —Sweet's syndrome
- Purpuric eruptions
  —Acute and chronic meningococcemia
  —Disseminated gonococcal infection
  —Enteroviral petechial rash
  —RMSF
  —Thrombotic thrombocytopenic purpura

EPIDEMIOLOGY

- Rash has been described in half of travelers with dengue.
- During the first stage of Lyme disease, a characteristic skin rash develops at the site of the tick bite in 80% of the cases.

Clinical Manifestations

- Rash is the hallmark of Rocky Mountain spotted fever (RMSF) and appears on day 4 (range, 1–15 days) of the illness. Initially, the rash consists of small pink or red macules that blanche with pressure. Over time, the rash evolves into petechia and purpura. Gangrenous areas may develop on the fingers, toes, nose, ears, scrotum, or vulva. Involvement of the scrotum or vulva is a diagnostic clue.
- Rash may be absent in about 10% of cases. "Spotless fever" has a relatively poor prognosis because of the difficulty in making a diagnosis.
- Acute meningococcemia and meningococcal meningitis are caused by *Neisseria meningitidis*, an encapsulated gram-negative diplococcus. Skin lesions are common and are an important early diagnostic clue to this rapidly progressive illness. Classically, the rash appears as a petechial eruption that is scattered on the trunk and extremities and then evolves into the pathognomonic palpable purpura with gun-metal gray necrotic centers. Urticarial, macular, and papular lesions also may occur. Clusters of petechia may develop at areas of pressure, such as under blood pressure cuffs or elastic bands. Adults with meningococcal disease are less likely to have cutaneous findings.
- Fulminant meningococcemia (Waterhouse-Friderichsen syndrome) can be complicated by purpura fulminans, a cutaneous manifestation of disseminated intravascular coagulation. This is a dramatic scenario in which large ecchymoses and hemorrhagic bullae appear, accompanied by ischemia of the digits and limbs.
- Although there is variability in the tempo and clinical manifestations of Lyme disease, it has been divided into three distinct stages: stage 1, a characteristic macular skin rash, erythema migrans, which resolves spontaneously within 4 weeks; stage 2, neurologic or cardiac involvement; and stage 3, arthritis.

Rash and Fever

- Headache and high fever are prominent in human ehrlichiosis. Rash appears to be variable in occurrence and most commonly is described as petechial or macular. A diffuse erythematous rash has also been described.
- The cutaneous signs of staphylococcal toxic shock syndrome include a sunburn-like, diffuse macular erythroderma, followed by desquamation, especially of the hands and feet, within 5 to 14 days. Conjunctival injection, mucosal hyperemia (oral and genital), and a strawberry tongue are important diagnostic signs. Less frequent manifestations are edema of the hands and feet, petechiae, and delayed loss of nails and hair.
- Streptococcal toxic shock syndrome occurs most commonly in the setting of invasive soft-tissue infections, such as necrotizing fasciitis, myonecrosis, and cellulitis; however, association with streptococcal pneumonia, sinusitis, and pharyngitis has also been reported. The pain is typically localized to an extremity and is often disproportionate to the findings on examination. A thorough examination of the skin often detects subtle evidence of a soft-tissue infection such as localized swelling, tenderness, or erythema or the more distinctive violaceous bullae that may be seen in necrotizing fasciitis.
- Among travelers with dengue, rash appears on the second to fifth day of the disease, and is usually maculopapular, involving also the palms of the hands.

Diagnosis

DIFFERENTIAL DIAGNOSIS

Desquamating erythroderma may be present in streptococcal toxic shock syndrome but is less common than in staphylococcal toxic shock syndrome.

LABORATORY

- Antibodies to *Rickettsia rickettsii* (RMSF) are detectable 7 to 10 days after the onset of illness, and they fall to nondiagnostic titers within 2 months. Early treatment may blunt or delay the increase in antibody levels.
- Diagnosis of meningococcal disease is made by Gram stain and culture of the blood and cerebrospinal fluid. Microbiologic analysis of the skin lesions may be a helpful diagnostic adjunct.
- In contrast to staphylococcal toxic shock syndrome, more than 60% of patients with streptococcal toxic shock syndrome have bacteremia.

Treatment

- The most important management tenet in streptococcal toxic shock syndrome is early and aggressive surgical exploration and debridement of any associated soft-tissue infection. Surgical exploration may also facilitate a definitive diagnosis through acquisition of tissue for culture, Gram stain, and histopathologic examination. Empiric treatment includes broad-spectrum antimicrobial coverage until the streptococcus is positively identified.
- Please see respective chapters for details on the treatment of other causes of skin eruptions caused by infectious causes.

COMPLICATIONS

The mortality rate of patients with RMSF untreated or treated with inappropriate antibiotics may be as high as 25% to 50%. With appropriate treatment, mortality falls to 3% to 5% and varies with severity of illness and time of onset of treatment.

Follow-Up

PREVENTION

When a patient presents with fever and petechiae, Waterhouse-Friderichsen syndrome must be considered, even when the patient has a nontoxic appearance. Due to the rapid progression and often devastating consequences, therapy should be instituted as soon as the diagnosis is suspected.

Selected Readings

Anonymous. Fever, nausea, and rash in a 37-year-old man. *Am J Med* 1998;104:596–601.

Aractingi S, Chosidow O. Cutaneous graft-versus-host disease. *Arch Dermatol* 1998;134:602–612.

Drage LA. Life-threatening rashes: Dermatologic signs of four infectious diseases. *Mayo Clin Proc* 1999;74:68–72.

Faul JL, Doyle RL, Kao PN, Ruoss SJ. Tickborne pulmonary disease: Update on diagnosis and management. *Chest* 1999;116:222–230.

Kaye ET, Kaye KM. Fever and rash. In:. Fauci AS, Braunwald E, Isselbacher KJ, et al., eds. *Harrison's principles of medicine,* 14th ed. New York: McGraw-Hill, 1998:90–97.

Schwartz E, Mendelson E, Sidi Y. Dengue fever among travelers. *Am J Med* 1996;101:516–520.

Red Eye

Basics

DEFINITION
- Serious sight conditions of the eye can present with redness of the eye.
- *Scleritis* is inflammation of the sclera that can be limited to a thin layer of connective tissue between the conjunctiva and sclera (episcleritis), or it can refer to a deeper, more severe inflammatory process. It may occur alone or with keratitis or uveitis.
- *Uveitis* is inflammation involving the anterior structures of the eye and can be anterior (iritis or iridocyclitis) or posterior or involve both the anterior and posterior segments of the eye (panuveitis).
- Please also see the Section II chapters, "Keratitis" and "Conjunctivitis," for details on these infections.

APPROACH TO THE PATIENT
- Conjunctivitis is the most common cause of a red eye. However, red eye may indicate more urgent conditions.
- Key features for the evaluation of patients with red eye include the following:
  —Acuity
  —Discharge
  —Extent and type of redness
  —Pain
  —Photophobia
  —Preauricular adenopathy
- Patients with conjunctivitis usually present with discharge and irritation and have normal vision, clear cornea, and normal pupil.
- Chronic, unilateral red eye can be due to meibomian gland carcinoma or Kaposi's sarcoma of the conjunctiva.
- Patients with red eye should be evaluated by an ophthalmologist, except those with a typical case of mild conjunctivitis.

ETIOLOGY
- Noninfectious causes of uveitis
  —Ankylosing spondylitis
  —Behçet's disease
  —Inflammatory bowel disease
  —Juvenile rheumatoid arthritis
  —Psoriasis
  —Reiter's syndrome
  —Sarcoidosis
- Infectious causes of uveitis
  —Aspergillosis
  —Brucellosis
  —Candidiasis
  —Coccidioidomycosis
  —Cryptococcosis
  —Cysticercosis
  —Histoplasmosis
  —Leprosy
  —Lyme disease
  —Onchocerciasis (infection due to *Onchocerca volvulus*, one of the eight filarial species that infect humans)
  —*Pneumocystis carinii* infection
  —Syphilis
  —Toxoplasmosis
  —Tuberculosis
  —Viral infections (due to herpes, cytomegalovirus, etc.)
  —Whipple's disease
- Scleritis is frequently associated with a connective tissue disease.
- Infectious scleritis is uncommon and may be endogenous or exogenous (due to trauma or surgery). All pathogens (including *Pseudomonas aeruginosa*) that involve the cornea and conjunctiva can spread to the sclera. Other possible pathogens include *Nocardia* spp, *Aspergillus* spp, *Pseudallescheria boydii*, and *Fusarium* spp.
- Three types of allergic conjunctivitis:
  —Hay fever conjunctivitis has a seasonal incidence and presents with itching, redness, and edema.
  —Vernal conjunctivitis is also seasonal. It affects exclusively children or adolescents. The cause is unknown, but air-borne antigens are thought to trigger symptoms. Itching, photophobia, epiphora, and mucous discharge are typical.
  —Atopic conjunctivitis occurs in subjects with atopic dermatitis or asthma.
- Most cases of episcleritis are idiopathic, but some occur in the setting of an autoimmune disease.

EPIDEMIOLOGY

Incidence
- *O. volvulus* infects an estimated 18 million individuals and is the second leading cause of infectious blindness worldwide. About one million of these people are blind or have severe visual impairment.
- Onchocerciasis is more common in the equatorial region of Africa, extending from the Atlantic coast to the Red Sea. A smaller number of patients live in Central and South America and Saudi Arabia.

Risk Factors
- Subconjunctival hemorrhage can be spontaneous or from the following:
  —An underlying bleeding disorder
  —Blunt trauma
  —Coughing
  —Eye rubbing
- In large series, seronegative spondyloarthropathy accounts for 28% of the patients with anterior uveitis, but spondyloarthropathy is not a common cause of posterior uveitis.
- Eye involvement occurs in approximately 25% of patients with sarcoidosis, and it can cause blindness. The usual lesions involve the uveal tract, iris, ciliary body, and choroid.

Clinical Manifestations

SYMPTOMS
- In anterior forms of scleritis, the patient complains of severe ocular tenderness and pain. With posterior scleritis, the pain and redness may be less marked.
- In conjunctivitis, pain is minimal.
- Uveitis usually presents with photophobia and visual loss.
- Episcleritis resembles conjunctivitis but is a more localized process and discharge is absent.
- Conjunctivitis due to adenovirus infection causes a watery discharge, mild foreign-body sensation, and photophobia.

Red Eye

- Conjunctivitis due to bacterial infection tends to produce a more mucopurulent exudate.
- In onchocerciasis, lesions may develop in all parts of the eye. The most common early finding is conjunctivitis with photophobia. Anterior uveitis can develop in about 5% of infected persons.
- In some patients, acute angle-closure glaucoma can present with nausea, vomiting, or headache, and minimal ocular symptoms are overshadowed by these, prompting a fruitless work-up for abdominal or neurologic disease.

SIGNS

- Bright red is usually due to subconjunctval hemorrhage, and limited redness involving only the corneal limbus suggests iridocyclitis, keratitis, or angle closure.
- Diffuse conjunctival hyperemia is nonspecific.
- The cornea is usually clear in conjunctivitis and uveitis, but can be edematous and cloudy in acute angle-closure glaucoma.
- The pupil is usually irregular and immobile in acute angle-closure glaucoma, but is usually normal in conjunctivitis.

Diagnosis

DIFFERENTIAL DIAGNOSIS

- Visual acuity
  —Conjunctivitis: slightly reduced
  —Subconjunctival hemorrhage: normal
  —Uveitis: normal or slightly reduced
- Intraocular pressure
  —Conjunctivitis: normal
  —Subconjunctival hemorrhage: normal or mildly elevated
  —Uveitis: markedly elevated

DIAGNOSTIC/TESTING PROCEDURES

- The diagnosis of anterior uveitis requires slit-lamp examination to identify inflammatory cells floating in the aqueous humor or deposited upon the corneal endothelium (keratic precipitates).

- The diagnosis of acute angle-closure glaucoma is made by measuring the intraocular pressure during an acute attack or by performing gonioscopy to reveal the narrowed chamber angle by means of a specially mirrored contact lens.
- Posterior uveitis is diagnosed by observing inflammation of the vitreous, retina, or choroid on fundus examination.

Treatment

- Symptoms caused by allergic conjunctivitis can be alleviated with cold compresses, topical vasoconstrictors, topical nonsteroidal antiinflammatory agents, antihistamines, and mast-cell stabilizers. Topical glucocorticoid solutions can provide symptomatic relief, but their long-term use has been associated with glaucoma, cataract, and secondary infection.
- Episcleritis and scleritis should be treated with nonsteroidal antiinflammatory agents. If these agents fail, topical or even systemic glucocorticoid therapy may be necessary, especially if an underlying autoimmune process is active.
- In uveitis, treatment with the judicious use of topical steroids is aimed at reducing inflammation and scarring.
- Acute angle-closure glaucoma is treated with oral or intravenous acetazolamide, topical beta blockers, and pilocarpine to induce miosis. If these measures fail, a laser can be used to create a hole in the peripheral iris to relieve pupillary block.
- Ivermectin (150 g/kg single dose, either yearly or semiannually) is the first-line agent for the treatment of onchocerciasis.

COMPLICATIONS

- Acute angle-closure glaucoma is a medical emergency. Also, uveitis, conjunctivitis, and other infectious and noninfectious causes of red eye may lead to vision loss if left untreated.

- In onchocerciasis, complications of the anterior uveal tract may cause secondary glaucoma.

Follow-Up

PREVENTION

- Individuals who wear contact lenses have an impaired ability to fight conjunctivitis and are at high risk for developing vision-threatening complications.
- All patients above age 50 should have eye examinations every 2 years to check for glaucoma. Patients over age 65 should have annual examinations. Testing can start earlier in patients with a positive history.

Selected Readings

Abiose A, Jones BR, Cousens SN, et al. Reduction in incidence of optic nerve disease with annual ivermectin to control onchocerciasis. *Lancet* 1993;341(8838):130–134.

Horton JC. Disorders of the eye. In: Fauci AS, Braunwald E, Isselbacher KJ, et al., eds. *Harrison's principles of internal medicine*, 14th ed. New York: McGraw-Hill, 1998:159–172.

O'Brien TR, Green WR. Conjunctivitis. In: Mandell GL, Bennett JE, Dolin R, eds. *Principles and practice of infectious diseases*, 4th ed. New York: Churchill Livingstone, 1995:1103–1110.

Rickman LS, Freeman WR, Green WR, et al. Brief report: Uveitis caused by *Trophermyma whippleii* (Whipple's bacillus). *N Engl J Med* 1995;332:363–366.

Rosenbaum JT, Holland GN. Uveitis and the Tower of Babel [Editorial]. *Arch Ophthalmol* 1996;114:604–605.

Rhinorrhea

Basics

DEFINITION

Rhinorrhea is the discharge of thin nasal mucus.

APPROACH TO THE PATIENT

- For the evaluation of rhinorrhea, the most helpful diagnostic approach is to elicit a thorough history and perform a physical examination.
- The history should distinguish patients with seasonal sensitivity or perennial sensitivity.
- The concomitant presence of watery and itchy eye symptoms can indicate allergic rhinitis or a nonallergic rhinitis with eosinophilia.
- Searching for triggers of the symptoms is important. If specific allergens are recognized, the disorder is likely allergic.
- Symptoms that may increase the likelihood of sinusitis include fever, malaise, cough, nasal congestion, maxillary toothache, purulent nasal discharge, little improvement with nasal decongestants, and headache or facial pain exacerbated by bending forward.
- A history of sudden onset should raise a suspicion of cerebrospinal fluid (CSF) rhinorrhea.
- If unilateral rhinorrhea has no obvious cause, a CSF fistula should be sought.
- The loss of or decrease in the sense of smell is an important symptom, implying involvement of the roof of the nasal cavity and the ethmoid sinus area.
- Dryness of the eyes suggests disorders related to the sicca syndrome. Unilateral epistaxis and nasal obstruction may indicate angiofibroma in young male patients or malignant disease in elderly patients. In children with nasal polyps, cystic fibrosis must be considered.
- Pulmonary symptoms should be sought, because asthma and other pulmonary disorders may be present.
- A physical examination helps to confirm the initial impression. The external appearance of the nose may demonstrate deviation of the septum or collapse of the nasal valve with inspiration. The appearance and color of the inferior and middle turbinates and the color of the mucosa may suggest a specific cause. Clinicians should note the type and color of the nasal secretions. Clear unilateral secretions may indicate a CSF leak, whereas bilateral purulent drainage usually indicates sinusitis. Inverted papilloma or nasal polyps are commonly visible on anterior rhinoscopy. Other areas that must be thoroughly evaluated include the conjunctiva, pharynx, tympanic membranes, and lungs.
- Referral to specialists in allergy or otorhinolaryngology (or both) is needed when simple and appropriate measures do not result in improvement, when complications occur, or when progression in the severity is noted.

ETIOLOGY

- The presence of rhinorrhea implies a secretory or excretory disorder:
  —Allergic rhinitis
  —Nonallergic rhinitis
  —Vasomotor rhinitis
  —Infectious rhinitis
  —Sinusitis
- In rhinorrhea without major obstruction, CSF leaks must be considered, especially if the rhinorrhea is unilateral and the patient has had head trauma or surgical treatment.
- CSF rhinorrhea can be either traumatic, nontraumatic (spontaneous), or iatrogenic.
- Spontaneous CSF rhinorrhea is either primary or secondary. Primary spontaneous rhinorrhea is poorly understood and much less common. The CSF is thought to pass through the cribriform plate via abnormally long prolongations of the subarachnoid space around the olfactory neurofilaments, which burst upon a sudden rise in CSF pressure caused by coughing or straining. Secondary spontaneous rhinorrhea is caused by a lesion such as hydrocephalus or cancer.

EPIDEMIOLOGY

- An estimated 40 million Americans have nasal disorders that result in 33 million annual office visits.
- The medications used to treat nasal obstruction cost about $5 billion annually, and surgical intervention is estimated to cost approximately $60 billion annually.
- Allergic rhinitis affects about 20% of the U.S. population.
- The incidence of CSF leakage after a basilar skull fracture is 15% to 20%; spontaneous cases represent between 4% and 33% of all cases of CSF rhinorrhea.

Clinical Manifestations

- Among patients with sinusitis, maxillary toothache, poor response to nasal decongestants, abnormal transillumination, and colored nasal discharge by history or examination are the most useful clinical findings. When all four features are present, the odds of sinusitis rise sharply, and when none is present, sinusitis is virtually ruled out.
- Vasomotor rhinitis is a vaguely defined syndrome. Patients complain of nasal obstruction, rhinorrhea, and postnasal drainage. In such patients, neither sneezing nor pruritus is a typical finding. The triggers seem to be nonspecific, including irritants (strong odors and fumes), temperature changes, humidity, and air conditioning. Psychologic factors have a major role.
- Among patients with allergic rhinitis, the symptoms usually involve the nose and cause bilateral obstruction, sneezing, and nasal pruritus. Frequent eye symptoms include irritation, lacrimation, and pruritus. Associated symptom complexes can include eustachian tube dysfunction, asthma, and atopic dermatitis. Patients with perennial allergic rhinitis may have subtle symptoms, including nasal obstruction and postnasal drainage. The physical findings are primarily an erythematous conjunctiva in association with pale, boggy, bluish nasal mucosa and clear to slightly discolored nasal secretions.

Diagnosis

DIFFERENTIAL DIAGNOSIS

- The list of differential diagnoses for patients with nasal congestion or discharge is long, but a handful of conditions encompass the vast majority of cases.
- Prolonged bilateral rhinorrhea is usually due to allergic or vasomotor rhinitis, or nasal polyposis.
- Intermittent loss of the sense of smell is noted in patients with allergic rhinitis, infections, and rhinitis medicamentosa. A more constant loss of the sense of smell occurs in patients with nasal polyposis, atrophic rhinitis, and immunologic disorders such as Wegener's granulomatosis or sarcoidosis.
- In vasomotor rhinitis, allergy skin-test results are negative, and other diagnoses must be excluded. Treatment includes patient education, a trial regimen of intranasal corticosteroid spray, and symptomatic therapy with antihistamines and decongestants.
- Unilateral rhinorrhea is generally caused by a foreign body or tumor.

LABORATORY

- For patients with possible allergic rhinitis, determination of specific IgE antibodies to allergens is best demonstrated by allergy skin testing, especially the prick method.
- Many of the disorders that cause nasal or sinus symptoms can be identified by nasal cytologic studies, because certain disorders, especially allergic- and eosinophilic-related disorders, tend to produce a high concentration of eosinophils in nasal secretions. In contrast, in infectious disorders, the concentration of neutrophils is high.

IMAGING

- The role of plain sinus roentgenograms in the management of sinusitis has changed substantially. Complete opacification of one sinus or presence of an air–fluid level suggests a sinus infection. At many institutions, routine sinus roentgenograms have been replaced by limited computed tomographic scans (5-mm slices).
- Transillumination and ultrasonography of the sinuses have low sensitivity and specificity and are unable to provide valuable information on the ethmoid sinuses or the ostiomeatal complex.

DIAGNOSTIC/TESTING PROCEDURES

- Fiberoptic nasal endoscopy has been helpful in evaluating the anatomic and pathologic features of the nose. The examination requires topically applied anesthesia and is well tolerated.
- The gold standard for diagnosing infectious sinusitis is sinus aspiration and culture. Its use is particularly appropriate for guiding antibiotic choice in patients with complicated or refractory sinusitis.

Treatment

- Anticholinergic agents, specifically the quaternary salt of atropine, are currently being recommended for chronic rhinitis and the common cold. Atropine sulfate, 50 or 75 μg four times daily, is effective in reducing rhinorrhea and postnasal drip within 2 weeks and may be an alternative therapy for the rhinorrhea component of rhinitis.
- Strategies for avoiding offending agents are important in management of allergic rhinitis. In intermittent disease, antihistamines and/or decongestants are first prescribed. More continuous symptoms may mandate intranasal steroids. Immunotherapy is often helpful for patients who respond poorly to pharmacotherapy and avoidance.

COMPLICATIONS

Bacterial meningitis is the major cause of morbidity and mortality in patients with CSF fistulas. Brain abscess and encephalitis occur much less frequently. The most common genus of infecting organisms in meningitis that occurs in the presence of a CSF fistula is *Pneumococcus,* followed by *Streptococcus* and *Haemophilus influenzae.*

Follow-Up

The reported incidence of meningitis in patients with posttraumatic CSF fistulas varies markedly, from 2% to more than 50%. Multiple factors, including duration of CSF leakage, delayed onset of CSF leakage, site of the fistula, and concomitant infection, are responsible for the significant variation in incidence.

PREVENTION

- Patients with CSF rhinorrhea should be warned to sneeze through their mouths and told not blow their noses, to avoid meningitis. The efficacy of prophylactic antibiotic therapy remains controversial.
- If conservative management of CSF fistulas (i.e., lumbar drains, bed rest, etc.) fails to close the fistulas within 7 to 10 days, surgical intervention, as opposed to long-term antibiotic therapy, is indicated.

Selected Readings

Brodie HA. Prophylactic antibiotics for posttraumatic cerebrospinal fluid fistulae. A meta-analysis. *Arch Otolaryngol Head Neck Surg* 1997;123:749–752.

Georgitis JW. Nasal atropine sulfate: Efficacy and safety of 0.050% and 0.075% solutions for severe rhinorrhea. *Arch Otolaryngol Head Neck Surg* 1998;12:916–920.

Guarderas JC. Rhinitis and sinusitis: Office management. *Mayo Clinic Proc* 1996;71:882–888.

Naclerio R, Solomon W. Rhinitis and inhalant allergens. *JAMA* 1997;278:1842–1848.

Prior AJ, Kenyon GS. A running nose. *Lancet* 1997;350:634.

Williams JW Jr, Simel DL. Does this patient have sinusitis? Diagnosing acute sinusitis by history and physical examination. *JAMA* 1993;270:1242–1246.

Sepsis Syndrome

Basics

DEFINITION

- *Bacteremia* (fungemia) is the presence of viable bacteria (fungi) in the blood.
- *Septicemia* is a systemic illness caused by the spread of microbes or their toxins via the bloodstream.
- *Systemic inflammatory response syndrome* (SIRS) is characterized by at least two of the following:
  — Oral temperature of >38°C or <36°C
  — Respiratory rate of >20 breaths/min or $PaCO_2$ of <32 mm Hg
  — Heart rate of >90 beats/min
  — Leukocyte count of >12,000/L or <4,000/L or >10% bands
- SIRS that has a proven or suspected microbial etiology is characterized as *sepsis*.
- *Sepsis syndrome* (or "severe sepsis") is sepsis with one or more signs of organ dysfunction, hypoperfusion, or hypotension, such as metabolic acidosis, acute alteration in mental status, oliguria, or adult respiratory distress syndrome
- *Septic shock* is sepsis with hypotension (i.e., systolic blood pressure <90 mmHg, or 40 mmHg less than the patient's baseline blood pressure) that is unresponsive to fluid resuscitation plus organ dysfunction or perfusion abnormalities.

APPROACH TO THE PATIENT

- Sepsis is a medical emergency. Successful management requires urgent measures to treat local infection, provide hemodynamic and respiratory support, and eliminate the offending microorganism.
- The outcome is also influenced by the patient's underlying disease, which should be managed aggressively.
- Noninfectious etiologies of SIRS that need to be considered include adrenal insufficiency, anaphylaxis, burns, bleeding, cardiac tamponade, dissecting or ruptured aortic aneurysm, drug overdose, myocardial infarction, pancreatitis, postcardiopulmonary bypass syndrome, and pulmonary embolism.
- The skin and mucosae should be examined carefully and repeatedly for lesions that might yield diagnostic information.
- Antimicrobial chemotherapy should be initiated as soon as samples of blood and specimens from other relevant sites have been cultured.
- The choice of initial antimicrobial therapy is based on knowledge of the likely pathogens at specific sites of local infection. Available information about patterns of antimicrobial susceptibility among bacterial isolates from the community, the hospital, and the patient also should be taken into account.
- Maximal recommended doses of antimicrobial drugs should be given by the parenteral route.

ETIOLOGY

- In sepsis, the lung is the most common site of infection, followed by the abdomen and the urinary tract.
- Blood cultures yield bacteria or fungi in approximately 20% to 40% of cases of severe sepsis and in 40% to 70% of cases of septic shock.
- Gram-negative sepsis and endotoxic shock are complicated pathophysiologic entities that are major triggers for the septic syndrome. Both gram-positive organisms such as *Staphylococcus aureus* and gram-negative species elaborate proteinaceous exotoxins, which appear to act through a similar molecular pathway to that of endotoxin.
- A key element in sepsis is cytokines, which are host-produced, pleomorphic immunoregulatory peptides. The most widely investigated cytokines are tumor necrosis factor, interleukin-1, and interleukin-8, which are generally proinflammatory, and interleukin-6 and interleukin-10, which tend to be antiinflammatory. A trigger, such as a microbial toxin, stimulates the production of tumor necrosis factor and interleukin-1, which in turn promote endothelial cell–leukocyte adhesion, release of proteases and arachidonate metabolites, and activation of clotting.
- Interleukin-8, a neutrophil chemotaxin, may have an especially important role in perpetuating tissue inflammation. Interleukin-6 and interleukin-10, which are counterregulatory, inhibit the generation of tumor necrosis factor, augment the action of acute-phase reactants and immunoglobulins, and inhibit T-lymphocyte and macrophage function.
- Evidence now implicates nitric oxide, produced by inducible nitric oxide synthase, as a mediator of septic shock.

EPIDEMIOLOGY

Incidence

- Each year, sepsis develops in more than 500,000 patients in the United States, with a mortality rate of 35% to 45%.
- Approximately two-thirds of cases occur in patients hospitalized for other illnesses.

Risk Factors

- Factors that predispose to bacteremia and sepsis include advanced HIV infection, burns, cirrhosis of the liver, hematologic malignancies and neoplasms, high dose of glucocorticoids or other immunosuppressive agents, injecting drug use (mainly gram-positive pathogens), mechanical ventilation, neutropenia, and presence of indwelling mechanical devices (especially for hemodialysis).
- Fungemia occurs most often in immunosuppressed patients with neutropenia.

Clinical Manifestations

SYMPTOMS

- The septic response can be variable.
- Nonspecific mental status changes and hyperventilation are often early findings.
- Gastrointestinal manifestations such as nausea, vomiting, diarrhea, and ileus can be present.
- Cholestatic jaundice, with elevated levels of serum bilirubin (mostly conjugated) and alkaline phosphatase, may precede other signs of sepsis.

SIGNS

- While most septic patients have fever, some have a normal temperature or are hypothermic.
- Tachypnea and tachycardia are common signs.
- Hypotension and disseminated intravascular coagulopathy, which can complicate sepsis, predispose to cyanosis and ischemic necrosis of peripheral tissues. Other skin lesions may be suggestive of specific pathogens (e.g., ecthyma

Sepsis Syndrome

gangrenosum, which is a bullous lesion with central hemorrhage and necrosis and can be present in neutropenic patients with infection due to *Pseudomonas aeruginosa*).

Diagnosis

- Cardiac output is initially normal or elevated in sepsis and helps in distinguishing septic shock from cardiogenic, extracardiac obstructive, and hypovolemic shock.
- A definitive etiologic diagnosis requires the isolation of the microorganism from the blood or a local site of infection.
- At least two, and probably three, sets of blood samples (10 mL each) should be obtained.
- Buffy-coat smears of peripheral blood is a quick and inexpensive method and can assist in more effective therapy in patients with overwhelming bacteremia.
- In early sepsis, abnormalities may include leukocytosis (leukopenia may develop in some cases), left shift (with or without toxic granulations), thrombocytopenia, hyperbilirubinemia, blood lactate levels, and proteinuria.
- Detection of endotoxin in blood by the limulus lysate test may portend a poor outcome, but this assay is not useful for diagnosing gram-negative bacterial infections.
- Cytokine assays are poorly standardized and currently have limited clinical value.

Treatment

MAIN TREATMENT

- Depletion of intravascular volume is common in septic patients, and the initial management of hypotension should include the administration of intravenous fluids.
- Empiric antibiotic therapy (all agents should be administered intravenously)
  —Nonimmunocompromised adult:
    —Ticarcillin–clavulanate (3.1 g q4h) or piperacillin–tazobactam (3.375 g q4h) plus gentamicin or tobramycin (1.7 mg/kg q8h)
    —Imipenem (0.5 g q6h)
    —Meropenem (1 g q8h)
    —Ampicillin (30 mg/kg q4h) plus gentamicin or tobramycin (1.7 mg/kg tid) plus metronidazole (500 mg q8h)
    —If the patient is allergic to beta-lactam agents: fluoroquinolone (e.g., ciprofloxacin 400 mg q12h) plus metronidazole (500 mg q8h) or clindamycin (900 mg q8h).
  —Injecting drug user:
    —Nafcillin or oxacillin (2 g qid i.v.) and gentamicin or tobramycin (1.7 mg/kg q8h)
  —Splenectomized patient:
    —Cefotaxime (2 g q4h), or
    —Ceftriaxone (2 g q12h)
  —Neutropenic patient:
    —Ceftazidime (2 g q8h)
    —Imipenem (0.5 g q6h)
    —Piperacillin–tazobactam (3.375 g q4h) or ticarcillin–clavulanate (3.1 g q4h) plus gentamicin or tobramycin (1.7 mg/kg q8h)
    —Cefepime (2 g q8h)
- In immunocompromised patients, vancomycin (15 mg/kg q12h) should be used if coagulase-negative staphylococci are suspected; if the patient has an infected vascular catheter, has received quinolone prophylaxis, or has received intensive chemotherapy causing mucosal damage; or if the institution has a high incidence of methicillin-resistant *S. aureus*.
- In splenectomized (and some nonimmunocompromised) patients, vancomycin (15 mg/kg q12h) should be added if the local prevalence of cephalosporin-resistant pneumococci is high.
- Removal of indwelling intravenous catheters and removal or drainage of a focal source of infection are essential.
- The duration of treatment is influenced by factors such as the site of tissue infection, the adequacy of surgical drainage, the patient's underlying disease, and the antimicrobial susceptibility of the pathogen(s).

COMPLICATIONS

- Adult respiratory distress syndrome develops in up to half of patients with sepsis.
- Depression of myocardial function develops within 24 hours in most patients with advanced sepsis.
- Renal failure in sepsis occurs due to acute tubular necrosis induced by hypotension or capillary injury, although some patients also have glomerulonephritis, renal cortical necrosis, or interstitial nephritis.
- Thrombocytopenia occurs in up to one-third of patients.
- Prolonged or severe hypotension may induce acute hepatic injury or ischemic bowel necrosis.

Follow-Up

Late deaths in sepsis often result from poorly controlled infection, complications of intensive care, failure of multiple organs, or underlying disease.

PREVENTION

- Prompt and aggressive management of patients with early sepsis is imperative.
- Approaches that are under study may help prevent deaths among patients with sepsis, and include the following:
  —Drugs that neutralize bacterial endotoxin and that thereby may benefit the septic patients who have gram-negative bacterial infections
  —Drugs that interfere with one or more mediators of the inflammatory response and may benefit all patients with sepsis

Selected Readings

Horn KD. Evolving strategies in the treatment of sepsis and systemic inflammatory response syndrome (SIRS). *Q J Med* 1998;91:265–277.

Munford RS. Sepsis and septic shock. In:. Fauci AS, Braunwald E, Isselbacher KJ, et al., eds. *Harrison's principles of internal medicine,* 14th ed. New York: McGraw-Hill, 1998:776–780.

Wheeler AP, Bernard GR. Treating patients with severe sepsis. *N Engl J Med* 1999;340:207–214.

Sexual Assault

Basics

DEFINITION

Sexual assault is defined as any sexual act performed by one person on another without that person's consent. Components of this violent act include the use or threat of force and/or the inability of the victim to give appropriate consent.

APPROACH TO THE PATIENT

- The management of a sexual assault case should be done with compassion and professionalism.
- Informed consent must be obtained before the physical and forensic examination of an assault victim in the emergency room.
- The duties of the examining physician include the following:
  —Treating injuries
  —Performing appropriate tests to detect, prevent, and treat sexually transmitted infections
  —Detecting pregnancy, and preventing or terminating it, according to the woman's wishes
- An initial assessment for unstable vital signs, altered consciousness, peritoneal injury, and pain will alert physicians to severe lacerations, fractures, or internal injuries.
- After the assessment and treatment of acute injuries, a focused history should be taken and a physical examination performed. When the examining physician is a man, a female caregiver should be present.
- The site and time of the assault; the race, identity, and number of assailants; and the nature of the physical contacts, weapons, and restraints should be noted.
- Bathing, douching, wiping, dental hygiene, bowel movements, and changes of clothing should be documented.
- A history of previous gynecologic conditions should be recorded, including infections, contraceptive use, and dates of the last menstrual period and the last episode of consensual intercourse.
- The physician should identify all injuries.
- Photographs of major injuries should be taken if feasible. Careful pelvic examination (with colposcopy if indicated) should be performed. It is important to use only saline for lubrication (for appropriate collection of forensic specimens).
- A rectal examination should be considered if anal penetration occurred or if signs of trauma are identified.
- Standard rape kits are available in most emergency departments and contain the necessary equipment for the collection of forensic specimens from the rape victim.

ETIOLOGY

- Spousal rape is often more violent, and it is less commonly reported.
- Two-thirds of the sexual assaults in an urban locale are committed by people known to the victims, and over two-thirds of these assaults are associated with physical trauma.

EPIDEMIOLOGY

- Sexual assault is one of the most increasingly occurring violent crimes in the United States. In 1990, the Department of Justice reported that the annual incidence of sexual assault was 80 per 100,000 women, accounting for 7% of all violent crimes. Although the incidence of rape peaks among girls and women 16 to 19 years old in the United States, more than 60,000 rapes of women older than 50 years of age are reported annually.
- The frequency of date rape is reportedly as high as 20% among adolescent girls, peaking in the 16- to 19-year-old age group.
- Up to 5% of rape victims have major nongenital physical injuries.
- Approximately 1% of victims have moderate or severe genital injury requiring surgical intervention.
- In 0.1% of assaulted women, the injuries sustained are fatal.
- The incidence of sexual assaults against men has not been studied extensively. Of a sample of 1,480 men in Los Angeles, 7% reported being "pressured or forced to have sexual contact" after the age of 16. In a cross-sectional survey conducted in the United Kingdom among 2,474 men, 3% reported nonconsensual sexual experiences as adults.
- Over 5% of men report sexual abuse as children; nonconsensual sexual experiences as a child are predictive of nonconsensual sexual experiences as an adult.

Clinical Manifestations

- A victim of sexual assault suffers psychological injury in addition to physical harm.
- Usual injuries are upper vaginal lacerations that present with profuse vaginal bleeding and pain.
- Genital trauma is common, even in rape victims who are asymptomatic.
- Bite marks on the genitalia and breasts are common.
- The assault is often followed by a "rape trauma syndrome." The short-term phase may last for hours or days and consists of the emotional shock, disbelief, and despair caused by a life-threatening event. The long-term phase of the syndrome, during which the victim attempts to restructure her life and relationships, may last months or years.

Diagnosis

LABORATORY

- Baseline serologic tests for syphilis and hepatitis B, ABO blood typing, and measurement of serum human chorionic gonadotropin (for women of reproductive age) should be performed after the physical examination. Other tests include the following:
  —HIV testing (repeat at 6 weeks, 3 months and 6 months)
  —Gonorrhea, chlamydia, and syphilis tests
  —Wet mount for *Trichomonas*
  —Pregnancy test (if indicated)
  —Hepatic enzyme tests (repeat as indicated)
  —Complete blood count (repeat as indicated)

Sexual Assault

- Swabs for gonorrhea and chlamydia cultures should be obtained from the cervix and from the rectum (if there was rectal penetration).
- Studies have demonstrated HIV antibodies in vaginal washings following unprotected intercourse with an HIV-infected male partner who has ejaculated. However, the frequency of false-negative results with vaginal washings, together with the low prevalence of HIV infection in perpetrators of sexual assaults, makes the predictive value of HIV testing of vaginal washings too low to be useful as a screening tool.

Treatment

In most patients, only limited injury to the rectum is evident on proctoscopy; spontaneous hemostasis is common, requiring no intervention. However, one-third sustain deep lacerations that require transanal suture repair, hospital admission, and treatment with broad-spectrum antibiotics.

COMPLICATIONS

- Rape may increase the risk of HIV transmission compared with consensual sex, because trauma is more likely.
- Intraperitoneal extension of a vaginal laceration is rare but, when present, requires exploratory laparotomy and broad-spectrum antibiotic therapy.
- The most common infections acquired from assault are *Trichomonas* infection, bacterial vaginosis, and *Chlamydia* infection. The Centers for Disease Control and Prevention estimate that the risk of an adult rape victim's acquiring gonorrhea as a result of sexual assault is 6% to 12%. The risk of *Chlamydia* infection is 4% to 17%, and the risk of syphilis 0.53%. Although seroconversion for HIV antibody has been reported among persons whose only known risk factor was sexual assault, the risk of acquiring this infection is less than 1%.

Follow-Up

- A follow-up plan should be established for both medical and psychological evaluation.
- In general, the patient should be seen for medical follow-up after 2 to 4 weeks. If the patient did not receive antibiotic prophylaxis, cultures for gonorrhea and chlamydia and examination of slides of vaginal secretions for trichomonas and bacterial vaginosis should be repeated at 2 weeks. Repeated serologic tests for syphilis at 4 to 6 weeks are recommended. An initial vaccination against hepatitis B should be done, and repeat doses scheduled 1 and 6 months later.
- A study reviewed the follow-up appointments from adolescent and adult victims. Only 31% of all sexual assault victims returned for a follow-up visit. Physical complaints were reported by 42.6%, but 98.0% had normal findings at a general examination, and 94.8% had a normal result of gynecologic examination. Since the assault, 49.2% had been sexually active, 10.0% with multiple partners and 73.3% without consistent condom use. Disturbances in sleep, sexual function, and appetite and assault-related fears were commonly reported among victims.

PREVENTION

- Prophylactic antibiotic therapy for sexually transmitted diseases should be prescribed if the assailant is known to be infected, if the victim has signs or symptoms of infection, or if prophylaxis is requested. If the patient is known to have been pregnant at the time of the assault, erythromycin or azithromycin may be substituted for doxycycline, and metronidazole should be administered only after the first trimester.
- Tetanus prophylaxis is appropriate for unimmunized patients with trauma.
- If the patient is found to be at risk for pregnancy as the result of assault, "morning-after" prophylaxis should be offered.
- Clinicians caring for rape survivors may recommend postexposure prophylaxis. When the choice is made to take medications to prevent HIV infection, treatment should be initiated as soon as possible. Usual prophylactic regimens for postexposure prophylaxis for HIV include the following:
  - Zidovudine 300 mg PO bid or 200 mg PO tid and lamivudine 150 mg PO bid for 28 days
  - Didanosine 200 mg PO bid and stavudine 40 mg PO bid (consider adding nelfinavir 750 mg PO tid or indinavir 800 mg PO tid) for 28 days

Selected Readings

Bamberger JD, Waldo CR, Gerberding JL, Katz MH. Postexposure prophylaxis for human immunodeficiency virus (HIV) infection following sexual assault. *Am J Med* 1999;106:323–326.

Coxell A, King M, Mezey G, Gordon D. Lifetime prevalence, characteristics and associated problems of nonconsensual sex in men: Cross sectional survey. *BMJ* 1999;318, 846–850.

Hampton HL. Care of the woman who has been raped. *N Engl J Med* 1995;332:234–237.

Holmes MM, Resnick HS, Frampton D. Follow-up of sexual assault victims. *Am J Obstet Gynecol* 1998;179:336–342.

Lurie P, Miller S, Hecht F, et al. Postexposure prophylaxis after nonoccupational HIV exposure: Clinical, ethical, and policy considerations. *JAMA* 1998;280:1769–1773.

Sore Throat

Basics

DEFINITION

- *Sore throat* is a commonly used term for inflammation with pain in the throat, especially on swallowing.
- The most common infectious causes of sore throat are discussed in separate Section II chapters in this book ("Pharyngitis/Tonsillitis," "Laryngitis/Laryngotracheobronchitis (Croup)," and "Infectious Mononucleosis"). In this chapter, the focus is on distinguishing features and other causes.

APPROACH TO THE PATIENT

- The first steps in evaluating patients with sore throat is to assess whether the process compromises the airway and to identify whether the symptoms are due to a localized or systemic (usually viral) process.
- The duration and type of symptoms and the presence of hoarseness or fever should be investigated. Based on the clinical situation, the history can include questions regarding other family members with similar symptoms, the presence of weight loss or other symptoms suggestive of noninfectious causes (neoplasms, etc.), or oral–genital sexual contact.
- Certain clinical findings (e.g., marked tonsillar exudate, enlarged tonsils, tender anterior cervical adenopathy and myalgias) and epidemiologic findings (e.g., age, season of the year, and prevalence of streptococcal colonization in the community) strongly suggest the diagnosis of streptococcal pharyngitis.
- The presence of conjunctivitis is suggestive of a viral illness.
- When epidemiologic and clinical data suggest the presence of gonococcal pharyngitis or diphtheria, specific microbiologic techniques are indicated and appropriate therapy should be instituted promptly.
- Laryngitis, croup, and other causes of sore throat and hoarseness must be differentiated from epiglottitis.
- Acute pharyngitis can occur during primary infection with HIV.
- In most cases, the pertinent issue is distinguishing group A streptococcal infection from nonstreptococcal causes. The time-honored method of diagnostic confirmation is the throat culture. Commercially produced kits are now available for rapid identification.

ETIOLOGY

- Most cases of acute pharyngitis are viral in etiology (e.g., rhinoviruses, coronaviruses, influenza A and B, and parainfluenza) and involve the pharynx as well as other portions of the respiratory tract.
- Most cases of acute laryngitis are caused by viruses (e.g., rhinovirus, influenza virus, parainfluenza virus, coxsackievirus, adenovirus, or respiratory syncytial virus).
- Certain viral infections causing sore throat exhibit clinical manifestations that are distinctive. Examples include enteroviruses (herpangina due to coxsackie A), Epstein-Barr virus (infectious mononucleosis), cytomegalovirus (cytomegalovirus mononucleosis), adenovirus (pharyngoconjunctival fever, acute respiratory disease of military recruits), and herpes simplex virus (pharyngitis, gingivitis, and stomatitis).
- Primary herpesvirus type 1 infection is a cause of acute pharyngitis. Herpesvirus type 2 can cause a similar illness as a consequence of oral–genital sexual contact.
- The most important bacterial cause of pharyngitis is group A streptococcus. Other bacterial causes of pharyngitis include the following:
  —Groups C and G streptococcus
  —*Neisseria gonorrhoeae*
  —*Arcanobacterium haemolyticum*
  —*Yersinia enterocolitica*
  —*Corynebacterium diphtheriae* (diphtheria)
  —*Mycoplasma pneumoniae*
  —*Chlamydia pneumoniae*
- Sore throat has also been described during the course of Lyme disease, acute toxoplasmosis, plague, brucellosis, and leptospirosis. It can accompany infection with *Treponema pallidum* (affecting 15% to 30% of patients with secondary syphilis), *Yersinia enterocolitica, Yersinia pestis,* and *Francisella tularensis*.
- *Histoplasma* and *Blastomyces* may cause nodules on the larynx, with or without ulcerations. *Candida* may cause sore throat, along with thrush, in immunosuppressed patients or in those with chronic mucocutaneous candidiasis.
- In Africa, and recently in the eastern United States, West Nile virus is a cause of febrile disease, usually without CNS involvement. Headache, sore throat, nausea and vomiting, and arthralgia are common accompaniments.
- Lemierre syndrome can present with sore throat (see Section II chapter, "Anaerobic Infections").
- Sore throat can be due to abscess formation in the parapharyngeal area:
  —Infection in the lateral pharyngeal space may follow tonsillitis, pharyngitis with adenoid involvement, parotitis, mastoiditis, or periodontal infection.
  —Infection in the retropharyngeal space may result from the spread of lateral pharyngeal space infection or from the lymphatic spread of infection. Retropharyngeal abscess may also follow trauma to the posterior pharynx or may result from anterior extension of infection from cervical osteomyelitis.
- Sore throat with foul breath, fever, and a sensation of choking can accompany acute necrotizing infections of the pharynx. These infections usually occur in association with ulcerative gingivitis.
- Ludwig's angina, a periodontal infection usually arising from the tissues surrounding the third molar, produces submandibular cellulitis that results in marked local swelling of tissues, with pain, trismus, and superior and posterior displacement of the tongue. Submandibular swelling of the neck can result in sore throat and, if untreated, can impair swallowing and cause respiratory obstruction.
- Periodic fever, aphthous stomatitis, pharyngitis, and cervical adenitis (PFAPA) syndrome can affect children and is characterized by periodic episodes (usual interval, <4 weeks) of unheralded onset, with a brisk rise to high fever (>39°C) that is sustained over 3 to 6 days and is unaccompanied by other symptomatology.

EPIDEMIOLOGY

- The group A streptococcus is the most common bacterial cause of acute pharyngitis.

Sore Throat

- The peak incidence of streptococcal pharyngitis is in children aged 5 to 15 years, and it accounts for more than 15% to 20% of cases of acute pharyngitis in this age group.
- Streptococci of Lancefield groups C and G have caused well-documented epidemics of acute pharyngitis, often associated with contaminated foods.
- A *hemolyticum* has a predilection for adolescents and young adults.
- Parainfluenza virus infection occurs most frequently among children.

Clinical Manifestations

- With parapharyngeal space infections, most patients appear toxic and have fever, sore throat, pain on swallowing, and leukocytosis. Rigidity of the neck or torticollis toward the opposite side may develop. Advanced cases include dyspnea and stridor.
- In acute necrotizing infections of the pharynx, the tonsillar pillars are swollen, red, ulcerated, and covered with a grayish membrane that peels easily. Lymphadenopathy is common.
- In infectious mononucleosis, pharyngitis is most prominent during the first 2 weeks of the illness.
- Herpangina, caused by the coxsackievirus, is characterized by fever, sore throat, myalgias, and a vesicular enanthem on the soft palate between the uvula and the tonsils.
- In tuberculous laryngitis, lesions include mucosal hyperemia and thickening, nodules, and ulcerations.

Diagnosis

DIFFERENTIAL DIAGNOSIS

- In most viral cases of pharyngitis, patients have a scratchy or sore throat as well as coryza and cough. The pharynx is inflamed and edematous, but exudate is not usually present. However, exudative pharyngitis may be seen in adenovirus infection and infectious mononucleosis.
- Most patients with sore throat due to *M. pneumoniae* are less ill, have less evidence of pharyngitis, and have prominent symptoms of tracheobronchitis.

LABORATORY

In most patients, group A beta-hemolytic streptococcal pharyngitis cannot be clinically diagnosed with accuracy. Throat cultures clearly are the standard laboratory test, yet rapid antigen testing as an aid to clinical diagnosis can be useful (see Section II chapter, "Pharyngitis/Tonsillitis").

IMAGING

Retropharyngeal space infections may be confirmed by a lateral neck soft-tissue x-ray. However, most parapharyngeal space infections should be confirmed by computed tomography with contrast.

DIAGNOSTIC/TESTING PROCEDURES

In tuberculous laryngitis, biopsy reveals granulomas with acid-fast bacilli. Cultures should be performed to confirm the diagnosis and evaluate the sensitivities of the pathogen.

Treatment

Parapharyngeal space infection treatment includes securing of the airway, surgical drainage in the operating room, and administration of intravenous antibiotics active against streptococci and oral anaerobes (e.g., penicillin 4 μ q4h i.v. and metronidazole 500 mg tid i.v. or cefoxitin 2 g tid i.v. or ampicillin–sulbactam).

COMPLICATIONS

- A peritonsillar abscess may follow untreated streptococcal pharyngitis. Examination reveals pronounced unilateral peritonsillar swelling and erythema, causing deviation of the uvula.
- Potential complications of parapharyngeal space infections include airway obstruction; intraoral rupture of the abscess, causing aspiration pneumonia; jugular vein thrombophlebitis; erosion into the carotid artery; and mediastinitis.

Follow-Up

- Chronic fatigue syndrome, which may follow a viral infection, can present with debilitating fatigue, fever, sore throat, painful lymphadenopathy, myalgia, arthralgia, sleep disorder, and headache
- Streptococcal infection from group A streptococci requires appropriate antimicrobial therapy and monitoring to achieve the following:
  —Prevent acute rheumatic fever, glomerulonephritis, and toxic shock, as well as suppurative complications
  —Minimize the possibility of secondary spread
  —Truncate the course of the illness
- Sore throat can be part of the prodrome of nonspecific constitutional symptoms that lead to viral encephalitis.

PREVENTION

- Remove patients with streptococcal pharyngitis from close contact with others.
- Counsel the patient to follow safe sex practices.

Selected Readings

Bisno AL. Acute pharyngitis: Etiology and diagnosis. *Pediatrics* 1996;97:949–954.

Durand M, Joseph M, Baker AS. Infections of the upper respiratory tract. In: Fauci AS, Braunwald E, Isselbacher KJ, et al., eds. *Harrison's principles of internal medicine,* 14th ed. New York: McGraw-Hill, 1998:179–184.

Pichichero M. Cost-effective management of sore throat: It depends on the perspective. *Arch Pediatr Adolesc Med* 1999;153:672–674.

Shulman ST. Evaluation of penicillins, cephalosporins, and macrolides for therapy of streptococcal pharyngitis. *Pediatrics* 1996;97:955–959.

Trauma-related Infections

Basics

DEFINITION
Trauma-related infections, while not strictly defined, generally refers to infections that directly or indirectly result from wounds or injuries.

APPROACH TO THE PATIENT
- The diagnosis of infection is difficult in trauma patients because of the following:
  — In this setting, patients can have fever due to noninfectious causes.
  — The physical examination is often limited.
  — The performance of diagnostic tests can be difficult.
- Documentation of the injured site and the colonizing organism are the first steps in diagnosing infection in trauma patients. What is more difficult is to interpret whether the culture results represent colonization or infection.
- Careful attention to indwelling devices, surgical wounds, and the respiratory system is needed.
- Consideration of the indigenous nosocomial pathogens is necessary.
- Drainage of fluid collections, complete debridement of necrotic tissues, and mobilization of respiratory secretions are very important.
- Documentation of tetanus and pneumococcal vaccination (or administering the vaccines as indicated) and appropriate nutritional support are essential.

ETIOLOGY
- Trauma patients are at increased risk for infection for a number of reasons:
  — Crush injury and other severe trauma can result in tears of the major vessels and damage to the microcirculation, with resultant ischemia, edema, compartment syndromes, and tissue necrosis.
  — Circulating plasma endotoxin lipopolysaccharide may be a trigger for increased proinflammatory cytokine production and may play a role in the septic syndromes seen in a substantial portion of trauma patients.
  — Immunoglobulin response after trauma may be depressed, depending on the type of injury, presence of infection, splenic function, and type of immunoglobulin.
  — Splenectomy, if performed, sharply reduces IgM response to infection at 7 and 14 days compared with nonsplenectomized infected posttraumatic patients.
  — Corticosteroid administration necessitated by head trauma may further impair immunity.
- Most common sites of infection in multiply traumatized patients include the following:
  — Lower respiratory tract (pneumonia and empyema)
  — Urinary tract
  — Intravenous line associated
  — Intraabdominal
  — Primary bacteremia
  — Sinuses

EPIDEMIOLOGY
- The age, hospital length-of-stay, and the percentage of deaths due to infection were determined in a population-based sample of patients hospitalized for more than 2 days for motor vehicle injuries. The incidence rate of fatal pulmonary infection was highest among those with hospital stays of 7 to 28 days and among those 70 years of age or older. Incidence rates varied substantially by age and length of hospital stay, from a low of 8 deaths per 100,000 patient-days for adult female patients with stays longer than 28 days to a high of 102 deaths per 100,000 patient-days for elderly men with stays of 7 to 28 days.
- Infection is the leading cause of morbidity and mortality occurring more than 48 hours after penetrating abdominal injury.
- Predominantly gram-negative enteric organisms, group D streptococci, and anaerobic organisms are isolated in cultures of specimens obtained from wounds among children injured in farm settings.

Clinical Manifestations

- The usual signs and symptoms of infection lose much of their predictive value in the multiply traumatized patient.
- Fever, tachycardia, and hypotension are frequently present after serious injury without an ongoing infection.

Diagnosis

DIFFERENTIAL DIAGNOSIS
Among patients with extensive trauma, signs of infection can be due to the following:
- Atelectasis
- Deep vein thrombosis
- Drug fever
- Hypovolemia
- Massive hematoma
- Noninfectious inflammation
- Pulmonary contusion
- Transfusion reactions

IMAGING
While computed tomography (CT) has proved useful in demonstrating sites of thoracic infections in septic trauma victims, the presence of concurrent thoracic pathology (particularly loculated hemothorax or hemopneumothorax and traumatic lung cysts with hemorrhage or surrounding parenchymal consolidation) introduces sources of diagnostic error. CT also has proved helpful in guiding appropriate revisions of malpositioned and occluded thoracostomy tubes.

Treatment

- Judicious surgical management of local factors, such as open fractures, is often more important than antibiotic therapy.
- Among trauma patients, hemodynamic instability in the absence of hypovolemia mandates consideration of empiric antibiotic therapy, even in the absence of other signs of infection.

Trauma-related Infections

- Empirical regimens should combine an antistaphylococcal agent with broad gram-negative coverage. When intraabdominal abdominal injury is present, anaerobic coverage should be added.

COMPLICATIONS

- Septic shock
- Pulmonary insufficiency
- Peritonitis and abdominal abscess
- Osteomyelitis
- Brain abscess
- Trauma can cause both septic and nonseptic olecranon bursitis. Clinical features are helpful in separating septic from nonseptic olecranon bursitis, but there may be local erythema in both. Aspiration should be carried out in all cases, and if the presence of infection is still in doubt, microscopy, Gram staining, and culture of the aspirate will resolve the issue. Septic olecranon bursitis should be treated by aspiration, which may need to be repeated, and a long course of antibiotics. Some cases will need admission, and a few will need surgical treatment. Nonseptic olecranon bursitis can be managed with aspiration alone. Nonsteroidal antiinflammatory drugs probably hasten symptomatic improvement. Intrabursal corticosteroids produce a rapid resolution, but concern remains over their long-term local effects. Recovery from septic olecranon bursitis can take months.
- Acute acalculous cholecystitis is a recently recognized entity that may present in the trauma patient, usually with fever.

Follow-Up

The risk of early serious infection in adults after splenectomy for trauma is low when isolated splenic injury is present, but this risk is increased by both the degree of injury and the presence of certain associated injuries. Encapsulated bacteria are frequent pathogens in both early and late infections. The mortality rate related to an early septic episode is high, but the risk of late serious infection is low and is not related to identifiable factors that decrease host defenses.

PREVENTION

- With the exception of patients with open fractures, the use of antibiotics for severely injured patients with bacterial contamination has not been evaluated in a placebo-controlled, prospective, randomized trial. However, antibiotics are used empirically for victims of penetrating chest or abdominal trauma and severe head wounds.
- Topical antibiotics are also used routinely in emergency rooms to treat corneal trauma, although no published evidence supports this treatment.
- In a recent retrospective analysis of 18 clinical reports on a total of 2,679 patients with penetrating trauma or open fractures, patients who received multiple days of antibiotics had the same infection rate as those treated for 1 day. Furthermore, a recent prospective randomized study of patients with penetrating abdominal trauma compared the efficacy of a 24-hour regimen to a 5-day regimen and reported no difference in major infection or death rate.
- Prophylactic antibiotic regimens in trauma patients may be significantly altered by large fluid shifts and hyperdynamic physiologic responses. Data suggest that high doses given for a short duration are more effective than long courses of antibiotics in reducing infections in trauma patients undergoing laparotomy.
- Emphasis should be placed on protecting from blood-borne diseases the health-care providers who take care of trauma patients.
- The use of antibiotics for the prevention of infection in patients with cerebrospinal fluid leak is discussed in the chapter, "Rhinorrhea."

Selected Readings

Ericsson CD, Fischer RP, Rowlands BJ, et al. Prophylactic antibiotics in trauma: The hazards of underdosing. *J Trauma* 1989;29:1356–1361.

Fife D, Kraus J. Infection as a contributory cause of death in patients hospitalized for motor vehicle trauma. *Am J Surg* 1988;155:278–283.

Fiore AE, Joshi M, Caplan ES. Approach to infection in the multiply traumatized patient. In: Mandell GL, Bennett JE, Dolin R, eds. *Principles and practice of infectious diseases*. New York: Churchill Livingstone, 1995:2756–2761.

Hadjiminas D, Cheadle WG, Spain DA, et al. Antibiotic overkill of trauma victims? *Am J Surg* 1994;168:288–290.

Hershman MJ, Cheadle WG, George CD, et al. The response of immunoglobulins to infection after thermal and nonthermal injury. *Am Surg* 1988;54:408–411.

Kelly JL, O'Sullivan C, O'Riordain M, et al. Is circulating endotoxin the trigger for the systemic inflammatory response syndrome seen after injury? *Ann Surg* 1997;225:530–541; discussion, 541–543.

Malangoni MA, Dillon LD, Klamer TW, Condon RE. Factors influencing the risk of early and late serious infection in adults after splenectomy for trauma. *Surgery* 1984;96:775–783.

Mirvis SE, Rodriguez A, Whitley NO, Tarr RJ. CT evaluation of thoracic infections after major trauma. *AJR* 1985;144:1183–1187.

Stell IM. Septic and nonseptic olecranon bursitis in the accident and emergency department—An approach to management. *J Accid Emerg Med* 1996;13:351–353.

Urethritis and Urethral Discharge

Basics

DEFINITION

- *Urethritis* is the inflammation of the urethra.
- *Urethral discharge* is the purulent or mucopurulent excretion from the male or female urethra.
- The terms *urethral syndrome* and, if pyuria is present, *dysuria with sterile pyuria syndrome* are used to describe women with dysuria and frequency but few bacteria in the urine.

APPROACH TO THE PATIENT

- Among patients with urethritis or urethral discharge, symptoms can vary from occasional discomfort to continuous irritation with discharge.
- Physicians must inquiry about the following:
  —The nature, onset, and duration of dysuria or other symptoms
  —The presence and characteristics of urethral discharge
  —The presence of generalized symptoms suggestive of a systemic disease
  —Previous sexually transmitted diseases
- During the physical examination, the entire genital area must be evaluated.
- Alternative diagnoses should be evaluated during history and physical examination. The testes and spermatic cord should be palpated for masses, and epididymitis should be excluded.
- When symptoms are suggestive for dysuria without urethral discharge, patients should be tested for cystitis, and men should be evaluated for prostatitis.
- Urethral discharge must be "milked" (using the gloved thumb and the forefinger) after the patient has not voided for several hours, preferably overnight (see also section, "Diagnosis").

ETIOLOGY/CAUSES

- Infectious urethritis
  —*Neisseria gonorrhoeae*
  —*Chlamydia trachomatis*
  —*Ureaplasma urealyticum*
  —*Mycoplasma genitalium*
  —*Trichomonas vaginalis*
  —Herpes simplex virus
- Noninfectious urethritis
  —Stevens-Johnson syndrome
  —Wegener's granulomatosis
  —Urethral irritation (chemicals, alcohol, etc.)
  —Reiter's syndrome

EPIDEMIOLOGY

Incidence

- Urethritis is more common in men and is the most commonly recognized sexually transmitted disease in this population.
- During the past decade, the incidence of gonococcal urethritis has fallen in nearly all industrialized countries, while that of nongonococcal urethritis remains high.
- More than one-third of the cases of nongonococcal urethritis are caused by *C. trachomatis*.
- Gonorrhea is the most common reportable infectious disease in the United States, with about 500,000 cases annually. The true incidence is probably at least one million cases annually.

Risk Factors

- The risk of acquiring infection depends on the type of contact with an infected person. Up to 80% of women in contact with men with urethral gonorrhea develop gonococcal cervicitis, while only one-third of men having sex with infected women develop gonorrhea.
- The highest incidence of gonorrhea is found in young (15 to 30 years of age) single persons of low socioeconomic and educational status.

Clinical Manifestations

SYMPTOMS

- Seventy-five percent of men acquiring urethral gonorrhea develop symptoms within 4 days, and up to 90% within 2 weeks.
- The incubation period for nongonococcal urethritis is usually 7 to 14 days.
- Dysuria is present in 50% to 75% of patients with nongonococcal urethritis, and in up to 90% of patients with gonorrhea.
- Acute urethral syndrome presents with dysuria, frequency, and urgency.

SIGNS

The urethral discharge is described as purulent in most cases of gonorrhea urethritis, but in less than one-third of patients with nongonococcal urethritis.

Diagnosis

DIFFERENTIAL DIAGNOSIS

- A brief history and examination should exclude systemic complications, such as disseminated gonococcal infection and Reiter's syndrome.
- Bacterial prostatitis and cystitis should be excluded by appropriate testing.
- Among women with acute dysuria and frequency, costovertebral pain and tenderness or fever suggests acute pyelonephritis.
- The finding of a single conventional urinary pathogen, such as *E. coli* or *Staphylococcus saprophyticus*, in a concentration $>10^2$ per milliliter in a properly collected specimen from a symptomatic woman with pyuria indicates probable bacterial urinary tract infection. However, pyuria with $<10^2$ conventional uropathogens per milliliter of urine ("sterile" pyuria) suggests acute urethral syndrome due to *C. trachomatis* or *N. gonorrhoeae*.

Urethritis and Urethral Discharge

LABORATORY

- Whether or not an abnormal discharge is evident, inflammation should be evaluated by examination of a Gram-stained smear after passage of a small swab 2 to 3 cm into the urethra; the presence of five or more neutrophils per high-power field in areas containing cells suggests urethritis.
- Gonorrhea is diagnosed by the demonstration of typical gram-negative diplococci within neutrophils, and a preliminary diagnosis of nongonococcal urethritis is warranted if gram-negative diplococci are not found.
- A Gram stain of urethral discharge is 95% sensitive in cases of gonococcal urethritis.
- Alternatively, the centrifuged sediment of the first 20 to 30 mL of voided urine can be examined for inflammatory cells.
- Culture or genomic detection tests for *N. gonorrhoeae* and culture, antigen, or genomic detection tests for *C. trachomatis* should be routinely used in most clinical settings. Genetic amplification using ligase chain reaction or polymerase chain reaction appears to be sensitive and highly specific for either organism; such tests are available for diagnostic testing for chlamydial infection and gonorrhea. Diagnostic testing for *C. trachomatis* is recommended, even if empirical treatment for chlamydial infection is planned, because the results predict the patient's prognosis and guide the counseling given to the patient and the management of the patient's sexual partner(s).
- *Candida* can be recovered from normal patients, but some investigators consider *Candida* as a possible pathogen among men with urethritis and no other obvious pathogens recovered.

DIAGNOSTIC/TESTING PROCEDURES

- Obtaining endourethral cultures or cultures of first-void urine sediment is the preferred method for diagnosis of trichomoniasis in men.
- Examination of a saline suspension of urethral exudate occasionally may reveal motile trichomonas.

Treatment

MAIN TREATMENT

- Patients with gonococcal urethritis should also receive treatment for chlamydial infection.
- Gonococcal urethritis: ceftriaxone 125-mg intramuscular injection (single dose)
- Nongonococcal urethritis: doxycycline (100 mg orally twice daily for 7 days) or azithromycin (1 g orally once)

ALTERNATIVE TREATMENT

- Gonococcal urethritis: cefixime (400 mg orally) or ciprofloxacin (500 mg orally) or ofloxacin (400 mg orally) (all antibiotics given once)
- Nongonococcal urethritis: erythromycin (500 mg orally four times daily for 7 days) or ofloxacin (300 mg twice daily orally for 7 days)

TREATMENT FAILURE

- *Neisseria gonorrhoeae* strains resistant to fluoroquinolones have been reported in Asia and certain areas in the United States.
- Patients with nongonococcal urethritis that do not respond to doxycycline can be infected with doxycycline-resistant *U. urealyticum* or *Trichomonas*. Empiric treatment with a single 2-g dose of metronidazole, followed by erythromycin 500 mg orally four times daily for 7 days, may be warranted in such cases.
- Patients with recurrent episodes of nongonococcal urethritis occasionally respond to a 3-week course of erythromycin, and require evaluation for prostatic involvement or possible anatomic abnormalities.

COMPLICATIONS

- *Chlamydia trachomatis* can lead to acute salpingitis or bartholinitis.
- Babies born from to women infected with *C. trachomatis* may develop chlamydial ophthalmia neonatorum or pneumonia.
- Carriage of *U. urealyticum* is associated with infertility.
- *Neisseria gonorrhoeae* and *C. trachomatis* can cause acute epididymitis.

Follow-Up

- If patients present with hematuria, especially when it persists after treatment of urethritis, a thorough urologic evaluation is needed.
- Patients who suffer from persistence or recurrence of symptoms after therapy for acute gonococcal urethritis could be experiencing one or more of the following:
  —Coinfection with *Chlamydia* or other bacteria causing nongonococcal urethritis
  —Gonococcal reinfection
  —Treatment failure

PREVENTION

- Condoms prevent most sexually transmitted diseases.
- Certain contraceptive foams have antigonococcal activity but are of unproved clinical efficacy.
- Sexual partners of patients with gonococcal or nongonococcal urethritis should be evaluated and treated to prevent reinfection and complications to both partners.
- Women with symptoms of urinary tract infection who do not have bacteriuria should have urethral cultures for *N. gonorrhoeae*.
- Patients with urethritis should be screened for other sexually transmitted diseases.

Selected Readings

Burstein GR, Gaydos CA, Diener-West M, et al. Incident *Chlamydia trachomatis* infections among inner-city adolescent females. *JAMA* 1998;280:521–526.

Holmes KK, Handsfield HH. Sexually transmitted diseases: Overview and clinical approach. In: Fauci AS, Braunwald E, Isselbacher KJ, et al., eds. *Harrison's principles of internal medicine,* 14th ed. New York: McGraw-Hill, 1998:801–812.

McCormack WM, Rein WF. Urethritis. In: Mandell GL, Bennett JE, Dolin R, eds. *Principles and practice of infectious diseases,* 4th ed. New York: Churchill Livingstone, 1995:1063–1074.

Vaginal Discharge/Vaginitis

Basics

DEFINITION
- Physiologic or normal vaginal discharge (also referred to as *leukorrhea*) generally consists of cervical mucus and desquamated epithelial cells.
- Usually, the term *vaginal discharge* is used in conjunction with a vaginal infection. Such infections are characterized by the following:
  — Abnormal color of discharge, caused by increased concentration of polymorphonuclear leukocytes
  — Dyspareunia
  — Increased volume of discharge
  — Vaginal malodor, and/or
  — Vulvar pruritus, irritation, burning, or dysuria
- Please also see Section I chapter, "Genital Lesions," and Section II chapters, "Cervicitis/Mucopurulent Cervicitis" and "Pelvic Inflammatory Disease."

APPROACH TO THE PATIENT
- Physicians should inquire about the characteristics of the discharge (color, odor, etc.) and the presence of other local or systemic symptoms. Previous similar symptoms and a complete sexual history can aid in the diagnosis.
- Examination of the vaginal fluid, using the following tests, can diagnose most cases:
  — Measuring pH, using pH paper that reads from 4.0 to 6.0
  — Detecting an amine ("fishy") odor, which is released upon alkalinizing vaginal fluid by adding one drop of KOH (10%) solution
  — Searching for clue cells (vaginal epithelial cells that are so overladen with adherent bacteria that the cell border is obscured) and for trichomonads and white blood cells in a saline preparation under the microscope
  — Examining a KOH preparation under the microscope for hyphae and mycelia of Candida
- Investigation of vaginal discharge in sexually active adult women should involve the collection of both endocervical and high vaginal swabs. High vaginal swabs should be placed in transport medium to prevent drying and to allow the survival of anaerobes.
- Harvesting of endocervical cells from the squamocolumnar junction is required for chlamydial culture, detection of chlamydial antigen, or chlamydial DNA by polymerase chain reaction.
- It is convenient to divide specimens into those requiring a full culture and those requiring a screening culture. A screening culture will include selective plates for *Neisseria gonorrhoeae*, *Candida* spp, and beta-haemolytic streptococci, and microscopy for *Trichomonas vaginalis* and bacterial vaginosis.

ETIOLOGY
- Physiologic discharge accounted for 10% of women attending a private practice with vaginal complaints.
- Three etiologies account for over 90% of cases of vaginitis:
  — *Trichomonas* (*T. vaginalis*) (25%)
  — *Candida* (25%)
  — Bacterial vaginosis (40%)
- Bacterial vaginosis is associated with multiple sexual partners and recent intercourse with a new partner. The prevalence and concentrations of *Gardnerella vaginalis*, *Mycoplasma hominis*, and several anaerobic bacteria are greater in vaginal fluid of women with bacterial vaginosis than in that of women without this syndrome. It is diagnosed when three out of four of the following are present:
  — Abnormal, thin, homogeneous vaginal discharge
  — Vaginal pH > 4.5
  — Positive amine test
  — Presence of clue cells
- Vaginal discharge may be the presenting manifestation of genital herpes and occasionally reflects mucopurulent cervicitis or pelvic inflammatory disease caused by gonorrhea or chlamydial infection.
- Vaginitis may be an early and prominent feature of toxic shock syndrome.

EPIDEMIOLOGY
Bacterial vaginosis is the most common cause of vulvovaginal symptoms in most clinical settings; it is closely followed in frequency by vulvovaginal candidiasis. Trichomoniasis is much less common in most settings in developed countries.

Clinical Manifestations

- Although the clinical signs and symptoms are often nonspecific, certain features can suggest the diagnosis of candidal vaginitis:
  — Vulvar pruritus and burning
  — Abnormal vaginal discharge; only 25% have the "typical" thick, curdy discharge.
  — Burning on urination at the urethral orifice
  — Vaginal erythema; white or yellow adherent plaques (in 40%)
- Findings and characteristics of the vaginal discharge:
  — Symptomatic trichomoniasis: characteristically produces a profuse, yellow, purulent, homogeneous vaginal discharge and vulvar irritation
  — Vulvovaginal candidiasis: The vaginal discharge typically is white and scant and sometimes takes the form of white thrushlike plaques or cottage cheese–like curds adhering loosely to the vaginal mucosa.
  — *Trichomonas vaginalis* usually manifests with malodorous vaginal discharge (often yellow), vulvar erythema and itching, dysuria or urinary frequency (in 30% to 50% of cases), and dyspareunia. These manifestations, however, do not clearly distinguish trichomoniasis from other types of infectious vaginitis.

Diagnosis

- Detection of motile trichomonas by microscopy of wet preparations of vaginal or prostatic secretions has been the conventional means of diagnosis:
  — For a wet preparation, vaginal fluid is added to a drop of saline on a slide, and covered with a coverslip. Wet preparations are checked for the presence of *T. vaginalis*, yeast cells, pus cells, epithelial cells, and clue cells.
  — Clue cells are vaginal epithelial cells covered with numerous, short coccobacilli. In addition, lactobacilli will be absent or reduced in number when clue cells are present. If clue cells are seen on the wet preparation, a confirmatory Gram stain is made.

Vaginal Discharge/Vaginitis

- —The relative numbers of epithelial and pus cells can be helpful.
- —Culture for *T. vaginalis* will yield few additional positives.
- Wet preparations provide an immediate diagnosis. Its sensitivity for the detection of *T. vaginalis* is only about 60% in routine evaluations of vaginal secretions (up to 70% to 80% among symptomatic patients). Direct immunofluorescent antibody staining is more sensitive (up to 90%) than wet-mount examinations. Culture of the parasite is the most sensitive means of detection; however, the facilities for culture are not generally available, and detection of the organism takes 3 to 7 days.
- The diagnosis of vulvovaginal candidiasis involves the demonstration of fungi by microscopic examination of vaginal fluid in saline or 10% KOH or by Gram stain. Culture does identify *C. albicans* in some women with symptoms and signs of vulvovaginal candidiasis in conjunction with negative results upon microscopic examination, but it also commonly detects coincidental colonization in women without such symptoms or signs. The pH of vaginal secretions is usually 4.5, and no amine odor is produced when vaginal secretions are mixed with 10% KOH.

Treatment

- For vaginal trichomoniasis, a single 2-g oral dose of metronidazole is the treatment of choice, and is as effective as more prolonged regimens.
- The standard regimen for the treatment of bacterial vaginosis has been metronidazole (500 mg orally, twice daily for 7 days). Clindamycin (300 mg orally, twice daily for 7 days) is also effective. Intravaginal treatment with 2% clindamycin cream (one applicator each night for 7 nights) or 0.75% metronidazole gel (one applicator twice daily for 5 days) is also effective.
- In most circumstances, therapy for candidal vaginal infection is indicated only if the patient is symptomatic or has signs of vulvovaginitis.

- Intravaginal products, many of which are available over the counter, are the treatments of choice. They should be applied at bedtime.
  - —Clotrimazole, 1% vaginal cream, 5 g for 7 to 14 days; 100-mg vaginal tablet, single tablet for 7 days or two tablets for 3 days; or 500-mg vaginal tablet, single application
  - —Miconazole, 2% vaginal cream, 5 g for 7 days; 200-mg vaginal suppository for 3 days; or 100-mg vaginal suppository for 7 days
  - —Butoconazole, 2% vaginal cream, 5 g for 3 days
  - —Terconazole, 80-mg vaginal suppository for 3 days
  - —In pregnancy, intravaginal clotrimazole, miconazole, or terconazole may be used for symptomatic women, but their use should be deferred until the second trimester.
  - —The newer azoles, fluconazole and itraconazole, can be used as a single oral dose, but they are more expensive than older treatments. For azole-resistant *Candida* strains, nystatin and boric acid can be used, but these products are not first-line treatments.
- About 10% of women will have another, or several, attacks of *Candida* vaginitis after what should be an appropriate treatment course. The definition of "recurrent candidiasis" is four or more episodes per year.

COMPLICATIONS

- Vaginal trichomoniasis and bacterial vaginosis early in pregnancy are independent predictors of premature onset of labor.
- The full significance of bacterial vaginosis is gradually unfolding, and is currently recognized as a risk factor in the following:
  - —Bacterial infection of the upper genital tract
  - —Endometritis following caesarean section
  - —Neonatal sepsis
  - —Preterm labor/late miscarriage
  - —Vaginal cuff cellulitis following abdominal hysterectomy

Follow-Up

Recurrent or chronic vulvovaginal candidiasis develops with increased frequency among women with systemic illnesses, such as diabetes mellitus or HIV infection.

PREVENTION

- Prevention suggestions for vaginal infections:
  - —Practice safe sex.
  - —Limit the number of sex partners.
  - —Treat infected partners, as indicated.
- Weekly oral fluconazole has been found effective in preventing vulvovaginal candidiasis among patients with advanced HIV infection, but this approach is rarely needed and should be based on selective criteria.

Selected Readings

Anonymous. 1998 Guidelines for treatment of sexually transmitted diseases. Centers for Disease Control and Prevention. *MMWR Morbid Mortal Wkly Rep* 1998;47(RR1):1–111.

Holmes KK, Handsfield H. Sexually transmitted diseases: Overview and clinical approach. In: Fauci AS, Braunwald E, Isselbacher KJ, et al., eds. *Harrison's principles of internal medicine*, 14th ed. New York: McGraw-Hill, 1998:801–812.

Macsween KF, Ridgway GL. The laboratory investigation of vaginal discharge. *J Clin Pathol* 1998;51:564–567.

Mylonakis E, Flanigan TP. Antifungal prophylaxis with weekly fluconazole for patients with AIDS [Editorial]. *Clin Infect Dis* 1998;27:1376–1378.

SECTION II
Specific Infections and Diseases

Acne Vulgaris

Basics

DEFINITION
Acne vulgaris (also called common acne), located on the face, chest, and back, is a chronic inflammation disease of the sebaceous follicles, which are special pilosebaceous units.

ETIOLOGY
- Several factors contribute to the pathogenesis of acne, including abnormal follicular differentiation, infection with *Propionibacterium acnes,* inflammation, and sebum formation.
- *P. acnes* is an anaerobic, gram-positive bacterium that populates the androgen-stimulated sebaceous follicle and is a normal constituent of the cutaneous flora. It is absent from the skin before the onset of puberty. Sebaceous follicles containing microcomedones provide an anaerobic, lipid-rich environment in which these bacteria flourish.
- Inflammation is a direct or indirect result of the proliferation of *P. acnes* through complement activation and release of other hydrolytic enzymes, such as proteases. Follicular rupture and extension of the inflammatory process into the surrounding dermis results in the formation of the inflammatory lesions of acne vulgaris: papules, pustules, and nodules.
- Sebum, the lipid-rich secretion product of sebaceous glands, has a central role in the pathogenesis of acne and provides a growth medium for *P. acnes*.

EPIDEMIOLOGY
Incidence
- Acne vulgaris is among the most common skin diseases, affecting nearly 80% of persons at some time between the ages of 11 and 30 years.
- The first signs of acne vulgaris commonly occur during puberty, but may appear as early as ages 7 to 9 years.

Risk Factors
- Enlargement of the sebaceous glands and increased production of sebum are stimulated by the increase in production of adrenal and gonadal androgens that precedes the clinical onset of puberty.
- Some women with acne have raised serum concentrations of testosterone, dehydroepiandrosterone sulphate, or androstenedione. In men, the association of acne with high androgen concentrations is less consistent.

Clinical Manifestations

SYMPTOMS
- Progressive enlargement of microcomedones gives rise to clinically visible comedones, the noninflammatory lesions of acne.
- The clinical hallmark of acne vulgaris is the comedone, which may be closed (whitehead) or open (blackhead).
- Inflammatory lesions usually accompany comedones.
- Acne is generally limited to the parts of the body that have the largest and most abundant sebaceous glands: the face, neck, chest, upper back, and upper arms.

SIGNS
- Closed comedones appear as 1- to 2-mm pebbly, white papules, which are accentuated when the skin is stretched.
- Open comedones (blackheads) appear as flat or slightly raised brown to black plugs that distend the follicular orifices.
- Other features that may be present, in addition to the typical lesions of acne, include scarring and hyperpigmentation.

Diagnosis

The morphology of acne vulgaris is usually characteristic; however, in some cases it can be confused with other skin lesions, such as molluscum contagiosum. When morphology is unclear or when there is no response to treatment, evaluation by a dermatologist is indicated.

Treatment

MAIN TREATMENT
- Treatment of acne vulgaris is directed toward elimination of comedones, strict skin hygiene, decreasing the number of microorganisms, and decreasing inflammation.
- Tretinoin is the most effective available topical comedolytic agent. This drug reverses the process of abnormal follicular keratinization, thereby reducing microcomedo formation. Tretinoin has the beneficial effect of lightening postinflammatory hyperpigmentation in Black patients.
- Topical application of tretinoin can lead to local irritation. Thus, therapy usually starts with the lowest strength preparation (0.025% cream), and formulations of increasing strength and efficacy are given, as tolerated, in the following sequence: 0.01% gel, 0.05% cream, 0.025% gel, 0.01% cream, and 0.05% solution.
- Maximum clinical improvement from the use of tretinoin may not be clinically evident for 3 to 4 months.
- Other topical agents, such as retinoic acid, benzoyl peroxide, tetracycline, erythromycin, clindamycin, or salicylic acid, may alter the pattern of epidermal desquamation, preventing the formation of comedones and aiding in the resolution of preexisting cysts.

Acne Vulgaris

- Most topical acne medications are applied twice daily. Once-daily or alternate-day therapy can be used if there is irritation; these schedules of application are commonly used for tretinoin.
- The medication should be applied to the entire area rather than simply to individual acne lesions.
- Skin type and the patient's preference determine the choice of vehicle in a topical medication. Gels are nongreasy and have a drying effect, which may be desirable for individuals with oily skin. Creams and lotions are cosmetically pleasing, moisturizing preparations that most patients find acceptable. Solutions, although drying, may be useful for application to large areas of skin.
- Oral antibiotics are indicated for patients with the following:
  —Inflammatory acne
  —Moderate to severe disease
  —Failed topical antibiotic therapy
  —Involvement of areas where the patient may have difficulty in adequately applying topical antibiotics
  —A potential for scarring or substantial pigmentary changes
- Oral antibiotics used in the treatment of acne include tetracyclines (tetracycline in doses of 250 to 1,000 mg daily, doxycycline, or minocycline), erythromycin, or cotrimoxazole.
- The tetracyclines and erythromycin have antiinflammatory properties in addition to their antibacterial action.

ALTERNATIVE TREATMENT

- Severe nodulocystic acne not responsive to oral antibiotics and topical therapy may be treated with the synthetic retinoid isotretinoin. It is used at doses of 0.5 to 2.0 mg/kg as a single daily dose for 15 to 20 weeks.
- Adapalene is a synthetic derivative of naphthoic acid with retinoid-like activity. It has comedolytic and antiinflammatory effects.
- Salicylic acid is a less effective option for patients who cannot tolerate tretinoin. Various products, including solutions, cleansers, and soaps, are available.
- Therapy can be started at the lowest dose and gradually increased, as tolerated, to the highest end of this range. Some patients who undergo retreatment may require a higher dose of isotretinoin (1.5–2.0 mg/kg daily), but others with less severe but refractory disease may respond to doses as low as 5 mg/d. The usual duration of treatment is 20 weeks.
- Hormonal treatment improves acne by decreasing androgen-induced sebum production.
- Spironolactone blocks androgen receptors, inhibits androgen synthesis, and is effective against lesions of inflammatory acne.
- Estrogens decrease serum concentrations of free androgens by suppressing ovarian hormonal production and increasing the concentration of sex hormone–binding globulin.
- Corticosteroids are used in the treatment of acne to suppress adrenal and ovarian androgens. They may be indicated when other hormonal therapy has failed. A low dose of prednisone (2.5–7.5 mg) or dexamethasone (0.125–0.500 mg) taken at night suppresses the morning surge of corticotropin secretion and produces a clinical improvement in some patients.

TREATMENT FAILURE

Tender nodules and cysts can be treated with intralesional injections of corticosteroids to reduce the size and inflammation of lesions quickly. Especially purulent nodules and cysts can be incised and drained.

COMPLICATIONS

- Acne can persist for years and result in disfigurement and permanent scarring, and it can have serious adverse effects on psychosocial development.
- Hyperpigmentation occurs more commonly and more prominently in patients with darker complexions.

Follow-Up

- Isotretinoin causes several adverse effects:
  —The drug is teratogenic.
  —Dryness or irritation of skin and mucous membranes occurs in more than 90% of patients and can be treated with emollients.
  —Pain or stiffness of bones, joints, and muscles
  —Hypertriglyceridaemia
  —Very high concentrations of triglycerides
  —Raised concentrations of cholesterol and decreased concentrations of high-density lipoprotein
  —About 15% of patients have mildly to moderately raised values on liver function tests.
  —Low counts of white and red blood cells occur rarely, but these abnormalities are not usually clinically significant.
- Female patients must be screened for pregnancy prior to initiating therapy with isotretinoin, must maintain a method of birth control during therapy, and must be screened for pregnancy during their treatment course. Patients receiving this medication develop extremely dry skin and cheilitis and must be followed for development of hypertriglyceridemia or hematologic abnormalities.

PREVENTION

Good skin hygiene might prevent some cases of acne.

Selected Readings

Brown SK, Shalita AR. Acne vulgaris. *Lancet* 1998;351(9119):1871–1876.

Leyden JJ. Therapy for acne vulgaris. *N Engl J Med* 1997;336:1156–1162.

Swerlick RA, Lawley TJ. Eczema, psoriasis, cutaneous infections, acne, and other common skin disorders. In: Fauci AS, Braunwald E, Isselbacher KJ, et al., eds. *Harrison's principles of internal medicine*, 14th ed. New York: McGraw-Hill, 1998:298–303.

Actinomycosis

Basics

DEFINITION

- A chronic, indolent, suppurative, tissue-destructive infection, presenting with lumps and sinus formation, usually involving the head and neck, although it can well affect other parts of the body, such as the thorax and abdomen

ETIOLOGY

- *Actinomyces* are microaerophilic/anaerobic, filamentous, branched, gram-positive, and acid-sensitive rods.
- Among several *Actinomyces* species, *Actinomyces israelii* is most commonly found in pus and tissues of patients suffering from actinomycosis.
- *Actinomyces naeslundii, Actinomyces meyeri, Actinomyces odontolyticus,* and *Propionibacterium propionica* (*Arachnia propionica* or *Actinomyces propionica*) have also been reported to cause human actinomycosis.
- *Actinomyces viscosus* has been established as a contributing factor to the etiology of periodontal disease.
- *Actinomyces* are oral and female genital tract commensals.
- Nevertheless, in most cases of actinomycosis, careful cultures yield polymicrobial isolates, mostly including anaerobic members of the normal oral flora. These might act as copathogens in the pathologic process.

EPIDEMIOLOGY

Incidence

- The reported incidence in the general population is about 1:300,000 in the United States, and about 1:100,000 in Europe.
- Infection occurs at all ages, with a peak incidence in the middle decades.
- The male-to-female ratio is 3:1.

Risk Factors

- Poor oral hygiene, dental procedures, oral surgery, and trauma
- Intrauterine contraceptive devices (all types; increased risk if in place for more than 2 years)
- Abdominal surgery, intraabdominal inflammatory processes (diverticulitis, appendicitis), foreign bodies
- Actinomycosis has been described in the setting of immunodeficiency (HIV infection, chronic steroid use).

INCUBATION PERIOD AND NATURAL HISTORY

- The natural reservoir of human actinomycosis pathogens is the human.
- The organisms usually grow as saprophytes in the mouth (mainly in dental plaque and tonsillar crypts).
- Transmission probably occurs from person to person by contact.
- Extraction of teeth or other trauma of the oral mucosa may precipitate actual local infection by *Actinomyces* species.
- The pathogens are probably aspirated and occasionally cause lung actinomycosis.
- Most cases of abdominal actinomycosis originate in the appendix.
- Although the exact incubation period is not known, diagnosis is usually done after long periods of time. Although an acute form has been recognized, chronic disease accounts for the majority of cases.
- Disruption of the mucosal barrier seems to be necessary for the initial establishment of the infection. It subsequently spreads contiguously and/or hematogenously. Aspiration or contiguous spread from the cervical area leads to pulmonary involvement. Foreign bodies and/or bowel perforation secondary to appendicitis or diverticulitis lead to the pathologic process in the abdominal and pelvic disease.
- Depending on the part of the body affected, oral/cervicofacial, thoracic, abdominal, pelvic, CNS, and a disseminated form of the disease are recognized. Muscle and bone involvement is due to direct spread by adjacent tissue infection or (less frequently) follows trauma or dissemination of infection.

Clinical Manifestations

SYMPTOMS

- Pain, vaginal discharge and/or bleeding (pelvic disease)
- Headache, focal symptoms
- Symptoms dependent on the extent of the lesions and the organ/system involved
- Possible pain, low-grade fever, weight loss
- Trismus (oral/cervicofacial disease)
- Chest pain, cough (productive or not), gradually increasing shortness of breath (thoracic disease)
- Abdominal pain, change in bowel habits (abdominal disease)
- Low abdominal neurologic symptoms in CNS disease

SIGNS

- Formation of space-occupying lesions of varying sizes, with varying degrees of suppuration and/or fibrosis, is the hallmark of the disease.
  - Spread to the adjacent tissues may occur, as well as drainage to adjacent cavities or to the skin via sinus formation.
  - Sinuses can be self-limited and recurrent.
  - Pus characteristically contains (usually) yellowish "sulfur granules," which may be seen macroscopically or microscopically.
- Cervicofacial/oral disease
  - The perimandibular region is most commonly affected, but every part of the head, neck, and oral cavity can be involved, including soft tissues, bones, salivary glands, thyroid, eyes (postoperative canaliculitis and endophthalmitis), and ears (chronic, myringotomy-resistant otitis media).
  - The overlying skin may be purple/red/bluish.
- Thoracic disease
  - Follows aspiration or (more rarely) contiguous spread from the cervical region. Signs are those of a space-occupying lesion or/and pneumonitis, with pleural involvement (thickening, effusion, empyema) in more than 50% of cases.
  - The presence of multiple cavities and the involvement of the chest wall (soft tissues and bones with sinus formation) support the diagnosis.
  - Mediastinal involvement (mainly cardiac structures), as well as spine involvement, may be present.
- Abdominal disease
  - Signs are those of a firm/hard mass lesion, most commonly in the right iliac fossa (following perforated appendicitis).

Actinomycosis

- Left iliac fossa disease follows diverticulitis.
- Perirectal or perianal disease presents as chronic, recurrent abscesses and sinus/fistula formation in the relevant region.
- Peritonitis is rare.
- Pelvic disease
  - Presents as pelvic masses and abscesses of varying extension, or is diagnosed as frozen pelvis, due to the indolent course of the disease
- CNS disease
  - Focal neurologic signs and/or signs of chronic meningitis

Diagnosis

DIFFERENTIAL DIAGNOSIS

- Malignant tumors
- Nocardiosis
- Botryomycosis
- Tuberculosis
- Histoplasmosis
- Blastomycosis
- Cryptococcosis

CLINICAL

- There is a high degree of suspicion when space-occupying lesions are combined with pus-draining sinus formation and soft-tissue/bone involvement.
- Inspect the bandage covering a draining sinus for sulfur granules.
- Take the specimen before initiating any antimicrobial therapy.

MICROBIOLOGY

- Identification of filamentous, gram-positive, acid-sensitive organisms in sulfur granules (slide examination) or in material obtained from a normally sterile site (not in sputum, bronchial washings, or vaginal secretions)
- A Gram stain of the specimen is more sensitive than culture.
- Swab cultures not recommended.
- Anaerobic processing of specimens is necessary.

IMMUNOFLUORESCENCE

Direct immunofluorescence (IF) using specific antisera against actinomycosis agents is highly specific and sensitive. It has been mainly used in diagnosis and prevention of intrauterine devices-related disease.

IMAGING

- X-rays and computerized tomography may be helpful in defining the extent of the disease, and the adjacent tissue involvement.
- The open bronchus sign—the presence of an aerobronchogram within a mass lesion—is highly suggestive of lung disease.
- A saw-toothed appearance and complete involvement of bones are characteristic of bone disease.
- Single (actinomycetoma) or multiple round or irregular multiloculated brain lesions, surrounded by edema and low-attenuation areas, are the usual mode of CNS disease presentation.

PATHOLOGY

- Presence of macroscopic or microscopic "sulfur granules" in pus and/or tissue material (other than tonsils), obtained by fine-needle aspiration or biopsy. Tissue Gram and Giemsa stains will reveal the organisms at the periphery of the granule.

Treatment

MAIN TREATMENT

- Penicillin G, 10 to 24 million units/d i.v. for 2 to 6 weeks, followed by penicillin V, 2 to 4 g/d PO for 6 to 12 months, or
- Ampicillin 50 mg/kg/d i.v. for 2 to 6 weeks, followed by amoxicillin, 1.5 g/d PO for 6 to 12 months
- Antibiotic treatment may need to be combined with surgical intervention.

ALTERNATIVE TREATMENT

- Tetracycline (Minocycline)
- Erythromycin (alternative if patient allergic or pregnant)
- Clindamycin

TREATMENT FAILURE

- Usually excellent response to antibiotics, no *Actinomyces* resistance. In the case of failure, there is a high possibility of an undrained abscess or a resistant bacterial copathogen.

COMPLICATIONS

- Disseminated actinomycosis
- Bowel obstruction due to extensive abdominal/pelvic actinomycosis

Follow-Up

- Emphasize the need for compliance to treatment (long-term drug treatment).
- Observe for drug toxicity.

PREVENTION

- Keep good oral hygiene, including removal of dental plaque.
- Gupta bodies or ALOs (actinomyces-like organisms) present in Papanicolaou cervicovaginal smears may be of help in preventing the development of advanced pelvic disease in women with long-term intrauterine contraceptive devices and symptoms of possible early pelvic actinomycosis, such as pain, abnormal bleeding, or abnormal discharge. Removal of the intrauterine device and a 2- to 3-week course of antibiotics is recommended in these cases.
- There is no need for patient isolation.

Selected Readings

Belmont MJ, Behar PM, Wax MK. Atypical presentations of actinomycosis. *Head Neck* 1999;21:264–268.

Burns BV, al-Ayoubi A, Ray J, et al. Actinomycosis of the posterior triangle: A case report and review of the literature. *J Laryngol Otol* 1997;111:1082–1085.

Lippes J. Pelvic actinomycosis: A review and preliminary look at prevalence. *Am J Obstet Gynecol* 1999;180:265–269.

Smego RA Jr, Foglia G. Actinomycosis. *Clin Infect Dis* 1998;26:1255–1261.

Zitsche RP III, Bothwell M. Actinomycosis: A potential complication of head and neck surgery. *Am J Otolaryngol* 1999;20:260–262.

Adenovirus Infections

Basics

DEFINITION

- Adenovirus infections are caused by complex DNA viruses that measure 70 to 80 nm in diameter.
- Human adenoviruses belong to the genus *Mastadenovirus,* which includes almost 50 serotypes.

ETIOLOGY

- Adenoviruses have a characteristic morphology consisting of an icosahedral shell composed of 20 equilateral triangular faces and 12 vertices.
- Human adenoviruses have been divided into six subgenera (A through F) on the basis of the homology of DNA genomes and other properties.
- The adenovirus genome is a linear double-stranded DNA that codes for structural and nonstructural polypeptides. The replicative cycle of adenovirus may result either in lytic infection of cells or in the establishment of a latent infection.
- Some adenovirus types can induce oncogenic transformation, and tumor formation has been observed in animals.

EPIDEMIOLOGY

Incidence

- Eighty percent of cases of acute respiratory illnesses are caused by viruses, most commonly rhinovirus, and less often, adenovirus.
- Infections are most common from fall to spring.

Risk Factors

- Adenovirus infection can be transmitted by inhalation of aerosolized virus, by inoculation of virus into conjunctival sacs, and, probably, by the fecal–oral route as well.
- Adenoviruses account for up to 5% of acute respiratory infections in children, but for fewer than 2% of respiratory illnesses in adults.
- Certain adenovirus serotypes are associated with outbreaks of acute respiratory disease in military recruits in winter and spring.
- Antibodies develop after infection and are associated with protection against infection with the same serotype.
- Adenoviruses also have been implicated in disseminated disease and pneumonia in immunosuppressed patients, including patients with AIDS and recipients of solid-organ or bone marrow transplants.

Clinical Manifestations

- In children, adenoviruses cause a variety of clinical syndromes. The most common is an acute upper respiratory tract infection with prominent rhinitis.
- On occasion, lower respiratory tract disease, including bronchiolitis and pneumonia, occurs.
- Adenoviruses can cause pharyngoconjunctival fever, a characteristic acute febrile illness of children that occurs in outbreaks, most often in summer camps. Low-grade fever is frequently present for the first 3 to 5 days, followed by rhinitis, sore throat, and cervical adenopathy. The illness generally lasts for 1 to 2 weeks and resolves spontaneously.
- Pharyngitis also has been associated with adenovirus infection.
- In adults, the most frequently reported illness has been acute respiratory disease. This illness is marked by a prominent sore throat and the gradual onset of fever, which often reaches 39°C. Cough is almost always present, and coryza and regional lymphadenopathy are frequently seen.
- Physical examination may show pharyngeal edema, injection, and tonsillar enlargement with little or no exudate.
- Adenoviruses can also cause nonrespiratory tract diseases:
  —Acute diarrheal illness in young children
  —Hemorrhagic cystitis
  —Epidemic keratoconjunctivitis
- Immunocompromised patients with adenovirus pneumonia can present with the abrupt onset of fever, rigors, malaise, nonproductive cough, nausea, vomiting, diarrhea, abdominal pain, headache, and arthralgia. Physical examination is often unremarkable.

Adenovirus Infections

Diagnosis

DIFFERENTIAL DIAGNOSIS

In most cases, illnesses caused by adenovirus infection cannot be differentiated from those caused by a number of other viral respiratory agents and *Mycoplasma pneumoniae*.

LABORATORY

- A definitive diagnosis of adenovirus infection is established by culture or detection of the virus from sites such as the conjunctiva and oropharynx or from sputum, urine, or stool.
- Virus may be detected in tissue culture by cytopathic changes, and specifically identified by immunofluorescence or other immunologic techniques.
- Adenovirus types that have been associated with diarrheal disease in children require special tissue-culture cells for isolation or are identified by direct ELISA of stool.
- Serum antibody rises can be demonstrated by complement-fixation or neutralization tests, ELISA, or radioimmunoassay.

IMAGING

In adenovirus pneumonia, the chest roentgenogram usually shows bilateral, diffuse, interstitial infiltrates and, occasionally, pleural effusions.

Treatment

MAIN TREATMENT

- Only symptom-based treatment and supportive therapy are available for adenovirus infections.
- Live vaccines have been developed against adenovirus types 4 and 7 (live, unattenuated virus administered in enteric-coated capsules) and are used to control epidemics in military recruits.
- The treatment of adenovirus infections in immunocompromised hosts is usually supportive and symptomatic.
- Severe adenovirus infections in immunocompromised patients can respond to treatment with ganciclovir and a single dose of intravenous immunoglobulin.
- Intravenous gamma globulin (IVIG) has been used in the treatment of adenovirus infections in transplant patients and immunocompromised hosts, and type-specific antibody may play a role in the treatment of this infection.
- Ribavirin has been used successfully for the treatment of adenovirus infections in immunocompromised and immunocompetent hosts.
- More research is needed before zinc can be recommended for the treatment of adenoviral infections.

COMPLICATIONS

In transplant recipients and immunocompromised patients, adenovirus pneumonia is associated with significant morbidity and mortality, which may exceed 60%.

Follow-Up

PREVENTION

Vaccines prepared from purified subunits of adenovirus are being investigated.

Selected Readings

Dolin R. DNA and RNA respiratory viruses. In: Fauci AS, Braunwald E, Isselbacher KJ, et al., eds. *Harrison's principles of internal medicine,* 14th ed. New York: McGraw-Hill, 1998:1100–1105.

Duggan JM, Farrehi J, Duderstadt S, et al. Treatment with ganciclovir of adenovirus pneumonia in a cardiac transplant patient. *Am J Med* 1997;103:439–440.

Gadomski A. A cure for the common cold? Zinc again. *JAMA* 1998;279:1999–2000.

Macknin ML, Piedmonte M, Calendine C, et al. Zinc gluconate lozenges for treating the common cold in children: A randomized controlled trial. *JAMA* 1998;279:1962–1967.

Amebiasis

Basics

DEFINITION
Amebiasis is a protozoal infection caused by pathologic strains of *Entamoeba histolytica* or *Entamoeba dispar*. Infection with these organisms leads to ulceration of the colon and diarrhea and, on occasion, liver abscess.

ETIOLOGY
- Amebiasis is a protozoal infection caused by *E. histolytica* and, on occasion, *E. dispar*.
- Cysts can survive for weeks in the environment.
- Trophozoites develop within the colon.
- Most people with the organism have no significant invasion of the colonic mucosa and are asymptomatic. These are called "cyst passers."
- Patients with symptomatic disease have flask-shaped colonic ulcers. This is associated with invasive disease.

Incidence
- Invasive disease occurs in 50 million people worldwide each year.
- It is estimated that infection with *E. histolytica* accounts for 100,00 deaths a year.

EPIDEMIOLOGY
- Disease is worldwide in distribution, but much more prevalent in underdeveloped nations with poor sanitation.
- Contaminated water or vegetables are often the source for infection in humans.
- Cysts are not eradicated with chlorine; boiling of water is necessary for decontamination.
- Disease is seen at all ages.
- Disease is relatively equally distributed in men and women.
- Prevalence of disease in the United States is less than 4%.

Risk Factors
In developed countries:
- Institutionalized patients
- Men who have sex with men

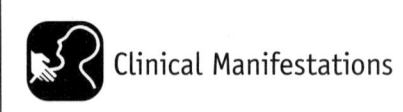

Clinical Manifestations

INCUBATION PERIOD
- Patients develop symptoms with invasive disease within 3 weeks of ingestion of the cysts.
- Amebic liver abscess formation takes about 3 months to develop.
- Some patients apparently carry the organisms for prolonged periods before developing significant clinical manifestations.

NONINVASIVE
Symptoms of noninvasive disease are mild, with diarrhea only.

INVASIVE
- Invasive disease is associated with crampy abdominal pain and bloody, mucoid diarrhea.
- Fevers occur in one-third of patients.
- Fulminant disease with peritonitis and perforation as well as toxic megacolon is rare but well described.
- Amebomas are mass lesions of the colon, often in the cecum or on the right side, caused by inflammation of amebic colitis. They may present with obstruction, and can masquerade as colon cancer.

AMEBIC LIVER ABSCESS
- This may present with fevers, right upper quadrant pain, and tenderness to palpation over the liver. Diarrhea and active amebic colitis are often not present at the time of abscess discovery.
- Rare rupture of the abscess may lead to peritonitis.
- Rupture of the liver abscess into the pleural space leads to empyema. Patients present with fevers, shortness of breath, and pleuritic chest pains.

Amebiasis

Diagnosis

- All patients with invasive disease have blood in the stools.
- Cysts or trophozoites should be visible on microscopic evaluation of the stool.
- Colonic biopsy specimens reveal organisms.
- Antiamebic antibodies can be sought and are positive in patients with invasive disease only. This is often the most reliable test in countries of low prevalence.
- Leukocytosis without eosinophilia is often seen in patients with invasive amebic disease.
- Elevated liver function tests can be seen in cases of liver involvement.
- Aspiration of a liver abscess often fails to recover the organism, since it lives in the walls of the abscess.

DIFFERENTIAL DIAGNOSIS

- Ulcerative colitis
- Carcinoma of the colon
- Crohn's disease with fistula formation
- Diverticulitis
- Abdominal abscess
- Irritable bowel syndrome

With Liver Abscess

- Pyogenic abscess
- Hepatoma
- Echinococcal cyst

IMAGING

Ultrasound or CT scan of the abdomen reveals liver cysts, usually in the right lobe in the upper, posterior segment.

Treatment

ASYMPTOMATIC CYST PASSER WITHOUT INVASIVE DISEASE

- Iodoquinol 650 mg orally three times per day for 20 days
- Paromomycin 500 mg orally three times per day for 7 days

DYSENTERY

- Metronidazole 750 mg orally three times per day for 10 days, followed by either of the following:
  —Iodoquinol 650 mg orally three time per day for 20 days
  —Paromomycin 500 mg orally three times per day for 7 days

LIVER ABSCESS

- Metronidazole 750 mg orally or intravenously three times per day for 10 days, followed by iodoquinol 650 mg orally three times per day for 20 days
- For a large abscess (>3 cm), aspiration and needle drainage is indicated. Smaller abscesses resolve with medical treatment.

COMPLICATIONS

- Toxic megacolon
- Amebomas
- Liver abscess
- Perforation of the diaphragm with a liver abscess, leading to pleural or pericardial disease
- Cerebral disease

Follow-Up

Patients treated for liver abscess should have follow-up ultrasounds to document cyst resolution, which may take several months.

PREVENTION

- Avoid fecal-oral contact during sexual activity.
- Boil water that may be contaminated.
- Make sure vegetables are washed well with water that does not contain cysts.
- For men having sex with men, practice safe sex.

Selected Readings

Adams EB, MacLeod IN. Invasive amebiasis. I. Amebic dysentery and its complications. *Medicine (Baltimore)* 1977;56:315–323.

Grisby W. Surgical treatment of amebiasis. *Surg Gynecol Obstet* 1969;128:609–627.

Nanda R, Baveja U, Anand BS. *Entamoeba histolytica* cyst passers: Clinical features and outcome in untreated subjects. *Lancet* 1984;2:301–303.

Reed SL, Wessel DW, Davis CE. *Entamoeba histolytica* infection and AIDS. *Am J Med* 1991;90:269.

Anaerobic Infections

Basics

DEFINITION
- Anaerobic infections are caused by bacteria that grow in the complete or almost complete absence of oxygen.
- Facultative bacteria can grow in the presence or absence of air.
- Anaerobes associated with human infections are relatively aerotolerant. They can survive for as long as 72 hours in the presence of oxygen.

ETIOLOGY
- Major reservoirs of anaerobic bacteria are the mouth, gastrointestinal tract, skin, and female genital tract.
- In the colon, the proportion of anaerobes is increased significantly, as is the overall bacterial count.
- Over 400 species of anaerobic bacteria have been identified as part of the normal flora of humans, but relatively few species are isolated commonly from human infection.
- Anaerobic bacterial infections usually occur when an anatomic barrier becomes disrupted and constituents of the local flora enter a site that was previously sterile. Therefore, tissue ischemia, trauma, surgery, perforated viscus, shock, and aspiration provide environments conducive to the proliferation of anaerobes.
- Actinomycosis accounts for most anaerobic infections in bone, except in the head and neck regions. Other anaerobes isolated from infected bone and joint are *Bacteroides* spp, anaerobic cocci, *Fusobacterium* spp, *Propionibacterium acnes,* and *Clostridium* spp.

EPIDEMIOLOGY
- Since the 1970s, various authorities reported isolation of obligate anaerobes in up to 25% of blood cultures; however, recent studies suggest a decrease in the incidence to less than 5%, probably related to earlier use of effective antibodies.
- If optimal bacteriologic techniques are employed, up to 85% of brain abscesses yield anaerobic bacteria, most often anaerobic gram-positive cocci and *Fusobacterium* and *Bacteroides* spp.
- Anaerobic infections of bone and joint frequently arise adjacent to soft-tissue infections. Conditions predisposing to anaerobic bone infections are vascular disease, bites, contiguous infection, peripheral neuropathy, hematogenous spread, and trauma. The predominant anaerobes associated with cellulitis are *Peptostreptococcus* spp, *Bacteroides fragilis* group, *Prevotella* and *Porphyromonas* spp, and *Clostridium* spp.
- Trauma has been associated with cellulitis due to *Clostridium* spp and *Bacteroides* spp with diabetes.
- *B. fragilis* has been isolated from up to 28% of patients with chronic otitis media.
- Gastrointestinal *Clostridium difficile* is discussed elsewhere in the book. Extraintestinal *C. difficile* has been isolated from intraperitoneal sites, blood cultures, perianal abscess, and prosthetic hip joint.

Clinical Manifestations

- Gingivitis is mainly caused by mouth anaerobes. It presents with tender bleeding gums, foul breath, and a bad taste. Patients, especially the immunocompromised, may develop fever, cervical lymphadenopathy, and leukocytosis.
- Ludwig's angina is a periodontal infection usually arising from the tissues surrounding the third molar. It presents with pain, trismus, and superior and posterior displacement of the tongue. Submandibular swelling of the neck can impair swallowing and cause respiratory obstruction.
- Lemierre's syndrome is characterized by nasopharyngitis or peritonsillar abscess, followed 4 to 12 days later by high fever and rigors, swelling of the lymph glands below the maxillary angle, tenderness along the lateral aspect of the sternocleidomastoid muscle (representing thrombophlebitis of the internal jugular vein), distant metastatic abscess formation, especially in the lung, and icterus or subicterus, associated with isolation of *Fusobacterium necrophorum* from blood. Because of difficulties associated with isolation and speciation of *Fusobacterium,* the diagnosis should be considered even in the absence of isolation of the organism from blood culture. *F. necrophorum* is generally sensitive to either penicillin or clindamycin, and persistent fever despite appropriate antibiotic coverage is common. Surgical drainage of abscess cavities should be considered.
- Anaerobic lung abscesses present usually with malaise, weight loss, fever, chills, and foul-smelling sputum, perhaps over a period of weeks.
- In empyema, patients may present with constitutional symptoms, pleuritic chest pain and chest-wall tenderness.
- The clinical presentation of bacteremia due to anaerobes may be quite similar to that seen in sepsis involving aerobic gram-negative bacilli.
- In cellulitis, certain clinical findings have been correlated with the following organisms:
  — Swelling and tenderness with *Clostridium* spp and *Prevotella* spp
  — Regional adenopathy with *B. fragilis* group
  — Gangrene and necrosis with *Peptostreptococcus* spp, *B. fragilis* group, and *Clostridium* spp
  — Foul odor with *Bacteroides* spp
  — Gas in tissues with *Peptostreptococcus* spp, *B. fragilis* group, and *Clostridium* spp

Diagnosis

- Because of the time and difficulty involved in the isolation of anaerobic bacteria, diagnosis of these infections must frequently be based on presumptive evidence.
- A foul odor is often indicative of anaerobes.
- The presence of gas in tissues is highly suggestive, but not diagnostic, of anaerobic infection.
- Anaerobic abscesses must be distinguished from those associated with tuberculosis, neoplasia, and septic emboli.
- In aspiration pneumonia, chest radiographs reveal consolidation in dependent pulmonary segments, more commonly on the right side.

Anaerobic Infections

- Specimens for the evaluation of possible anaerobic infections must be collected by avoidance of contamination with the normal flora, air must be expelled from the syringe used to aspirate the abscess cavity, and the needle must be capped with a sterile rubber stopper.
- Diagnostic radiologists now are able to drain a number of abscess sites percutaneously.

Treatment

- Successful therapy for anaerobic infections involves a combination of appropriate antibiotics, surgical resection, debridement, and drainage.
- Facultative bacteria, such as *Escherichia coli,* are responsible for acute peritonitis and sepsis associated with bowel perforation. Anaerobes, particularly *B. fragilis,* play the seminal role in subsequent abscess formation. Treatment of only the facultative bacteria, without adequate antibiotic coverage for anaerobic bacteria, leads to clinical failures, with complications of abscess formation. Such therapeutic misadventures have been witnessed in the treatment of mixed infections with cephalosporins and penicillins that lack significant activity against anaerobes. Similarly, use of metronidazole or clindamycin as a single agent is associated with failures caused by infection with facultative bacteria. Mixed infections involve complex interactions between facultative bacteria and strict anaerobes, many of which possess intrinsic pathogenicity. The best therapeutic results are realized with antimicrobial drugs that are active against both types of microorganisms.
- Anaerobic infections arising below the diaphragm should be treated with specific therapy directed at *B. fragilis*. Organisms belonging to the *B. fragilis* group are resistant to penicillin.
- Rates of resistance of *B. fragilis* and non-*fragilis* species of the *B. fragilis* group are increasing. In a 5-year (1990–1994) prospective, eight-center survey, there was a significant decline in cefoxitin, cefmetazole, and clindamycin activity over time against these strains. Among *B. fragilis* isolates, virtually no resistance was seen to imipenem, meropenem, ampicillin/sulbactam, piperacillin/tazobactam, or ticarcillin/clavulanate.
- Clindamycin appears to be superior to penicillin for the treatment of lung abscesses.
- Life-threatening infections involving the anaerobic flora of the mouth, such as space infections of the head and neck, should be treated empirically as if penicillin-resistant anaerobes are involved. Less serious infections involving the oral microflora can be treated with penicillin alone; metronidazole can be added (or clindamycin can be substituted) if the patient responds poorly to therapy.
- Other supportive measures in the management of anaerobic infections include careful attention to fluid and electrolyte balance (because extensive local edema may lead to hypoalbuminemia); hemodynamic support for septic shock; immobilization of infected extremities; maintenance of adequate nutrition during chronic infections by parenteral hyperalimentation; relief of pain; and anticoagulation with heparin for thrombophlebitis. Hyperbaric oxygen therapy is advocated by some experts for clostridial infections, but is of no proven value.

COMPLICATIONS

Contiguous craniad spread of anaerobic head and neck infections may lead to osteomyelitis of the skull or mandible or intracranial infections.

Follow-Up

Acute necrotizing infections of the pharynx can complicate ulcerative gingivitis. Symptoms include sore throat, foul breath, bad taste, and fever. Examination of the pharynx demonstrates that the tonsillar pillars are swollen, red, ulcerated, and covered with a grayish membrane that peels easily. Lymphadenopathy and leukocytosis are common. The disease may last for only a few days or, if not treated, may persist for weeks.

PREVENTION

Aspiration precautions should be applied in patients who have a depressed gag reflex, altered state of consciousness, impaired swallowing, or a tracheal or nasogastric tube.

Selected Readings

Brook I, Frazier EH. Anaerobic osteomyelitis and arthritis in a military hospital: A 10-year experience. *Am J Med* 1993;94:21–28.

Brook I, Frazier EH. Clinical features and aerobic and anaerobic microbiological characteristics of cellulitis. *Arch Surg* 1995;130:786–792.

Gorbach SL. Antibiotic treatment of anaerobic infections. *Clin Infect Dis* 1994;18[Suppl 4]:5305–5310.

Kasper DL. Infections due to mixed anaerobic organisms. In: Fauci AS, Braunwald E, Isselbacher KJ, et al., eds. *Harrison's principles of medicine,* 14th ed. New York: McGraw-Hill, 1998:9917.

Leugers CM, Clover R. Lemierre syndrome: Postanginal sepsis. *J Am Board Fam Pract* 1995;8:384–391.

Snydman DR, McDermott L, Cuchural GJ Jr, et al. Analysis of trends in antimicrobial resistance patterns among clinical isolates of *Bacteroides fragilis* group species from 1990 to 1994. *Clin Infect Dis* 1996;23[Suppl 1]:554–565.

Wolf LE, Gorbach SL, Granowitz EV. Extraintestinal *Clostridium difficile:* 10 years' experience at a tertiary-care hospital. *Mayo Clin Proc* 1998;73:943–947.

Anorectal Infections

Basics

DEFINITION

- Anorectal infections involve the anus and rectum (the distal part of the large intestine beginning anteriorly to the third sacral vertebra).
- Under the eponym Fournier's gangrene is included any necrotizing infection of the external genitalia and perineum.
- Solitary rectal ulcer syndrome is a rare disorder characterized by erythema or ulceration of the rectal wall, associated with typical histologic features and disturbed defecatory behavior, with the passage of blood and mucus.

ETIOLOGY

- Most common anorectal infections include bacterial and parasitic infections (e.g., abscesses or soft-tissue infection) and sexually transmitted diseases. Most of these infections are also discussed in other chapters of the book.
- Among women and men who had sex with men, primary anal or rectal infection develops after receptive anorectal intercourse. In women, rectal infection with lymphogranuloma venereum (or non-LGV) strains of *Chlamydia trachomatis* presumably can also arise by the contiguous spread of infected secretions along the perineum (as in rectal gonococcal infections in women) or perhaps by spread to the rectum via the pelvic lymphatics.
- Both herpes simplex viruses 1 and 2 can cause symptomatic or asymptomatic rectal and perianal infections. Herpes infection proctitis is usually associated with rectal intercourse. However, subclinical perianal shedding of herpes simplex virus (HSV) is detected both in heterosexual men and in women who report no rectal intercourse.
- The pathogenesis of solitary rectal ulcer varies in different patients; it includes trauma from straining, direct digital trauma, and, possibly, primary neuromuscular pathology. The histologic findings of extension of the muscularis mucosa between crypts and muscularis propria disorganization on full-thickness specimens are characteristic.
- Perianal warts are common among men who have sex with men, but they develop in heterosexual men as well.
- Perirectal abscesses often represent the tracking down into the anal area of purulent material escaping from the rectosigmoid. Diverticulitis, Crohn's disease, ulcerative colitis, or previous surgery may be the underlying cause.
- In contrast to Fournier's original report, according to which the causative agent of the syndrome was unknown, it is now possible to identify one or more specific etiologic factors in almost all cases. Aerobic bacteria are found in the majority of cases, but at times the infection is complicated by anaerobic infections (mixed infections).

EPIDEMIOLOGY

Incidence

Among organ transplant recipients, the prevalence of external anogenital lesions is 1.5% to 2.3%, and women are more often involved. Most of the lesions are due to anogenital warts, followed by bowenoid papulosis, giant condyloma, and *in situ* carcinoma.

Risk Factors

- In Fournier's gangrene, frequently there is a recent history of urinary infection and/or urologic instrumentation, or long-standing colorectal disease. Furthermore, most patients are affected by heavy comorbidity conditions such as diabetes, alcoholism, or intravenous drug abuse, which hinder immunologic defense.

- Among men who had sex with men, most common causes of anorectal infection include the following:
  — Anorectal gonococcal infection
  — HSV
  — Infections with enteric pathogens, usually *Giardia lamblia*, *Entamoeba histolytica* or *Campylobacter* spp, and *C. trachomatis*
  — Syphilis
- Rectal lesions are common in HIV-infected patients, particularly the perirectal ulcers and erosions due to the reactivation of HSV infection. Other rectal lesions more commonly seen in HIV-infected patients include condyloma acuminatum, Kaposi's sarcoma, and intraepithelial neoplasia.

Clinical Manifestations

- Symptoms of herpes simplex proctitis include anorectal pain, anorectal discharge, tenesmus, and constipation.
- The main manifestations of anogenital warts are cauliflower-like condylomata acuminata that usually involve moist surfaces; keratotic and smooth papular warts, usually on dry surfaces; and subclinical "flat" warts, which can be found on any mucosal or cutaneous surface.
- Fournier's gangrene is characterized by localized gangrene and massive swelling of the scrotum and penis, with extension into the perineum or the abdominal wall and legs.

Diagnosis

DIFFERENTIAL DIAGNOSIS

- Perianal donovanosis may resemble condylomata lata of secondary syphilis. Other venereal diseases, particularly syphilis, frequently coexist with donovanosis. In countries where

Anorectal Infections

donovanosis is endemic, the persistence of suspected condylomata lata after appropriate penicillin therapy for syphilis is highly suggestive of donovanosis.
- The differential diagnosis of anogenital warts includes condylomata lata of secondary syphilis, molluscum contagiosum, hirsutoid papillomatosis (pearly penile papules), fibroepitheliomas, and neoplasms.

LABORATORY

Anorectal swab samples can help in diagnosing *C. trachomatis* infections with the use of PCR.

DIAGNOSTIC/TESTING PROCEDURES

In anorectal infection with HSV, sigmoidoscopy reveals ulcerative lesions of the distal 10 cm of the rectal mucosa. Rectal biopsies show mucosal ulceration, necrosis, polymorphonuclear and lymphocytic infiltration of the lamina propria, and (in occasional cases) multinucleated intranuclear inclusion-bearing cells.

Treatment

- Cryotherapy can be very successful in clearing warts that have failed to respond to podophyllin. Perianal warts, however, do not respond so well. Interferons have been used as adjuvant to other therapy.
- Conservative therapy with local or systemic antibiotics seems appropriate for perianal abscess. For granulomatous lesions, spontaneous resolution is unlikely, and surgery should be the treatment of choice.
- Early and aggressive surgical exploration is essential in patients with Fournier's gangrene and should aim at removing necrotic tissue, reducing compartment pressure, and obtaining material for Gram staining and for aerobic and anaerobic cultures. Empirical antibiotic treatment for mixed aerobic–anaerobic infections could consist of clindamycin (900 mg intravenously tid) ampicillin or ampicillin/sulbactam (2–3 g intravenously qid), plus gentamicin (1.0–1.5 mg/kg tid). Hyperbaric oxygen treatment may also be useful in gas gangrene due to clostridial species. Duration of therapy varies, but antibiotics should be continued until all signs of systemic toxicity have resolved and all devitalized tissue has been removed.

COMPLICATIONS

- Epidermodysplasia verruciformis is a rare autosomal recessive disease characterized by the inability to control human papilloma virus infection. Patients are often infected with unusual human papilloma virus types and frequently develop cutaneous squamous cell malignancies, particularly in sun-exposed areas. The lesions resemble flat warts or macules similar to those of pityriasis versicolor.
- The complications of warts include itching and, occasionally, bleeding. In rare cases, warts become secondarily infected with bacteria or fungi. Large masses of warts may cause mechanical problems, such as obstruction of the birth canal.
- Perianal sepsis must always be kept in mind as a possible focus among HIV-infected patients, especially among those with low CD4 lymphocyte counts.
- Fournier's gangrene can result in septicemia and carries mortality rates as high as 22% to 66%.

Follow-Up

The presence of anal warts and HIV infection are independent risk factors for the development of cytologic abnormalities. Those at highest risk for anal abnormalities include men with anal human papilloma virus infection and a history of intravenous drug use. Some authorities suggest that these groups as well as organ transplant recipients infected with oncogenic human papilloma should be strongly considered as candidates for anal cytology screening to identify and treat potentially precancerous anal disease.

PREVENTION

When immunocompromised patients present with abscesses, perianal sepsis must be considered as a possible focus. Perianal fistulas in such patients should be laid open or treated by fistulectomy, and perianal abscesses require adequate drainage, in order to avoid necrotizing gangrene and metastatic abscesses.

Selected Readings

Consten EC, Slors JF, Danner SA, et al. Severe complications of perianal sepsis in patients with human immunodeficiency virus. *Br J Surg* 1996;83:778–780.

Euvrard S, Kanitakis J, Chardonnet Y, et al. External anogenital lesions in organ transplant recipients. A clinicopathologic and virologic assessment. *Arch Dermatol* 1997;133:175–178.

Frisch M, Olsen JH, Bautz A, et al. Benign anal lesions and the risk of anal cancer. *N Engl J Med* 1994;331:300–302.

Handsfield HH. Clinical presentation and natural course of anogenital warts. *Am J Med* 1997;102(5A):16–20.

Mylonakis E, Nizam R, Freeman N. Periurethral abscess: Complication of UTI. *Geriatrics* 1997;52:86–88.

Pizzorno R, Bonini F, Donelli A, et al. Hyperbaric oxygen therapy in the treatment of Fournier's disease in 11 male patients. *J Urol* 1997;158:837–840.

Vaizey CJ, van den Bogaerde JB, Emmanuel AV, et al. Solitary rectal ulcer syndrome. *Br J Surg* 1998;85:1617–1623.

Anthrax

Basics

DEFINITION
- Anthrax is a gram-positive bacillus that can lead to a constellation of illnesses, ranging from necrotic skin lesions to fatal pneumonia and severe gastrointestinal hemorrhage.
- Dermal infection accounts for the majority of cases.

ETIOLOGY
- *Bacillus anthracis* is an aerobic gram-positive, spore-forming organism.
- The organism, because of its lethality, is felt to be a prime candidate for the use in germ warfare.

EPIDEMIOLOGY

Incidence/Prevalence
- Anthrax is a zoonotic disease of herbivores.
- The organism in spore form remains dormant, at times for years, in the soil.
- Epidemics, though rare in humans, occur in association with disease in animals, mainly in developing countries.
- Cutaneous disease has been associated with imported animal hair or fur.
- Food-borne outbreaks have been documented and related to ingestion of tainted meat.
- The major concern at this time is exposure of large populations to the organism via a terrorist attack.

Risk Factors
- In developing countries, the major risk is with exposure to contaminated soil or sick animals.
- In urban locations, the major risk is through exposure to contaminated hides and animal hairs.

INCUBATION PERIOD
- Cutaneous disease: 3 to 10 days
- Pulmonary disease: 3 to 5 days

Clinical Manifestations

Disease can manifest as cutaneous, respiratory, or gastrointestinal, but cutaneous is the most common form.

SYMPTOMS AND SIGNS
- Cutaneous disease begins as an ulcerating papule. Small vesicles may develop around this lesion. A circular eschar (1–3 cm) forms the classic lesion. This may progress to sepsis and death if not treated.
- Respiratory disease has been described as biphasic. Mild, viral-like upper respiratory illness lasts 2 to 4 days, followed by a severe fulminant pneumonitis leading to death.
- Gastrointestinal disease causes abdominal pain, nausea, vomiting, and fever, and it is associated with hematemesis and hematochezia.

Diagnosis

- A typical skin lesion should cause suspicion of anthrax, especially in a patient with exposure to sick or dead herbivores or animal hides or hairs.
- The diagnosis of pneumonia or gastroenteritis is difficult to establish due to the nonspecific nature of the illness. In the late stage of pulmonary disease, the mediastinum widens on chest x-ray.

Anthrax

DIFFERENTIAL DIAGNOSIS

- Cutaneous
  - Tularemia
  - *Staphylococcus aureus*
  - Spider bite
  - Burn lesion
- Pulmonary
  - Wide array of bacterial and viral processes
- Gastrointestinal
  - *Shigella*
  - *Yersinia*
  - *Campylobacter*

LABORATORY

- Cultures and Gram stains of vesicular lesions should reveal the organism, a large, encapsulated, gram-positive rod in short chains.
- Blood cultures are usually positive in febrile, acutely ill patients with pulmonary or gastrointestinal disease.
- Stool cultures reveal the organism in gastrointestinal disease.

IMAGING

Chest x-ray often reveals diffuse infiltrates and effusions. Widening of the mediastinum is sometimes seen late in the disease.

Treatment

- Primary skin lesions should be treated with penicillin G 6 to 8 million units per day, divided every 6 hours intravenously, or penicillin VK 500 mg every 6 hours orally.
- Sepsis should be treated with penicillin G 24 million units per day, divided every 6 hours intravenously.
- Erythromycin, ciprofloxacin, and tetracycline or doxycycline are alternatives in penicillin-allergic patients.

COMPLICATIONS

- Pulmonary disease and gastrointestinal disease are almost always fatal.
- Cutaneous disease often leaves a scar in the area of the eschar.

Follow-Up

Patients should be followed for evidence of recurrence of disease after therapy.

PREVENTION

- Vaccination of livestock is indicated in endemic areas.
- Decontamination of imported hides and animal hair would reduce risk.
- Anthrax vaccine is available to individuals with potential exposure to the organism. These include military personnel, veterinarians, and people exposed to imported hides or animal hairs.

Selected Readings

Inglesby TV, Henderson DA, Bartlett JG, et al. Anthrax as a biological weapon: Medical and public health management. Working Group on Civilian Biodefense. *JAMA* 1999;281(18):1735–1745.

Little SF, Ivins BE. Molecular pathogenesis of *Bacillus anthracis* infection. *Microbes Infect* 1999;1(2):131–139.

Antibiotic- and *Clostridium difficile*-associated Diarrhea and Colitis

Basics

DEFINITION

- The *term antibiotic-associated diarrhea and colitis* is used to describe a variety of clinical syndromes that occur during or within 4 to 6 weeks after antibiotic therapy that alters the bowel flora. Diagnosis requires that there is no other identifiable cause for diarrhea.
- Based on the degree of colonic involvement, it is divided in four categories:
  —Normal colonic mucosa
  —Mild erythema with some edema
  —Granular, friable, or hemorrhagic mucosa
  —Pseudomembrane formation

ETIOLOGY

- *Clostridium difficile,* a gram-positive, spore-forming anaerobic bacillus, is the most common identifiable pathogen causing antibiotic-associated diarrhea and colitis.
- Possible pathogens of antibiotic-associated diarrhea in *C. difficile*–negative patients include the following:
  —*Salmonella*
  —*Clostridium perfringens*
  —*Candida albicans*
  —*Staphylococcus aureus*
- In most cases of antibiotic-associated diarrhea in which *C. difficile* is not detected, no etiologic agent is identified.

PATHOGENESIS

- The first step in development of *C. difficile* colonization is disruption of the normal flora of the colon, usually caused by antibiotics or, in unusual cases, by certain antineoplastic drugs.
- The antibiotics most frequently associated with *C. difficile* infection are clindamycin, ampicillin, amoxicillin, and the cephalosporins. However, all broad-spectrum antibiotics can lead to the infection.
- Some strains of *C. difficile* are nontoxinogenic, but the majority make two protein exotoxins: toxin A and toxin B.
- Toxin A is mainly responsible for the disease, but toxin B is a much more potent cytotoxin in tissue culture.

EPIDEMIOLOGY

- *C. difficile* causes about three million cases of diarrhea and colitis in the United States every year. Most cases occur in hospitals or long-term care facilities, while the incidence of this infection in the outpatient setting is low, but not negligible.
- Transmission of the organism occurs from patient to patient, and the organism can be cultured from many environmental surfaces in rooms of infected patients and from the hands, clothing, and stethoscopes of health care workers.
- Hospital personnel may carry the bacteria from room to room and promote the infection, but fecal carriage by staff is rare.
- Toxinogenic *C. difficile* is isolated from stool specimens in approximately 3% of healthy adults, but colonization frequently occurs during hospitalization, and about a third of patients colonized with *C. difficile* develop clinical symptoms.

Clinical Manifestations

SYMPTOMS AND SIGNS

Diarrhea and Colitis Due to Clostridium difficile

- The clinical presentation is variable and includes diarrhea, colitis without pseudomembranes, pseudomembranous colitis, and fulminant colitis.
- Mild to moderate infection is usually accompanied by lower abdominal cramping pain, but no systemic symptoms or physical findings.
- Moderate or severe colitis usually presents with profuse diarrhea, abdominal distention with pain, and, in some cases, occult colonic bleeding. Also, systemic symptoms such as fever, nausea, anorexia, and malaise are usually present.
- A minority of patients have disease primarily in the cecum and right colon, presenting with marked leukocytosis and abdominal pain but little or no diarrhea.

Antibiotic-associated Diarrhea Not Related to Clostridium difficile

- Diarrhea is dose-related, usually mild, and not accompanied by abdominal pain or fever.
- There is often history of diarrhea with the same antibiotic, and symptoms usually resolve quickly after discontinuation of the inciting antibiotic.

Diagnosis

MICROBIOLOGY

C. difficile can be isolated by anaerobic stool culture, but this test is seldom used because it takes 2 to 3 days to complete and does not distinguish toxinogenic from nontoxinogenic strains.

IMAGING/ENDOSCOPY

- Diffusely thickened or edematous colonic mucosa may sometimes be seen by abdominal CT scan and may be very suggestive of the *C. difficile*–associated diarrhea or colitis.
- Endoscopy for *C. difficile*–associated diarrhea and colitis is reserved for special situations, such as when other diseases need to be ruled out, rapid diagnosis is necessary, or a stool sample cannot be obtained because the patient develops ileus.
- The results of sigmoidoscopy may be normal in patients with mild disease.
- Ten percent of episodes of colitis involve only the right colon and may be missed by flexible sigmoidoscopy.

OTHER TESTS

- Leukocytosis with a left shift and fecal leukocytes in about 50% to 60% of cases
- The average peripheral count is 12,000 to 20,000/mm^3, but occasionally the peripheral count is higher and cases of leukemoid reaction have been described.
- Gram stain of fecal specimens is of no value in diagnosing *C. difficile*–associated diarrhea.
- The most sensitive (94%–100%) and specific (99%) test for diagnosis of *C. difficile* infection is a tissue culture assay

Antibiotic- and *Clostridium difficile*–associated Diarrhea and Colitis

for the cytotoxicity of toxin B. However, the test takes 1 to 3 days to complete and requires tissue culture facilities.
- Enzyme-linked immunosorbent assays have been developed and have a sensitivity of 71% to 94% and a specificity of 92% to 98%. Because of the rapidity of testing and ease of performance, these tests are now used most frequently by clinical laboratories for diagnosis of *C. difficile* infection.
- Approximately 20% of patients may require more than one stool assay to detect *C. difficile* toxin. When *C. difficile* infection is suspected, a single stool specimen should be sent. If the results are negative and diarrhea persists, one or two additional stool samples could be sent.

Treatment

MAIN TREATMENT

- The inciting antibiotic should be discontinued if possible.
- Supportive therapy with fluids and electrolytes should be instituted, as needed.
- Antibiotic-associated diarrhea will resolve without specific antimicrobial therapy in up to one-fourth of patients with infection and in almost all cases of non-*C. difficile*–associated diarrhea due to antibiotics.
- Antiperistaltic and opiate drugs should be avoided in patients with *C. difficile*–associated diarrhea, because they mask symptoms and may worsen the course of the disease.
- Antibiotic therapy is indicated for patients with moderate or severe infection with *C. difficile*, and antimicrobial therapy can be instituted even before the laboratory results are available.
- Oral metronidazole (500 mg tid or 250 mg qid orally) or vancomycin (125 mg qid orally) is the antibiotic most commonly used. The duration of initial therapy is usually 10 to 14 days (or therapy may be continued until 1 week after completion of the inciting antibiotic, if that cannot be stopped earlier).
- Because of lower cost and avoidance of selective pressure for vancomycin-resistant organisms such as vancomycin-resistant enterococci, initial therapy with metronidazole is currently the preferred initial therapy for *C. difficile* colitis. Some authorities prefer initial therapy with vancomycin in the most severely ill patients, or in women who are pregnant or in children less than 10 years of age, in whom metronidazole should be avoided if possible.

ALTERNATIVE TREATMENT

- Oral bacitracin (20,000 to 25,000 U qid)
- For critically ill patients who are unable to take oral antimicrobials, treatment is empirical and may include intravenous metronidazole (given as 500 mg i.v. q8h), administration of vancomycin by rectal enema or through long catheters in the small intestine, or, occasionally, surgery (usually subtotal colectomy).

TREATMENT OF RELAPSES

- Mild relapses can be managed without further antibiotic treatment.
- Because the relapses are not related to development of resistance, another 10- to 14-day course of either oral metronidazole or vancomycin can be administered (i.e., you can just repeat the same treatment for the same duration).
- In cases of recurrent *C. difficile*–associated diarrhea, most clinicians employ tapering oral doses of vancomycin over a 6-week period:
  —Week 1: vancomycin 125 mg qid
  —Week 2: vancomycin 125 mg bid
  —Week 3: vancomycin 125 mg qd
  —Week 4: vancomycin 125 mg qod
  —Weeks 5 and 6: vancomycin 125 mg every 3 days

COMPLICATIONS

- *C. difficile* diarrhea and colitis can complicate idiopathic inflammatory bowel disease or lead to the following:
  —Hyperpyrexia
  —Fulminant colitis
  —Ileus
  —Perforation
  —Toxic megacolon
  —Reactive arthritis
  —Chronic diarrhea
  —Hypoalbuminemia with anasarca

Follow-Up

TYPICAL PROGRESSION AND PROGNOSIS

- Approximately 2% to 3% of patients develop fulminant colitis, with ileus, toxic megacolon, perforation, and death.
- The relapse rate among patients with *C. difficile* infection is 10% to 20%. A smaller number of patients have multiple relapses.

PATIENT FOLLOW-UP

- No diagnostic testing at the end of treatment or during follow-up is needed, unless symptoms recur.
- Clinicians should monitor patients for the development of complications of *C. difficile* infection.
- The development of life-threatening complications (ileus, toxic megacolon, perforation, etc.) might be accompanied by a decrease in diarrhea due to loss of colonic muscular tone and ileus.

PREVENTION

- Enteric isolation precautions are recommended for patients with *C. difficile*–associated diarrhea or colitis, and patients should be moved to a private room, if possible.
- Educate personnel to use gloves when in contact with patients with *C. difficile* infection and for the handling of body substances.
- Avoid nonessential antibiotic prescription.

Selected Readings

Bartlett JG. Antibiotic-associated diarrhea. *Clin Infect Dis* 1992;15:573–581.

Johnson S, Gerding DN. *Clostridium difficile*–associated diarrhea. *Clin Infect Dis* 1998;26:1027–1036.

Kelly CP, LaMont JT. *Clostridium difficile* infection. *Annu Rev Med* 1998;49:375–390.

Mylonakis E, Ryan ET, Calderwood SB. *Clostridium difficile*-associated diarrhea. A review. *Arch Intern Med* 2001;161:525–533.

Appendicitis

Basics

DEFINITION
- Appendicitis is inflammation of the appendix. If the inflammation compromises the blood supply to the organ, it is called *gangrenous appendicitis;* and if it leads to perforation, it is called *perforating appendicitis*.
- When the appendicitis is triggered by obstruction of the lumen of the organ, the term *obstructive appendicitis* is used.

ETIOLOGY
- Luminal obstruction has always been thought to be the first step in the development of appendicitis. However, recent studies have shown that ulceration of the mucosa is the initial event in the majority of cases.
- Obstruction, when present, is most commonly caused by the following:
  —A fecalith
  —Enlarged lymphoid follicles associated with viral infections (e.g., measles)
  —Worms
  —Tumors (e.g., carcinoid or carcinoma)
- Luminal bacteria multiply and invade the appendiceal wall, as venous engorgement and subsequent arterial compromise result from the high intraluminal pressures.
- Finally, gangrene and perforation occur.
- If the process evolves slowly, a localized abscess can develop.
- Rupture of primary appendiceal abscesses may produce fistulas between the appendix and other organs.
- Occasionally, acute appendicitis may be the first manifestation of Crohn's disease.
- In relatively uncommon cases, recurrent acute appendicitis with complete resolution of inflammation and symptoms between attacks can occur. Also, chronic infection of the appendix with tuberculosis, amebiasis, and actinomycosis may occur.

EPIDEMIOLOGY

Incidence
- Each year in the United States there are at least 250,000 new cases of appendicitis, requiring hospital admission for more than 1 million patient-days.
- A similar number of patients with suspected appendicitis are hospitalized but are found to have other conditions.
- The appendix is normal in 15% to 40% of patients who undergo emergency appendectomy.
- In at least 20% of patients with appendicitis, the correct diagnosis is not made. Missed appendicitis is the most frequently successful malpractice claim against emergency department physicians.

Risk Factors
- Acute appendicitis can occur at any time of life, but the maximum incidence occurs in the second and third decades of life.
- Perforation is relatively much more common in infancy and in the aged.
- Males and females are equally affected, except between puberty and age 25, when the ratio is 3:2.

Clinical Manifestations

SYMPTOMS
- The abdominal pain in the beginning is usually poorly localized in the periumbilical or epigastric region. As inflammation spreads to the parietal peritoneal surfaces, the pain becomes somatic, steady, and more severe, aggravated by motion or cough, and usually located in the right lower quadrant.
- There is often an accompanying urge to defecate or pass flatus, neither of which relieves the distress.
- Anorexia is so frequent that the presence of hunger should arouse suspicion of the diagnosis of acute appendicitis.
- Nausea and vomiting occur in 50% to 60% of cases, but vomiting is rarely profuse and protracted.
- The development of nausea and vomiting before the onset of pain is extremely rare.
- Urinary frequency and dysuria occur if the appendix lies adjacent to the bladder.

SIGNS
- Physical findings vary with time after onset of the illness and according to the location of the appendix.
- While tenderness is sometimes absent in the early visceral stage of the disease, it ultimately develops and is found in any location corresponding to the position of the appendix.
- Percussion, rebound tenderness, and referred rebound tenderness are often present. These signs are most likely to be absent early in the illness. Flexion of the right hip and guarded movement by the patient are due to parietal peritoneal involvement.
- The temperature is usually normal or slightly elevated, but a temperature above 38.3°C (101°F) should always suggest the presence of perforation.
- The presence of rigidity, a positive psoas sign, fever, and rebound tenderness are signs on physical examination indicating an increased likelihood of appendicitis.

Diagnosis

DIFFERENTIAL DIAGNOSIS
- The absence of right lower quadrant pain, the absence of the classic migration of pain, and the presence of similar pain previously are powerful symptoms in the history that make appendicitis less likely. In the physical examination, the lack of right lower quadrant pain, rigidity, or guarding makes appendicitis less likely.
- When acute appendicitis is erroneously diagnosed, the most common conditions

Appendicitis

discovered at operation are the following:
- Acute cholecystitis
- Acute diverticulitis
- Acute gastroenteritis
- Acute pancreatitis
- Acute pelvic inflammatory disease
- Endometriosis
- Mesenteric lymphadenitis
- Perforated ulcer
- Pyelonephritis
- Ruptured graafian follicle or corpus luteum cyst
- Ruptured tubal pregnancy
- Strangulating intestinal obstruction
- Twisted ovarian cyst
- Ureteral calculus

- It is also necessary to consider the possibility of Munchausen's syndrome or even Munchausen's syndrome by proxy.
- The differential diagnosis of acute appendicitis is discussed in more detail in the Section I chapter, "Abdominal Pain and Fever."

LABORATORY

- Leukocytosis of 10,000 to 18,000 cells per milliliter with a left shift is frequent, but the absence of leukocytosis does not eliminate the possibility of acute appendicitis.
- Urinalysis is most useful in excluding genitourinary conditions that may mimic acute appendicitis.

IMAGING

- Of the noninvasive diagnostic aids, appendiceal computed tomography (CT) has proved more precise, with an accuracy of more than 90%.
- The highest accuracy has been reported with the use of helical CT after the instillation of 3% diatrizoate meglumine (Gastrografin)–saline solution into the colon.
- Appendiceal CT is safe, can be performed in approximately 15 minutes, and requires only one-third of the radiation exposure of standard CT of the abdomen and pelvis.
- Routine appendiceal CT performed in patients who present with suspected appendicitis improves patient care and reduces the use of hospital resources.

- Ultrasound is most useful to exclude ovarian cysts, ectopic pregnancy, or tuboovarian abscess.
- Normal ultrasonographic findings should not deter the surgeon from performing an appendectomy if the history is indicative of appendicitis and unequivocal tenderness is present in the right lower quadrant.

Treatment

MAIN TREATMENT

- The management options available to physicians evaluating patients with suspected appendicitis include hospital observation, diagnostic imaging, laparoscopy, and appendectomy.
- Cathartics and enemas should be avoided if appendicitis is under consideration, and antibiotics should not be administered when the diagnosis is in question, because they will only mask the presence or development of perforation.
- The treatment is early operation and appendectomy as soon as the patient can be prepared.
- Appendectomy is increasingly accomplished laparoscopically, but there is no demonstrable value of this technique over open operation, except where a diagnostic dilemma exists.
- If a palpable mass is present 3 to 5 days after the onset of symptoms, operation should be delayed, because a phlegmon rather than a definitive abscess will be found. Such patients should be treated with broad-spectrum antibiotics, parenteral fluids, and rest. Appendectomy can and should be done safely 3 months later. Should the mass enlarge or the patient become more toxic, drainage of the abscess is necessary.
- The antibiotic management is the same as in other intraabdominal infections and is detailed in the Section II chapters, "Peritonitis" and "Intraabdominal Abscess."

COMPLICATIONS

- Delay in the diagnosis increases the risk of appendiceal perforation, which increases the risk of postoperative complications to 39%, as compared with 8% for simple appendicitis.
- The mortality rate has decreased steadily in Europe and the United States to less than 1 per 100,000.
- Perforation is rare before 24 hours after onset of symptoms, but the rate may be as high as 80% after 48 hours.
- For a perforated appendicitis, there is an overall mortality rate of 3%, a figure that increases to 15% in the elderly.
- The development of intraabdominal abscesses usually follows perforation with generalized peritonitis and can be avoided by early diagnosis of the disease.

Follow-Up

Because no finding on the clinical examination can effectively rule out appendicitis, close follow-up of patients with abdominal pain who do not receive further diagnostic testing is indicated.

PREVENTION

N/A

Selected Readings

McColl I. More precision in diagnosing appendicitis. *N Engl J Med* 1998;338:190–191.

Rao PM, Rhea JT, Novelline RA, et al. Effect of computed tomography of the appendix on treatment of patients and use of hospital resources. *N Engl J Med* 1998;338:141–146.

Silen W. Acute appendicitis. In: Fauci AS, Braunwald E, Isselbacher KJ, et al., eds. *Harrison's principles of internal medicine*, 14th ed. New York: McGraw-Hill, 1998:1658–1660.

Wagner JM, McKinney WP, Carpenter JL. Does this patient have appendicitis? *JAMA* 1996;276:1589–1594.

Aspergillosis

Basics

DEFINITION

- The term *aspergillosis* has been used to describe a wide range of illnesses, from simple colonization or allergic provocation to localized or disseminated invasive disease.
- Although any organ can be involved, the infection usually affects the lungs, and less often the paranasal sinuses and the central nervous system.

ETIOLOGY

- *Aspergillus* is a ubiquitous mold with septate hyphae.
- Disease in humans is usually due to *Aspergillus fumigatus* or *Aspergillus flavus* (second most common, usually causing invasive disease in immunocompromised patients and involving the paranasal sinuses), and less often due to *Aspergillus niger, Aspergillus terreus,* and others.

EPIDEMIOLOGY

- Aspergilloma (mycetoma or fungus ball) grow in preexisting cavities, usually from antecedent tuberculosis.
- Invasive aspergillosis is second in frequency to candidiasis among invasive mycoses in most immunosuppressed groups of patients.
- The most common predisposing factors for invasive infection are the following:
  —Granulocytopenia (probably the most significant predisposing factor)
  —Acquired immunodeficiency syndrome (AIDS) (almost always in patients with CD4 counts of 50 cells/mm^3 or less)
  —Prolonged corticosteroid or cytotoxic therapy
  —Bone marrow transplantation
  —Hematologic malignancy
  —Prolonged use of antibiotics
  —Liver failure
  —Diabetes mellitus
  —Chronic granulomatous disease of childhood

Clinical Manifestations

SYMPTOMS AND SIGNS

Hypersensitivity Lung Diseases

- Extrinsic asthma: inhalation of spores, causing IgE-mediated reaction
- Extrinsic allergic alveolitis (Farmer's lung): Sensitized individuals develop cough, dyspnea, fever, and diffuse pulmonary infiltrates after inhalation of spores.
- Allergic bronchopulmonary aspergillosis: Exposure can be from colonization in the respiratory tract or from the environment. Patients usually present with bronchospasm that may be accompanied by fever or cough with brown sputum.

Noninvasive Pulmonary Aspergillosis

Aspergilloma: cough and/or hemoptysis; less often weight loss, fatigue, chest pain, and fever are the most common symptoms. Some patients are asymptomatic (incidental finding on chest radiograph).

Invasive Aspergillosis

- Lung
  —Fever, cough, and dyspnea are the most common symptoms, but only a minority of patients have all three of these on presentation.
  —Other symptoms include pleuritic chest pain, generalized malaise, weight loss, and hemoptysis. The same clinical features are seen in necrotizing bronchitis with pseudomembrane formation that is a variant of the invasive infection, usually seen in patients with AIDS and in patients with tracheobronchitis due to *Aspergillus*.
- Sinus
  —Fever
  —Local pain and tenderness
  —Nasal or ear discharge
  —Headache
- Central nervous system
  —Symptoms include seizure activity or focal neurologic deficits and vary based on the location of the lesion. Meningitis is uncommon.
- Other forms of invasive aspergillosis
  —Disseminated or localized invasive aspergillosis can affect virtually any organ.
  —Involvement of the external ear canal and pinna (otomycosis) is usually benign.
  —Endocarditis on a native or prosthetic valve or in a mural location resembles bacterial endocarditis and is characterized by negative blood cultures and peripheral embolization.
  —Multiple cutaneous erythematous papules and pustules or, usually, necrotic lesions can occur as a result of hematogenous spread.

Diagnosis

- Hypersensitivity lung diseases
  —Allergic bronchopulmonary aspergillosis: Clues to the diagnosis are the following:
    —Peripheral eosinophilia
    —Immediate reaction to skin testing with *Aspergillus*
    —Elevated total serum IgE and IgG
    —Fleeting pulmonary infiltrates (also noted in extrinsic allergic alveolates)
  —Bronchiectasis
- Noninvasive pulmonary aspergillosis
  —Chest radiograph shows the fungus ball, often surrounded by the air-crescent shadow.
  —The radiologic findings are better seen by CT or MRI.
  —Usually, patients have intermittently positive sputum (smear and culture) and high titers of IgG antibody to *Aspergillus*.
- Invasive aspergillosis

MICROBIOLOGY

- Definitive diagnosis can be made by finding tissue invasion on histology *and* culture.
- In the appropriate clinical scenario, aggressive antifungal therapy should be initiated, pending definitive diagnosis.
- Blood cultures are almost always negative, even among patients with endocarditis.
- Isolation of *Aspergillus* from sputum cultures is of limited value, because the fungus can be colonizing the respiratory tract without causing invasive disease.

Aspergillosis

- Examination of bronchoalveolar lavage or transbronchial, percutaneous transthoracic, or open lung biopsy is used to confirm the diagnosis.
- Isolation of aspergilli from nasal cultures and antibody testing by a variety of techniques are under evaluation.

IMAGING

- Cavitation of the pulmonary lesion is absent in the majority of cases.
- CT and especially MRI can help by demonstrating target-like lesions, but are not pathognomonic and are mainly used in evaluation of the extent of the lesion and for follow-up of the lesion.

SPECIFIC TESTS

Serologic tests have no established value in the diagnosis of invasive disease.

Treatment

- Extrinsic alveolitis
  - Main treatment
    - Avoidance of the stimulus
- Other hypersensitivity lung diseases
  - Main treatment
    - Corticosteroids during exacerbations
  - Alternative treatment
    - Itraconazole might be beneficial.
- Noninvasive pulmonary aspergillosis
  - Main treatment
    - Management is individualized. Surgery has a role, especially in patients with recurrent, significant hemoptysis.
  - Alternative treatment
    - Bronchial artery embolization and less often intracavitary amphotericin B or itraconazole are used.
- Invasive aspergillosis
  - Main treatment
    - Surgical drainage or debridement whenever possible
    - Amphotericin B in daily dosages of up to 1 mg/kg (total dose of at least 30 mg/kg) or even higher is still the therapy of choice. Combination with flucytosine and, especially, rifampin does not seem to be beneficial.
  - Alternative treatment
    - Liposomal formulations of amphotericin B (liposomal amphotericin B, lipid complex, and colloidal dispension) in daily doses at least three times higher than that of regular amphotericin B can be used in patients who cannot tolerate the regular form.
    - Itraconazole (no intravenous form available) is approved by the Food and Drug Administration as a second-line agent for patients who are intolerant of or who have failed amphotericin B therapy.

COMPLICATIONS

- Bronchiectasis can complicate allergic bronchopulmonary aspergillosis.
- Pulmonary fibrosis can complicate both allergic bronchopulmonary aspergillosis and extrinsic allergic alveolitis.
- Hemoptysis (sometimes massive, especially for lesions located close to the hilum) can complicate both invasive and noninvasive pulmonary aspergillosis.
- Pneumothorax might occur in immunocompromised individuals and is usually associated with improvement of the immune system.
- Introduction of aspergilli to the pleural space (due to pneumothorax or the development of bronchopleural fistula) can lead to empyema.
- In all cases of pulmonary and extrapulmonary invasive aspergillosis, relentless dissemination to other organs and an increase of the lesion can occur, especially among immunocompromised individuals.
- Patients with CNS involvement can have cerebral vessels occluded by *Aspergillus*.

Follow-Up

TYPICAL PROGRESSION AND PROGNOSIS

- The prognosis of allergic bronchopulmonary aspergillosis and extrinsic allergic alveolitis is variable. Patients can experience no loss of pulmonary function, but allergic bronchopulmonary aspergillosis might lead to bronchiectasis or pulmonary fibrosis.
- Up to one-fourth of patients with aspergillomas, treated without surgery, die, usually due to hemoptysis. The average surgical mortality is 7%.
- Mortality among patients with invasive disease is very high. It is associated with the course of the underlying disease and can be up to 80%, or even higher among certain populations of immunosuppressed patients.

PATIENT FOLLOW-UP

- Patients with hypersensitivity lung diseases should be monitored for relapses and for the development of pulmonary fibrosis or bronchiectasis.
- Patients with aspergillomas that do not undergo surgery need clinical and radiographic monitoring for extension of the lesion and development of hemoptysis. Patients that undergo surgery for aspergilloma need to be monitored for relapse of the infection, even after initial surgical success.
- Patients with invasive disease need to be monitored for relapses, especially when they become neutropenic.

PREVENTION

Possible preventive measures include the following:

- Environmental control measures, especially during construction activities, to prevent conidia from reaching patients at risk
- Air-flow units with high-efficacy particulate air filters
- Prophylactic use of amphotericin B: might be considered in patients with previous invasive disease who could become neutropenic
- Ketoconazole and fluconazole: no effect in prophylaxis

Selected Readings

Denning DW, Stevens DA. The treatment of invasive aspergillosis. *Rev Infect Dis* 1990;12:1147.

Mylonakis E, Barlam TF, Flanigan T, et al. Pulmonary aspergillosis in the acquired immunodeficiency syndrome: Review of 342 cases. *Chest* 1998;114:251–262.

Mylonakis E, Rich J, Skolnik P, et al. Invasive *Aspergillus* sinusitis in patients with human immunodeficiency virus infection. Report of two cases and review. *Medicine (Baltimore)* 1997;76:249–255.

Mylonakis E, Paliou M, Sax PE, Skolnik PR, Baron MJ, Rich JD. Central nervous system aspergillosis in patients with human immunodeficiency virus infection. *Medicine (Baltimore)* 2000;79:269–280.

Atypical Mycobacteria

Basics

DEFINITION

Many mycobacterial species can produce disease in humans. These include skin and soft-tissue infections, lymphadenitis, pulmonary disease, and disseminated disease, as seen in patients with AIDS. In general, atypical mycobacteria are not spread from human to human. Of concern is the fact that many species of mycobacteria are drug resistant.

ETIOLOGY

Large numbers of pathogens are divided up by the rate of growth in culture.

- Rapid-growing organisms include the following:
  - *Mycobacterium fortuitum* complex
  - *Mycobacterium chelonei/abscessus*
  - *Mycobacterium smegmatis*
- Intermediate-growing organisms include the following:
  - *Mycobacterium marinum*
  - *Mycobacterium gordonae*
  - *Mycobacterium haemophilum*
  - *Mycobacterium ulcerans*
- Slow-growing organisms include the following:
  - *Mycobacterium avium* complex (MAC)
  - *Mycobacterium kansasii*
  - *Mycobacterium xenopi*
  - *Mycobacterium scrofulaceum*

EPIDEMIOLOGY

MYCOBACTERIUM AVIUM COMPLEX

- MAC organisms are ubiquitous, found in water, soil, and air.
- Disseminated MAC infection is the most common systemic bacterial infection in AIDS patients.

MYCOBACTERIUM KANSASII

- The reservoir of *M. kansasii* is not known. It has been noted to be in the water supply.
- Prevalence is highest in the midwestern portion of the United States and in Great Britain.
- Disease is often clustered in cities.

MYCOBACTERIUM MARINUM

The organism resides in fresh and salt water.

MYCOBACTERIUM ULCERANS

M. ulcerans is present in Mexico, Australia, and Africa.

Clinical Manifestations

SKIN AND SOFT-TISSUE INFECTIONS

- Most skin infections related to atypical mycobacteria are caused by *M. marinum*.
- *M. marinum* is contracted by immersion of the skin within a fish tank or nonchlorinated swimming pool, or after skin injury in a saltwater locale (swimming pool granulomata, fish-handler's nodules).
- Incubation takes up to 3 weeks.
- Patients note small, often purple papular lesions, usually on the extremities. These lesions may ulcerate or spread locally.
- Ulcerative or nodular skin infection with *M. marinum* or *M. haemophilum* often spreads extensively in patients with HIV or in patients on immunosuppressants.

DIFFERENTIAL DIAGNOSIS

- Other mycobacterial organisms that can lead to similar-looking skin infections include the following:
  - *M. abscessus*
  - *M. chelonae*
  - *M. fortuitum*
- These often occur in the setting of skin trauma.

- At times, nosocomial spread can occur within surgical wounds or within arteriovenous fistulas or central catheters.
- *Mycobacterium bovis* infection following cystic infusion for bladder carcinoma has been described as having caused an implantable defibrillator pocket infection.

PULMONARY INFECTIONS

- Atypical mycobacterial infections often occur in patients with preexisting lung disease, such as cystic fibrosis, silicosis, healed tuberculosis, bronchiectasis, or chronic obstructive lung disease.
- Reports of atypical mycobacterial disease in healthy patients are rare, but present.
- Patients note chronic cough, low-grade fevers, and, on occasion, weight loss.
- Patients' ages are often in the middle or older years.
- Organisms isolated from the sputum include MAC, *M. kansasii*, *M. xenopi*, or *M. abscessus*, *M. fortuitum*, and *M. chelonae*.
- Chest x-ray in patients with atypical mycobacterial pulmonary disease may reveal upper lobe cavitary disease, nodular or reticulonodular disease, or adenopathy.
- Effusions are rare.
- At times, it is hard to distinguish between underlying pulmonary disease and atypical mycobacterial infection.
- *M. kansasii* can produce extensive upper lobe cavitary disease.
- At times, surgery is needed to remove badly diseased lung tissue.

LYMPHADENITIS

- Atypical mycobacteria should be considered in patients with unilateral cervical lymphadenitis.
- Most commonly, this infection occurs in children ages 1 through 5 years.
- Swelling often occurs around the affected nodes, usually in the anterior cervical chain. The adenitis may enlarge rapidly, and fistula formation through the skin is common. Enlarged nodes are often painless.

Atypical Mycobacteria

- Systemic symptoms are rare.
- Most symptoms are caused by MAC; *M. scrofulaceum* and *M. tuberculosis* are also encountered, but less frequently.

DISSEMINATED INFECTION

- Disseminated infection occurs in the setting of profound immunosuppression.
- In patients with AIDS, it is seen when the CD4 count dips below 100 cells/mm^3.
- Disease in this population is caused by MAC, but, at times, *M. kansasii* can cause disseminated infection.
- Most organs are affected, and bone marrow cultures and blood cultures are frequently positive.
- The time between initial contact with the organism (gastrointestinal tract or lung) and development of dissemination in AIDS patients is 6 to 12 months.

Diagnosis

- There is cross-reaction on the purified protein derivative (PPD) test with *M. kansasii* and *M. tuberculosis*.
- Cultures for mycobacteria should be obtained from skin, sputum, or blood/bone marrow. Cultures of *M. marinum, M. chelonae,* and *M. haemophilum* should be plated at 28°C.
- RNA probes can help with early diagnosis of *M. tuberculosis,* MAC, and *M. kansasii*.

DIFFERENTIAL DIAGNOSIS

M. tuberculosis needs to be ruled out in most instances.

Treatment

MYCOBACTERIUM AVIUM *INFECTIONS*

- Clarithromycin 500 mg orally twice per day (azithromycin 500 mg PO qd) plus ethambutol 15 mg/kg orally once per day
- Rifampin 600 mg orally every day should also be considered.
- Pulmonary disease should be treated until the sputum cultures remain negative for 1 year.
- Disseminated disease in AIDS patients should be treated for life.

MYCOBACTERIUM MARINUM *SKIN INFECTIONS*

- All regimes should be given for a minimum of 3 months.
- Clarithromycin 500 mg orally twice per day
- Alternatives: Minocycline 100 mg orally twice per day or a combination of rifampin 600 mg/d and ethambutol 15 mg/kg/d

MYCOBACTERIUM KANSASII *PNEUMONIA*

- Isoniazid 300 mg once per day with rifampin 600 mg/d and ethambutol 600 mg/d
- Treatment should be for at least 18 months, and sputum cultures should be negative for at least 12 months prior to discontinuing medications. Ethambutol can be stopped after 9 to 12 months.

COMPLICATIONS

Complications are often secondary to the slow progression of these diverse illnesses and arise from the effects of the often toxic medications needed for treatment.

Follow-Up

Because of the drug resistance of these indolent organisms, specialists with knowledge of these infections are needed for treatment. At times, patients require years of therapy.

PREVENTION

- In patients with AIDS, filtering water or drinking bottled water can decrease the likelihood of infection with MAC.
- In patients with CD4 counts less than 100 cells/mm^3, weekly azithromycin 1,200 mg orally, or daily clarithromycin 500 mg orally bid, or rifabutin 300 mg orally once per day has been shown to be effective in preventing disseminated MAC.

Selected Readings

American Thoracic Society. Diagnosis and treatment of disease caused by nontuberculous mycobacteria. *Am Rev Respir Dis* 1990;142:940.

Kalayjian R, Toossi Z, Tomachefski J, et al. Pulmonary disease due to infection by *Mycobacterium avium* complex in patients with AIDS. *Clin Infect Dis* 1995;20:1186.

O'Brien RJ, Geiter LJ, Snider DE. The epidemiology of nontuberculous mycobacterial diseases in the United States: Results from a national survey. *Am Rev Respir Dis* 1987;135:1007.

Babesiosis

Basics

DEFINITION
- Febrile illness with many similarities to malaria, caused by the protozoa *Babesia*

ETIOLOGY
- *Babesia microti, Babesia divergens,* and *Babesia bovis*

EPIDEMIOLOGY
Incidence and Prevalence
- There is a complex life cycle in this zoonotic illness.
- The white-footed mouse is a major reservoir of infection in the United States. The vector to humans is the *Ixodes* tick.
- Most cases are from the New England coastal regions, but there are other cases from Washington State.
- Seroprevalence in areas of risk are about 4% to 5%.

Risk Factors
- Exposure to ticks is the main risk factor.
- Incidence of severe disease increases with the following:
  - Age over 50
  - Asplenia
  - Immunodeficiency
- One must always consider coinfection with *Borrelia burgdorferi*.

Incubation
- One to 3 weeks after tick bite

Clinical Manifestations

- Most infections are unnoticed.
- Fever
- Chills
- Headache
- Photophobia
- In patients with overwhelming parasitemia, acute respiratory distress syndrome, hemolytic anemia, and shock may occur.

Diagnosis

DIFFERENTIAL DIAGNOSIS
- Viral syndromes
- Malaria

LABORATORY
- White blood counts are normal or elevated.
- Thrombocytopenia is common.
- Anemia may be a result of hemolysis.
- LDH may be elevated.
- Thin or thick smears should reveal intraerythrocytic organisms.
- A serologic test confirms previous exposure and is available from the Centers for Disease Control and Prevention.

Babesiosis

Treatment

- In patients with severe disease, clindamycin 600 mg i.v. every 6 hours and quinine 650 mg every 6 hours for 7 days
- Exchange transfusions are useful in patients with high levels of parasitemia.
- For less severe disease, the clindamycin and quinine can be given orally.

COMPLICATIONS

On rare occasions, infection can lead to death.

Follow-Up

PREVENTION

- High-risk individuals (aging, asplenia, immunodeficiency) should take the most precautions when entering an endemic area.
- Prevent tick bites with restrictive clothing and insect repellant.

Selected Readings

Jacoby GA, Hunt JV, Kosinski KS, et al. Treatment of transfusion-transmitted babesiosis by exchange transfusion. *N Engl J Med* 1980;303:1098–1100.

Krause PJ, Spielman A, Telford SR III, et al. Persistent parasitemia after acute babesiosis. *N Engl J Med* 1998;339:160–165.

Ruebush TK II, Juranek DD, Chrisholm ES, et al. Human babesiosis on Nantucket Island: Evidence of self-limited and subclinical infections. *N Engl J Med* 1977;297:825–827.

Bacillary Angiomatosis/Peliosis Hepatica

Basics

DEFINITION

- Rare, vascular proliferative infectious disease of the skin and viscera, most commonly seen in the immunosuppressed (T-cell deficiencies), especially HIV-positive individuals
- The term *bacillary angiomatosis* mainly describes the cutaneous/disseminated form, while the term *peliosis hepatica* describes the visceral form of this febrile illness related to *Rochalimaea* (*Bartonella*) species.

ETIOLOGY

- *Rochalimaea henselae* (mainly bacillary angiomatosis) and *Rochalimaea quintana* (mainly bacteremia)
- *Rochalimaea* (now renamed *Bartonella*) species are gram-negative organisms of the alpha Proteobacteria family.
- Cats are the main animal reservoir for *R. henselae*; *R. quintana* can be transmitted via the body louse.
- Cat scratches seem to be the usual mode of transmission of *R. henselae*.

EPIDEMIOLOGY

This globally encountered disease is rare; isolated cases have been described from all areas of the world.

Risk Factors

- HIV infection (CD4 < 200)
- Other forms of immunosuppression
- Poor sanitary conditions, contact with cats

Incubation Period and Natural History

- The incubation period is at least 1 week.
- Manifestations range from isolated bacteremia to skin and visceral (peliosis hepatica) disease, as well as multiple organ (skin, bones, CNS) involvement.
- If untreated, it can be fatal.

Clinical Manifestations

SYMPTOMS

- Bacillary angiomatosis
  - Constitutional: fever, malaise, weight loss, anemia
- Peliosis hepatica
  - Constitutional: persistent fever, malaise, weight loss, abdominal pain
  - Gastrointestinal symptoms: nausea, vomiting
- Other organ/system symptoms depend on the specific part of the body affected (i.e., bone pain, neurologic deficits, etc.).

SIGNS

- Bacillary angiomatosis
  - Cutaneous manifestations (93% of patients)
    - Elevated, bright red papules, from one to hundreds in number and from 1 mm to several centimeters in size, in two-thirds of patients
    - Smaller lesions can be covered with an attenuated epidermis, while larger ones tend to erode and bleed easily.
    - A surrounding collarette is common.
    - Subcutaneous nodular lesions (in one-fourth of patients) are usually large, and there may be no overlying skin change.
    - Cellulitic plaque-like lesions (in 5%–10% of patients) often overlie deeper osseous lesions.
    - Ulcerations and folliculitis lesions are rare.
    - Lesions occur in any part of the body; several forms develop concurrently or sequentially.
    - Extracutaneous manifestations: These are mainly bone and visceral (liver, spleen) lesions, but several other organ/system involvements have been reported, with or without vascular proliferation changes, painful or painless lymphadenopathy, and CNS abscesses. Bone disease can begin with pain only and can be accompanied, or not, by overlying skin lesions.
- Peliosis hepatica
  - Massive hepatomegaly, developing over weeks or months
  - Splenomegaly
  - Possible skin or other organ involvement

Diagnosis

DIFFERENTIAL DIAGNOSIS

- Bacillary angiomatosis
  - Kaposi's sarcoma
  - Pyogenic granulomas
  - Angiomas
  - Verruga peruana (bartonellosis, endemic in South America)
- Peliosis hepatica
  - Kaposi's sarcoma
- Extracutaneous manifestations
  - Other space-occurring lesions
  - The possibility of coexistence with Kaposi's sarcoma should always be considered.

MICROBIOLOGY

- Diagnosis is made by demonstration of causative organisms in hematoxylin and eosin–stained tissue sections (granular purple material); it also may be made by the Warthin-Starry or Brown-Hopp's tissue stains.
- Organisms appear individually or in clumps and tangles.
- Obtaining culture is difficult and time consuming.
- PCR can be used to identify the precise *Bartonella* type.
- Serology is not helpful.

Bacillary Angiomatosis/Peliosis Hepatica

PATHOLOGY

- Skin, liver, and lymph node biopsy or fine-needle aspiration specimens are usually used.
- The pathologic pattern depends on the organ involved.
- Skin: "epithelioid hemangioma" appearance of lesions, demonstration of organisms
- Peliosis hepatica: In liver biopsy specimens, markedly dilated, blood-filled cystic spaces can be seen within the parenchyma. They are often associated with a myxoid stroma. Foci of necrosis can be seen in advanced cases.

BIOCHEMISTRY/HEMATOLOGY

- Mild elevation of transaminases (average ×2 of normal), moderate to severe elevation of alkaline phosphatase (average ×5 of normal), normal or slightly elevated bilirubin
- Mild to moderate pancytopenia may occur in the visceral type of the disease.

IMAGING

- Bone disease: plain bone x-rays show well-circumscribed lytic areas or ill-defined regions of extensive cortical destruction with aggressive periosteal reaction.
- CT scans can show hepatosplenomegaly and intraabdominal and/or retroperitoneal lymph node enlargement. Visceral parenchyma can appear heterogeneous in consistency.

Treatment

MAIN TREATMENT

- An initial evaluation is needed to determine the extent of organ involvement.
- Erythromycin 500 mg PO q6h for 8 weeks initially
- HIV-positive patients with osteolytic lesions need at least 4 months of treatment, and patients with visceral disease need at least 3 months of treatment.
- Patients can usually be treated on an outpatient basis; inpatient care and intravenous antibiotics are needed for patients with extensive skin disease, lytic bone lesions, and/or visceral lesions or fulminant disease.
- Patients may experience a Jarisch-Herxheimer reaction and should be pretreated with antipyretic agents for the first 72 hours of therapy.
- After initiation of treatment (about 4–7 days of therapy), significant improvement of skin and visceral/other organ lesions is noted frequently.
- There is usually complete resolution by 3 to 4 weeks.
- Relapses occur in approximately 15% of cases.

ALTERNATIVE TREATMENT

- For erythromycin intolerance: doxycycline 100 mg q12h for 8 weeks
- Tetracycline and/or rifampicin
- Ciprofloxacin

TREATMENT FAILURE

- On relapse, 4 months or continuous suppressive treatment

COMPLICATIONS

The visceral form of the disease can be complicated by anaemia, pancytopenia due to hypersplenism, and splenic rupture with haemoperitoneum.

Follow-Up

- Clinical monitoring is essential.
- Serial biochemical tests (i.e., liver function tests) may help in monitoring response to treatment of visceral disease.
- Use x-rays or bone scans to monitor bone disease.
- The possibility of coexistence with Kaposi's sarcoma should be considered if imaging findings will not reverse after appropriate antibiotic treatment.

PREVENTION

- In HIV-positive or otherwise immunocompromised patients, regarding cats: It is best to obtain a cat over 1 year of age and in good health. The patient should observe careful handwashing after litter box cleaning. Avoid bites and scratches; handwash if they happen. Declawing or testing a cat is not suggested.
- The possible necessity of secondary prophylaxis or life-long continuation of treatment in HIV-positive patients has not been defined.

Selected Readings

Gasquet S, Maurin M, Brouqui P, et al. Bacillary angiomatosis in immunocompromised patients. *AIDS* 1998;12(14):1793–1803.

Huh YB, Rose S, Schoen RE, et al. Colonic bacillary angiomatosis. *Ann Intern Med* 1996;124:735–737.

Spach DH, Koehlet JE. *Bartonella*-associated infections. *Infect Dis Clin North Am* 1998;12(1):137–155.

Tappero JW, Koehler JE, Berger TG, et al. Bacillary angiomatosis and bacillary splenitis in immunocompetent adults. *Ann Intern Med* 1993;118:331–336.

Bacterial Vaginosis

Basics

DEFINITION
- Vaginal discharge with an offensive odor
- Although linked epidemiologically with sexual activity, bacterial vaginosis (BV) is not considered a classic sexually transmitted disease (STD) because no specific pathogenic microbes are found in the sex partner, and treatment of the male consort does not prevent recurrences.

ETIOLOGY
- Previous studies observed *Haemophilus vaginalis* in 50% to 95% of women with BV, and in approximately 50% of healthy, asymptomatic women. After this organism was disqualified as the pathogen, the condition became known as "nonspecific vaginitis," now known as BV.
- Flora shift from normal predominance of peroxidase-producing lactobacilli to a polymicrobial, mainly anaerobic, consisting of *Bacteroides, Peptostreptococcus,* and *Mobiluncus,* along with *Haemophilus* and *Mycoplasma.*

EPIDEMIOLOGY

Incidence and Prevalence
- Fifty percent of diagnosed women are asymptomatic.
- BV is more common in non-White women and is typically found in the following:
  - 5% of asymptomatic college students
  - 15% to 20% of sexually active women
  - 10% to 30% of pregnant women
  - 30% to 60% of women seen at STD clinics

Risk Factors
- Sexual activity
- New sex partner
- Use of antibiotics
- Concurrent trichomoniasis
- Use of an intrauterine device

Clinical Manifestations

- Neither presenting symptoms nor the appearance of the vulva or vagina on direct inspection can separate vaginitis caused by BV, *Candida,* or *Trichomonas.*
- BV usually presents with the following:
  - Increased vaginal discharge
  - Offensive, "fishy" vaginal odor, which is worse after coitus
  - Mild or absent vulvovaginal irritation

Diagnosis

- Clinical diagnosis is based on the presence of any three of the four characteristics of vaginal discharge:
  - Thin, homogenous, milky, noninflammatory appearance
  - Clue cells (vaginal epithelial cells so overladen with bacteria that cell border is obscured)
  - pH greater than 4.5 (measure pH, using pH paper, which measures from 4.0 to 6.0)
  - Release of amine "fishy" odor upon mixing alkalinizing vaginal fluid with one drop of KOH (10%) solution
- Culture of vaginal fluid for *Haemophilus* or anaerobes is not advised.

DIFFERENTIAL DIAGNOSIS
- Other forms of vaginitis (e.g., *Candida, Trichomonas,* and herpes)

Bacterial Vaginosis

Treatment

- There is an 80% to 90% cure rate with appropriate antimicrobial drugs, administered either orally or intravaginally.
- Metronidazole is the preferred drug, administered 500 mg bid orally for 7 days. A 2-g single dose can be used but has lower cure rate.
- Clindamycin cream 2%, one full applicator of 5 g intravaginally at bedtime for 7 days
- Metronidazole gel 0.75%, one full applicator of 5 g intravaginally at bedtime for 5 days. Avoid during the first trimester of pregnancy.
- Clindamycin 300 mg bid for 7 days; safe to use throughout pregnancy
- Amoxicillin–clavulanic acid 250 mg tid for 7 days
- Oral regimens with little or no efficacy are the following:
  - Ampicillin
  - Cephalosporins
  - Quinolones
  - Tetracycline and erythromycin
  - Intravaginal sulfa creams
  - Povidone–iodine gel

COMPLICATIONS

- Adverse outcomes in pregnancy:
  - Preterm, low-birth-weight babies
  - Amniotic fluid retention
  - Chorioamnionic infection
  - Premature rupture of membranes
  - Postoperative infection following cesarean section
- Increased risk of postoperative infection following vaginal or abdominal hysterectomy
- Postabortion pelvic inflammatory disease

Follow-Up

There is a high risk of recurrence. Patients should be followed with periodic checkups and pelvic exams.

PREVENTION

- Safe-sex practices

Selected Readings

Flynn CA, Helwig AL, Meurer LN. Bacterial vaginosis in pregnancy and the risk of prematurity: A meta-analysis. *J Fam Pract* 1999;48(11):885–892.

Joesoef MR, Schmid GP, Hillier SL. Bacterial vaginosis: Review of treatment options and potential clinical indications for therapy. *Clin Infect Dis* 1999;28[Suppl 1]:S57–S65.

Sobel JD. Bacterial vaginosis. *Annu Rev Med* 2000;51:349–356.

Soper DE. Gynecologic sequelae of bacterial vaginosis. *Int J Gynaecol Obstet* 1999;67[Suppl 1]:S25–S28.

Balanitis

Basics

DEFINITION
- Inflammation and/or infection on the glans penis

ETIOLOGY
- Infectious
  - *Candida albicans*
  - *Trichomonas*
  - Anaerobic bacteria/*Bacteroides* spp
  - *Chlamydia*
  - *Mycoplasma*
- Noninfectious
  - Irritants, such as soaps

EPIDEMIOLOGY
Incidence and Prevalence
- Sexual exposure; increased incidence in men who have women sexual partners with candida vaginitis

Risk Factors
- Uncircumcised men
- Diabetes, especially new-onset diabetes
- Broad-spectrum antibiotics
- Immunodeficiency
- Poor hygiene

Clinical Manifestations

SYMPTOMS AND SIGNS
- Erosions
- Erythema
- Pustules
- With anaerobic infections, foul smell of the glans penis

Diagnosis

DIFFERENTIAL DIAGNOSIS
- Paget's disease
- Psoriasis
- Lichen planus
- Reiter's disease
- Squamous cell carcinoma

LABORATORY
- Fungal preps usually indicate *Candida*.
- Wet mount may show *Trichomonas*.

Balanitis

Treatment

- Search for and control underlying diabetes.
- Practice good hygiene, with foreskin retraction and gentle washing of the glans penis.
- Treat sexual partner(s) simultaneously for *Candida* or *Trichomonas*.
  - *Candida* responds to fluconazole.
  - *Trichomonas* respond to metronidazole.

COMPLICATIONS

- Phimosis
- Fissure of prepuce

Follow-Up

Patients should be followed by a physician for evidence of recurrence or development of diabetes.

PREVENTION

- Circumcision
- Good hygiene
- Treatment of sexual partner(s) if they are diagnosed as having *Candida* vaginitis or *Trichomonas*

Selected Reading

Edwards S. Balanitis and balanoposthitis: A review. *Genitourin Med* 1996;72:155–159.

Bartonellosis (Oroya Fever and Verruga Peruana)

Basics

DEFINITION

- An endemic infection caused by *Bartonella bacilliformis,* which presents in endemic areas in two distinct forms:
  — Nonimmune persons present with an acute febrile illness associated with profound anemia (Oroya fever).
  — After a variable period of time from resolution, a chronic, benign cutaneous form can develop, characterized by angioproliferative skin lesions (verruga peruana). The latter show a striking similarity to bacillary angiomatosis lesions, caused by *Rochalimaea henselae* and *Rochalimaea quintana.*

ETIOLOGY

- *B. bacilliformis* is a small, gram-negative bacillus of the class Proteobacteria, closely related to *B. (Rochalimaea) quintana.*
- It is transmitted via an arthropod (sandfly, *Phlebotomus*) vector.
- *Bartonella* spp invade the erythrocytes and endothelial cells.
- They multiply into intracellular vacuoles within the erythrocytes. The latter are subsequently phagocytosed and destroyed by the reticuloendothelial system.

EPIDEMIOLOGY

- The disease is exclusively endemic to the Andes River valleys at altitudes from 600 to 2,500 meters (Peru, Ecuador, Colombia).
- Rare cases have been reported in the United States.

Risk Factors

- Life in endemic areas and exposure to the sandfly vector

Incubation Period and Natural History

- The incubation period of the acute illness (Oroya fever) is about 3 weeks (up to 100 days).
- The onset of symptoms, mainly resulting from high fever and profound anemia, can be either acute or subacute.
- The acute phase is succeeded by a convalescence phase.
- Verruga skin lesions (nodules) develop in crops over 1 to 2 months, after a variable time from resolution of Oroya fever.

Clinical Manifestations

SYMPTOMS

Acute Form (Oroya Fever)

- Subacute onset (low-grade fever, malaise, headache, anorexia)
- Sudden onset (high fever, chills, diaphoresis, headaches, and changes in mental status, followed by sudden development of severe anemia)
- Muscle and joint pains
- Dyspnea, angina; the patient may have the feeling that the cardiac pulse is transmitted to the head and ears.
- Insomnia, delirium, decreased level of consciousness, coma
- During the subsequent convalescent (critical) phase, fever declines and anemia symptoms reverse.

SIGNS

Oroya Fever

- High fever
- Signs of profound anemia
- Generalized, nontender lymphadenopathy
- Splenomegaly not usual; if present, may indicate concurrent infection
- Thrombocytopenic purpura

Verruga Peruana

- Nodular lesions, usually at the skin and subcutaneous tissues of exposed parts of the body, can also affect mucous membranes and internal organs.
- Color varies from red to purple, as well as the size (from tiny to several centimeters in diameter).
- Lesions at varying stages of evolution can be concurrently present.
- There is no local tenderness, unless the patient is secondarily infected.

Diagnosis

DIFFERENTIAL DIAGNOSIS

- The acute phase can be easily differentiated from other endemic febrile illnesses (i.e., malaria) by examination of peripheral blood smears.
- Verruga peruana lesions resemble those of bacillary angiomatosis and Kaposi's sarcoma, lymphoproliferative diseases, and other neoplasms. The main diagnostic clue is epidemiology.

Bartonellosis (Oroya Fever and Verruga Peruana)

HEMATOLOGY

- In the acute phase, diagnosis is made by demonstration of numerous organisms adhered to red blood cells, by the cosin/thiazin (Diff-Quik, Merz, Dade) stain, in peripheral blood smears. The number of bacteria declines abruptly during convalescence.
- Also, in peripheral blood smears, macrocytosis, poikilocytosis, Howell-Jolly bodies, nucleated red blood cells, and immature myeloid cells may be found. The leukocyte differential shifts to the left, and the total count may be normal.
- Profound anemia; negative Coombs' test
- In the subacute form, initial peripheral blood smears can be negative; diagnosis can be made by positive blood cultures.
- In the chronic form, diagnosis can be done by the demonstration of the causative agent in cultured material from skin lesions and bone marrow cultures.
- Blood cultures can be positive in apparently healthy individuals.

SEROLOGY

IgM antibodies are of no help, as they can be positive in healthy patients or in patients with the chronic form of the disease.

PATHOLOGY

- Skin biopsy, bone marrow aspiration, and biopsy specimens from other affected organs are used.
- Increased angiogenesis, Rocha-Lima inclusions in endothelial cells
- PCR to detect *B. bacilliformis* is under development.

Treatment

MAIN TREATMENT

- The appropriate health care setting is inpatient in the acute form, and outpatient in chronic form.
- Choice of antibiotics can be influenced by concurrent infectious complications. *B. bacilliformis* is usually sensitive to chloramphenicol, tetracyclines, penicillin, and streptomycin.
- Chloramphenicol is usually used at a dose of 2 g or more daily for at least 7 days, as salmonellosis is the most common bacterial superinfection.
- Supportive and symptomatic treatment is also necessary in the acute form; use blood transfusion support to reverse anemia.

ALTERNATIVE TREATMENT

- Tetracyclines
- Penicillin
- Streptomycin

TREATMENT FAILURE

Large and secondarily infected skin nodules may need surgical excision.

COMPLICATIONS

- Oroya fever, if untreated, can lead to death in greater than 50% to 88% of cases. Fever disappears within 24 hours after appropriate antibiotic treatment, although bacteremia may persist for longer periods of time.
- Verruga lesions show variable response to antibiotic treatment.
- Bacterial secondary infections, including salmonellosis and other enteric infections, malaria, and tuberculosis are common (45%) during the convalescent phase of Oroya fever.
- Verruga lesions can be secondarily infected and pustulate, or ulcerate and bleed.

Follow-Up

- Monitor hydration status and full blood count during the acute phase.
- Monitor signs of other infections: splenomegaly, recurrence of fever with leukocytosis in the convalescent phase, diarrheas.
- Monitor verruga lesions for signs of secondary infections.

PREVENTION

Prevention requires control of the sandfly vector: the spraying of interiors and exteriors of houses with DDT, use of insect repellents, use of bed netting.

Selected Readings

Arias-Stella J, Lieberman PH, Erlandson RA, et al. Histology, immunohistochemistry, and ultrastructure of the verruga in Carrion's disease. *Am J Surg Pathol* 1986;10:595–610.

Arias-Stella J, Lieberman PH, Garcia-Caceres U, et al. Verruga peruana mimicking malignant neoplasms. *Am J Dermatopathol* 1987;9:279–291.

Benson LA, Kar S, McLaughlin G, et al. Entry of *Bartonella bacilliformis* into erythrocytes. *Infect Immun* 1986;54:347–353.

Gray GC, Johnson AA, Thornton SA, et al. An epidemic of Oroya fever in the Peruvian Andes. *Am J Trop Med Hyg* 1990;42:215–221.

Bell's Palsy

Basics

DEFINITION
- Acute, idiopathic, unilateral paralysis of the facial nerve

ETIOLOGY
- Herpes simplex
- Herpes zoster, including herpes zoster oticus
- HIV infection
- Lyme disease
- Otitis media and mastoiditis
- Syphilis
- Sarcoidosis
- Skull trauma

EPIDEMIOLOGY

Incidence and Prevalence
- Rates average 25 in 100,000 in the United States.
- Incidence is highest in persons aged 20 to 35 years and over 70 years.
- There is an equal distribution of males and females.
- The disease is more common in HIV-infected patients, especially those with HIV seroconversion.

Risk Factors
- Recent head trauma
- HIV seroconversion

Clinical Manifestations

SYMPTOMS AND SIGNS
- Rapid progression of partial or total unilateral paralysis of the facial nerve
- Decreased tear production on the ipsilateral side
- Hyperacusis
- Dysgeusia
- Retroauricular pain

Diagnosis

DIFFERENTIAL DIAGNOSIS
- Cerebral aneurism
- Tumor of the parotid gland
- Meningioma

Bell's Palsy

- Carcinomatous meningitis
- Granulomatous meningitis of unknown etiology

LABORATORY

- Tests performed to rule out specific causes:
  - —HIV antibody
  - —Lyme serology
  - —RPR or VDRL
  - —Angiotensin converting enzyme

IMAGING

A CT scan or MRI scan may be required to rule out intracerebral pathology or middle ear disease in complicated cases.

Treatment

- Steroids (controversial): Start with prednisone 30 mg bid for 5 days and then taper over the next 5 days.
- Antiviral agents against HSV (controversial): Treat with acyclovir 400 mg PO 5 times a day for 10 days.
- Protection of the ipsilateral eye with artificial tears, and lubricants at night

COMPLICATIONS

- Incomplete recovery in one-third of patients
- Keratitis and corneal abrasions

Follow-Up

- If serology for Lyme disease and HIV is initially negative, these should be repeated in 3 months.
- If the patient is at high risk for acute HIV infection, further testing, including HIV viral load measurements, should be obtained as soon as possible.

PREVENTION

At present, there is no way to prevent Bell's palsy.

Selected Readings

Spruance SL. Bell palsy and herpes simplex virus. *Ann Intern Med* 1994;120:1045.

Valne A, Edstrom S, Arstila P, et al. Bell's palsy and herpes simplex virus. *Arch Otolaryngol* 1981;107:72.

Blastomycosis

Basics

DEFINITION

Blastomycosis is a disease of humans and animals caused by inhalation of airborne spores from *Blastomyces dermatitidis*, a dimorphic fungus found in soil.

ETIOLOGY

- Blastomycosis is caused by inhalation of spores into the lungs, where they transform into yeasts and elicit a characteristic pyogranulomatous response. From here, the organism can disseminate to a variety of extrapulmonary sites.
- Humans and canines are the primary targets of disease.

EPIDEMIOLOGY

Incidence

- The endemic area in North America includes the southeastern and south central states, especially those bordering on the Mississippi and Ohio River basins; the midwestern states and Canadian provinces that border the Great Lakes; and a small area in New York and Canada that follows the St. Lawrence River.
- In states where blastomycosis is reportable (e.g., Wisconsin and Mississippi), the annual incidence of disease is 1.3 to 1.4 per 100,000 population; in areas where it is endemic, smaller areas of hyperendemicity can have rates of up to 41.9 cases per 100,000 persons.
- Occasional cases have also been reported in Africa, Central and South America, India, and the Middle East.

Risk Factors

- Middle-aged men with outdoor occupations that expose them to soil are at greatest risk for blastomycosis.
- In acquired immunodeficiency syndrome (AIDS) patients, central nervous system (CNS) complications of blastomycosis are more common.

Clinical Manifestations

SYMPTOMS

- Analysis of point-source outbreaks indicates that only about one-half of infected individuals develop symptomatic disease and that the median incubation period is 30 to 45 days.
- The spectrum of clinical manifestations of blastomycosis includes acute pulmonary disease, subacute and chronic pulmonary disease (most common presentations), and disseminated extrapulmonary disease (cutaneous manifestations are most common, followed by involvement of the bone, the genitourinary tract, and central nervous system).
- Skin lesions from infection with *B. dermatitidis* are classically of two types: verrucous or ulcerative. The verrucous form begins as a small papule that, over a period of weeks to months, progresses to a warty, crusted lesion with an elevated, serpiginous, sharply sloping border. Less commonly, the lesion may be of the ulcerative type, beginning as a small pustule that rapidly forms into a superficial ulceration with a granulomatous base. Both types of lesions may coexist, as in our patient.
- The clinical manifestations of pulmonary disease are those of chronic pneumonia, including productive cough, hemoptysis, weight loss, and pleuritic chest pain. Fever, if present, tends to be of low grade. The radiologic findings in these patients are variable. Lobar or segmental alveolar infiltrates, with or without cavitation, are most frequently reported.
- Forty percent to 80% of all cases of pulmonary blastomycosis will result in cutaneous lesions during the course of the disease.
- Skin disease is the most common extrapulmonary manifestation of blastomycosis.
- Two different types of skin lesions may be seen. The first is the more characteristic verrucous lesions that usually appear on exposed body areas. These often begin as small papulopustular lesions and slowly spread to form crusted, heaped-up lesions that can vary in color from gray to a violaceous hue. Older lesions may show central clearing, with scar formation and depigmentation.
- The second type of lesion is described as ulcerative, in which the initial pustule spreads as a superficial ulcer or slightly raised lesion, with a bed of red granulation tissue that bleeds easily.
- A well-circumscribed osteolytic lesion is typical of bone involvement due to blastomycosis.
- From 10% to 30% of the cases in men have been reported to involve the genitourinary tract, primarily the prostate and epididymis. Prostatic involvement is most common and is usually manifested by symptoms of obstruction; an enlarged, tender prostate; and pyuria.
- CNS blastomycosis is reported to be almost invariably associated with involvement of other organs and is most often the result of dissemination from a pulmonary source.
- Epidural, cranial, or spinal abscesses and acute or chronic meningitis characterize CNS involvement.
- Blastomycosis may infrequently involve the liver, spleen, gastrointestinal tract, thyroid, pericardium, adrenal glands, and other sites.

Diagnosis

DIFFERENTIAL DIAGNOSIS

- Blastomycosis should be considered in the differential diagnosis of subacute lobar or segmental pneumonia, especially in residents of or visitors to areas with endemic blastomycosis. The pulmonary disease may be acute or chronic and can mimic infection with pyogenic bacteria, tuberculosis, other fungi, and malignancy.
- Radiographic findings often resemble changes seen in bronchogenic carcinoma and granulomatous processes such as tuberculosis, sarcoidosis, histoplasmosis, and silicosis.

LABORATORY

- Diagnosis of blastomycosis may be based on isolation of *B. dermatitidis* from specimens obtained from sputum, skin, or tissue biopsy (cultures should be held for at least 4 weeks), or the demonstration of characteristic broad-based budding yeast cells by direct microscopic examination of wet unstained clinical specimens, cytology preparations, or histopathology slides.
- When blastomycosis is a possible diagnosis, sputum or pus could be examined by wet preparation.

Blastomycosis

- Bronchial washings and postbronchoscopy sputum samples should be sent for cytology as well as smear and culture.
- Any material obtained should be placed on Sabouraud's or, preferably, more enriched agar (Sabhi, brain-heart infusion, Gorman's media, etc.).
- The immunodiffusion test is more sensitive and specific than the complement fixation test.
- *B. dermatitidis* colonies can be identified early by using recently developed DNA probes and exoantigen technology.

IMAGING

- Chest radiograph findings usually show areas of local consolidation or masslike lesions. Patterns of diffuse alveolar infiltrates or diffuse miliary infiltrates are next most common.
- Pleural thickening and small pleural effusions may occur, but large pleural effusions are uncommon.

DIAGNOSTIC/TESTING PROCEDURES

- Meningitis is frequently difficult to diagnose. Evaluation of the cerebrospinal fluid is usually nondefinitive, and cultures are generally negative. Ventricular fluid has been associated with higher positive culture rates.
- The diagnosis may be confirmed by a 10% potassium hydroxide preparation of sputum or skin lesion exudate, which reveals an 8- to 15-μm broad-based budding yeast with a characteristic doubly refractile cell wall.
- Urine cultures, especially after prostatic massage, are often positive in prostatic involvement.

Treatment

MAIN TREATMENT

- The decision to withhold therapy for patients with acute pulmonary blastomycosis is difficult and controversial. Although it is true that in some patients blastomycotic pneumonia may resolve without therapy, there is no way of determining which patients will later present with extrapulmonary disease, often with serious sequelae.
- Amphotericin B remains the drug of choice for patients with life-threatening disease and/or CNS involvement, and for patients with compromised immune function. Most authors, therefore, recommend a total dose of 1.5 to 2.5 g of amphotericin B. In seriously ill patients, 0.3 to 0.6 mg/kg (usually not exceeding 50 mg) should be administered daily until objective evidence of improvement is noted.

ALTERNATIVE TREATMENT

The newer imidazole antifungals, including ketoconazole and, more recently, itraconazole, have been used for mild to moderate disease. A multicenter trial assessing the efficacy of itraconazole at doses of 200 to 400 mg per day achieved a success rate of 95% when treatment was continued for at least 2 months.

COMPLICATIONS

Overwhelming infection with *B. dermatitidis* can cause diffuse pneumonitis and the adult respiratory distress syndrome, even in immunocompetent hosts.

Follow-Up

Most authorities recommend a minimum of 6 months of therapy with the azole antifungals until further data are available.

PREVENTION

- The risk for exposure to blastomycosis remains small, even in areas where the disease is endemic. Protective measures include the following:
  - Use of a CDC-approved N-95 disposable half-facepiece filtering respirator (or equivalent) and protective clothing and shoe covers by all persons engaged in soil-disturbing activities during prairie dog relocation
  - Employer-provided instruction of all persons with potential to be engaged in these activities in the proper fitting and wearing of the recommended face mask
  - Implementation of a respiratory-protection program for employees
  - Education of workers about clinical signs and symptoms of disease and screening and treatment options

Selected Readings

Anonymous. Blastomycosis—Wisconsin, 1986–1995. From the Centers for Disease Control and Prevention. *JAMA* 1996;276:444.

Anonymous. From the Centers for Disease Control and Prevention. Blastomycosis acquired occupationally during prairie dog relocation—Colorado, 1998. *JAMA* 1999;282:21–22.

Chapman SW. Blastomyces dermatitidis In: Mandell GL, Bennett JE, Dolin R, eds. *Principles and practice of infectious diseases*, 5th ed. New York: Churchill Livingstone, 2000, 2733–2746.

Cohen LM, Golitz LE, Wilson ML. Widespread papules and nodules in a Ugandan man with acquired immunodeficiency syndrome. African blastomycosis. *Arch Dermatol* 1996;132:821–822, 824.

Cummins RE, Romero RC, Mancini AJ. Disseminated North American blastomycosis in an adolescent male: A delay in diagnosis. *Pediatrics* 1998;102:977–979.

Meyer KC, McManus EJ, Maki DG. Overwhelming pulmonary blastomycosis associated with the adult respiratory distress syndrome. *N Engl J Med* 1993;329:1231–1236.

Rabatin JT, Utz JP. 55-year-old man with a lung lesion and hemidysesthesia. *Mayo Clin Proc* 1999;74:515–518.

Vasquez JE, Mehta JB, Agrawal R, et al. Blastomycosis in northeast Tennessee. *Chest* 1998;114:436–443.

Weil M, Mercurio MG, Brodell RT, et al. Cutaneous lesions provide a clue to mysterious pulmonary process. Pulmonary and cutaneous North American blastomycosis infection. *Arch Dermatol* 1996;132:822, 824–825.

Blepharitis and Chalazion

Basics

DEFINITION

- Blepharitis is infection of the eyelid and inflammation of lid margins. It includes the following:
  - Superficial and deep marginal
  - Angular
  - Alternative
  - Granulomatous
- Chalazion is a painless, granulomatous inflammation of a meibomian gland that produces a nodule within the eyelid.

ETIOLOGY

- Almost all infections that affect the skin and colonize the eyelids from nearby areas such as the scalp and nares can cause infectious diseases of the eyelid.
- The most common causes are *Staphylococcus* spp, particularly *S. aureus*. Other pathogens include the following:
  - *Bacillus anthracis*
  - *Bacillus cereus*
  - *Blastomyces dermatitidis*
  - *Candida* spp
  - *Clostridium* spp
  - *Cryptococcus neoformans*
  - *Haemophilus ducreyi*
  - Herpes simplex virus
  - Herpes zoster virus
  - *Moraxella* spp
  - *Mycobacterium tuberculosis*
  - *Mycobacterium leprae*
  - *Phthirus pubis*
  - Poxvirus spp
  - *Proteus mirabilis*
  - *Pseudomonas* spp
  - *Streptococcus* spp
  - *Vaccinia* virus

EPIDEMIOLOGY

- Marginal blepharitis is usually associated with rosacea and seborrheic dermatitis.
- More than three-fourths of patients with the blepharitis of atopic dermatitis have a positive culture for *S. aureus*. However, a positive culture does not necessarily mean that there is an ongoing infection, and clinical correlation is important.
- Angular blepharitis caused by *Moraxella* spp is usually seen in adolescents, particularly in warmer climates.

Clinical Manifestations

SYMPTOMS

- Usual symptoms include chronic irritation, a burning sensation, mild redness, and occasional pruritus.
- Patients with crab louse of the eyebrow usually present with pruritus.

SIGNS

- In acute blepharitis, there are usually collections of pus and an ulcerative margin.
- In chronic blepharitis, there is usually a loss or misdirection of lashes, telangiectasia, and a swollen lid margin.
- Superficial lid involvement is the most common expression of staphylococcal lid disease and usually presents with hyperemia and telangiectasia of the lid margin.
- Lymphadenopathy is usually more pronounced in streptococcal disease, and the erythema surrounding the skin lesions spreads more rapidly.
- Patients with crab louse of the eyebrow have erythema of the lid margin, excoriation, and toxic follicular conjunctivitis caused by the organism's feces. Oval nits firmly adherent to the lashes can be easily recognized.

Blepharitis and Chalazion

Diagnosis

- The lid margin is examined with the slit-lamp for evidence of folliculitis.
- Culture of the lid margin requires "scrubbing" with a swab soaked in sterile broth and plating out directly on blood agar and a selective medium for *S. aureus*.

Treatment

MAIN TREATMENT

- Usually, treatment of blepharitis consists of warm compresses, strict eyelid hygiene, and topical antibiotics.
- Firm massage, using a 50:50 mixture of baby shampoo and water and a cotton-tipped applicator, enhances the flow of oily secretions from the meibomian glands.
- Topical ophthalmic preparations for staphylococcal blepharitis include bacitracin or erythromycin (bid or qid for 2 weeks), gentamicin, and 1% mercuric oxide.
- In chronic cases of blepharitis, cultures should be obtained when patients have smoldering blepharitis not responding to topical antibiotics. Systemic antibiotics that can be used in such cases are dicloxacillin (500 mg qid), quinolones, or azithromycin.
- In the uncommon cases of necrotizing fasciitis that involves the eyelids, prompt surgical debridement is needed.
- Oral acyclovir (800 mg orally qid) is recommended for patients with severe primary ocular herpes involving the eyelid.
- Patients with crab louse of the eyebrow and all affected family members and sexual contacts require treatment with 1% gamma benzene hexachloride lotion or shampoo, which is applied to the infected areas and adjacent hairy parts, left on for 24 hours, and repeated 1 week later. An alternative is 1% yellow mercuric oxide ointment once or twice a day for several days. The nits should be removed mechanically.
- For chalazion, if it persists and is nontender, incision and curettage can be done. Removal of the inflammatory debris can be done by making a vertical or, if necessary, a horizontal conjunctival incision. In the absence of an infection, intralesional injection of corticosteroids may be given.

COMPLICATIONS

An external hordeolum (stye) is caused by staphylococcal infection of the superficial accessory glands of Zeis or Moll, located in the eyelid margins. An internal hordeolum occurs after suppurative infection of the oil-secreting meibomian glands within the tarsal plate of the eyelid.

Follow-Up

Basal cell, squamous cell, or meibomian gland carcinoma should be suspected for any nonhealing, ulcerative lesion of the eyelids.

PREVENTION

N/A

Selected Readings

Alvarez H, Tabbara KF. Infections of the eyelid. In: Tabbara KF, Hyndiuk RA, eds. *Infections of the eye*. Boston: Little, Brown and Company, 1996:559–570.

Horton JC. Disorders of the eye. In: Fauci AS, Braunwald E, Isselbacher KJ, et al, eds. *Harrison's principles of medicine,* 14th ed. New York: McGraw-Hill, 1998:159–172.

Orbit, lids and lacrimal system. In: Seal DV, Bron AJ, Hay J, eds. *Ocular infection: Investigation and treatment in practice*. St. Louis: Mosby–Year Book and Martin Duitz Ltd. Publishers, 1998:25–36.

Botulism

Basics

DEFINITION
- Syndrome produced by neurotoxins liberated by *Clostridium botulinum*
- Disease may be secondary to toxins
  —Produced in food
  —Liberated by infection of wounds
  —Liberated by organisms colonizing the stomach or intestinal tract in children

ETIOLOGY
- *C. botulinum* is an anaerobic gram-positive rod that produces spores and potent neurotoxins.
- The organism is typed A to G by nature of the antibodies to the neurotoxin produced.
- Disease in humans is associated with toxin types A, B, E, and F.
- Type A is often found in the western United States and in China.
- Type B is found in the eastern United States and in Europe.
- Type F is found in Alaska, is worldwide, and is often associated with fish products.
- Spores are found in soil and in marine sediment.
- Spores are resistant to boiling.

EPIDEMIOLOGY

Incidence
- Small outbreaks due to either commercially or home-canned foods occur infrequently.
- In the United States, an average of 100 cases occur per year: 72% in infants, 25% from foods, and 3% from wounds.

Risk Factors
- Homemade fermentation of foods with home canning leads to increased risks.
- Age is a risk factor for poor outcome, with a fatality rate of 30% in patients over the age of 60 years.
- Ingestion of honey by infants is a risk factor for gastrointestinal colonization and production of toxins.

Incubation
Symptoms develop 12 to 36 hours after ingestion of the toxin.

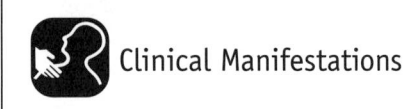

Clinical Manifestations

SYMPTOMS AND SIGNS
- Bilateral cranial neuropathies
- Bilateral descending weakness
- Absence of fever
- The patient remains awake and alert as the syndrome progresses.
- No sensory abnormalities

Botulism

Diagnosis

DIFFERENTIAL DIAGNOSIS
- Myasthenia gravis
- Eaton-Lambert syndrome
- Tick paralysis
- Miller Fisher variant of Guillain-Barré syndrome
- Stroke

LABORATORY
- Detection of the toxin in serum, stool, or food sample

Treatment

- Supportive care
- Antitoxin available (covers toxin types A, B, and E)
- Antibiotic treatment for wound botulism

Follow-Up

Patients often need long-term follow-up with rehabilitation following a case of botulism.

PREVENTION
- Observe careful food preparation, especially when canning food at home.
- Ensure that care is taken when canning low-acidic foods such as corn, asparagus, beans, and beets.
- If foods have been home canned, boil them for 10 minutes prior to eating.
- Avoid giving honey to infants less than 1 year of age.
- Perform a rapid screening of possible cases in order to stop potential outbreaks.
- Avoid the use of food stored in bulging cans.

Selected Readings

Cherington M. Botulism. *Semin Neurol* 1990;10:27–31.

Chia JK, Clark JB, Ryan CA, et al. Botulism in an adult associated with food borne intestinal infection with *Clostridium botulinum*. *N Engl J Med* 1986;315:239–241.

Shapiro RL, Hatheway CL, Swerdlow DL. Botulism in the United States: A clinical and epidemiologic review. *Ann Intern Med* 1998;129:221–228.

Brain Abscess

Basics

DEFINITION
Brain abscess is a collection of purulent material within the brain parenchyma caused by an infectious source of bacteria, fungi, or protozoa. The structure can have a defined abscess wall or consist of an inflammatory process ("cerebritis").

ETIOLOGY
- Infection can reach the brain by the following:
  - Direct spread from the sinus, orbit, tooth, mastoid, middle ear, and meninges
  - Post trauma or neurosurgery
  - Hematogenous spread
- The nature of the organisms found in the infection often relates to the mode of transmission:
  - Middle ear, sinus
    - Mixed infections with anaerobes, microaerophilic streptococci
  - Trauma and postoperative
    - *Staphylococcus aureus*
    - *Pseudomonas*
    - Other gram-negatives
  - Hematogenous
    - *S. aureus*
    - *Salmonella*
    - *Listeria*
    - Streptococci
    - Fungi

EPIDEMIOLOGY
- Rare infection, occurring in 0.2% to 1.3% of large autopsy series, and in 1 of 10,000 hospital admissions
- Median age of infection: age 30 to 45 years

Risk Factors
- Sinusitis
- Otitis media
- Poor dental hygiene
- Endocarditis
- Bacteremia from indwelling central lines and intravenous drug use
- Osler-Weber-Rendu disease
- Preexisting brain injury
- Immunodeficiency, especially with tuberculosis or cryptococcus

Clinical Manifestations

- Usual symptoms include headache, mental status changes, nausea, and vomiting.
- Low-grade fevers may be present.
- Seizures may be the initial cause for CT scanning.

Diagnosis

- Diagnosis depends on the location of the abscess, the organism, and the preexisting disease causing it.
- CT scans and MRI scans are the best way to diagnose possible brain abscess.
- Lumbar punctures are dangerous and help with the microbiologic diagnosis only infrequently.
- Microbiologic diagnosis
  - Blood cultures positive
  - Direct aspiration of abscess

Brain Abscess

DIFFERENTIAL DIAGNOSIS

- Brain tumor
- Infarcts
- Hematoma
- Radiation Necrosis
- Cytomegalovirus (in AIDS)
- Toxoplasmosis (in AIDS)

IMAGING

- CT and MRI are important diagnostic tools.
- Imaging the sinuses and contiguous bones helps find the cause of the lesions.
- Serial scans need to be performed, especially when empiric treatment is given.
- Ring lesions can persist for 3 to 4 months despite adequate therapy.

DIAGNOSTIC PROCEDURES

- Stereotactic aspiration: the procedure of choice if the abscess is easily accessible and greater than 2.5 cm in size
- Craniotomy with aspiration in areas where direct visualization of blood vessels is needed and the abscess is greater than 2.5 cm in size

Treatment

- Culture and sensitivity of any isolated organism should help with the choice of antibiotic.
- Empiric treatment with cefotaxime 2 g i.v. q4h or ceftriaxone 2 g i.v. q12h *and* metronidazole 7.5 mg/kg i.v. q6h.
- Alternative drugs include penicillin G 24 million units qd in divided doses q4h *and* metronidazole 7.5 mg/kg i.v. q6h.
- Postsurgical infections should be empirically treated with nafcillin 2 g i.v q4h or vancomycin 1 g i.v. q12h *and* a third-generation cephalosporin such as cefotaxime or ceftriaxone.
- Treat with the highest dose possible.
- Four to 8 or more weeks of intravenous therapy is needed, with follow-up of CT scans.

COMPLICATIONS

High morbidity is associated with residual neurologic deficits in patients with prior brain abscesses.

Follow-Up

Patients often require serial CT scans or MRI scans for at least a year following completion of antibiotics.

PREVENTION

- Sinusitis and otitis should be treated in all patients.
- Good dental hygiene is needed with treatment of apical abscesses, especially in the upper molars.

Selected Readings

Haplan K. Brain abscess. *Med Clin North Am* 1985;69:345–360.

Mamelak AN, Mampalam TJ, Obana WG, et al. Improved management of multiple brain abscesses: A combined surgical and medical approach. *Neurosurgery* 1995;36:76–86.

Mathisen GE, Johnson JP. Brain abscess. *Clin Infect Dis* 1997;25:763–781.

Bronchiolitis

Basics

DEFINITION
- Acute bronchiolitis is a disease of the lower respiratory tract and results from inflammatory obstruction of the small bronchioles.
- Bronchiolitis refers to the inflammatory disease primarily involving the terminal and respiratory bronchioles, but in some cases, extending to the adjacent alveolar ducts and alveolar spaces.

ETIOLOGY
- Bronchiolitis is most commonly caused by the respiratory syncytial virus (in more than 50% of cases).
- Other viruses, such as parainfluenza, influenza, rhinovirus, rubeola, mumps, parvovirus, enterovirus, coronavirus, coxsackievirus, and varicella zoster, are occasionally isolated.
- In adults, there are occasional reports of viral- or bacterial (*Mycoplasma pneumoniae* and *Legionella pneumophila*)-induced bronchiolitis.
- The histologic appearance of bronchiolitis includes inflammatory (cellular) bronchiolitis, constrictive bronchiolitis obliterans, and a proliferative bronchiolitis.

EPIDEMIOLOGY

Incidence
- The incidence of bronchiolitis has been shown to be as high as 11 cases per 100 children per year for both the first and second 6 months of life. In the first 6 months of life, 6 children per 1,000 are hospitalized with bronchiolitis per year in the United States. The care of hospitalized infants with bronchiolitis is estimated to cost up to $300 million each year.
- In the United States, there are at least 675,000 ambulatory and 75,000 hospitalized children (younger than 2 years of age) with bronchiolitis each year.
- In 1995 in New York State, bronchiolitis accounted for 17% of all infant hospitalizations (nine admissions per 1,000 child-years).
- Bronchiolitis is the most common cause of hospitalization of infants.
- Bronchiolitis occurs in a seasonal pattern, with peak incidence in the winter to spring months.

Risk Factors
- Bronchiolitis usually occurs during the first 2 years of life, with a peak incidence at approximately 6 months of age.
- Bronchiolitis is most common among male infants between 3 and 6 months of age who have not been breast fed and who live in crowded conditions.
- Infants whose mothers smoke cigarettes are more likely to develop bronchiolitis.
- Known causes of bronchiolitis include toxic fume inhalation, tobacco smoke, mineral dust inhalation, penicillamine, collagen vascular diseases, and infections. Bone marrow, heart–lung, and lung transplantation have also been associated with this complication.

Clinical Manifestations

SYMPTOMS
- Bronchiolitis is characterized by the following:
  —Air trapping
  —Coryza
  —Cough
  —Expiratory wheezing
  —Fever
  —Grunting
  —Increased respiratory effort
  —Retractions
  —Tachypnea
- Infants with bronchiolitis first have a mild upper respiratory tract infection with serous nasal discharge and sneezing. These symptoms usually last several days and may be accompanied by diminished appetite.
- The fever usually ranges between 38.5°C and 39.0°C.

SIGNS
- Air-flow obstruction is a major clinical finding in patients with constrictive bronchiolitis. Wheezing is expected, but crackles are more common, especially during the first 15% of inspiration.
- An examination reveals a tachypneic infant often in extreme respiratory distress.

Diagnosis

DIFFERENTIAL DIAGNOSIS
- The condition most commonly confused with acute bronchiolitis is asthma. Other entities that should be included in the differential include congestive heart failure, foreign body in the trachea, pertussis, organophosphate poisoning, cystic fibrosis, and bronchopneumonias.
- Infants with bronchiolitis are wheezing for the first time, unlike those with asthma, in whom wheezing is recurrent.

LABORATORY
The white blood cell and differential cell counts are usually within normal limits.

IMAGING
Chest radiograph usually reveals hyperinflation of the lungs and an increased anteroposterior diameter on lateral view.

Bronchiolitis

Treatment

MAIN TREATMENT

- The traditional approach to symptomatic management of bronchiolitis has been supportive care with attention to oxygen therapy, hydration, and respiratory support as needed.
- Infants with respiratory distress should be hospitalized. The patients are commonly placed in an atmosphere of cool, humidified oxygen.
- Studies evaluating the effects of bronchodilators on pulmonary mechanics in infants with bronchiolitis have shown mixed results. None of these studies has evaluated the efficacy of patients receiving nebulized albuterol treatments beyond 4 hours or has advocated the use of bronchodilators as a means of reducing hospitalizations or length of stay.
- In the outpatient setting, short-term benefit from nebulized beta-adrenergic bronchodilators has been demonstrated through improvements in oxygen saturation or clinical respiratory scores.

ALTERNATIVE TREATMENT

Ribavirin has been available for the treatment of respiratory syncytial virus infection since 1985. Its use has been recommended for infants with congestive heart failure and bronchopulmonary dysplasia. However, its use remains controversial.

COMPLICATIONS

- The case fatality rate is below 1%.
- The mortality rate among infants with high-risk conditions (e.g., congestive heart failure, immune deficiency, cystic fibrosis, etc.) is less than 3.5%.

Follow-Up

- Some infants may progress to respiratory failure and require ventilatory support.
- A significant proportion of infants with bronchiolitis have hyperactive airways in late childhood.

PREVENTION

N/A

Selected Readings

Anonymous. Case records of the Massachusetts General Hospital. Weekly clinicopathological exercises. Case 11-1998. A 35-year-old woman with obstructive pulmonary disease and cystic changes on CT scans of the chest. *N Engl J Med* 1998;338:1051–1058.

Chan ED, Kalayanamit T, Lynch DA, et al. *Mycoplasma pneumoniae*-associated bronchiolitis causing severe restrictive lung disease in adults: Report of three cases and literature review. *Chest* 1999;115:1188–1194.

Kellner JD, Ohlsson A, Gadomski AM, et al. Efficacy of bronchodilator therapy in bronchiolitis. A meta-analysis. *Arch Pediatr Adolesc Med* 1996;150:1166–1172.

Miyashita N, Niki Y, Nakajima M, et al. *Chlamydia pneumoniae* infection in patients with diffuse panbronchiolitis and COPD. *Chest* 1998;114:969–971.

Orenstein DM. Bronchiolitis. In: Behrman RE, Kliegman RM, Arvin AM, eds. *Nelson textbook of pediatrics*. Philadelphia: WB Saunders, 1996:1211–1213.

Welliver RC. Therapy for bronchiolitis: Help wanted. *J Pediatr* 1997;130:170–172.

Bronchitis

Basics

DEFINITION

Bronchitis is a lower respiratory tract infection. Inflammation of the bronchi is classified as acute or chronic. *Chronic bronchitis* is defined as chronic productive cough for 3 months in each of 2 successive years. (Other causes of chronic cough have been excluded.)

ETIOLOGY

- Acute purulent bronchitis is typically caused by viral organisms:
  —Influenza
  —Parainfluenza
  —Coronavirus
  —Rhinovirus
  —*Mycoplasma pneumoniae* (rare)
  —*Chlamydia pneumoniae* (rare)
  —*Bordetella pertussis* (rare)
- Chronic bronchitis
  —*Streptococcus pneumoniae*
  —*Haemophilus influenzae*
  —Air pollutants
  —Cigarette smoke pollutants
  —Subclinical asthma
  —Viral infections
  —Allergies

EPIDEMIOLOGY

- Fourteen million office visits per year
- Second leading cause of work disability
- Five hundred thousand hospitalizations per year

Risk Factors

- For chronic bronchitis
  —Smoking
  —Air pollution
  —Exposure to dust and gases
  —Asthma
  —Upper respiratory tract infections

Clinical Manifestations

SYMPTOMS AND SIGNS

- Acute
  —Cough with sputum
  —Absence of chronic bronchitis
  —Absence of crackles on auscultatory examination
  —Chest x-ray negative for acute infiltrate
- Chronic (acute exacerbation of chronic bronchitis [ACEB])
  —Increased dyspnea
  —Increased sputum production
  —Increased sputum purulence

Diagnosis

PHYSICAL EXAMINATION

- Acute
  —Often negative examination; possibility of occasional wheezes or rhonchi
- ACEB
  —Occasional wheezes or rhonchi
  —Deterioration in respiratory function
  —Fever and leukocytosis uncommon

DIFFERENTIAL DIAGNOSIS

- Infectious
  —Pneumonia
- Noninfectious
  —Pulmonary embolism with infarction
  —Congestive heart failure
  —Wegener's granulomatosis
  —Sarcoid
  —Atelectasis
  —Chemical pneumonitis

LABORATORY

- Pulmonary function tests (FEV, peak flow, arterial oxygen saturation)
- Chest x-ray
- Bronchoscopy

Bronchitis

Treatment

MAIN TREATMENT

- Acute: no treatment unless there is the presence of the following:
  - Influenza A
    - Amantadine—14 to 64 years: 100 mg PO bid; over 65 years: 100 mg per day PO
    - Rimantadine—14 to 64 years: 100 mg PO bid; over 65 years: 100 to 200 mg per day PO (50 mg qid)
  - Pertussis
    - Erythromycin: 50 mg PO qid
- Chronic: Clinical trials show variable results with antibiotics. Patients with moderate to severe episodes (FEV <50%) do benefit.
  - Doxycycline: 100 mg PO bid
  - Amoxicillin: 500 mg PO tid
  - Ciprofloxacin: 250 to 500 mg every 12 hours × 7 days
  - Levofloxacin: 500 mg once per day × 7 days
  - Moxifloxacin: 400 mg once per day × 5 days
  - Gatifloxacin: 400 mg once per day × 7 days
  - Clarithromycin: 500 mg bid × 7 days
  - Azithromycin: 250 mg once daily × 5 days

COMPLICATIONS

- Failure to respond to treatment as a result of the following:
  - Disease too far advanced or treatment delayed too long
  - Wrong diagnosis
  - Inadequate dose of antibiotic
  - Compromised or debilitated host
  - Presence of resistant bacteria, e.g., Pseudomonas

Follow-Up

PREVENTION

- Smoking cessation
- Prophylactic antibiotics have not proven successful in preventing recurrences.

Selected Readings

Grossman RF. Management of acute exacerbation of chronic bronchitis. *Can Respir J* 1999;6[Suppl A]:40A–45A.

Read RC. Infection in acute exacerbations of chronic bronchitis: A clinical perspective. *Respir Med* 1999;93(12):845–850.

Sethi S. Infectious exacerbations of chronic bronchitis: Diagnosis and management. *J Antimicrob Chemother* 1999;43[Suppl A]:97–105.

Brucellosis

Basics

DEFINITION
- Brucellosis is a zoonotic infectious disease of both wild and domestic animals.
- Humans are the accidental host of the pathogen and develop a systemic disease of acute or insidious onset.

ETIOLOGY
- Brucellosis is caused by *Brucella* species, which are small, nonmotile, gram-negative coccobacilli.
- Brucella species that infect humans:
  - *Brucella melitensis*
  - *Brucella abortus*
  - *Brucella suis*
  - *Brucella canis*

EPIDEMIOLOGY

Incidence and Prevalence
- Brucellosis has a worldwide distribution.
- The infection is endemic in the Mediterranean countries of Europe, in Asia, and in Africa, as well as in Central and South America and central Asia and India.
- The responsible *Brucella* species varies from area to area.
- Although the reported incidence in the United States is less than 120 cases per year, it is thought that the infection is generally underdiagnosed and underreported worldwide.

Risk Factors
- Brucellosis is an occupational disease. The infection is more common in the following populations:
  - Farm and ranch workers
  - Abattoir workers
  - Veterinarians
  - Meat inspectors
  - Laboratory personnel
- Ingestion of unpasteurized milk or milk products also is a significant risk factor in endemic areas.
- The incubation period is variable and difficult to ascertain. It is usually considered to be 1 week to 2 months, although an incubation period of several months has been observed in occasional cases.

Clinical Manifestations

SYMPTOMS AND SIGNS
- Brucellosis presents with the following:
  - Fever
  - Chills
  - Rigor
  - Malaise
  - Headache
  - Weight loss
  - Sweating
  - Generalized aches
  - Arthralgias
- Depression is also a common symptom.
- Hepatomegaly, splenomegaly, and lymphadenopathy may be found.
- A significant proportion of patients (20%–50%) have osteoarticular involvement. (Sacroiliitis is the most common manifestation.)
- Symptoms due to orchitis and/or epididymitis also may be manifestations of brucellosis in a considerable proportion (5%–25%) of patients with the infection.
- Brucellosis may affect any organ of the body and present occasionally as a localized infection.
- Endocarditis is an especially severe manifestation of brucellosis, with very high case-fatality rate.

Diagnosis

DIFFERENTIAL DIAGNOSIS
- Brucellosis should come to the mind of a physician when he or she sees a patient from an endemic area with a febrile illness of acute or insidious onset, especially if there are manifestations of osteoarticular involvement.
- Differential diagnosis should be made from several other infectious diseases.
- Brucellosis may present as fever of unknown origin.

LABORATORY
- Definitive diagnosis of brucellosis is made with the culture of the pathogen from blood, bone marrow, or other tissue specimens.
- The laboratory personnel should be told by the clinician that brucellosis is a diagnostic possibility when cultures are sent. This is because some media that support the growth of *Brucella* species require an environment with 5% to 10% CO_2 for optimal isolation of the pathogen.
- Cultures should be kept for at least 4 weeks when brucellosis is a possibility.
- Serologic tests are also helpful. However, interpretation of the results of these tests should be done carefully.
- False-negative serologic tests for brucellosis may be due to the prozone phenomenon.
- False-positive results may be obtained due to cross-reactions with antibodies to other infections, such as *Yersinia enterocolitica*, *Vibrio cholera*, and *Francisella tularensis*.
- Attention also should be paid to the fact that IgG antibodies against *Brucella* species may be found in all forms of the infection: acute, recurrent, or chronic brucellosis.

Brucellosis

Treatment

MAIN TREATMENT

- Doxycycline 100 mg PO every 12 hours, combined with rifampin 600 to 900 mg/d PO for 6 weeks, is the recommended regimen for most cases of brucellosis.
- Streptomycin (1 g/d IM) should be given instead of rifampin (in combination with doxycycline) for the first 3 weeks of treatment in case of brucellosis with osteomyelitis, meningitis, or endocarditis.
- Replacement of the heart valve is usually necessary in cases of *Brucella* endocarditis.
- Prednisone has been used when there is central nervous system involvement.

ALTERNATIVE TREATMENT

Trimethoprim–sulfamethoxazole and fluoroquinolones also have efficacy against *Brucella* species.

COMPLICATIONS

- Recurrence of symptoms is a common problem in brucellosis. It is attributed to the difficulty of eradicating the pathogen due to its sequestration in areas where antibiotics do not accomplish high concentrations, and not to the development of resistance of the pathogen to antimicrobial agents.
- Antibiotic regimens of longer duration (several months) must be used in such cases.
- The case-fatality rate for brucellosis is about 2% and is mainly attributable to endocarditis.
- A Jarisch-Herxheimer–like reaction may be seen occasionally, shortly after the initiation of treatment with antibiotics.

Follow-Up

- Careful follow-up is crucial for patients with brucellosis due to the considerable probability of recurrence of symptoms.
- Renal function should be monitored in patients who receive aminoglycoside antibiotics for treatment of brucellosis.
- Patients should be advised to watch for adverse reactions to doxycycline and rifampin.

PREVENTION

- Efforts should be made to eradicate *Brucella* species from cattle, goats, swine, and other animals.
- Milk and dairy products should be pasteurized. If pasteurization of milk is not possible, boiling also is effective.

Selected Readings

Acocella G, Bertrand A, Beytout J, et al. Comparison of three different regimens in the treatment of acute brucellosis: A multicenter multinational study. *J Antimicrob Agents Chemother* 1989;23:433–439.

Ariza J, Gudiol F, Pallares R, et al. Treatment of human brucellosis with doxycycline plus rifampin or doxycycline plus streptomycin. *Ann Intern Med* 1992;117:25–30.

Arnow PM, Smaron M, Ormiste V. Brucellosis in a group of travellers to Spain. *JAMA* 1984;251:505–507.

Jacobs F, Abramowicz D, Vereerstraeten P, et al. *Brucella* endocarditis: The role of combined medical and surgical treatment. *Rev Infect Dis* 1990;12:7404.

Kolman S, Maayan MC, Gotesman G, et al. Comparison of the BACTEC and lysis concentration methods for recovering *Brucella* species from clinical specimens. *Eur J Clin Microbiol Infect Dis* 1991;10:647–648.

Lang R, Rubinstein E. Quinolones for the treatment of brucellosis. *J Antimicrob Chemother* 1992;29:357–363.

Lulu AR, Araj GF, Khateeb MI, et al. Human brucellosis in Kuwait: A prospective study of 400 cases. *Q J Med* 1988;66:39–54.

Madkour MM, Sharif HS, Abed MY, et al. Osteoarticular brucellosis: Results of bone scintigraphy in 140 patients. *AJR* 1988;150:1101–1105.

McLean Dr, Russell N, Khan MY. Neurobrucellosis: Clinical and therapeutic features. *Clin Infect Dis* 1992;15:580–590.

Peiris V, Faser S, Fairhust M, et al. Laboratory diagnosis of *Brucella* infection: Some pitfalls. *Lancet* 1992;339:1415–1416.

Taylor JP, Perdue JN. The changing epidemiology of human brucellosis in Texas, 1977–1986. *Am J Epidemiol* 1989;130:160–165.

Bursitis

Basics

DEFINITION
- Bursitis is inflammation of the bursae due to a number of causes, including pyogenic infections, crystal release secondary to trauma or gout, or arthritis.
- There are over 150 bursae in the body.

ETIOLOGY
- The most common organism isolated in bursitis is *Staphylococcal aureus*.
- The second most common organism, leading to 5% to 30% of cases, is *Streptococcus*.
- Disease due to gram-negatives or fungi is rare.

EPIDEMIOLOGY
N/A

Clinical Manifestations

- There may be painful swelling and erythema of the bursae.
- Fevers may be present.
- Evidence of cellulitis may extend from the bursae.

Diagnosis

DIFFERENTIAL DIAGNOSIS
- Cellulitis/fasciitis
- Arthritis and septic arthritis
- Gout
- Crystal-induced bursitis
- Trauma

LABORATORY
- Bursal fluid contains a low white blood cell count, often below 10,000 cells/mm.
- Gram stain and cultures are positive when bacterial infection is present.
- Crystal analysis should be negative in bacterial bursitis, but both crystal-induced and bacterial bursitis may occur at the same time.

DIAGNOSTIC PROCEDURE
- Aspiration of the affected bursae

Treatment

- Aspiration by needle and syringe, on a frequent, even daily, basis until the bursa is no longer fluctuant

Bursitis

- Antibiotics
  - The choice of antibiotics depends on the culture and sensitivity of the aspirated material. For *S. aureus*, oxacillin or nafcillin (2 g q6h i.v.) or dicloxacillin (500 mg q6h PO) is given. If the organism is methicillin-resistant, vancomycin (750–1,000 mg q12h i.v.) is indicated.
  - Antibiotics should be given for at least 14 days.
  - Use of parenteral versus oral antibiotics depends on the severity of the clinical situation and the amount of systemic toxicity associated with the infection.
  - Empiric treatment should be directed against *S. aureus*.
- Immobilization of affected bursae

- If antibiotics do not control the infection, and swelling and pain persist, surgical incision and drainage is indicated. Excision of the bursa is done when the infection is chronic and the fluid has become loculated.

COMPLICATIONS
N/A

Follow-Up

Patients require follow-up with rehabilitation services so that limitation of joint movement does not occur.

PREVENTION
N/A

Selected Readings

Pioro MH, Mandell BF. Septic arthritis. *Rheum Dis Clin North Am* 1997;23:239–258.

Shemerling RH, Delbanco TL, Tosetson ANA, et al. Synovial fluid tests. *JAMA* 1990;264:1009–1014.

Campylobacter Infections

Basics

DEFINITION
Campylobacteriosis refers to the group of infections caused by gram-negative bacteria of the genus *Campylobacter*.

ETIOLOGY
- *Campylobacter* species are motile, non–spore-forming, gram-negative rods.
- *Campylobacter* species cause both diarrheal and systemic illnesses.
- The prototype for enteric infection is *Campylobacter jejuni,* and for extraintestinal infection is *Campylobacter fetus.*

EPIDEMIOLOGY
- Campylobacteriosis is a worldwide zoonosis, and *Campylobacter* enteritis is a common form of acute gastroenteritis in North America.
- *Campylobacter* bacteria are efficiently spread through contaminated drinking water and unpasteurized milk. Sporadic cases are usually associated with the preparation of contaminated food.
- *C. jejuni* infections occur year-round in the United States and other developed countries but with a sharp peak in summer and early fall.
- About 90% of broiler chickens are contaminated with *Campylobacter,* and the infective dose is low.
- Meat originating from infected poultry or animals frequently becomes contaminated with intestinal contents during the slaughtering process.
- Consumption of undercooked poultry is estimated to be responsible for 50% to 70% of sporadic *Campylobacter* infections in developed countries.
- The epidemiology of infection in developing countries is markedly different. In these settings, *C. jejuni* is often isolated from asymptomatic persons, and is especially common during the first 5 years of life.
- HIV-infected patients are at increased risk of infection.

Clinical Manifestations

- Acute enteritis is the most common presentation of *C. jejuni* infection.
- Symptoms may last from 1 day to 1 week or longer.
- Often there is a prodrome with fever, headache, myalgia, and malaise.
- The most common symptoms are the following:
  - Abdominal pain (usually cramping)
  - Diarrhea
  - Fever (usually of low grade but can be up to 40°C or more)
  - Malaise
- Diarrhea may vary from loose stools to massive watery stools or grossly bloody stools.
- *C. fetus* infections may cause intermittent diarrhea or nonspecific abdominal pain without localizing signs.
- *C. fetus* also may cause a prolonged relapsing illness characterized by fever, chills, and myalgias, without a source of the infection being demonstrated.

Diagnosis

DIFFERENTIAL DIAGNOSIS
The diagnosis can be suspected on the basis of symptoms and is easily confirmed by stool culture. See also Section I chapter, "Diarrhea and Fever."

LABORATORY
- Confirmation of the diagnosis of *C. jejuni* infection is based on a positive stool culture or, occasionally, a positive blood culture.
- *Campylobacter* species are isolated from fecal specimens, using microaerobic incubation conditions and selective techniques that reduce the growth of competing microorganisms.
- Bacteremia is noted in less than 1% of patients with *C. jejuni* infection.

Treatment

- Fluid and electrolyte replacement are essential.
- *In vitro, C. jejuni* is susceptible to a wide variety of antimicrobial agents (erythromycin, tetracyclines, aminoglycosides, chloramphenicol, quinolones, nitrofurans, and clindamycin).
- There is a clear benefit from early treatment. In contrast, other studies, in which initiation of treatment was delayed for several days until *C. jejuni* was isolated, did not show a therapeutic effect.
- The preferred treatment is ciprofloxacin, 500 mg PO bid for 5 to 7 days. However, resistance of *Campylobacter* to quinolones is increasing.
- Erythromycin is an alternative treatment. The recommended dosage for adults is 250 mg PO qid for 5 to 7 days; the recommended dosage for children is 30 to 50 mg/kg/d in divided doses for the same period.
- Most *C. jejuni* and *Campylobacter coli* isolates are not susceptible to cephalosporins or penicillin, and these agents should not be used.
- Susceptibility to sulfonamides and metronidazole is variable. Unlike *Salmonella* infections, treatment with

Campylobacter Infections

- antimicrobial agents does not prolong carriage of *C. jejuni*; on the contrary, treatment eliminates carriage within 72 hours in most patients.
- *Campylobacter* strains acquired in developing countries are more likely to be resistant to erythromycin and tetracycline.
- Use of an antimotility agent can prolong the duration of symptoms, unless it is combined with an antibiotic.
- The necessity for treating septic or bacteremic episodes with agents other than ciprofloxacin has not been established. For those patients who are very toxic-appearing, treatment with gentamicin or imipenem is indicated.
- Patients with endovascular infections due to *C. fetus* require at least 4 weeks of therapy, and gentamicin is probably the agent of choice. Treatment with ampicillin or third-generation cephalosporins is another alternative.
- Infections of the CNS should be treated with third-generation cephalosporins, ampicillin, or chloramphenicol for 2 to 3 weeks.

COMPLICATIONS

- Among immunocompromised patients, *Campylobacter* infections can be fatal.
- *C. jejuni* may cause septic abortion.
- There have been infrequent reports of *C. jejuni* infections manifesting with acute cholecystitis, pancreatitis, and cystitis.
- *C. fetus* infections appear to have a tropism for vascular sites; vascular necrosis occurs in patients with endocarditis and pericarditis.
- CNS infections with *C. fetus* occur in neonates and adults. The prognosis is poor for premature infants, but some full-term neonates have survived infection. Infection is manifested as a meningoencephalitis with a cerebrospinal fluid polymorphonuclear pleocytosis.

- The clinical manifestations of infection due to other enteric *Campylobacter* species overlap substantially with those of *C. jejuni*.
- Among immunocompromised patients, especially those with AIDS, bacteremia by the "atypical" *Campylobacter* species appears relatively commonly, and it can continue indefinitely without antibiotic therapy.

Follow-Up

- Relapses may be seen in 5% to 10% of untreated patients with *C. jejuni* infection.
- A reactive arthritis may occur up to several weeks postinfection in persons with the HLA-B27 histocompatibility antigens.
- The Guillain-Barré syndrome is an uncommon consequence of *C. jejuni* infection that usually occurs 2 to 3 weeks after the diarrheal illness.

PROGNOSIS

- The vast majority of patients recover fully after *C. jejuni* infection, either spontaneously or after appropriate antimicrobial therapy.
- *C. fetus* infection may be lethal to patients with chronic compensated diseases such as cirrhosis or diabetes mellitus.
- *Campylobacter* infections are the most important recognized antecedent of Guillain-Barré syndrome.

PREVENTION

- In the United States, the increase in quinolone-resistant *C. jejuni* infections is largely due to infections acquired during foreign travel. However, the number of quinolone-resistant infections acquired domestically has also increased, largely because of the acquisition of resistant strains from poultry.

- *Campylobacter* can be killed by cooking poultry and other meats to an internal temperature of 82°C (180°F). This is the temperature at which the meat is no longer pink and the juice runs clear.
- Poultry and other meats must be prepared separately from other foods, both in restaurants and at home.
- Countertops, utensils, towels, and aprons used in the preparation of poultry and other meats should be washed with hot water and soap before they are used for other foods, particularly foods that will not be cooked.
- Handwashing is also essential.
- Suspected cases, particularly when associated with other cases among family members or acquaintances, should be reported promptly to the local health department.

Selected Readings

Anonymous. Campylobacter enteritis: It could happen to you. *Can Med Assoc J* 1998;158:1056–1057.

Blaser MJ. Campylobacter and related species. In: Mandell GL, Bennett JE, Dolin R, eds. *Principles and practice of infectious diseases.* New York: Churchill Livingstone, 1995:1948–1956.

Smith KE, Besser JM, Hedberg CW, et al. Quinolone-resistant *Campylobacter jejuni* infections in Minnesota, 1992–1998. Investigation Team. *N Engl J Med* 1999;340:1525–1532.

Wegener HC. The consequences for food safety of the use of fluoroquinolones in food animals [Editorial]. *N Engl J Med* 1999;340:1581–1582.

Candida Vaginitis

Basics

DEFINITION
Candida vaginitis is a fungal yeast infection that produces an odorless, thick, white vaginal discharge with the consistency of cottage cheese. Yeast infections usually cause the vagina and the vulva to be very itchy and red.

ETIOLOGY
- *Candida albicans* is the cause in 90% of patients.
- *C. albicans* is found in the normal vaginal flora of 15% to 25% of asymptomatic women of childbearing years.
- *Candida glabrata, Candida krusei, Candida tropicalis,* and *Candida pseudotropicalis* produce infection in recurrent cases and in women with HIV infection.

EPIDEMIOLOGY
Incidence and Prevalence
- Yeast vaginitis occurs in 75% of women during their lifetimes.
- Fifty percent of women have two or more episodes that are clinically apparent just before the onset of a menstrual period.
- *C. albicans* is found in the normal vaginal flora of 15% to 25% of asymptomatic women during childbearing years. This organism colonizes the intestinal tract of most women.

Risk Factors
- Frequent intercourse (highest risk, seven or more times per week)
- Vaginal contraceptives
- Passive oral–genital contact
- Use of antibiotics, corticosteroids, and immunosuppressives
- Diabetes mellitus, particularly with glycosuria
- Pregnancy
- Obesity
- Excessive warmth, perspiration, and moisture in the groin area

Clinical Manifestations

- Vulvar pruritus and burning
- Abnormal vaginal discharge
- Burning on urination at the urethral orifice
- Vaginal erythema; white or yellow adherent plaques in 40%

Diagnosis

- Examination under microscope shows hyphae or mycelia in the KOH preparation.
- If microscopic examination is negative, vaginal discharge culture usually yields *Candida*.
- Culture is the most reliable method of diagnosis, but unnecessary if the KOH preparation is positive in a symptomatic woman.
  - Clue cells (vaginal epithelial cells so overladen with bacteria that the cell border is obscured)
  - pH greater than 4.5 (measure pH, using pH paper, which measures from 4.0 to 6.0)
  - Release of amine "fishy" odor upon mixing alkalinizing vaginal fluid with one drop of KOH (10%) solution
- Culture of vaginal fluid for *Haemophilus* or anaerobes is not advised.

DIFFERENTIAL DIAGNOSIS
- Other forms of vaginitis (e.g., *Trichomonas*, herpes, and bacterial vaginosis)

Treatment

MAIN TREATMENT
- Removal of predisposing factors is the first consideration.
- Intravaginal products are the treatment of choice and should be applied at bedtime:
  - Clotrimazole
    - 1% vaginal cream, 5 g for 7 to 14 days
    - 100-mg vaginal tablet, one tablet for 7 days or 2 tablets for 3 days
    - 500-mg vaginal tablet, single application

Candida Vaginitis

- Miconazole
  - 2% vaginal cream, 5 g for 7 days
  - 200-mg vaginal suppository for 3 days
  - 100-mg vaginal suppository for 7 days
- Butoconazole
  - 2% vaginal cream, 5 g for 3 days
- Terconazole, 80-mg vaginal suppository for 3 days
- Fluconazole and itraconazole can be used as a single oral dose.
- Nystatin and boric acid can be used for azole-resistant strains.
- Intravaginal clotrimazole, miconazole, or terconazole may be used for symptomatic pregnant women, but should be deferred until the second trimester.

RECURRENCES

- About 10% of women will have one or more attacks of *Candida* vaginitis following treatment.
- The reservoir of these *Candida* strains appears in the intestinal tract. It is not clear whether these episodes are due to recurrence (same strain) or reinfection (different strain).
- Management of recurrent candidiasis includes the following:
  - Reculture vaginal fluid to prove *Candida*.
  - Identify species and do sensitivity tests against azoles to search for resistant strains.
  - Remove predisposing causes:
    - Caution patient on the use of antibiotics.
    - Avoid the use of vaginal contraceptives.
    - Treat the male partner for balanitis, if present, with topical medication (consider altering sexual practices).
  - Treat intermittently or continuously with oral ketoconazole (100 mg) or fluconazole (100 mg) or with weekly intravaginal clotrimazole or another azole.
  - Consume yogurt with lactobacillus acidophilus, 4 oz, twice daily.

COMPLICATIONS

N/A

Follow-Up

Because of frequent recurrences, patients should have periodic pelvic examinations and cultures.

PREVENTION

Avoid the previously mentioned risk factors.

Selected Readings

Ries AJ. Treatment of vaginal infections: Candidiasis, bacterial vaginosis, and trichomoniasis. *J Am Pharm Assoc (Wash)* 1997;NS37(5):563–569.

Ringdahl EN. Treatment of recurrent vulvovaginal candidiasis. *Am Fam Physician* 2000;61(11):3306–3312, 3317.

Rodgers CA, Beardall AJ. Recurrent vulvovaginal candidiasis: Why does it occur? *Int J STD AIDS* 1999;10(7):435–439.

Sobel JD. Vaginitis. *N Engl J Med* 1997;337(26):1896–1903.

Candidiasis

Basics

DEFINITION
- *Candida* organisms are yeasts (fungi that exist predominantly in a unicellular form).
- Both sexual and asexual forms exist. They are small (4–6 mm), thin-walled, ovoid cells (blastospores) that reproduce by budding.

ETIOLOGY
- The organism stains gram-positive.
- There are more than 150 species of *Candida*. The most common species are the following:
  - *C. albicans*
  - *C. glabrata* (formerly classified as *Torulopsis glabrata*)
  - *C. guilliermondi*
  - *C. krusei*
  - *C. lusitaniae*
  - *C. parapsilosis*
  - *C. pseudotropicalis*
  - *C. tropicalis*

EPIDEMIOLOGY
- Candidemia currently accounts for 10% to 15% of hospital-acquired infections of the bloodstream. A growing number of patients are at risk, among them those with severe underlying diseases such as cancer, those undergoing organ transplantation or extensive surgical procedures, those with AIDS, and those with major burns.
- The majority of *Candida* infections are of endogenous origin. Predisposing factors include the following:
  - Immune suppression
  - Prolonged use of broad-spectrum antibiotics
  - Use of hyperalimentation fluid
  - Use of indwelling intravenous catheter
- Hepatosplenic candidiasis is an important clinical problem in immunocompromised hosts.
- Antibiotics, diabetes mellitus, and Foley catheters have been associated with candiduria.
- *Candida* vaginitis is most frequently seen in the following settings:
  - Antibiotic therapy
  - Diabetes mellitus
  - Pregnancy
- There is a significantly higher risk of vulvovaginal candidiasis in women who use oral contraceptives.
- Seventy-five percent of women have an episode of candidal vaginitis during their lifetimes.
- By age 25, half of all college women will have experienced at least one physician-diagnosed episode of vulvovaginal candidiasis.
- Defined as four or more episodes of infection per year, recurrent vulvovaginal candidiasis occurs in less than 5% of healthy women.
- Inhaled steroids has been associated with oral thrush.

Clinical Manifestations

- The term *thrush* is applied to a specific form of oral candidiasis characterized by creamy white, curdlike patches on the tongue and on other oral mucosal surfaces, which are removable by scraping and leave a raw, bleeding, and painful surface.
- The most common symptoms of *Candida* esophagitis include the following:
  - Nausea
  - Painful swallowing
  - Substernal chest pain
  - Vomiting
- The clinical signs and symptoms of vulvovaginal candidiasis include vulvovaginal pruritus, irritation, soreness, dyspareunia, burning on micturition, and whitish, cheesy discharge. Unfortunately, none of these symptoms, either individually or collectively, is pathognomonic; a reliable diagnosis, therefore, cannot be made on the basis of the history and physical examination without the corroborative evidence of laboratory tests.
- Intertriginous candidiasis affects any site where skin surfaces are in close proximity. It begins as vesicopustules, which enlarge and rupture, causing maceration and fissuring. The area of involvement has a scalloped border with a white rim consisting of necrotic epidermis, which surrounds an erythematous, macerated base.
- *Candida* is one of the most common causes of diaper rash in infants and paronychia in all age groups.
- Chronic mucocutaneous candidiasis describes a heterogeneous group of *Candida* infections of the skin, mucous membranes, hair, and nails that has a protracted and persistent course.
- *Candida* can infect parenchymal brain tissue or the meninges. Also, it can infect the eye either by hematogenous spread or by direct inoculation, especially during eye surgery.
- *Candida* intravascular infection can involve both peripheral and deep vascular structures and implanted prosthetic vascular materials.

Diagnosis

- The diagnosis of *Candida* esophagitis is based on the clinical presentation and endoscopic appearance of white patches resembling thrush.
- *Candida* spp grow well in vented routine blood culture bottles and on agar plates and do not require special fungal media for cultivation.
- Many patients with *Candida* endocarditis have negative blood cultures.
- The presence of *Candida* in the urine does not necessarily indicate renal tract infection.
- CT scans, ultrasound, or MRI may visualize liver or splenic abscesses.
- The diagnosis of vulvovaginal candidiasis is easily established by the finding of a normal vaginal pH (4.0–4.5) and positive results on saline or 10% potassium hydroxide microscopy. Because of the poor sensitivity of these tests and the lack of specificity of clinical signs, vulvovaginal candidiasis is still possible despite negative microscopical results in patients with a compatible clinical presentation and normal pH; in such cases, a vaginal culture should be obtained.

Candidiasis

Treatment

- Nystatin has been the primary agent used for mucous membrane and cutaneous candidiasis. The usual adult dose is 4 to 6 mL of the fluid qid.
- Clotrimazole is approximately equally as effective as nystatin but is generally much better tolerated. Usually, 7 to 10 days of therapy is sufficient; the patient should be treated for 48 hours after becoming asymptomatic.
- Most common therapy of chronic mucocutaneous candidiasis is an azole followed by transfer factor.
- Ketoconazole (400 mg/d orally for up to 9 months) or fluconazole has been effective for chronic mucocutaneous candidiasis.
- For oral thrush, fluconazole (100 mg/d orally for 5–14 days) or itraconazole oral solution (100 mg orally twice daily for 7–14 days). A 14-day course is usually suggested for patients with AIDS and thrush or esophagitis. A last resort is low-dose (10–20 mg/d) intravenous amphotericin B.
- Management of *Candida* diaper rash has been successful with nystatin powder or cream in combination with a corticosteroid.
- For bloodstream infections, amphotericin B (usually 0.5 mg/kg/d, up to 1 mg/kg/d for septic patients) or fluconazole (400–800 mg/d) can be used.
- If the patient is neutropenic or the course is consistent with an acute sepsis, causing the patient to be in an unstable or rapidly worsening condition, amphotericin B is usually selected for initial therapy. Depending on the severity of the situation, 5-fluorocytosine (5-FC) (37.5 mg/kg orally every 6 hours) can be added to the regimen to provide rapid attainment of therapeutic blood levels. Bone marrow suppression or diarrhea may be complications of simultaneous use of these agents.
- However, fluconazole may be used even in neutropenic patients, unless the candidaemia is caused by fluconazole-resistant organisms, such as *C. glabrata* or *C. krusei*. Removal of the vascular catheter is recommended, because catheter retention allows the candidaemia to persist.
- The failure rate for cure of hepatosplenic candidiasis has been high with both amphotericin B alone and in combination with 5-FC. Reports of cures with liposomal amphotericin have appeared and are promising. Successful results also have been obtained with fluconazole.
- Oral azoles are contraindicated in pregnancy.

COMPLICATIONS

- Perforation of the esophagus due to esophageal candidiasis is very rare. Other complications include bleeding and dissemination.
- Papillary necrosis, fungus ball formation, and perinephric abscess can result from ascending infection, particularly in the presence of urinary tract obstruction, renal stones, or diabetes mellitus.
- *Candida* intravascular infection can cause superior cava obstruction, mural endocarditis of the right atrium, tricuspid endocarditis, and pulmonary venous thrombosis.

Follow-Up

- Recurrent vulvovaginal candidiasis is a form of complicated vulvovaginal candidiasis and is defined as four or more episodes of proved infection during a 12-month period.
- Some patients with cardiac valvular candidiasis have had relapses years after surgery.

PREVENTION

- In a cohort of marrow transplant patients, prophylactic fluconazole resulted in a significant reduction in infection caused by *Candida* species and an increase in mold infections.
- Consider fluconazole prophylaxis for AIDS patients with esophageal candidiasis.

Selected Readings

Edwards JE Jr. Candida species. In: Mandell GL, Bennett JE, Dolin R, eds. *Principles and practice of infectious diseases*. New York: Churchill Livingstone, 1995:2289–2306.

Mylonakis E, Flanigan TP. Antifungal prophylaxis with weekly fluconazole for patients with AIDS. *Clin Infect Dis* 1998;27:1376–1378.

Raad I. Intravascular-catheter-related infections. *Lancet* 1998;351:893–898.

Rex JH, Bennett JE, Sugar AM, et al. A randomized trial comparing fluconazole with amphotericin B for the treatment of candidemia in patients without neutropenia. Candidemia Study Group and the National Institute. *N Engl J Med* 1994;331:1325–1330.

Sobel JD, Faro S, Force RW, et al. Vulvovaginal candidiasis: Epidemiologic, diagnostic, and therapeutic considerations. *Am J Obstet Gynecol* 1998;178:203–211.

Sobel JD. Vaginitis. *N Engl J Med* 1997;337:1896–1903.

van Burik JH, Leisenring W, Myerson D, et al. The effect of prophylactic fluconazole on the clinical spectrum of fungal diseases in bone marrow transplant recipients with special attention to hepatic candidiasis. An autopsy study of 355 patients. *Medicine* 1998;77:246–254.

Cat-Scratch Disease

Basics

DEFINITION

- Cat-scratch disease is usually a self-limited acute illness associated with lymphadenopathy, fatigue, headache, and anorexia, usually caused by *Bartonella henselae*.
- Disseminated infection by *Bartonella quintana* and *B. henselae* may be manifested by bacillary angiomatosis, bacillary peliosis, a spectrum of inflammatory lesions, or a combination of these. Such infections may not become evident until well after the bacteremic events from which they presumably arise.

ETIOLOGY

Isolation of *Afipia felis* from cat-scratch disease lesions prompted initial interest in this organism as the major cause of the syndrome. Current evidence suggests that *A. felis* causes few, if any, cases of cat-scratch disease, and most cases are caused by *B. henselae* (a gram-negative bacterium).

EPIDEMIOLOGY

Incidence

- Cat-scratch disease occurs worldwide. In temperate climates, it is seasonal, with most cases occurring between August and January.
- *B. quintana* is believed to be globally endemic and causes trench fever.
- Cat-scratch disease occurs in immunocompetent patients of all ages, with 80% being younger than 21 years of age.
- Cat-scratch disease is a common disease (0.77–0.86 case per 100,000 population), and it is considered the most common cause of chronic, benign adenopathy in children and young adults, with an estimated 24,000 cases recognized each year.

Risk Factors

- Patients are more likely to have at least one kitten 12 months of age or younger (odds ratio, 15), to have been scratched or bitten by a kitten (odds ratio, 27), and to have at least one kitten with fleas (odds ratio, 29).
- A history of contact with cats is found in 90% of patients, and antecedent cat scratch in 60%.
- Originally described involving the liver and sometimes spleen in HIV-infected persons, some of whom also had concurrent bacillary angiomatosis, it has since been identified in other types of immunosuppressed persons, and found to involve lymph nodes as well.

Clinical Manifestations

- Often, the initial symptom of cat-scratch disease is the formation of a small erythematous papule or pustule at the site of the scratch that persists for several weeks. Subsequently, lymph nodes draining the site of inoculation become enlarged and tender.
- Patients with cat-scratch disease do not always have fever. Low-grade fever and malaise are seen in 30% of patients.
- Patients with cat-scratch disease can experience rash, hepatosplenomegaly, lytic bone lesions, granulomatous conjunctivitis, pneumonitis, and central nervous system involvement. This process usually lasts 2 to 4 months and resolves spontaneously.
- Trench fever's natural course in normal hosts has been well summarized. Incubation after inoculation may span 3 to 38 days before the usually sudden onset of chills and fevers. Afebrile infection is the least common form. Associated symptoms and signs (e.g., headache, vertigo, retro-orbital pain, conjunctival infection) are all nonspecific.
- *B. henselae* bacteremia in HIV-infected persons is associated with insidious development of fatigue, malaise, body aches, weight loss, recurring fevers of progressively greater duration and elevation, and sometimes headache. Associated hepatomegaly may occur.
- Characteristic of the gross morphology of bacillary angiomatosis, skin lesions are subcutaneous or dermal nodules, and/or single or multiple dome-shaped, skin-colored or red to purple papules, any of which may display ulceration, serous or bloody drainage, and crusting. Visceral lesions can be quite dramatic as well, in both their number and heterogeneity of gross appearance.
- Bacillary peliosis involves organs that contain numerous blood-filled cystic structures, the sizes of which can range from microscopic to several millimeters.
- Endocarditis due to *B. quintana*, *B. henselae*, and *B. elizabethae* has been reported.

Diagnosis

DIFFERENTIAL DIAGNOSIS

- The diagnosis of cat-scratch disease is suggested by the following:
  —Contact with a cat and the presence of a scratch or primary lesion
  —A positive skin test
  —A compatible clinical picture, usually with unilateral regional lymphadenitis and negative studies for other causes of lymphadenopathy
  —Characteristic histopathologic findings (the presence in a lymph node biopsy specimen of multiple microabscesses or granulomas)
  —Exclusion of other identifiable causes, especially mycobacterial

LABORATORY

- Acute lymphadenitis due to bacteria generally develops over 3 to 4 days. Sonography may be helpful to detect early suppuration of the bubo and to direct needle aspiration, when indicated. Early in

Cat-Scratch Disease

the disease, a total white blood cell count may show mild leukocytosis and an increased number of polymorphonuclear cells, with eosinophilia in 10% to 20% of patients.
- *B. henselae* and *B. quintana* can be isolated from blood if lysis-centrifugation blood cultures are used, but both species, as well as *B. elizabethae*, have also been isolated with use of the BACTEC blood culture system.
- Serologic tests (indirect fluorescent antibody) for *B. henselae* are becoming standardized. The enzyme immunoassay also is reportedly more sensitive than the indirect fluorescent-antibody test for the diagnosis of cat-scratch disease.

Treatment

MAIN TREATMENT

- The literature is full of contradictory statements about the role and selection of antibiotics for cat-scratch disease. Azithromycin (500 mg orally once and 250 mg once daily for the following 4 days) can be used.
- If suppuration occurs, aspiration should be considered to relieve the pain and hasten recovery. Needle aspiration is generally preferred to incision and drainage. After washing the skin with an iodophor skin cleanser, aspiration may be accomplished by inserting an 18- or 19-gauge needle tangentially through normal skin at the base of the node. Rarely, reaspiration may be necessary.
- For bacillary angiomatosis involving only the skin, 8 to 12 weeks of oral therapy with erythromycin 500 mg four times daily or doxycycline 100 mg orally twice daily is recommended. Lesions often begin to recede within a week, but usually take considerably longer to involute completely and may leave residual hyperpigmentation. If not resolved by 12 weeks, therapy should be extended.
- For bacteremia, at least 4 weeks of therapy is indicated. Treatment of longer duration (2–3 months) is appropriate in the HIV-infected patient, if fever is persistent or recurrent in the HIV-uninfected patient, and in the setting of endocarditis.

- In endocarditis, hemodynamic considerations may require valve replacement (see also chapters in Section II on endocarditis).

ALTERNATIVE TREATMENT

Despite *in vitro* findings suggesting likely susceptibility, treatments with a variety of β-lactams, with trimethoprim–sulfamethoxazole, and with fluoroquinolones have had inconsistent, and often unfavorable, results. The use of rifampin and aminoglycosides, which may have some beneficial effect in cat-scratch disease, requires further investigation.

COMPLICATIONS

- Unusual manifestations of cat-scratch disease include Parinaud's oculoglandular syndrome (in 6% of patients), encephalopathy (in 2%), and conjunctivitis (in 5%).
- Encephalopathy usually develops several weeks after the acute illness. Seizures and status epilepticus may herald encephalopathy but are self-limited, with rapid improvement, usually within several days. The cerebrospinal fluid is usually normal, although pleocytosis may occur. The cause of the encephalopathy is uncertain, but direct infection, a toxin, and an autoimmune process have been implicated.
- Inflammatory reactions to *B. henselae* infection in persons with AIDS, without associated angiomatosis or peliosis, have been reported involving liver, spleen, lymph nodes, heart, and bone marrow.
- *B. henselae* bacteremia can evolve into long-term asymptomatic persistence.

Follow-Up

- The lymphadenopathy of cat-scratch disease usually resolves spontaneously within a period of several months.
- One episode of cat-scratch disease appears to confer lifelong immunity. Rarely, a recurrence of sinus tract drainage from the nodes originally involved may occur. If the adenopathy is massive (>5 cm), chronic adenopathy may persist for 1 to 2 years.

- Remission of fever among patients with bacteremia is usually prompt in non–HIV-infected persons, but may take up to several weeks in the HIV-infected patient. Within a week of starting therapy, bacteremia is usually no longer detectable, even if fever persists.

PREVENTION

- Three strategies for cats could be considered:
  —Flea control
  —Treatment of established *R. henselae* infections of cats
  —Vaccination of cats to prevent infection

Selected Readings

Adal KA, Cockerell CJ, Petri WA Jr. Cat scratch disease, bacillary angiomatosis, and other infections due to *Rochalimaea*. N Engl J Med 1994;330:1509–1515.

Anonymous. Case records of the Massachusetts General Hospital. Case 1-1998. An 11-year-old boy with a seizure. N Engl J Med 1998;338:112–119.

Dolan MJ, Wong MT, Regnery RL, et al. Syndrome of *Rochalimaea henselae* adenitis suggesting cat scratch disease. Ann Intern Med 1993;118:331–336.

Fisher GW. Cat scratch disease. In: Mandell GL, Bennett JE, Dolin R, eds. *Principles and practice of infectious diseases*. New York: Churchill Livingstone, 1995:1310–1312.

Margileth AM, Hayden GF. Cat scratch disease. From feline affection to human infection [Editorial]. N Engl J Med 1993;329:53–54.

Tompkins DC, Steigbigel RT. *Rochalimaea*'s role in cat scratch disease and bacillary angiomatosis. Ann Intern Med 1993;118:388–390.

Tompkins LS. *Rochalimaea* infections. Are they zoonoses? JAMA 1994;271:553–554.

Zangwill KM, Hamilton DH, Perkins BA, et al. Cat scratch disease in Connecticut. Epidemiology, risk factors, and evaluation of a new diagnostic test. N Engl J Med 1993;329:8–13.

Cervicitis/Mucopurulent Cervicitis (MPC)

Basics

DEFINITION
- Sexually transmitted disease manifested as inflammation of the endocervix

ETIOLOGY
- *Chlamydia trachomatis*
- *Neisseria gonorrhoeae*

EPIDEMIOLOGY

Incidence
- Frequent in sexually active adolescent girls under the age of 20 years
- Also found in young adults aged 20 to 24 years

Risk Factors
- New sex partner within past 3 months
- More than one sex partner within past 6 months
- Sex partner with multiple other sex partners
- Inconsistent use of barrier contraceptives

Clinical Manifestations

SYMPTOMS AND SIGNS
- Frequently asymptomatic
- Abnormal vaginal discharge or vaginal bleeding, particularly after intercourse
- Yellow exudate visible in endocervical canal or on an endocervical swab specimen
- Cervical friability

Diagnosis

- Appearance of cervix on direct inspections
- Culture of cervical discharge

LABORATORY
- Gram stain
- Culture for gonococcus
- *Chlamydia* testing
- Cytologic examination of endocervical mucus specimens
  —Detection of gram-negative, intracellular diplococci in endocervical mucus is highly specific for gonococcal infection.
  —It is only 50% sensitive in MPC, in contrast to 95% sensitive in gonococcal urethritis.
- Microscopic examination of ectocervical fluid specimens using normal, wet-mount saline and KOH
- If cervical ulcers or necrotic lesions are present, test for genital herpes.

TESTING PROCEDURES
Wipe the ectocervix clean with a swab before obtaining the endocervical mucus specimen.

Treatment

Presumptive treatment should be undertaken if there is a high prevalence of *C. trachomatis* and *N. gonorrhoeae* in the local population and there is little likelihood that the patient will comply with return visits. Awaiting test results before treatment is initiated is recommended if prevalence of *C. trachomatis* and *N. gonorrhoeae* is low and compliance with return visits is likely.

Cervicitis/Mucopurulent Cervicitis (MPC)

MAIN TREATMENT

- Presumptive
- Gonococcal: ceftriaxone 125 mg i.m., single dose
- *C. trachomatis*: doxycycline 100 mg PO bid for 7 days

ALTERNATIVE TREATMENT

- Alternatives to ceftriaxone
  - Cefixime 400 mg PO, single dose
  - Ciprofloxacin 500 mg PO, single dose
  - Ofloxacin 400 mg PO, single dose
- For patients who cannot take cephalosporins or fluoroquinolones
  - Spectinomycin 2 g i.m., single dose
  - Spectinomycin rarely effective in gonococcal pharyngitis
- Alternatives to doxycycline
  - Azithromycin 1 g PO, single dose
  - Ofloxacin 300 mg PO bid for 7 days
  - Erythromycin 500 mg PO qid for 7 days
- Pregnancy
  - Fluoroquinolones contraindicated
  - Tetracyclines contraindicated
  - Azithromycin effectiveness not established
  - Ceftriaxone recommended
  - Spectinomycin recommended in patients allergic to cephalosporins
  - Erythromycin base or ethylsuccinate (not estolate) recommended

SEX PARTNERS

- Examination, treatment
- Presumptive treatment if prevalence of *C. trachomatis* or *N. gonorrhoeae* is high or if compliance with return visits deemed unlikely

COMPLICATIONS

- Pelvic inflammatory disease
- Ectopic pregnancy
- Infertility
- Chorioamnionitis
- Premature rupture of membranes
- Puerperal infections

Follow-Up

- Rescreen for *C. trachomatis* or *N. gonorrhoeae* several months after treatment.
- Note: Follow-up testing should not be done immediately after clinical resolution: Nonculture tests for chlamydia performed within 3 weeks of completion of successful treatment may be false-positive as a result of continued excretion of dead organisms.

PREVENTION

- Safe sex practices

Selected Reading

Molodysky E. Urethritis and cervicitis. *Aust Fam Physician* 1999;28(4):333–338.

Sweet RL. The enigmatic cervix. *Dermatol Clin* 1998;16(4):739–745, xii.

Chancroid

Basics

DEFINITION
Chancroid is a sexually-transmitted disease manifested as genital lesions or, later, genital ulcers. The primary lesion is typically a group of excavated papules or pustules 2 to 20 mm diameter with undermined, ragged, or irregular edges.

ETIOLOGY
- *Haemophilus ducreyi*

EPIDEMIOLOGY
Incidence
- Prevalent in
  - Africa
  - Asia
  - Latin America
  - United States, lower socioeconomic groups

Risk Factors
- Sex with multiple partners
- Sex with partner infected with *H. ducreyi*
- Sex with persons in countries where chancroid is endemic

INCUBATION
- One to 14 days

Clinical Manifestations

SYMPTOMS AND SIGNS
- Tender papules that become pustular, eroded, and ulcerated within 1 to 2 days
- Several lesions can coalesce to form a large ulcer wider than 2 cm.
- Tender inguinal nodes in approximately 40% of patients
- Inguinal lymph nodes occasionally suppurate and rupture spontaneously.
- Combined painful genital ulcer with suppurative inguinal lymphadenopathy

Diagnosis

Initial diagnosis is based on epidemiologic factors and the characteristics of the lesions. History and physical examination alone often lead to misdiagnosis, making laboratory examination of utmost importance.

DIFFERENTIAL DIAGNOSIS
Infectious
- Isolation of *H. ducreyi* to provide definitive diagnosis of chancroid
- Genital herpes
- Syphilis
- Acute HIV infection
- Lymphogranuloma venereum
- Granuloma inguinale or donovanosis
- Mycobacteria
- Fungi
- Parasites
- Venereal warts
- Scabies
- Molluscum contagiosum
- Folliculitis

Noninfectious
- Malignancy
- Trauma
- Fixed drug eruption
- Erythema
- Dermatitis herpetiformis
- Behçet's syndrome

Chancroid

LABORATORY

- Culture for *H. ducreyi* (80% sensitivity)
- No evidence of syphilis by dark-field examination, immunofluorescence test, or a serologic test performed more than 7 days after the onset of ulcers
- No evidence of genital herpes based on clinical presentation or herpes simplex virus culture or antigen test

TESTING PROCEDURES

- Gently abrade the lesion with sterile gauze pad to provoke oozing, but not gross bleeding.
- Squeeze the lesion between a gloved thumb and forefinger to increase exudate from lesion.
- Apply exudate directly onto a microscope slide if used for dark-field and direct immunofluorescence tests.

Treatment

MAIN TREATMENT

- Azithromycin 1 g PO, single dose
- Ceftriaxone 250 mg i.m., single dose
- Erythromycin base 500 mg PO qid for 7 days; preferred regimen in HIV-infected patients

ALTERNATIVE TREATMENT

- Amoxicillin/clavulanic acid 500/125 mg PO tid for 7 days
- Ciprofloxacin 500 mg PO bid for 3 days

SEX PARTNERS

Evaluate and treat partners who have had sexual intercourse with the patient within 10 days of onset of the patient's symptoms. Use the same drugs and dosages as above.

COMPLICATIONS

- Inaccurate diagnosis
- Coinfection with another sexually transmitted disease (e.g., syphilis)
- Reinfection
- HIV infection. *Note:* Transmission of and susceptibility to HIV infection is increased during intercourse in patients with chancroid.
- Poor patient compliance with treatment
- Antimicrobial resistance

Follow-Up

- Reexamine within 3 to 7 days of initial treatment for signs of improvement of ulcers.
- Fluctuant lymphadenopathy improves more slowly and may require needle aspiration through adjacent intact skin.

PREVENTION

- Avoid sexual contact with a person infected with chancroid or a person who has genital lesions or ulcers.
- Observe safe-sex practices.

Selected Readings

Lewis DA. Diagnostic tests for chancroid. *Sex Transm Infect* 2000;76(2):137–141.

Schmid GP. Treatment of chancroid, 1997. *Clin Infect Dis* 1999;28[Suppl 1]:S14–S20.

Chickenpox

Basics

DEFINITION
- Chickenpox is a febrile, highly contagious illness of the early childhood (usually), worldwide in distribution, and characterized by a maculopapular rash in varying stages of evolution.
- It is due to primary infection by varicella zoster virus (VZV), and occurs in epidemics during late winter and early spring.

ETIOLOGY
- Varicella zoster virus (HHV-3, DNA virus, family: Herpesviridae)
- There is no known animal reservoir for VZV. Transmission occurs via person-to-person contact; the virus is spread by the respiratory route and replicates in the nasopharynx or the upper respiratory tract.
- The incubation period is 10 to 14 days (range, 10–20 days).
- The primary attack rate in susceptible individuals is 90%, and secondary attack rate in the same household is 70% to 90%.
- Systems affected: skin, disseminated/viraemia, CNS, respiratory, other viscera

EPIDEMIOLOGY
Incidence
- Three to 4×10^6 cases per year in the United States

Risk Factors
- Close contact of a nonimmune person to a patient transmitting the virus
- Predominant age: 90% of cases in children less than 3 years old
- Ninety percent of individuals over 15 years of age are immune; 10% remain susceptible.
- Incidence in adults is increasing.
- Predominant sex: males equal to females

Clinical Manifestations

SYMPTOMS AND SIGNS
Immunocompetent Children
- *Prodromal symptoms* may occur 1 to 2 days prior to the rash: malaise, low-grade fever.
- *Constitutional symptoms*: low-grade fever, malaise, pruritus, anorexia, listlessness
- *Rash*: begins on the face and trunk and spreads centripetally
- Initially maculopapular; develops into vesicles, full of clear fluid
- Fluid turns purulent after a few hours.
- Lesions are round or oval, with an erythematous base, sized from 5 to 12 to 13 mm in diameter. Central umbilication appears as healing progresses.
- Crust formation follows and coexists with evolution of new lesions.
- All forms of lesions are concurrently present in varying stages of evolution.
- The successive crops of lesions generally appear over 2 to 4 days.
- The rash may involve mucous membranes.

Immunocompromised Patient
- More numerous lesions with haemorrhagic base
- Healing time three times longer
- At greater risk for visceral complications (30%–50% of cases; of those, 15% fatal)

Adults
- More severe illness
- At greater risk for visceral complications

Perinatal Varicella
- When chickenpox develops 5 days before to 48 hours after delivery, may result in progressive disease in the newborn, involving viscera, particularly the lung
- Death rate high (mortality 30%)

Congenital Varicella
Infection of the fetus during the first two trimesters of pregnancy may lead to severe malformations (skin scarring, hypoplastic extremities, eye abnormalities, CNS impairment).

Diagnosis

DIFFERENTIAL DIAGNOSIS
- Disseminated herpes simplex virus infection in patients with atopic dermatitis
- Disseminated rashes due to coxsackieviruses, echoviruses, atypical measles
- Rickettsialpox ("herald spot" at the site of mite bite, serology)

LABORATORY
- Diagnosis is mainly clinical.
- VZV isolation from material taken from the bottom of the lesions; needs about 1 week
- Serology: seroconversion or fourfold increase in antibodies to VZV membrane antigens in convalescent serum samples (ELISA test)

IMAGING
- Abnormalities in chest x-rays appear in 16% of chickenpox patients; only 10% of patients with positive chest x-rays develop clinical symptoms from the respiratory system.
- In pneumonitis, a nodular pattern or increased reticular shadowing can be seen.

SPECIAL TESTS
- Tzank smear from the bottom of a vesicle; shows multinucleated giant cells
- Detection of viral antigens in smears by direct immunofluorescence staining or other assays

Chickenpox

Treatment

- Appropriate health care is usually outpatient, unless complication occurs or the patient is at high risk for complications (i.e., pregnant woman, the immunosuppressed)
- General measures are careful bathing, astringent soaks, and closely cropped fingernails to prevent scratching.
- Topical administration of antipruritic drugs: Use acetaminophen for fever. *Do not use aspirin, as it predisposes to Reye's syndrome development.*
- Allow activity to the degree allowed by the clinical status.
- There are no specific recommendations for diet.
- The patient must be out of school until no longer contagious: A patient is infectious 48 hours prior to the appearance of the rash, until all vesicles are crusted.
- Oral acyclovir is recommended for adolescents, adults, premature children, and children with bronchopulmonary disease within 24 hours of onset of the disease.
- Children 2 to 16 years of age: 20 mg/kg q8h for 5 days; maximum, 800 mg q8h for 5 days
- Adolescents/Adults: 800 mg q8h for 5 days

COMPLICATIONS

- Mortality is less than 2 in 100,000 cases for a normal child, but increases by over 15-fold for adults.
- *Secondary bacterial infection*/gram-positive organisms, systemic infection in the neutropenic host
- *Varicella pneumonitis*, especially occurs in adults (1 in 400 cases), and immunocompromised individuals. It manifests with tachypnea, cough, dyspnea, and fever, usually 3 to 5 days after the onset of illness. It can be life-threatening in pregnant women during the second or third trimester. Chest x-ray shows nodular or interstitial pneumonitis. Chest x-ray changes can be apparent in the absence of clinical symptoms.
- *Cerebellar ataxia* appears in 1 in 4,000 cases, usually in patients younger than 15 years of age, as late as 21 days after the onset of rash, but usually within 1 week. Symptoms include ataxia, emesis, dysphasia, fever, vertigo, and tremor. Cerebrospinal fluid examination shows lymphocytosis and elevated protein. Usually, it is a benign complication and resolves within 2 to 4 weeks.
- *Encephalitis* can be life-threatening in adults; it appears in 0.1% to 0.2% of patients. It presents with decreased level of consciousness, headache, vomiting, altered thought patterns, fever, and seizures. Mortality ranges from 5% to 20%; neurologic sequelae can be detected in 15% of survivors. The duration is at least 2 weeks.
- *Meningitis, transverse myelitis*
- *Reye's syndrome* appears at the late stages of the illness, and has been epidemiologically associated with the administration of aspirin. It presents with vomiting, restlessness, irritability, progressive decrease in the level of consciousness, progressive cerebral edema, high blood ammonia, bleeding diathesis, hyperglycaemia, and elevated transaminases.
- Also, myocarditis, nephritis, bleeding diathesis, hepatitis (rarely)

Follow-Up

- The crusts fall off within 1 to 2 weeks of onset and leave a slightly depressed area of skin.
- Most cases are mild; monitor respiratory function (% O_2 saturation of haemoglobin) in high-risk groups.

PREVENTION

- *Passive immunization* with varicella zoster immunoglobulin (VZIG) should be given within 96 hours, preferably within 72 hours, of exposure to chickenpox or herpes zoster cases to immuno-compromised, susceptible children; to normal susceptible adults and adolescents, in particular pregnant women; newborn children of mothers with onset of chickenpox 5 days before or 2 days after delivery; and hospitalized premature infants (>28 weeks of gestation when mother has no history of chickenpox, and <28 weeks of gestation, and/or birth weight of <1,000 g, regardless of maternal history).
- *Live attenuated VZV vaccine* was recently licensed in the United States. It is recommended for children older than 12 months, susceptible immunocompetent adults, and immunocompromised patients.
  —Varicella (Varivax): 0.5 mL s.c.; repeat 4 to 8 weeks later. This treatment is for susceptible adolescents/adults who (1) are health care workers, (2) are the susceptible household contact of an immunocompromised person, (3) work in schools/day care centers, (4) are college students or in the military, and (5) are nonpregnant women of childbearing age.
  —Susceptible children may receive varicella vaccine (Var) during any visit after the first birthday, and unvaccinated persons who lack a reliable history of chickenpox should be vaccinated during the 11- to 12-year-old visit. Susceptible persons 13 years of age or older should receive two doses, at least 1 month apart.

Selected Readings

Echevarria JM, Martinea-Martin P, Tellez A, et al. Aseptic meningitis due to varicella-zoster virus: Serum antibody levels and local synthesis of specific IgG, IgM, and IgA. *J Infect Dis* 1987;155:959–967.

Kamiya H, Ito M. Update on varicella vaccine. *Curr Opin Pediatr* 1999;11:3–8.

Ljungman P, Lonnqvist B, Gahrton G, et al. Clinical and subclinical reactivations of varicella-zoster virus in immunocompromised patients. *J Infect Dis* 1986;153:840–847.

Wurtz R, Check IJ. Breakthrough varicella infection in a healthcare worker despite immunity after varicella vaccination. *Infect Control Hosp Epidemiol* 1999;20:561–562.

Cholecystitis/Cholangitis

Basics

DEFINITION

- Cholecystitis is the acute or chronic inflammation of the gallbladder.
- Cholangitis is the clinical diagnosis based on symptoms and signs of systemic sepsis originating in the biliary tract.
- Emphysematous (or gaseous) cholecystitis is inflammation of the gallbladder, characterized by gas in the gallbladder lumen that can infiltrate the gallbladder wall and/or the surrounding tissues.

ETIOLOGY

- The infecting organisms colonize the biliary tract, organizing in the bowel.
- Colonization of the bile is usually associated with advanced age (>70 years), previous biliary tract surgery, and common dust stones.
- When the biliary pressure is increased to 15 to 20 cm of water (normal, 8 to 12), clinical signs and symptoms of cholangitis occur as the bacteria spread from the bile ducts into the lymphatic structures and then, at higher pressures, into the bloodstream.
- Most infections are polymicrobial. The organisms most commonly cultured are the following:
  - *Escherichia coli*
  - *Klebsiella* spp
  - *Enterococcus* spp
  - *Enterobacter* spp
  - *Pseudomonas* spp
- *Staphylococcus* and *Pseudomonas* may be found after interventional endoscopy or a surgical procedure.
- Anaerobes are most commonly cultured in elderly patients and after biliary tract operations.
- Parasitic infections (e.g., *Clonorchis sinensis*) is associated with cholangitis due to obstruction of the biliary radials.
- Emphysematous cholecystitis is thought to begin with acute cholecystitis (calculous or acalculous), followed by ischemia or gangrene of the gallbladder wall and infection by gas-producing organisms. Bacteria most frequently cultured include anaerobes, such as *Clostridium*, and aerobes, such as *E. coli*.

EPIDEMIOLOGY

- The obstructive lesions that predispose to pyogenic bacterial cholangitis include the following:
  - Biliary stones or sludge
  - Biliary parasites. Parasites commonly associated with cholangitis are the trematodes *Clonorchis* and *Opisthorchis*; the nematodes *Ascaris* and, rarely, *Strongyloides*; and the cestodes (*Echinococcus granulosus* and *Echinococcus multicularis*).
  - Complications of endoscopic, surgical, and radiologic manipulations of the biliary system
  - Congenital intrahepatic biliary dilatation (Caroli's disease)
  - Iatrogenic bile duct injury
  - Ischemic cholangitis
  - Malignant strictures
  - Opportunistic infections in immunosuppressed patients (*Cryptosporidium*, *Microsporida*, cytomegalovirus) and in immunocompetent patients (tuberculosis)
  - Primary sclerosing cholangitis
- Emphysematous cholecystitis is more common in the elderly and in patients with diabetes mellitus.
- In 5% to 10% of patients with acute cholecystitis, calculi obstructing the cystic duct are not found at surgery. Acalculous cholecystitis is associated with the following:
  - Diabetes mellitus
  - Major surgical operations in the postoperative period
  - Obstructing adenocarcinoma of the gallbladder
  - Parasitic infestation of the bile duct and/or gallbladder
  - Parenteral hyperalimentation
  - Postpartum period following prolonged labor
  - Serious trauma or burns
  - Systemic diseases (sarcoidosis, cardiovascular disease, tuberculosis, syphilis, actinomycosis, etc.)
  - Torsion of the gallbladder
  - Vasculitis
- In over 50% of such cases, an underlying explanation for acalculous inflammation is not found.
- Calculous and acalculous cholecystitis have been well documented in patients infected with the human immunodeficiency virus. Opportunistic pathogens in this population include cytomegalovirus, *Cryptosporidium*, *Microsporidia*, *Mycobacterium avium* complex, *Candida albicans*, *Isospora belli*, and *Pneumocystis carinii*. Malignancies, including lymphoma and Kaposi's sarcoma, have also been associated with biliary tract disease in this population. However, in as many as 55% of cases, a potential cause cannot be identified.

Clinical Manifestations

SYMPTOMS

- Acute cholecystitis often begins as an attack of biliary colic and fever that progressively worsens. Approximately 60% to 70% of patients report having experienced prior attacks that resolved spontaneously.
- Charcot's classic triad of fever, pain, and jaundice is the hallmark of bacterial cholangitis but is fully present in only 70% of cases.
- The most common aspect of the triad is fever, which is detected in 95% of cases.
- Pain, usually in the right upper quadrant, may be mild and transient but can be elicited in 90% of cases, whereas jaundice (often detected only chemically) is noted in 80% of cases.
- The pain may radiate to the interscapular area, right scapula, or shoulder.
- The clinical manifestations of emphysematous cholecystitis are essentially indistinguishable from those of nongaseous cholecystitis, except that the patient may have high fever, shaking chills, and hypertension.
- Other symptoms of cholecystitis and cholangitis include anorexia, nausea, and vomiting.

SIGNS

- Peritoneal signs of inflammation may be apparent in both acute cholecystitis and cholangitis.
- Jaundice is unusual early in the course of acute cholecystitis but may occur when edematous inflammatory changes involve the bile ducts and surrounding lymph nodes.

Cholecystitis/Cholangitis

- In cholecystitis, an enlarged, tense gallbladder is palpable in one-fourth to one-half of patients. Deep inspiration or cough during subcostal palpation of the right upper quadrant usually produces increased pain and inspiratory arrest (Murphy's sign).
- Cholangitis presents with high fever, chills, and hypertension.

Diagnosis

DIFFERENTIAL DIAGNOSIS

The differential diagnosis of cholangitis and cholecystitis is discussed in the chapters on Abdominal Pain and Fever and Jaundice and fever.

LABORATORY

Leukocytosis with a left shift is found in acute cholecystitis, while the serum bilirubin is mildly elevated in half of patients, and 25% have modest elevations in serum aminotransferases.

IMAGING

- In acute cholecystitis, the radionuclide (e.g., HIDA) biliary scan may be confirmatory if bile duct imaging is seen without visualization of the gallbladder. Ultrasound will demonstrate calculi in 90% to 95% of cases.
- The diagnosis of emphysematous cholecystitis can be made on plain abdominal film by the finding of gas within the gallbladder lumen, dissecting within the gallbladder wall to form a gaseous ring, or in the pericholecystic tissues.

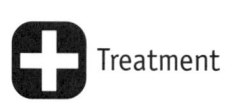

Treatment

- Although surgical intervention remains the mainstay of therapy for acute cholecystitis and its complications, a period of in-hospital stabilization may be required before cholecystectomy. Oral intake is eliminated, nasogastric suction is initiated, and extracellular volume depletion and electrolyte abnormalities are repaired. Meperidine or pentazocine are usually employed for analgesia.
- After blood cultures have been obtained, empiric intravenous antibiotic therapy should be directed against the most common organisms.
- Ticarcillin/clavulanate (3.1 g i.v. q6h) or piperacillin/tazobactam (3.375 g i.v. q6h) or ampicillin (2 g q6h) and gentamicin is appropriate for mild to moderate infections. Monotherapy with imipenem (500 mg qid) can be used for severe infections. Gentamicin or tobramycin should be used if *Pseudomonas* is suspected (e.g., after endoscopy or biliary tract surgery). The treatment regimen can be modified on the basis of culture results.
- Biliary decompression may be accomplished through percutaneous transhepatic, surgical drainage or endoscopic drainage, endoscopic cholangiography, and sphincterotomy for stone extraction.
- Urgent cholecystectomy or cholecystostomy is appropriate in patients in whom a complication of acute cholecystitis, such as empyema, emphysematous cholecystitis, or perforation, is suspected or confirmed.

COMPLICATIONS

- The incidence of severe acute cholangitis (with shock or mental confusion) is significantly higher in elderly patients than in younger patients.
- Hepatic abscess is a common complication, and an enlarged and tender liver attributable to the abscess may overshadow the underlying cholangitis.
- The complication rate for acalculous cholecystitis exceeds that for calculous cholecystitis.
- Empyema of the gallbladder carries a high risk of gram-negative sepsis and/or perforation.
- Fistulization into an adjacent organ adherent to the gallbladder wall may result from inflammation and adhesion formation.

Follow-Up

Of the 75% of patients with acute cholecystitis who undergo remission of symptoms, approximately one-fourth will experience a recurrence of cholecystitis within 1 year, and 60% will have at least one recurrent bout within 6 years.

PREVENTION

Appropriate antibiotics intra- and postoperatively are recommended in chronic inflammation, because colonization with these organisms may be associated with devastating septic complications following surgery.

Selected Readings

Benator DA, French AL, Beaudet LM, et al. *Isospora belli* infection associated with acalculous cholecystitis in a patient with AIDS. *Ann Intern Med* 1994;121:663–664.

Carpenter HA. Bacterial and parasitic cholangitis. *Mayo Clinic Proc* 1998;73:473–478.

Greenberger NJ, Isselbacher KJ. Diseases of the gallbladder and bile ducts. In: Fauci AS, Braunwald E, Isselbacher KJ, et al, eds. *Harrison's principles of medicine*, 14th ed. New York: McGraw-Hill, 1998:1725–1736.

Leiva JI, Etter EL, Gathe J Jr, et al. Surgical therapy for 101 patients with acquired immunodeficiency syndrome and symptomatic cholecystitis. *Am Surg* 1997;174:414–416.

Pol S, Romana CA, Richard S, et al. Microsporidia infection in patients with the human immunodeficiency virus and unexplained cholangitis. *N Engl J Med* 1993;328:95–99.

Sugiyama M, Atomi Y. Treatment of acute cholangitis due to choledocholithiasis in elderly and younger patients. *Arch Surg* 1997;132:1129–1133.

Cholera

Basics

DEFINITION
Cholera is an epidemic as well as endemic severe diarrheal disease caused by *Vibrio cholerae*.

ETIOLOGY
- *V. cholerae* is a motile gram-negative bacillus.
- Two biotypes are noted. The classic biotype causes symptomatic diarrhea in 50% of those infected, and the El Tor biotype causes disease in 1% to 20% of those infected.
- *V. cholerae* is a waterborne infection. The organism can live on algae and upon the shells of crustaceans.
- Disease is caused by secretion of a bacterial enterotoxin, which leads to massive secretion of fluids from the small bowel.

EPIDEMIOLOGY
- Cholera can be an endemic disease in some locations, and it can cause epidemic illness in other locations.
- There have been at least seven cholera pandemics worldwide in the last 200 years.
- Large outbreaks of illness occur commonly in Africa, Asia, and South America.
- People get infections after drinking contaminated water or eating contaminated food.
- Upon foods, the organism can survive up to 2 weeks.
- Boiling of water destroys the organism.

Incubation Period
Incubation periods depend on gastric acidity and inoculum ingested. In general, illness occurs between 12 and 72 hours after ingestion.

Clinical Manifestations

- Patients develop watery diarrhea, losing 1 to 3 L per day in the usual case, and up to 20 L in a severe case. The stool turns gray and mucoid ("rice-water").
- Dehydration can be extreme, and occurs rapidly.
- Patients note abdominal pain.
- High fever is rare.
- Patients are restless and, at times, in stupor.
- Skin turgor is increased, and the blood pressure can be low at times of severe dehydration.
- Mortality rates range from 1% when proper treatment is available to above 10% where treatment is lacking.
- Risk factors for poor outcome include elderly people and children.

Diagnosis

DIFFERENTIAL DIAGNOSIS
Few illnesses can cause such profound dehydration over such a short period of time. In milder cases, the illness cannot be distinguished from diarrhea caused by enterotoxigenic *E. coli* and, in children, rotavirus.

LABORATORY
- The stool is isotonic.
- WBCs and RBCs are absent in the stool.
- Serum electrolytes reflect severe dehydration, with azotemia and acidosis.
- Hemoconcentration is noted with dehydration.
- Stool samples sent for culture will grow the organism.
- Rapid diagnosis can be established with observation of motile gram-negative rods on dark-field microscopy.

Cholera

Treatment

- Rehydration is critical and can be done by oral rehydration fluid or, in severe cases, with an initial bolus of intravenous fluids.
- Attention should be given to restoring volume along with treatment of the acidosis that can develop.
- Hourly stool and urine output should be recorded during therapy.
- Antibiotics should be given after rehydration has been established.
- Resistance has been noted in many locations, and a knowledge of these patterns should be known prior to therapy.
- Doxycycline 300 mg orally × 1
- Tetracycline 500 mg orally qid for 3 days
- Ciprofloxacin 1 g orally × 1 or 250 mg/d for 3 days
- *In children*: Trimethoprim–sulfamethoxazole or ciprofloxacin is effective.

COMPLICATIONS

- In patients who survive but who were not rehydrated acutely, renal failure may develop.
- Miscarriage occurs in 50% of pregnant women affected.

Follow-Up

- Patients who survive require no long-term follow-up.
- Long-term bacterial shedding does not occur.

PREVENTION

- Cholera often occurs in developing countries, following wars or natural disasters. This is due to a breakdown in sanitation and the use of contaminated waters.
- Efforts to chlorinate water, or boil water, should be observed in epidemic settings.
- An effective, long-lasting vaccine for cholera does not yet exist.
- Prophylactic chemoprophylaxis in areas of outbreaks may be effective.
- For travelers, attention should be paid to consuming clean water and properly cooked foods; however, the disease is rare in travelers.

Selected Readings

Bennish ML, Azad AK, Rahman O, et al. Hypoglycemia during diarrhea. Prevalence, pathophysiology and therapy in Asiatic cholera. *N Engl J Med* 1990;322:1357.

Carpenter CJ. The treatment of cholera: Clinical science at the bedside. *J Infect Dis* 1992;166:2–14.

Swerdlow DL, Ries AA. *Vibrio cholerae* non-O1: The eighth pandemic? *Lancet* 1993;342:382.

Chorioretinitis (Uveitis and Retinitis)

Basics

DEFINITION

- Uveitis is the inflammation of the uvea, which is the vascular layer of the eye. It is divided into choroid, ciliary body, and iris and lies between the outer coat (sclera and cornea) and the inner coat (retina) of the eye.
- Uveitis is divided into
  - Anterior (iris and/or ciliary body)
  - Intermediate (pars plana)
  - Posterior (choroid with or without involvement of the retina)
- Although not a part of the uvea, the retina is often involved when there is inflammation of the choroid.

ETIOLOGY

- Infectious causes of uveitis include the following:
  - Bacterial
    - *Bartonella henselae* (cat-scratch disease)
    - Bejel
    - Brucellosis
    - Leptospirosis
    - Leprosy
    - Lyme disease
    - Nocardiosis
    - Syphilis
    - Tuberculosis
  - Viral
    - Cytomegalovirus (CMV)
    - Epstein-Barr virus
    - Herpes simplex virus (HSV)
    - Herpes zoster virus
    - Human immunodeficiency virus (HIV)
    - Rubella
    - Rubeola
  - Fungal
    - Aspergillosis
    - Candidiasis
    - Cryptococcosis
    - Histoplasmosis (presumed ocular histoplasmosis syndrome [POHS])
    - *Pseudallescheria boydii*
  - Parasitic
    - Cysticercosis
    - Onchocerciasis
    - Toxocariasis
    - Toxoplasmosis
- The anatomic location of uveitis can help in identifying the etiology. Most cases of anterior uveitis are idiopathic or autoimmune (ankylosing spondylitis, Behçet's disease, inflammatory bowel disease, juvenile rheumatoid arthritis, psoriasis, Reiter's syndrome, and sarcoidosis). HSV is the most common infectious pathogen.
- CMV is the most common cause of chorioretinitis; it is usually associated with advanced HIV infection.
- POHS usually presents with bilateral chorioretinal scars, macular disease, and peripheral atrophy. It is presumed to be due to histoplasmosis, but there is no proof yet.
- Intermediate uveitis is not due to infectious causes and is not discussed here.

EPIDEMIOLOGY

- In the United States, uveitis affects 1.2 million people and causes 10% of all blindness.
- Up to 10% of patients with candidemia have involvement of the choroid and/or the retina.
- Approximately 100,000 new cases of macular histoplasmosis occur annually in the United States.
- Frequency of uveitis by location
  - Anterior: 28%
  - Posterior: 38%
  - Intermediate: 15%
  - Panuveitis: 8%

Clinical Manifestations

SYMPTOMS

- Anterior uveitis presents with eye pain and photophobia, with or without decreased vision.
- Posterior uveitis is usually not accompanied by pain, but presents as progressive vision loss.
- POHS usually presents with blurred vision.

SIGNS

- Redness of the eye can be present in anterior uveitis, and a slit-lamp shows cells in the anterior chamber.
- In Lyme disease, endogenous infections of the retina and choroid occur 1 to 4 months after infection with diffuse, multifocal choroiditis and/or vitreitis.
- *Candida* chorioretinitis usually presents as focal white lesions.
- *Toxoplasma* chorioretinitis usually presents as large, smooth, yellow-white lesions. In immunosuppressed patients, lesions can be multiple and bilateral.
- In tuberculous uveitis, yellow-white choroidal nodules with indistinct borders and sizes up to one-half the disk diameter can be seen.

Diagnosis

LABORATORY

- Patients with posterior uveitis should undergo the following:
  - Complete blood count
  - Serology for syphilis (VDRL and FTAABS)
  - *Toxoplasma* titer
  - Evaluation for tuberculosis (PPD skin test and chest radiograph)
- IgM-positive and IgG-negative serology is helpful for diagnosis of primary toxoplasmosis, while, if both IgM and IgG are negative, the diagnosis of toxoplasmosis is unlikely.
- Diagnosis of *Nocardia asteroides* ocular infection can be made by identification of organisms microscopically on vitreous specimens or tissue specimens stained with Brown and Brenn modification of the Gram stain or Grocott methenamine silver stain.
- The diagnosis of CMV chorioretinitis is based on clinical data, and serology is unreliable. Modern technologies may help clinicians in the early diagnosis of the infection. Detection of the pp65 antigen and CMV PCR are the most promising of those new methods (see also the Section II chapter, "Cytomegalovirus Infections").

Chorioretinitis (Uveitis and Retinitis)

IMAGING/DIAGNOSTIC/TESTING PROCEDURES

- The diagnosis of anterior uveitis requires slit-lamp examination to identify inflammatory cells floating in the aqueous humor or deposited on the corneal endothelium (keratic precipitates).
- Lumbar puncture, computed tomography, or magnetic resonance imaging of the head can assist in the evaluation of certain patients (such as patients with possible toxoplasmosis, reticulum cell sarcoma, etc.).
- If these procedures do not provide a diagnosis, examination of the vitreous is the next step, especially when significant vitreitis is present on physical examination.

Treatment

- Treatment of anterior uveitis with judicious use of topical steroids is aimed at reducing inflammation and scarring. Dilation of the pupil reduces pain and prevents the formation of synechiae.
- Lyme, tuberculous, and syphilitic uveitis requires systemic treatment. In syphilitic disease, the duration of therapy depends on the duration of the infection and the results of the cerebrospinal fluid test (see relevant chapters).
- There is no general consensus for medical management of POHS. Systemic antifungal medications have not been useful. Corticosteroids and photocoagulation have been used with some success.
- Three antiviral agents (ganciclovir, foscarnet, and cidofovir) have been shown to be effective in the treatment of CMV retinitis. The systemic therapy for CMV is discussed in the relevant chapter.
- Resistant or relapsing CMV retinitis may be treated with local therapies, such as intraocular injections, or with a sustained-release ganciclovir implant.
- The time to first progression among patients with CW retinitis that received a ganciclovir intraocular implant is longer than that of any other treatment, making the implant the preferred choice, by most experts, for patients with immediately sight threatening disease. However, this approach requires intraocular surgery, which may lead to adverse effects. Many patients have immediate transient blurred vision that usually lasts for a few weeks.
- The implant is depleted of the drug after 5 to 8 months; then replacement is necessary. The outcome of several reimplantation procedures is still under investigation.
- Local therapy is ineffective in controlling dissemination of the CMV infection in other organs, especially in the other eye.
- Weekly or twice-weekly intravitreous injections of ganciclovir or foscarnet have appeared to slow the progression of retinitis in uncontrolled case series that mainly enrolled patients who could not tolerate systemic therapy or in whom CMV retinitis progressed despite systemic therapy.

COMPLICATIONS

- HSV, varicella zoster virus, and, rarely, CMV can cause a widespread, bilateral necrotizing retinitis referred to as the acute retinal necrosis syndrome. This syndrome is associated with pain, keratitis, and iritis. It is often associated with orolabial HSV or trigeminal zoster. Ophthalmologic examination with the use of an indirect ophthalmoscope reveals widespread, pale gray peripheral lesions. The peripheral retina is affected first, and this condition is often complicated by retinal detachment.
- Progressive outer retinal necrosis is a subset of acute retinal necrosis that occurs mainly among patients with advanced HIV infection. It can lead to rapid loss of vision.
- Neuroretinitis is characterized by swelling of the optic disk, peripapillary and macular hard exudates, and, often, vitreous cells. Initially thought to be idiopathic, *B. henselae* is a cause of neuroretinitis in cat-scratch disease. Doxycycline and rifampin appear to shorten the course of disease and hasten visual recovery. The long-term prognosis is good, but some individuals may acquire a mild postinfectious optic neuropathy.

Follow-Up

PREVENTION
N/A

Selected Readings

Donahue SP, Greven CM, Zuravleff JJ, et al. Intraocular candidiasis in patients with candidemia. Clinical implications derived from a prospective multicenter study. *Ophthalmology* 1994;101:1302–1309.

Henderly DE, Genstler AJ, Smith RE, et al. Changing patterns of uveitis. *Am J Ophthalmol* 1987;103:131–136.

Reed JB, Scales DK, Wong MT, et al. *Bartonella henselae* neuroretinitis in cat scratch disease. Diagnosis, management, and sequelae. *Ophthalmology* 1998;105:459–466.

Chronic Fatigue Syndrome

Basics

DEFINITION
Chronic fatigue syndrome (CFS) is a heterogeneous disorder with a constellation of somatic complaints associated with severe, debilitating fatigue, lasting at least 6 months.

ETIOLOGY
- There is no known specific etiology of CFS.
- Prolonged cases of fatigue following influenza, brucellosis, and Epstein-Barr virus infection have been well documented.
- Other infections have been implicated as the etiology of CFS, including cytomegalovirus (CMV), human herpesvirus-6, enterovirus, parvovirus, retroviruses other than the HIV virus, Lyme disease, and candida.
- Gilbert's disease is found in patients with CFS five times more frequently than in the general population.

EPIDEMIOLOGY
- CFS occurs in 3 to 11 in 100,000 people in the United States.
- The illness most commonly affects middle-aged women (ratio female to male, 7:1).
- Outbreaks with multiple cases have been reported on a college campus among orchestra members and at a resort hotel.

Clinical Manifestations

- CFS usually has a sudden onset, directly in association with or following a viral-like upper respiratory tract infection.
- Patients note weakness and muscle pains.
- Low-grade fevers are common.
- Patients note severe fatigue with, at times, inability to carry out functions of daily living, sore throat, pain behind the eyes, and jaw pain.
- Sleep disorders are common and range from insomnia to hypersomnia.
- Difficulty in concentrating and forgetfulness are common complaints.
- Spontaneous remissions occur.

Diagnosis

- The diagnosis of CFS is a diagnosis of exclusion.
- There are no diagnostic tests for the illness.
- Minor changes in hormone levels have been noted in affected patients.
- Low urinary-free cortisol levels are common, and an exaggerated response to corticotropin is noted, but these test results are variable.
- Minor changes in lymphocyte subtypes are, at times, noted in patients with CFS; the significance is not known.
- MRI scans can reveal unidentified bright objects in the brain of patients with chronic fatigue; the significance is not known.

DIFFERENTIAL DIAGNOSIS
- Depression
- CMV
- Epstein-Barr virus
- Brucellosis
- Postinfluenza

Chronic Fatigue Syndrome

- Lyme disease
- HIV infection
- Collagen-vascular disorders
- Tumors with paraneoplastic syndrome
- Brain tumor

Treatment

- Patients should be treated with tricyclic antidepressants (e.g., amitriptyline 20 mg q hs).
- Nonsteroidal antiinflammatory drugs are often helpful.
- Psychiatric support is helpful.
- Rehabilitation with a scheduled exercise program, up to tolerance, should be started.
- No specific therapy is yet available.
- The use of salt tablets is useful in some patients, in order to decrease the incidence of postural hypotension.

COMPLICATIONS

Morbidity associated with chronic fatigue syndrome is variable.

Follow-Up

Patients often need close follow-up with their primary care physician.

PREVENTION

- No etiology has been established for this illness; therefore, no prevention is available.

Selected Readings

Bates DW, Schmitt W, Buchwald D, et al. Prevalence of fatigue and chronic fatigue syndrome in a primary care practice. *Arch Intern Med* 1993;153:2759–2765.

Lerner MA, Zervos M, Dworkin HJ, et al. A unified theory of the cause of chronic fatigue syndrome. *Infect Dis Clin Pract* 1997;6:239–243.

Straus SE. History of chronic fatigue syndrome. *Rev Infect Dis* 1991;13[Suppl 1]):S2–S7.

Coccidioidomycosis

Basics

DEFINITION
Coccidioidomycosis pulmonary and/or extrapulmonary infection is caused by the fungus *Coccidioides immitis*.

ETIOLOGY
- The fungus *C. immitis* lives in soil.
- The optimal temperature for the growth of *C. immitis* is 30°C, but the fungus grows well at 37°C.

EPIDEMIOLOGY

Incidence
- It is estimated that, in the United States, about 100,000 people are infected annually.
- *C. immitis* is endemic to the southwestern United States (principally, California, Arizona, and Texas) and also to Mexico and Central and South America.
- Increasingly, cases are being recognized outside the endemic areas (travelers or reactivations).
- Periodically, there are sharp increases in the number of cases.

Risk Factors
- For patients with immunosuppressive conditions or therapies, such as AIDS, solid-organ transplantation, or lymphoma, it is important to be aware of even distant exposure to endemic regions, because late recrudescence of latent infection is possible in such patients.
- Among patients with AIDS, coccidioidomycosis is particularly likely in patients with CD4 counts under 250 cells/mm^3.
- People with diabetes or a compromised immune system are particularly susceptible to a chronic form of *C. immitis* infection characterized by the development of cavities in their lungs.
- Persons of African or Philippine descent may also have an increased risk for extrapulmonary complications.

Clinical Manifestations

- Symptoms develop 1 to 3 weeks after exposure. The typical presentation is a lower respiratory infection accompanied by systemic symptoms, such as the following:
  — Anorexia
  — Arthralgias
  — Chest pain
  — Cough
  — Fever
  — Sputum production
  — Sweating
  — Weakness
- Erythema nodosum or erythema multiforme may develop.
- About 5% of infected people have asymptomatic residual in their lungs, usually nodules or thin-walled cavities.
- Symptomatic extrapulmonary disease develops in about 1 of 200 people infected with *C. immitis*. The common sites are the meninges, bone and joints, skin, and soft tissues.
- Disease outside the lungs usually develops within a year after the initial infection, but may appear much later if immunity is impaired.
- Skin involvement may take a variety of forms, though wartlike nodules are the most common.
- Joint lesions are unifocal in over 90% of patients with joint involvement.

Diagnosis

- In endemic areas, prior *C. immitis* infection is frequently diagnosed when a lung nodule is resected because of suspected carcinoma.
- For patients outside of the endemic regions, prompt diagnosis of coccidioidal infection depends on obtaining an accurate travel history.
- To detect the presence of extrapulmonary infection, a careful review of symptoms and physical examination are usually adequate, because coccidioidal lesions are typically focal and produce localized symptoms, such as discomfort, swelling, or ulceration.
- The mainstays of diagnosis are culture, serologic testing, and positive coccidioidal skin test.
- Serologic testing is best performed in experienced laboratories. Serum IgM antibodies can be detected temporarily in 75% of people with primary infections. IgG antibody is present later and usually disappears in several months if the infection resolves. False-positive serologic tests are rare.
- Skin-test reactions to coccidioidal antigens become positive soon after the development of symptoms in virtually all people with primary infections, and cross-reactions with other infections are rare.
- Although cultures are often used to diagnose coccidioidomycosis in patients with disseminated infection, they are often not obtained in patients with primary infections.
- Chest radiographic findings may include infiltrates, a pleural effusion, and hilar adenopathy. Associated conditions that are particularly important risk factors include immunosuppressive diseases or therapies, pregnancy in the late stages, and diabetes.
- Meningitis usually involves the basilar meninges. Examination of the cerebrospinal fluid shows a mononuclear pleocytosis, with a low glucose level and an elevated protein level.

Treatment

- The value of antifungal therapy in patients with mild or moderate manifestations of early infections is not known, because randomized comparisons between antifungal and placebo regimens have not been done.
- Treatment may hasten symptom resolution. Thus, on a case-by-case basis, physicians should decide whether a patient's circumstances warrant therapy with available oral antifungal agents.

Coccidioidomycosis

- If treatment is initiated, reasonable dosages are 400 mg/d for ketoconazole, 400 mg/d for fluconazole, and 200 mg twice daily for itraconazole. Courses of typically recommended treatment would range from 3 to 6 months.
- Factors that should be weighed in favor of therapy include the following:
  - A negative skin test
  - Circumstances suggesting a high inoculum of the fungus
  - Concurrent noncoccidioidal disease
  - Elevated antibody titers
  - Inability to work
  - Increased susceptibility
  - Infiltrates involving more than half of one lung
  - Intense night sweats persisting longer than 3 weeks
  - Loss of body weight greater than 10%
  - Portions of both lungs
  - Prominent or persistent hilar adenopathy
  - Symptoms that persist more than 2 months
- In patients with disseminated disease, prolonged chemotherapy is always indicated.
- Pulmonary resection has a role in managing severe hemoptysis or cavities that rupture or enlarge during chemotherapy. Surgery is also indicated to drain empyemas, close persistent bronchopleural fistulas, or expand lungs that are restricted by residual disease.
- The traditional treatment of *C. immitis* meningitis consists of the administration of amphotericin B directly into the cerebrospinal fluid by the lumbar or cisternal route or into the ventricles or other sites through a reservoir. Amphotericin B should be given daily at first, then tapered (from every other day to once every 6 weeks) as clinical improvement occurs, as indicated by signs, symptoms, and cerebrospinal fluid leukocyte counts and antibody titers.
- The oral azoles offer a useful alternative treatment of meningeal disease.
- Even if *C. immitis* infection cannot be cured with azole therapy and lifelong suppression is required, the facts that these medications are well tolerated, do not have the toxic effects of amphotericin B, and do not require administration into the cerebrospinal fluid may represent important advantages in patients with an otherwise fatal illness.
- Once the disease has spread outside the lungs, chemotherapy is almost always indicated. With amphotericin B, doses of 1.0 to 1.5 mg/kg/d, tapering to 1.0 to 1.5 mg/kg three times weekly, to a total dose of 1.0 to 2.5 g intravenously, are usually used, with more prolonged courses if remission is not achieved.
- An intraarticular regimen of amphotericin that has been used is 15 to 50 mg (for large joints), depending on tolerance, three times a week for 2 weeks; weekly for 6 weeks; and biweekly for 4 months.

COMPLICATIONS

- The disease is enhanced in immunocompromised patients, particularly if they have extrapulmonary coccidioidal disease. Patients who have received organ transplants are at greatest risk for infection in the first year after the transplantation.
- Meningitis usually occurs within 6 months after the primary infection and may appear acutely almost coincident with it.
- The signs of meningeal irritation common in bacterial meningitis are usually absent. The most common symptom is headache. Fever, weakness, confusion, sluggishness, seizures, abnormal behavior, stiff neck, diplopia, ataxia, vomiting, and focal neurologic defects may occur.

Follow-Up

- Five percent to 10% of infections result in any residual sequelae, many of which have few long-term effects.
- In people with increased susceptibility to *C. immitis* infection, the serologic response to the fungus is usually at least qualitatively intact. A history of travel or residence in an area of endemic disease should alert the physician to the possibility of this diagnosis. Routine serologic testing can prevent a delayed diagnosis.
- Early diagnosis of meningitis is important; without treatment, 90% of patients die within 12 months.
- In some patients, the acute pneumonia does not resolve, but progresses to chronic pulmonary disease. Diabetic patients and patients with compromised immunity are disproportionately overrepresented in this group.

PREVENTION

- Occasionally, the acute pulmonary infection does not resolve, and a progressive pneumonia or chronic lung infection develops.
- Experience with organ transplantation suggests that antifungal therapy should be used in patients with a history of coccidioidomycosis, whether or not they have active infection, at the time of engraftment. Antifungal therapy also should be used in seropositive transplant recipients, even if they are asymptomatic, during episodes of acute rejection.
- Infections acquired during pregnancy are often aggressive.

Selected Readings

Arsura EL, Bellinghausen PL, Kilgore WB, et al. Septic shock in coccidioidomycosis. *Crit Care Med* 1998;26:62–65.

Catanzaro A, Galgiani JN, Levine BE, et al. Fluconazole in the treatment of chronic pulmonary and nonmeningeal disseminated coccidioidomycosis. NIAID Mycoses Study Group. *Am J Med* 1995;98:249–256.

Galgiani JN. Coccidioidomycosis: A regional disease of national importance. Rethinking approaches for control. *Ann Intern Med* 1999;130:293–300.

Stevens DA. Coccidioides immitis. In: Mandell GL, Bennett JE, Dolin R, eds. *Principles and practice of infectious diseases.* New York: Churchill Livingstone, 1995:1310–1312.

Stevens DA. Coccidioidomycosis. *N Engl J Med* 1995.332:1077–1082.

Common Cold

Basics

DEFINITION
- Upper respiratory viral infection (URTI)

ETIOLOGY

Viral
- Rhinovirus (25%–40%)
- Coronavirus
- Influenza
- Parainfluenza
- Less common: respiratory syncytial virus, adenovirus, enterovirus, reovirus, picornaviruses

Nonviral
- *C. pneumoniae*
- Less common: *M. pneumoniae*
- *Chlamydia*
- *Mycoplasma*

Noninfectious
- Vasomotor rhinitis
- Allergic rhinitis

EPIDEMIOLOGY

Incidence
- The average adult reports two to five colds per year.
- The overall incidence of URTIs is 1 billion annually.

Risk Factors
- Hand contact with infected person
- Winter season (due to people clustering indoors)
- Susceptibility increased by smoking and psychological stress

Incubation
Two to 4 days

Clinical Manifestations

SYMPTOMS AND SIGNS
- Rhinorrhea
- Sneezing
- Nasal obstruction

Diagnosis

Diagnosis based on clinical symptoms

DIFFERENTIAL DIAGNOSIS

Infectious
- Pneumonia
- Whooping cough
- Sinusitis

Noninfectious
- Allergic rhinitis

LABORATORY
- No laboratory tests are required unless symptoms persist more than 3 weeks.
- If symptoms persist longer than 3 weeks, consider the following:
  - Throat and/or sputum culture
  - Chest and/or sinus x-rays
  - Culture of nasal discharge

Common Cold

Treatment

MAIN TREATMENT
- No antiviral agents with established merits
- Aspirin, acetaminophen to relieve symptoms
- Ibuprofen to relieve symptoms
- Decongestants
  - Nasal: rebound effect with use greater than 3 days
  - Oral: benefits questionable
- Antihistamines: responsive to allergic form of infection
- Vitamin C: variable results, based on multiple studies
- Zinc: possible symptom improvement; some studies report no benefit
- Ipratropium bromide nasal spray: symptom relief of rhinorrhea and sneezing, but bloody nasal discharge in 10% to 20%
- Antibiotics: contraindicated for common cold
- Inhalation of hot, humid air: no benefit

COMPLICATIONS
- Serous otitis
- Otitis media
- Sinusitis
- Pharyngitis
- Acute bronchitis
- Exacerbation of chronic bronchitis, asthma, and obstructive sleep apnea

Follow-Up

A cough persisting greater than 3 weeks could be pneumonia.

PREVENTION
- Avoid hand-to-eye and hand-to-nose contact.
- Wash hands frequently.

Selected Readings

Hayden FG. Update on influenza and rhinovirus infections. *Adv Exp Med Biol* 1999;458:55–67.

Mossad SB. Treatment of the common cold. *BMJ* 1998;317(7150):33–36.

Mygind N, Gwaltney JM Jr, Winther B, et al. The common cold and asthma. *Allergy* 1999;54[Suppl 57]:146–159.

Pitkaranta A, Hayden FG. Rhinoviruses: Important respiratory pathogens. *Ann Med* 1998;30(6):529–537.

Conjunctivitis

Basics

DEFINITION
- Conjunctivitis is inflammation of the conjunctiva that usually presents with hyperemia and discharge.
- Trachoma is a chronic conjunctivitis associated with infection by *Chlamydia trachomatis* serovar A, B, Ba, or C.
- Inclusion conjunctivitis (or paratrachoma) is an acute ocular infection caused by sexually transmitted *C. trachomatis* strains (usually serovars D through K) in adults exposed to infected genital secretions and in their newborn offspring.

ETIOLOGY
Infectious Causes
- Bacteria
  - *Acinetobacter* spp
  - *Bartonella henselae*
  - *Chlamydia trachomatis*
  - *Corynebacterium diphtheriae*
  - *Francisella tularensis*
  - *Haemophilus influenzae, Haemophilus aegyptius,* and *Haemophilus ducreyi*
  - *Moraxella* spp
  - *Mycobacteria tuberculosis*
  - *Neisseria meningitidis* and *Neisseria gonorrhoeae*
  - *Proteus vulgaris*
  - *Shigella flexneri*
  - *Streptococcus* spp
  - *Staphylococcus* spp
  - *Treponema pallidium*
- Fungi
  - *Candida* spp
  - *Sporothrix schenckii*
- Viruses
  - Adenoviruses
  - Echoviruses
  - Enteroviruses
  - Epstein–Barr virus
  - Herpes simplex virus
  - Herpes zoster virus
  - Influenza A and B viruses
  - Measles
  - Molluscum contagiosum
  - Mumps
  - Vaccinia
- Parasites
  - *Loa loa*
  - *Microsporidium* spp
  - *Onchocerca volvulus*
  - *Toxocara canis*
  - *Wuchereria bancrofti*

Infectious Causes in Newborns
- *C. trachomatis*
- *N. gonorrhoeae*
- *H. influenzae*
- *S. pneumoniae*
- Herpes simplex virus

EPIDEMIOLOGY
Incidence
- Trachoma is responsible for an estimated 20 million cases of blindness throughout the world.
- Endemic trachoma is still the major cause of preventable blindness in northern Africa, sub-Saharan Africa, the Middle East, and parts of Asia.
- In the United States, endemic trachoma still occurs in Native American populations and in immigrants from areas where trachoma is endemic.
- Conjunctivitis is the most common cause of a red eye (see also relevant chapter in this book).
- The worldwide incidence and severity of trachoma have decreased during the past decades, mainly as a result of improving hygienic and economic conditions.
- The most common viral etiology is adenovirus infection.

Risk Factors
- Trachoma transmission is from eye to eye via hands, flies, towels, and other sources.
- Organisms of serovars D through K can be transmitted from the genital tract to the eye, usually causing only the inclusion conjunctivitis syndrome.
- Acute relapse of old trachoma can occur after treatment with cortisone eye ointment or in very old persons who were exposed in their youth.

Clinical Manifestations

SYMPTOMS
- The clinical findings and course of conjunctivitis is influenced by the causing pathogen.
- It usually presents with hyperemia and discharge. Pain is minimal and the visual acuity is reduced only slightly. The cornea can become involved, with inflammatory leukocytic infiltrations and superficial vascularization, especially in viral conjunctivitis.
- Both endemic trachoma and adult inclusion conjunctivitis is characterized by small lymphoid follicles in the conjunctiva.
- Adult inclusion conjunctivitis presents as the acute onset of unilateral follicular conjunctivitis and preauricular lymphadenopathy. If untreated, the disease may persist for years.
- In conjunctivitis due to *F. tularensis*, the conjunctiva is painful, with numerous yellowish nodules and pinpoint ulcers and regional lymphadenopathy. Because of debilitating pain, the patient may seek medical attention before regional lymphadenopathy develops.
- Adenovirus infection causes a watery discharge, mild foreign-body sensation, and photophobia.

SIGNS
- Secretion varies from purulent to serosanguineous, depending on the pathogen, and bacterial infection tends to produce a more mucopurulent exudate.
- Neonatal chlamydial conjunctivitis has an acute onset and often produces a profuse mucopurulent discharge.

Diagnosis

DIFFERENTIAL DIAGNOSIS
- In adult inclusion conjunctivitis, evidence of chlamydiae by Giemsa- or immunofluorescence-stained smears, by

Conjunctivitis

- isolation in cell cultures, or by newer nonculture tests constitutes definitive infection.
- In the newborn, chlamydial conjunctivitis generally has a longer incubation period (5–14 days) than gonococcal conjunctivitis (1–3 days).
- Noninfectious causes of conjunctivitis include allergic reaction, mucous membrane pemphigoid, and in graft-versus-host disease.

LABORATORY

- Intracytoplasmic chlamydial inclusions are found in 10% to 60% of Giemsa-stained conjunctival smears in such populations, but isolation in cell cultures, newer antigen detection testing, or chlamydial PCR is more sensitive.
- Serum antibody does not constitute evidence of chlamydial eye infection.
- Gram-stained smears may show gonococci or occasional small gram-negative coccobacilli in *Haemophilus* conjunctivitis, but smears should be accompanied by cultures for these agents.

DIAGNOSTIC/TESTING PROCEDURES

Smears and cultures are usually reserved for severe, resistant, or recurrent cases of conjunctivitis.

Treatment

MAIN TREATMENT

- Mild cases of infectious conjunctivitis usually are treated empirically with broad-spectrum topical ocular antibiotics, such as sulfacetamide 10%, polymixin–bacitracin–neomycin, or trimethoprim–polymixin combination.
- Adult inclusion conjunctivitis: doxycycline 100 mg orally bid for 13 weeks
- Trachoma: azithromycin 20 mg/kg orally, single dose
- Gonococcal: ceftriaxone 125 mg i.m./i.v.
- Herpes simplex: See Section II chapter, "Keratitis."
- Because concomitant pharyngeal infection is often present, neonatal chlamydial conjunctivitis should be treated with oral antimicrobials in order to prevent chlamydial pneumonia:
  — Gonococcal: ceftriaxone 25 to 50 mg/kg qid i.v. for 7 days
  — *C. trachomatis*: erythromycin syrup 10 to 15 mg/kg/day qid for 14 days
- Topical antibiotic treatment is not required for patients who receive systemic antibiotics.

ALTERNATIVE TREATMENT

- Adult inclusion conjunctivitis: erythromycin 250 mg orally qid daily for 13 weeks
- Trachoma: doxycycline 100 mg orally twice daily for 2 weeks
- Gonococcal neonatal conjunctivitis: penicillin G 25,000 U/kg/d qid for 7 days

COMPLICATIONS

- In trachoma, conjunctival scarring eventually distorts the eyelids, causing them to turn inward (trichiasis and entropion). Eventually, the corneal epithelium may ulcerate, with subsequent corneal scarring and blindness.
- Rarely, in inclusion conjunctivitis, the eye disease progresses, with the development of pannus and scars similar to those seen in endemic trachoma.

Follow-Up

In adult inclusion conjunctivitis, genital examination and tests for genital chlamydial infection are indicated.

PREVENTION

- Promote general hygienic measures associated with improved living standards.
- Patients with conjunctivitis should be advised to wash their hands frequently and not to touch their eyes.
- In adult inclusion conjunctivitis, treatment of all sexual companions of the patient is necessary.
- Public health control programs for endemic trachoma have consisted of the mass application of tetracycline or erythromycin ointment to the eyes of all children in affected communities for 21 to 60 days or on an intermittent schedule, or single-dose azithromycin therapy.

Selected Readings

Anonymous. From the Centers for Disease Control and Prevention. Acute hemorrhagic conjunctivitis—St. Croix, US Virgin Islands, September–October 1998. *JAMA* 1998;280:1737.

Horton JC. Disorders of the eye. In: Fauci AS, Braunwald E, Isselbacher KJ, et al, eds. *Harrison's principles of medicine*, 14th ed. New York: McGraw-Hill, 1998:159–172.

O'Brien TR, Green WR. Conjunctivitis. In: Mandell GL, Bennett JE, Dolin R, eds. *Principles and practice of infectious diseases*, 4th ed. New York: Churchill Livingstone, 1995:1103–1110.

Stamm WE. Chlamydial infections. In: Fauci AS, Braunwald E, Isselbacher KJ, et al, eds. *Harrison's principles of medicine*, 14th ed. New York: McGraw-Hill, 1998:1055–1064.

Creutzfeldt-Jakob Disease

Basics

DEFINITION

- The transmissible spongiform encephalopathies are chronic, progressive, and always fatal neurodegenerative disorders of animals and humans.
- Animal-transmissible spongiform encephalopathies include the sheep disease (scrapie) and the cow disease (bovine spongiform encephalopathy).
- Human-transmissible spongiform encephalopathies include Creutzfeldt-Jakob disease (CJD), kuru, and Gerstmann-Straussler-Scheinker syndrome.
- CJD is characterized by the following:
  —Degeneration of the pyramidal and extrapyramidal systems
  —Progressive dementia
  —Wasting of the muscles
  —Tremor
  —Athetosis
  —Spastic dysarthria
- In 1995, a novel form of CJD, named "new variant CJD" was described, and appears to be transmission of bovine spongiform encephalopathies to humans. Consumption of beef is indicated in this condition.

ETIOLOGY

- The pathologic hallmarks of CJD are spongiform changes (small, round vacuoles) within the neuropil, neuronal loss, hypertrophy and proliferation of glial cells, and absence of significant inflammation or white matter involvement.
- Pathologic changes are most severe in the cortex but are often prominent in the basal ganglia, cerebellum, and thalamus as well.
- The finding of prion rods or scrapie-associated fibrils, which may be seen in electron micrographs of prepared brain material, appears to be pathognomonic for prion diseases.

EPIDEMIOLOGY

- Most cases are sporadic, although some are familial, with an autosomal dominant pattern of inheritance.
- Regions of high incidence and prevalence resulting from the presence of families with CJD are scattered throughout the world, most prominently in parts of Libya and North Africa and in Slovakia.
- A recent summary of 300 cases of prion disease studied at the National Institutes of Health found that 79% of sporadic CJD cases were transmissible.
- Spread of the disease has occurred following transplantation of corneas, dural grafts, or improperly decontaminated neurosurgical instruments and stereotactic intracerebral depth electrodes.
- Approximately 50 cases have been reported in patients with panhypopituitarism who received supplemental cadaveric human growth hormone therapy and in patients who received cadaveric human gonadotropins for treatment of infertility.

Clinical Manifestations

SYMPTOMS

- Early in the course of the disease, most CJD patients exhibit rapidly progressive dementia, myoclonus, and pyramidal tract dysfunction.
- Mental impairment may be manifested as slowness in thinking, difficulty concentrating, impaired judgment, and memory loss. Mood changes and emotional lability may be combined with visual or other types of hallucinations.
- About one-third of patients present initially with prominent cerebellar or visual disturbances, which may initially overshadow the mental impairment.
- Sixty percent of patients present with ataxia, and 10% to 20% will have a purely ataxic illness.
- Almost any combination of cortical, subcortical, cerebellar, and spinal cord findings is possible.
- Myoclonus occurs in more than 90% of patients. Additional motor signs and symptoms can include tremor, clumsiness, and choreoathetosis.
- As the disease progresses, about two-thirds of patients develop a parkinsonian extrapyramidal syndrome with hypokinesia and rigidity. Hyperreflexia, spasticity, and extensor plantar responses occur in about half of patients.
- The clinical presentation of CJD associated with use of cadaveric human pituitary hormone therapy differs from that of classic CJD. Patients are typically younger and often present with a kuru-like illness, in which cerebellar features may be more prominent initially than dementia.
- Cases of a new variant form of CJD have recently been identified in certain countries in Europe (mainly the United Kingdom). Cases are linked to bovine spongiform encephalopathies, perhaps as a result of human consumption of or other exposure to bovine spongiform encephalopathies. Patients range in age from 19 to 41 years and developed a progressive illness leading to death within 7 to 23 months after onset. The clinical features include early and prominent behavioral disturbances and ataxia. Myoclonus and progressive dementia occur in most patients as later features.

Diagnosis

DIFFERENTIAL DIAGNOSIS

- The differential diagnosis of CJD includes a number of noninfectious conditions, such as Parkinson's disease and motor neuron disease.
- The differential diagnosis of dementia is extensive (Alzheimer's disease, vascular dementia, vitamin deficiencies, alcoholism, medications, etc.) and includes a number of infectious etiologies, such as the following:
  —HIV
  —Neurosyphilis
  —Progressive multifocal leukoencephalopathy
  —Tuberculosis
  —Whipple's disease

LABORATORY

- Definite diagnosis of all forms of CJD is still possible only by histological examination of the brain.

Creutzfeldt-Jakob Disease

- Cerebrospinal fluid (CSF) pleocytosis is unusual and should prompt a thorough search for other processes. It has been suggested recently that two-dimensional isoelectric focusing of CSF proteins may show abnormal protein species, two of which (proteins designated 130 and 131) may be typical of CJD. These proteins appear to be identical to a brain protein designated 14-3-3.
- Recent molecular genetic studies have established an unequivocal linkage between mutations in the *PRNP* gene and familial cases of CJD. Several mutations have been described, which may correlate with variations in the clinical phenotype of the disease in individual familial clusters. These include point mutations in codons 178, 200, and 210. Octarepeat inserts in the *PRNP* gene also occur in several families with CJD. No consistent *PRNP* gene mutation has been identified in cases of sporadic CJD.
- Patients with CJD have a median serum concentration of the brain-specific S 100 protein higher than that of controls.
- In the new variant CJD, the typical periodic EEG pattern usually associated with CJD does not occur. Neuropathologic features include spongiform change and plaques. The prion protein plaques resemble those seen in kuru and are often surrounded by a zone of spongiform change. Prion protein plaques are extensively distributed throughout the cerebrum and cerebellum. Laboratory tests are helpful in excluding other causes of rapidly progressing dementia. The CSF is typically unremarkable, although the protein level may be mildly elevated.

IMAGING

- CT and MRI may show evidence of generalized cortical atrophy, but, more typically, the degree of clinical dementia appears disproportionate to the amount of tissue loss seen on CT and MRI. In some patients, MRI has shown areas of high T2 signal intensity in the striatum.
- Reduced brain cortical perfusion in cases of variant CJD disease by single-photon emission CT (SPECT) analysis: Although this finding is nonspecific, it may help to raise the suspicion of disease in young adults presenting with psychiatric disorders where all other routine investigations have been useless.

DIAGNOSTIC/TESTING PROCEDURES

- The EEG may be quite useful in suggesting the diagnosis. The typical pattern of periodic sharp-wave complexes consists of a generalized slow background interrupted by bilaterally synchronous sharp-wave complexes occurring at intervals of 0.5 to 2.5 s and lasting for 200 to 600 ms.
- The classic EEG pattern is found in 75% to 95% of cases, although it may not be present very early or in the terminal stages of the disease.

Treatment

CJD is invariably fatal, and no specific therapy is available. A number of drugs, including amantadine, have been reported to slow disease progression in isolated anecdotal case reports; however, the results have not been reproducible.

COMPLICATIONS

N/A

Follow-Up

- In some patients, sequential studies performed at biweekly or monthly intervals may show rapidly progressing loss of brain tissue and ventricular enlargement.
- Sequential EEG studies may be useful if the initial recording fails to reveal the typical pattern.

PREVENTION

- The consensus is that the current risk of transmission of spongiform encephalopathies in the United States is minimal because of the following:
  —Spongiform encephalopathies have not been shown to exist in the United States.
  —Adequate regulations exist to prevent entry of foreign sources of spongiform encephalopathies into United States.
  —Adequate regulations exist to prevent undetected cases of BSE from uncontrolled amplification within the U.S. cattle population.
  —Adequate preventive guidelines exist to prevent high-risk bovine materials from contaminating products intended for human consumption.

Selected Readings

Pocchiari M. Early identification of variant Creutzfeldt-Jakob disease [Editorial]. *BMJ* 1998;316:563–564.

Tan L, Williams MA, Khan MK, et al. Risk of transmission of bovine spongiform encephalopathy to humans in the United States: Report of the Council on Scientific Affairs. American Medical Association. *JAMA* 1999;281:2330–2339.

Tyler KL. Aseptic meningitis, viral encephalitis, and prion diseases. In: Fauci AS, Braunwald E, Isselbacher KJ, et al, eds. *Harrison's principles of internal medicine*, 14th ed. New York: McGraw-Hill, 1998:2439–2451.

van Duijn CM, Delasnerie-Laupretre N, Masullo C, et al. Case-control study of risk factors of Creutzfeldt-Jakob disease in Europe during 1993–95. European Union (EU) Collaborative Study Group of Creutzfeldt-Jakob disease (CJD). *Lancet* 1998;351:1081–1085.

Cryptococcal Infections

Basics

DEFINITION
Cryptococcosis is a systemic infection caused by the yeastlike fungus *Cryptococcus neoformans*.

ETIOLOGY
C. neoformans is an encapsulated, yeastlike fungus that reproduces by budding. It is a saprobe in nature, with a worldwide distribution. Soil may also contain the fungus, especially if the soil is contaminated with bird droppings. The portal of entry is the lung.

EPIDEMIOLOGY
- AIDS is the major predisposing factor in cryptococcal infections.
- AIDS-associated cases usually occur when CD4+ T-lymphocyte counts fall below 200 cells/mm^3, usually below 100 cells/mm^3.
- Organ transplantation is the second most frequent risk factor, largely attributable to the use of corticosteroids and immunosuppressive drugs.
- The incidence of cryptococcosis is increased in patients with lymphoreticular malignancies (especially Hodgkin's disease), those on high-dose corticosteroids or other immunosuppressive agents, and patients with sarcoidosis or diabetes mellitus.
- About half of patients with cryptococcosis lack apparent predisposing factors.

Clinical Manifestations

SYMPTOMS
- The onset of CNS cryptococcosis may be acute or insidious.
- Those who have a more chronic course have waxing and waning manifestations over weeks or months, often with completely asymptomatic periods.
- Symptoms include the following:
  —Confusion
  —Dizziness
  —Headache
  —Irritability
  —Nausea
  —Obtundation
  —Seizures
  —Somnolence
  —Visual loss
- Some HIV-positive patients have minimal or no symptoms at the time of presentation.
- Patients are often afebrile or have a mildly elevated temperature.
- Most patients have minimal or no nuchal rigidity.
- Papilledema is noted in up to one-third of the cases.
- Pulmonary cryptococcosis may be asymptomatic or may cause production of only scant, sometimes blood-streaked, sputum. HIV-infected patients usually develop fever, cough, and dyspnea, often with pleuritic chest pain, sometimes with roentgenographic findings of lymphadenopathy or pleural effusions, most often with diffuse mixed interstitial and intraalveolar infiltrates.
- In most cases of CNS cryptococcosis in nonimmunosuppressed patients, pulmonary involvement is not apparent.
- Besides the respiratory system and the CNS, cryptococcosis may involve a number of other organs:
  —Adrenals
  —Bone (causing lesions that can be mistaken for neoplasms)
  —Eye
  —Heart (leading to pericarditis, myocarditis, or endocarditis)
  —Sinus
  —Skin (causing nonspecific lesions that could be the first signs of infection)
  —Urinary tract (as an unusual cause of pyelonephritis)

Diagnosis

DIFFERENTIAL DIAGNOSIS
- CNS cryptococcosis may resemble closely other mycoses and tuberculosis, as well as viral meningoencephalitis or meningeal metastases.
- Cryptococcosis may resemble chronic meningitis that is due to treatable infections (e.g., coccidioidomycosis, histoplasmosis, other mycoses, brucellosis, syphilis) or to noninfectious causes (e.g., sarcoidosis, chronic benign lymphocytic meningitis).
- The clinical findings of pulmonary cryptococcosis in HIV-infected patients can be indistinguishable from those of patients with acute pneumonia that is due to *Pneumocystis carinii* pneumonia, tuberculosis, or other organisms. Bronchoscopy usually is diagnostic.

LABORATORY
- The isolation of *C. neoformans* from respiratory specimens warrants attention from physicians. In some cases, the *C. neoformans* isolate can represent a pulmonary infection, either alone or in association with a disseminated disease; in other cases, it can represent an asymptomatic carriage. The distinction between disseminated cryptococcal disease, pulmonary cryptococcosis, and airway colonization with *C. neoformans* has important diagnostic and therapeutic implications.
- Except for infections in severely immunosuppressed patients, CNS cryptococcosis is almost always indicated by abnormalities in cerebrospinal fluid (CSF). Opening pressure is often elevated, glucose is depressed, protein concentration is usually increased, and leukocyte counts are 20 per millimeter or higher, with lymphocytes generally outnumbering neutrophils. Also, cryptococci grow in cultures.

Cryptococcal Infections

- Smears using India ink to define the organism can be valuable in supporting a presumptive diagnosis that guides the direction of further diagnostic efforts. Cryptococci are seen in 25% to 50% of the patients with cryptococcal meningitis.
- Negative cultures do not absolutely rule out cryptococcosis, because, often, only small numbers of organisms are present in some CSF and may be missed.
- Positive blood cultures occur most often in association with AIDS.
- Whenever cryptococcosis is documented at any site, this mandates a careful search for lesions elsewhere, both inside and outside the CNS.
- Latex agglutination detects antigen in CSF or serum (or both) from 90% or more of the HIV-infected patients with cryptococcal meningitis.

IMAGING

HIV-negative patients with cryptococcal meningitis tend to have radiographic findings different from those reported in patients with AIDS. Cryptococcal meningitis in this group is usually associated with pulmonary mass(es) or a normal chest radiograph, whereas a respiratory presentation is usually associated with air-space consolidation.

Treatment

- An effective regimen for CNS cryptococcosis among non-AIDS patients is a 6-week course of 0.3 mg/kg of amphotericin B i.v. plus 150 mg of flucytosine in four divided oral doses daily.
- In the era before effective antiretroviral therapy, cryptococcosis seldom was cured in HIV-positive patients, and lifespans of these patients were limited, so lifelong suppressive treatment was always indicated in this group.
- In a double-blind multicenter trial, patients with a first episode of AIDS-associated cryptococcal meningitis were randomly assigned to treatment with higher dose amphotericin B (0.7 mg/kg/d) with or without flucytosine (100 mg/kg/d) for 2 weeks (step 1), followed by 8 weeks of treatment with itraconazole (400 mg/d) or fluconazole (400 mg/d) (step 2). For the initial treatment of AIDS-associated cryptococcal meningitis, the use of higher dose amphotericin B plus flucytosine was associated with an increased rate of CSF sterilization and decreased mortality at 2 weeks, as compared with regimens used in previous studies. Consolidation therapy with fluconazole was associated with a higher rate of CSF sterilization.
- Higher doses of fluconazole (400 mg) may be used, if necessary; doses up to 800 mg/d have been well tolerated.

COMPLICATIONS

- Dementia may develop because of direct involvement of the brain by the infection. However, late recrudescence of symptoms may indicate the presence of hydrocephalus.
- CNS cryptococcosis may be complicated by hydrocephalus. This may be signaled by early or late clinical deterioration, with late development of increased intracranial pressure, or by a recrudescence of abnormalities after initial improvement. When hydrocephalus is suspected, computed tomography or magnetic resonance imaging is the preferred method for defining the ventricular system and confirming the diagnosis.

Follow-Up

- In nonimmunosuppressed patients, pulmonary cryptococcosis may progress or regress spontaneously or may remain stable for long periods.
- In patients with AIDS, cryptococcal pneumonia can be severe and rapidly progressive.
- After initial therapy, up to 20% to 25% of patients with cryptococcal meningitis relapse.
- When severe enough to require shunting, hydrocephalus has a bleak prognosis.
- Clinical judgment and periodic examinations of the CSF are required to determine whether treatment should deviate from standard regimens.

PREVENTION

Patients with cryptococcosis involving any site should be evaluated every few months for at least 1 year after therapy, even if they are asymptomatic.

Selected Readings

Aberg JA, Mundy LM, Powderly WG. Pulmonary cryptococcosis in patients without HIV infection. *Chest* 1999;115:734–740.

Diamond RD. Cryptococcus neoformans. In: Mandell GL, Bennett JE, Dolin R, eds. *Principles and practice of infectious diseases*. New York: Churchill Livingstone, 1995:2331–2341.

Mylonakis E, Merriman NA, Rich JD, et al. Use of cerebrospinal fluid shunt for the management of elevated intracranial pressure in a patient with active AIDS-related cryptococcal meningitis. *Diagn Microbiol Infect Dis* 1999;34:111–114.

Sarosi GA. Cryptococcal lung disease in patients without HIV infection [Editorial; Comment]. *Chest* 1999;115:610–611.

van der Horst CM, Saag MS, Cloud GA, et al. Treatment of cryptococcal meningitis associated with the acquired immunodeficiency syndrome. National Institute of Allergy and Infectious Diseases Mycoses Study Group and AIDS Clinical Trials Group. *N Engl J Med* 1997;337:15–21.

Cryptosporidiosis

Basics

DEFINITION
- Intracellular protozoan that is responsible for self-limited diarrhea in children and adults and protracted and even fatal diarrhea in patients with HIV infection

ETIOLOGY
- *Cryptosporidium* is an intracellular protozoan, able to infect cells of epithelial origin.
- Cells affected in humans include respiratory and gastrointestinal cells.
- The entire life cycle occurs within one person.
- Infection usually occurs by ingestion of oocysts from fecally contaminated water.
- Oocysts can survive as long as 18 months in the environment.
- Studies have shown that ingestion of less than 1,000 oocysts can lead to disease.

EPIDEMIOLOGY
- The organism is ubiquitous and worldwide in distribution.
- Seroprevalence rates are often as high as 25% in industrialized countries and as high as 75% in developing countries.
- In temperate climates, increased transmission is noted during warmer months.
- Large waterborne outbreaks associated with contaminated water supplies have recently been documented in the United States.
- Much of the contamination of water supplies has been due to dairy farms or other farms with livestock.
- Rates of oocyst shedding in the stool of animal hosts ranges from 1% in industrialized nations to 10% in the developing world.
- The organism is resistant to most water purification methods, such as chlorination.
- Filtration appears to be the best method of oocyst removal.
- Other means of infection include transmission via the following:
  — Pets
  — Childcare centers
  — Hospitals
  — Sexual contact
  — Swimming pools

Incubation
Incubation is between 7 and 10 days.

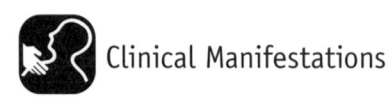

Clinical Manifestations

- Diarrhea in normal persons occurs at various degrees of severity from 2 days to 1 month.
- Patients may have crampy abdominal pains.
- Low-grade fevers may occur.
- In patients with immunosuppression, such as HIV infection, voluminous diarrhea with as much as 15 L/d can occur.

Diagnosis

DIFFERENTIAL DIAGNOSIS
- Enteric bacterial infections such as *salmonella, Shigella,* and *Campylobacter*
- *C. difficile*
- Mycobacterial infection
- Enteric protozoal infections such as *Giardia, Cyclospora, Isospora,* and Microsporidia
- Cytomegalovirus colitis

LABORATORY
- Stool specimens reveal oocysts with Giemsa stains or modified acid-fast stains.
- Fluorescent antibody stains for stool or tissue specimens are available.
- Leukocytosis is rare.
- Fecal leukocytes are not present.
- D-Xylose tests are abnormal in most patients.
- Fat absorption is impaired.
- Vitamin B12 levels may become low.

IMAGING
Radiographs may reveal an ileus pattern along with bowel wall edema. The findings are nonspecific.

Cryptosporidiosis

Treatment

- There is no effective treatment for this illness.
- Patients who are immunocompetent are likely to run a self-limited illness of several days to 6 weeks, for which supportive care is given.
- In HIV-infected individuals, supportive care is critical.
- Drugs that have been used with limited efficacy include the following:
  —Paromomycin
  —Clarithromycin
  —Metronidazole
- Octreotide has been shown to decrease the amount of watery stool produced, without eradication of the organism.
- For patients with HIV infection, starting highly active antiretroviral drugs has been shown to be effective in some patients.

COMPLICATIONS

- In patients with HIV infection, protracted diarrhea is common and may be life-threatening.
- The organisms can involve the bile ducts and the gallbladder, leading to cholecystitis and sclerosing cholangitis.
- Pancreatitis can occur.
- Tracheitis and bronchitis can occur when the respiratory tract is involved.

Follow-Up

- In patients who are immunocompetent, no special follow-up is required.
- In HIV-infected individuals or patients immunocompromised by other means, eradication of the organism is less common, and exacerbation and remission is common. Those patients need to be followed closely.

PREVENTION

- For persons with HIV infection, many precautions are recommended, including the following:
  —Avoidance of drinking from rivers, streams, or pools
  —Avoidance of swallowing water while swimming
- Contact with human or animal feces is contraindicated. Care must be taken especially when working with farm animals or with soil possibly contaminated with animal feces.
- Pets with diarrhea should have their stools examined for *Cryptosporidium*.
- Drinking water can be filtered to 1 μ or boiled for 1 minute.
- Bottled water may be safer than tap water, but the filtering process may vary with some brands of bottled water, and purity is not guaranteed.
- Carbonated drinks are safe.

Selected Readings

Flanigan T, Ramratnam B, Graeber C, et al. Prospective trial of paromomycin for cryptosporidiosis in AIDS. *Am J Med* 1996;100:370–372.

Juranek D. Cryptosporidiosis: Sources of infection and guidelines for prevention. *Clin Infect Dis* 1995;21:S57–S61.

MacKenzie W, Hoxie N, Proctor M, et al. A massive outbreak in Milwaukee of *Cryptosporidium* infection transmitted through the public water supply. *N Engl J Med* 1994;331:161–167.

Cysticercosis

Basics

DEFINITION
Cysticercosis is infection with larval cysts of *Taenia solium*. Although cysts can locate anywhere throughout the body, especially in striated muscles, the central nervous system (CNS) is the most significant site for infection.

ETIOLOGY
- The adult tapeworm is found in the small intestine of humans (definitive host).
- The pig (intermediate host) ingests the egg and larvae are formed. The larvae travel via the bloodstream throughout the pig and achieve high concentrations in the muscle.
- Ingestion of undercooked pork (muscle) leads to the evagination of the head, which then attaches to the bowel wall of the new host. This leads to classic tapeworm infection.
- Humans acquire cysticercosis, which is caused by the larval forms, when eggs excreted in the feces are ingested.
- The eggs develop into oncospheres that traverse the small intestine.
- Egg ingestion may occur as autoinfection in a patient with a preexisting tapeworm or from another human source with tapeworm infection.
- A single tapeworm can produce 40,000 eggs a day.
- Eggs may live for months in the soil.
- Cyst formation in humans is most common in the CNS.

EPIDEMIOLOGY
- *T. solium* is a pork tapeworm that is found in southern Europe, South and Central America, Africa, and in some parts of Southeast Asia and India.
- For the cyst life cycle to be maintained, pigs must have contact with human feces.

Incidence
- Cysticercosis is the most common parasite leading to CNS disease.
- It is the most common cause of seizures in developing countries.
- In Mexico, up to 10% of all CT scans in some institutions show evidence of neurocysticercosis.
- Autopsy studies in Mexico reveal an incidence of up to 3.6%.

Risk Factors
- In areas with poor sanitation, pigs may be in contact with human excrement.
- Ingestion of infected and undercooked pork leads to tapeworm infection.
- Ingestion of infected feces leads to cysticercosis.

Incubation
The average time from infection to development of symptoms is about 5 years.

Clinical Manifestations

- Seizures
- Headache
- Possible signs of hydrocephalus
- Symptoms depend on the number, size, and location of the lesions.
- Intraventricular disease leads to hydrocephalus.
- Subretinal or intravitreal disease may lead to blindness.
- Cysts may present in the orbit, leading to blindness.

Cysticercosis

Diagnosis

- The infection should be suspected when evaluating a patient from an endemic area who has CNS symptoms, including headache or seizures.
- Subcutaneous cysts may be palpated in skeletal muscles and are approximately 2 cm and rubbery upon palpation.

DIFFERENTIAL DIAGNOSIS

- Tuberculosis
- Fungal abscess
- Toxoplasmosis
- Tumor
- Paragonimiasis

LABORATORY

- Serologic tests are available.
- Eosinophilia is not present.

IMAGING

- A CT scan or an MRI show the cysts as rounded lesions.
- Calcifications of muscle cysts are seen on radiographs.

Treatment

FOR NEUROCYSTERCERCOSIS

- Praziquantel 50 mg/kg every day for 15 days
- Albendazole 15 mg/kg every day for 1 to 4 weeks
- Expect an inflammatory reaction to the medications; steroids are often given with treatment to alleviate inflammation in the CNS, which can cause headache and seizures.
- Antiseizure medications may be considered.

FOR TAPEWORM INFECTION ALONE

- Praziquantel 10 mg/kg, single dose.

COMPLICATIONS

- Hydrocephalus
- Seizures
- Blindness

Follow-Up

Patients should have frequent evaluations following therapy and follow-up CT scans to ensure resolution of lesions.

PREVENTION

- Good hygiene with adequate waste management
- Avoidance of exposure of pigs to human feces
- Treatment of all human cases of intestinal tapeworm infections

Selected Readings

Baily GG. In: Cook GC, ed. *Manson's tropical disease*, 20th ed. Philadelphia: WB Saunders, 1996:chapter 76.

Wilson ME. *World guide to infections*. Oxford Press, 1991.

Cystitis

Basics

DEFINITION
Cystitis is a lower urinary tract infection (UTI) involving the bladder that occurs in both women and men. Bacteria from the women's bowel flora are spread retrograde from the urethra. Cystitis is classified as an uncomplicated UTI.

ETIOLOGY
- *Escherichia coli*
- *Staphylococcus saprophyticus*
- *Klebsiella* (rare, 3%)
- *Proteus* (rare, 2%)
- *Enterococcus* (rare, 2%, typically found in complicated UTI)
- Combined infections

EPIDEMIOLOGY
Incidence
- More prevalent in young women than in young men (20% vs. 0.5%, respectively, ages 16 to 35 years)
- Seven million cases of UTI annually in United States

Risk Factors
- Women
  —Use of spermicides, antibiotics, diaphragm
  —Reduced estrogen levels
  —Gynecologic surgery
  —Bladder prolapse
  —Incontinence
  —Chronic catheterization
- Men
  —Prostatic hypertrophy
  —Urethral obstruction
  —Catheterization
  —Surgery
  —Incontinence

Clinical Manifestations

SYMPTOMS AND SIGNS
- Dysuria
- Urinary frequency
- Urinary urgency
- Abrupt onset
- Turbid urine, sometimes foul-smelling and bloody
- Suprapubic tenderness or low back pain in 10% of patients
- Children
  —Nonspecific symptoms (fever, vomiting, diarrhea, etc.)
- Elderly
  —Paucity of symptoms

Diagnosis

DIFFERENTIAL DIAGNOSIS
Infectious
- Pyelonephritis (upper UTI)
- Asymptomatic bacteriuria
- Urethritis
- Vaginitis

Noninfectious
- Stone
- Bladder tumor

Cystitis

LABORATORY

- Urine culture not needed for first attack; should be obtained for subsequent episodes
- Imaging: ultrasonography if suspicion of obstruction or renal involvement

Treatment

- Antibiotics (for uncomplicated cystitis)
  - Trimethoprim-sulfamethoxazole (TMP-SMX) 160 to 800 mg orally every 12 hours for 3 days
  - TMP 100 mg orally every 12 hours for 3 days
  - Norfloxacin 400 mg orally every 12 hours for 3 days
  - Ciprofloxacin 250 mg orally every 12 hours for 3 days
  - Levofloxacin 250 mg orally once per day for 3 days
- Pregnancy
  - Amoxicillin 250 mg every 8 hours for 3 days
  - Microcrystalline nitrofurantoin 100 mg qid for 3 days
  - Cefpodoxime 200 mg every 12 hours for 3 days
  - Also consider 7-day regimen if necessary
- Seven-day regimen considered for the following:
  - Pregnancy
  - Diabetes
  - Symptoms lasting longer than 7 days
  - Diaphragm use
  - Age over 65 years

COMPLICATIONS

- Pyelonephritis
- Bacteremia
- Recurrence caused by reinfection
  - Tend to occur more than 2 weeks after completion of therapy for the initial episode in 20% to 30% of patients
  - Caused by bacterial species different from that in the initial episode
- In pregnancy: premature and low-birth-weight babies
- In early childhood: Sometimes infection can cause renal failure.

PREVENTION

- Avoid diaphragm, if complicated.
- During pregnancy, obtain frequent screenings of urine in third trimester.
- In diabetes, avoid glycosuria.

Selected Readings

Roberts JA. Pathophysiology of bacterial cystitis. *Adv Exp Med Biol* 1999;462:325–338.

Sussman M, Gally DL. The biology of cystitis: Host and bacterial factors. *Annu Rev Med* 1999;50:149–158.

Tice AD. Short-course therapy of acute cystitis: A brief review of therapeutic strategies. *J Antimicrob Chemother* 1999;43[Suppl A]:85–93.

Weir M, Brien J. Adolescent urinary tract infections. *Adolesc Med* 2000;11(2):293–313.

Cytomegalovirus Infections

Basics

DEFINITION
- A group of infections of different systems and organs caused by cytomegalovirus (CMV)

ETIOLOGY
- CMV is a DNA virus that belongs to the herpesvirus group.
- Latent infection after primary infection is the rule with CMV, as with other herpes-group viruses.

EPIDEMIOLOGY

Incidence and Prevalence
- CMV is a common human pathogen that affects people worldwide.
- The proportion of a population with serologic evidence of past infection is related to age and socioeconomic factors.
- A big proportion of people, by the age of 20 years, are seropositive for CMV (have IgG antibodies against the virus).
- About 50% of adults in industrialized countries have evidence of past infection.
- About 90% of adults have evidence of past infection in some populations (especially in developing countries).

Risk Factors
- CMV may be passed from mother to fetus and newborn.
- In addition, CMV may be transmitted from donor to recipients of transplanted organs and tissues.
- Immunosuppression predisposes to severe manifestations of CMV infection during primary infection or during reactivation of the virus.

Clinical Manifestations

- CMV causes (usually) an asymptomatic infection in immunocompetent people.
- In a minority of immunocompetent people, CMV may cause an infectious mononucleosis-like syndrome.
- The virus may cause significant health problems in two distinct populations: fetuses and immunocompromised patients.
- Congenital CMV infection is the most common cause of congenital anomalies among all infectious agents during past decades in industrialized countries (after the decrease in incidence of rubella due to immunization).
- Congenital CMV infection may cause abortion and many problems to the fetus, including jaundice, anemia, and central nervous system damage.
- Primary CMV infection may cause severe clinical manifestations in immunocompromised patients of all ages.
- In addition, CMV may reactivate during phases of immunosuppression and cause severe disease in such patients.
- Specifically, the virus causes multiple and severe problems in bone marrow transplant recipients, solid-organ transplant recipients, patients infected with HIV, and patients with severe neoplasia-related cellular immunity suppression, such as those with lymphoma or leukemia.
- A syndrome with fever, malaise, hepatitis, thrombocytopenia, and atypical lymphocytes is commonly attributable to CMV in these populations. In addition, CMV may affect other organs and cause pneumonitis, esophagitis, colitis, and central nervous system manifestations in immunocompromised patients.
- CMV pneumonitis is a significant problem, especially in bone marrow recipients, both in terms of frequency and severity.
- CMV retinitis commonly affects patients with advanced HIV infection and subsequent severe immunosuppression (CD4 count less than 100/mm^3 of blood).
- CMV frequently causes disease in the transplanted organs. For example, CMV infection has been implicated as a pathogenetic factor in early coronary artery disease after heart transplantation.
- The virus has been thought by some investigators to contribute to atherosclerosis pathogenesis in immunocompetent people, but evidence is limited.

Diagnosis

- The only definite way to diagnose active CMV infection is histologic examination of affected tissues.
- However, serology, viral culture, and molecular biology tests may be of significant help to physicians in clinical practice.
- IgM antibodies against CMV may be found in an acute CMV infection. Reactivation of CMV infection may also lead to increased IgM antibodies, as well as to increased IgG antibodies by fourfold or more.
- Viral culture of the buffy coat of blood or specimens of other body fluids or tissues may lead to growth and isolation of CMV.
- In addition, identification of special CMV antigens in patients' serum or other body fluids or tissue specimens is helpful. Among CMV antigens, glycoprotein 55 is the most frequently used.
- Molecular biology techniques, including polymerase chain reaction (PCR), may also be needed for diagnosis of CMV infection. However, someone should try to discriminate between active and latent CMV infection, because a positive PCR test for CMV does not necessarily mean active CMV infection.

Cytomegalovirus Infections

Treatment

MAIN TREATMENT

- There is no need to treat CMV infection that causes an infectious mononucleosis-like syndrome. Such a syndrome is usually self-limited.
- Rest may be of benefit in unusual cases of CMV infection leading to prolonged malaise.
- CMV infection in immunocompromised patients that causes clinical manifestations should be aggressively treated using antiviral agents.
- Ganciclovir (5 mg/kg twice a day) intravenously is the best-studied treatment for symptomatic CMV infection in immunocompromised patients.
- Cytomegalovirus immune globulin (CMVIG) is protective and therapeutic against CMV infections.
- CMVIG may be used as a preventive measure in solid-organ and bone marrow transplant recipients.
- CMVIG also may be used in combination with ganciclovir for treatment of severe CMV infections, including CMV pneumonitis.

ALTERNATIVE TREATMENT

Foscarnet should be used in patients with infection due to CMV isolates that are resistant to ganciclovir.

COMPLICATIONS

- CMV infection may lead to death, especially in severely immunocompromised persons.
- Among the most severe forms of CMV infection is pneumonitis due to this virus, especially in bone marrow transplant recipients.
- CMV colitis may lead to perforation of the large bowel and, subsequently, to peritonitis and death.
- CMV encephalitis also may lead to death.
- HIV-infected patients may develop a special syndrome caused by CMV that affects the last part of the spinal cord and the spinal nerve roots. This condition is called cauda equina syndrome.

Follow-Up

Immunocompromised patients with CMV infection need careful follow-up after treatment of a primary or reactivated CMV infection.

PREVENTION

- Careful screening of blood donors and testing of blood units for antibodies to CMV will lead to reduction of the incidence of blood transfusion–related CMV infection. However, most hospitals do not observe this practice, because it would cause a significant reduction in the use of blood product units.
- Reduction of the level of the immunosuppression would decrease the possibility of reactivation of CMV infection in HIV patients. The modern management of HIV infection, including highly active antiretroviral treatment, has led to a significant reduction of CMV-related disease in this population.

Selected Readings

Behar R, Wiley C, McCutchan A. Cytomegalovirus polyradiculoneuropathy in acquired immune deficiency syndrome. *Neurology* 1987;37:557–561.

Falagas ME, Arbo M, Ruthazer R, et al. Cytomegalovirus disease is associated with increased cost and hospital length of stay among orthotopic liver transplant recipients. *Transplantation* 1997;63:1595–1601.

Falagas ME, Griffiths J, Worthington M, et al. Cytomegalovirus colitis mimicking colonic carcinoma in an HIV-negative patient with chronic renal failure. *Am J Gastroenterol* 1996;91:168–169.

Falagas ME, Snydman DR, Griffith J, et al. Effect of cytomegalovirus infection status on first year mortality rates among orthotopic liver transplant recipients. *Ann Intern Med* 1997;126:275–279.

Falagas ME, Snydman DR, Ruthazer R, et al. Surveillance cultures of blood, urine, and throat specimens are not valuable for predicting cytomegalovirus disease in liver transplant recipients. *Clin Infect Dis* 1997;24:824–829.

Ljungman P, Engelhard D, Link H, et al. Treatment of interstitial pneumonitis due to cytomegalovirus with ganciclovir and intravenous immune globulin: Experience of European Bone Marrow Transplant Group. *Clin Infect Dis* 1992;14:831–835.

Montgomery RL, Youngblood LA, Medearis DN Jr. Recovery of cytomegalovirus from the cervix in pregnancy. *Pediatrics* 1972;49:524–531.

Morgello S, Cho ES, Nielsen S. Cytomegalovirus encephalitis in patients with acquired immunodeficiency syndrome: An autopsy study of 30 cases and a review of the literature. *Hum Pathol* 1987;289–297.

Palestine AG, Polis MA, DeSmet MD, et al. A randomized, controlled trial of foscarnet in the treatment of cytomegalovirus retinitis in patients with AIDS. *Ann Intern Med* 1991;115:665–673.

Stago S, Pass RF, Dworsky ME, et al. Congenital and perinatal cytomegalovirus infections. *Semin Perinatol* 1983;7:31–42.

Dengue

Basics

DEFINITION
Dengue is a febrile illness due to a mosquito-borne virus. At times, the virus can cause a hemorrhagic fever–shock syndrome, with a patient fatality rate of 1% to 5%. Dengue is an emerging infection in the tropics.

ETIOLOGY
- Dengue virus is of the family Flaviviridae (SSRNA).
- There are four serotypes that are antigenically distinct (types 1–4).

EPIDEMIOLOGY
- The virus is present throughout the tropical and subtropical zones between 30 degrees North and 40 degrees South latitudes.
- Dengue hemorrhagic fever has not been seen in Africa.
- The virus is transmitted by the *Aedes aegypti* mosquito.
- There is increased transmission during the rainy season.
- Human and nonhuman primates are the only reservoirs of infection.

Risk Factors
Travel in urban or rural tropical regions where dengue and the *A. aegypti* mosquito are present is a risk factor.

Incubation
- Five to 8 days after mosquito bite

Clinical Manifestations

DENGUE FEVER
- Fever with headache, retro-orbital pains, chills, and myalgias
- Fevers occurring for a period of 5 to 6 days
- Skin rash may be fleeting and maculopapular; seen in about 10% of cases
- At the end of the febrile period, a petechial rash may develop on the extremities.
- Hemorrhagic complications are rare.

DENGUE HEMORRHAGIC FEVER–SHOCK SYNDROME
- This is a severe form of dengue, with hemorrhage and occasional shock.
- Severe plasma leakage leads to marked hemoconcentration.

Dengue

Diagnosis

- Mild cases are very hard to diagnose.
- Severe cases are diagnosed based on the following:
  - High fever for 2 to 7 days
  - Hemorrhage
  - Hepatomegaly
  - Shock

DIFFERENTIAL DIAGNOSIS

- Malaria
- Chikungunya fever
- Rickettsial illness

LABORATORY

- In severe cases, thrombocytopenia and hemoconcentration are seen.
- Serology (ELISA) for IgG and IgM antibodies

Treatment

- Symptomatic and supportive
- Hydration
- Avoid aspirin, due to the hemorrhagic nature of the illness.

COMPLICATIONS

N/A

Follow-Up

Patients who have had dengue should take extra care to avoid mosquito bites when traveling in endemic regions.

PREVENTION

- Control of mosquito vector in urban and rural locales
- Insect repellant

Selected Readings

Imported Dengue—United States, 1996. *MMWR Morbid Mortal Wkly Rep* 1998;47:544.

Ramirez-Ronda CH, Garcia CD. Dengue in the Western Hemisphere. *Infect Dis Clin North Am* 1994;8:107.

Diphtheria

Basics

DEFINITION

- Diphtheria is an upper respiratory tract infection caused by *Corynebacterium diphtheriae*.
- Major morbidity and mortality are related to an exotoxin that leads to pseudomembrane production in the throat, myocarditis, and neuropathy.

ETIOLOGY

- *C. diphtheriae* is a pleomorphic gram-positive rod.
- An exotoxin is produced in those strains harboring a lysogenic phage.
- The toxin inhibits cellular protein production.

EPIDEMIOLOGY

- Infection is spread by respiratory droplets.
- Preschool-age children have the highest attack rate.
- The organism may colonize the respiratory tract without causing disease.
- Disease is very rare in the United States as a result of immunization.
- Incidence of disease has increased in Russia over the last decade to as high as 8.7 to 17.0 per 100,000 in some large cities. Over 3,000 deaths have been reported in Russia from 1990 through 1999.

Incubation

- Generally thought to be about 2 to 4 days

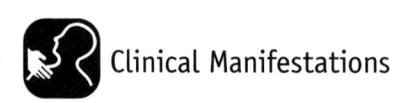

Clinical Manifestations

- Fever, sore throat as initial manifestations
- Plaques are gray and adherent.
- Membranes develop in the posterior pharynx. They emit a "mousy" odor.
- Swelling of the neck may occur and cause marked swelling along with cervical adenopathy.
- Stridor and airway obstruction may occur due to occlusion by the pharyngeal membrane. Paralysis of the palatal muscles may contribute to obstruction.
- Skin lesions, nasal lesions, otitis media, and corneal lesions may occur and produce marked destruction.
- Myocardial dysfunction in 10% to 25% of patients occurs 1 to 2 weeks after the initial sore throat.
- Neuropathy can develop 10 days to 3 months after the sore throat.
- Cranial neuropathy, peripheral sensory neuropathy, and motor neuropathy of the extremities occur.

Diphtheria

Diagnosis

- Generally, this will be a clinical diagnosis based on the characteristic appearance of the pseudomembrane.
- Swabs from under the membrane may be cultured on selective media, such as cysteine-tellurite. Loeffler's media or Tinsdale agar may also be used, if available.
- Gram stain shows typical organisms: club-shaped, slightly curved, frequently understained, assuming an angular "Chinese-letter" appearance.

DIFFERENTIAL DIAGNOSIS

- Streptococcal pharyngitis
- Mononucleosis
- Viral pharyngitis
- Epiglottitis
- Vincent's angina
- Herpes simplex virus

Treatment

- Erythromycin 20 to 25 mg/kg every 12 hours i.v. for 1 to 2 weeks
- Penicillin G is an alternative to erythromycin.
- Diphtheria antitoxin should be given as soon as possible. Because it is horse serum, it must be given carefully to prevent severe allergic reactions.
- Supportive care is needed, along with strict bed rest, in patients with carditis.

COMPLICATIONS

N/A

Follow-Up

Patients with myocarditis need follow-up with a cardiologist.

PREVENTION

- Immunization with toxoid as infant and child
  - Three doses before age 1 year and boosters at 15 to 18 months and at 4 to 6 years
  - Td given as booster every 10 years
- Persons in contact with diphtheria patients should be given a Td booster and treated with either erythromycin or an intramuscular injection of benzathine penicillin.

Selected Readings

Hardy IRB, Dittmann S, Sutter RW. Current situation and control strategies for the resurgence of diphtheria in newly independent states of the former Soviet Union. *Lancet* 1996;347:1739–1744.

Harnish JP, Tronca E, Nolan CM, et al. Diphtheria among alcoholic urban adults. A decade of experience in Seattle. *Ann Intern Med* 1989;111:71–82.

Tiley SM, Kociuba KR, Heron LG, et al. Infective endocarditis due to nontoxigenic *Corynebacterium diphtheriae:* Report of seven cases and review. *Clin Infect Dis* 1993;16:271–275.

Diverticulitis

Basics

DEFINITION

- A diverticulum is a pouch or sac that results from herniation of the mucous membrane through a defect in the muscular coat of a tubular organ.
- The terms *diverticulosis* and *diverticular disease* refer simply to the presence of uninflamed diverticula.
- Diverticulitis is inflammation of a diverticulum, most commonly involving the left side of the colon.
- The term *perforated diverticulitis* is reserved for cases in which a periverticular abscess has ruptured into the peritoneal cavity and caused a purulent peritonitis.

ETIOLOGY

- The etiology of diverticular disease is believed to be increased intraluminal pressure in the colon secondary to reduced stool bulk, possibly related to decreased intake of dietary fiber.
- Once diverticula are present, obstruction of the neck of a diverticulum can result from mucus secretion and overgrowth of normal colonic bacteria, leading to vascular compromise and subsequent perforation.
- The process is classified by the varieties of inflammatory conditions: Stage I includes patients with small, confined pericolonic abscesses; stage II involves larger collections; stage III represents patients with generalized suppurative peritonitis; and stage IV indicates fecal peritonitis.

EPIDEMIOLOGY

Incidence

- Although often considered a disease of the elderly, the incidence of diverticular disease is rapidly increasing in younger patients as well. Estimates of incidence in the young population ranged from 2% to 4% in the late 1960s, but more recently have climbed to 12% to 30%. By age 80, 70% of Americans have diverticular disease.
- Most of the elderly population with diverticulosis remain asymptomatic. It is estimated that only 10% to 25% of persons with diverticulosis will develop diverticulitis.
- Although 85% of cases of diverticulitis occur in the sigmoid and descending colon, diverticula may be found throughout the colon.

Risk Factors

- Epidemiologic studies have demonstrated an association with Western diets high in refined carbohydrates and low in dietary fiber.
- Immunocompromised persons tend to have more severe diverticulitis, although the incidence is no greater.
- Right-sided diverticulitis occurs with greater frequency in Asians.

Clinical Manifestations

SYMPTOMS

- Acute colonic diverticulitis is a disease of variable severity.
- The presentation is characterized by the following:
  - Fever
  - Abdominal pain (that usually begins in the hypogastrium and then localizes to the left lower quadrant)
- There may be alterations in bowel habits (diarrhea occurring more frequently than constipation).
- Dysuria, urinary frequency, and urinary urgency may occur if the affected colonic segment lies close to the urinary bladder.
- If a colovesical fistula is present, pneumaturia, fecaluria, or recurrent urinary tract infection occurs.

SIGNS

- Tenderness is usually localized to the left lower quadrant and is often accompanied by peritoneal irritation (muscle spasm, guarding, and rebound tenderness).
- When generalized peritonitis is present, either rupture of a periverticular abscess or free rupture of an uninflamed diverticulum has occurred.
- Rectal examination may reveal a tender mass if the area of inflammation is close to the rectum.
- Rectal bleeding, usually microscopic, is noted in 25% of cases; it is rarely massive.

Diagnosis

DIFFERENTIAL DIAGNOSIS

- Right-sided diverticulitis is easily confused with appendicitis, because it occurs at a somewhat younger age than does left-sided diverticulitis. Sigmoid diverticulitis also may mimic acute appendicitis if a redundant colon is positioned in the suprapubic region or right lower quadrant.
- On barium enema examination or CT study with oval contrast, multiple diverticula along with a segmental sigmoid narrowing or extravasation of contrast material suggest the presence of diverticulitis, although luminal narrowing and extravasation are also consistent with the diagnosis of Crohn's disease.
- See also the Section I chapter, "Abdominal Pain and Fever."

LABORATORY

Polymorphonuclear leukocytosis is common.

IMAGING

- Computerized tomography (CT) is the safest and most cost-effective diagnostic method, with additional potential for use in the treatment of abscesses. The sensitivity of CT ranges from 67% to 93%.
- Diverticula are easily demonstrated by contrast enema, but their presence alone does not establish or negate the presence of diverticulitis.
- The presence of a stricture or signs of extraluminal compression occasionally make differentiation from carcinoma difficult, but the clinical distinction between diverticulitis and nonperforating carcinoma is usually not subtle.
- Evidence of acute diverticulitis includes the following:
  - Inflammation of the pericolic fat
  - The presence of a single diverticulum or multiple diverticula
  - Thickening of the bowel wall to more than 4 mm
  - The finding of a periverticular abscess
- Several authors advocate the use of ultrasonography in the diagnosis and treatment of acute diverticulitis. However, ultrasonography is more

Diverticulitis

operator-dependent than is CT, abdominal tenderness may preclude the use of the requisite amount of external pressure to visualize the intraabdominal contents adequately, and the image quality is often poor in obese patients.
- CT with oral, intravenous, and/or rectal contrast might enhance the accuracy of positive findings.

DIAGNOSTIC/TESTING PROCEDURES

Sigmoidoscopy is of value in establishing the diagnosis of carcinoma or Crohn's colitis.

Treatment

MAIN TREATMENT

- In patients for whom the diagnosis of diverticulitis can be made with confidence by clinical examination, it is reasonable to begin empirical antibiotic treatment immediately.
- For a patient with a mild first attack, who is able to tolerate oral hydration, treatment may be initiated on an outpatient basis, consisting of a liquid diet and 7 to 10 days of oral broad-spectrum antimicrobial therapy, including coverage against anaerobic microorganisms. For example, ciprofloxacin 500 mg bid PO (or one double-strength tablet of trimethoprim–sulfamethoxazole twice daily PO) and metronidazole 500 mg PO qid.
- Intravenous regimens for the management of perforated diverticulitis or secondary peritonitis are discussed in the Section II chapter, "Peritonitis."
- Approximately 20% of patients with diverticulitis will require surgical treatment.
- The indications for emergency colonic resection include the following:
  —Acute clinical deterioration
  —Extracolonic contrast or gas, or a moderately dilated cecum mandates immediate surgery.
  —Generalized peritonitis
  —Marked tenderness of the right lower quadrant in the setting of a significantly dilated cecum
  —Signs of cecal necrosis (i.e., air in the bowel wall) on abdominal radiography
  —Uncontrolled sepsis
  —Visceral perforation
- It remains safest to carry out a two-stage procedure in the presence of peritonitis.

ALTERNATIVE TREATMENT

- Recent reports advocate the use of radiologically assisted percutaneous drainage as the initial therapeutic maneuver in patients with peridiverticular abscesses more than 5 cm in diameter.
- Current trends in the surgical management of diverticular disease include the laparoscopic approach to sigmoid resection, which has been used primarily in elective operations.
- Some authors suggest elective surgery after the first episode of diverticulitis in patients under age 40.

COMPLICATIONS

- Complications of diverticulitis include free perforation, which results in acute peritonitis, sepsis, and shock, particularly in the elderly.
- The perforation may be walled off by adherent omentum or neighboring structures such as the bladder or small bowel. If nearby organs become involved or if an abscess ruptures into a nearby organ, a fistula may result.
- Colonic obstruction, though relatively uncommon, may develop after repeated episodes of acute diverticulitis. Small-bowel obstruction occurs somewhat more frequently, especially in the presence of a large peridiverticular abscess.
- Severe pericolitis may cause a fibrous stricture around the bowel, which can be associated with colonic obstruction and may mimic a neoplasm.
- Pylephlebitis is a rare but serious complication of diverticular disease and should be suspected in patients with diverticulitis in whom jaundice or hepatic abscesses develop.

Follow-Up

- Once the acute attack has resolved, the patient should be instructed to maintain a diet high in fiber. Colonoscopy is advisable to exclude a diagnosis of cancer. Previous studies have shown a recurrence rate of at least 50%.
- About 20% to 30% of those patients who develop acute diverticulitis will eventually require surgical therapy. However, 70% of elderly patients who have a single uncomplicated episode of diverticulitis will have no recurrence.

PREVENTION

- Supplementation of dietary fiber has been shown to increase stool weight, alter gastrointestinal transit time, and decrease intraluminal pressures, leading to a decrease in the incidence of diverticulosis.

Selected Readings

Ambrosetti P, Grossholz M, Becker C, et al. Computed tomography in acute left colonic diverticulitis. *Br J Surg* 1997;84:532–534.

Cunningham MA, Davis JW, Kaups KL. Medical versus surgical management of diverticulitis in patients under age 40. *Am J Surg* 1997;174:733–735; discussion 735–736.

Ferzoco LB, Raptopoulos V, Silen W. Acute diverticulitis. *N Engl J Med* 1998;338:1521–1526.

Isselbacher KJ, Epstein A. Diverticular, vascular, and other disorders of the intestine and peritoneum. In: Fauci AS, Braunwald E, Isselbacher KJ, et al., eds. *Harrison's principles of internal medicine*, 14th ed. New York: McGraw-Hill, 1998:1648–1656.

Konvolinka CW. Acute diverticulitis under age forty. *Am J Surg* 1994;167:562–565.

Echinococcosis

Basics

DEFINITION
- Echinococcosis is an infection caused by *Echinococcus* species.
- Manifestations depend on the infecting *Echinococcus* species.

ETIOLOGY
- There are three *Echinococcus* species that cause disease in humans and animals:
  —*Echinococcus granulosus* causes unilocular or cystic hydatid disease.
  —*Echinococcus multilocularis* causes multilocular or alveolar hydatid disease.
  —*Echinococcus vogeli* causes polycystic hydatid disease.

EPIDEMIOLOGY

Incidence and Prevalence
- The domestic dogs and other canids are the definitive hosts for *E. granulosus*, the most common cause of echinococciasis.
- Herbivores (mainly sheep) are intermediate hosts of the parasite.
- Humans are the occasional intermediate host for *E. granulosus*.
- The incubation period (time from infection to manifestation of symptoms) is long (usually from 1 to many years).
- *E. granulosus* infections are common in several countries (including Mediterranean Sea countries).
- The adult *E. multilocularis* is found in wild animals such as foxes (and occasionally in dogs and cats) in central Europe, the former Soviet Union, northern Japan, Canada, and Alaska and the north central United States.
- The adult *E. vogeli* is found in bush dogs in Central and South America.

Risk Factors
- Living in endemic areas
- Children are more likely, compared with adults, to acquire infection with *Echinococcus* species, because they are more likely to have close contact with infected animals.

Clinical Manifestations

SYMPTOMS AND SIGNS
- Hydatid cysts enlarge slowly. They usually require several years to develop to a degree sufficient to cause problems.
- Symptoms usually appear when the cysts enlarge and cause mass effects.
- Specific symptoms and signs in echinococciasis depend mainly on which organ is affected.
- Cysts usually develop in the liver but also in other organs, including the lungs, kidneys, bones, spleen, and the central nervous system.
- There are scattered reports of hydatid cysts in almost every organ of the body presenting with protean manifestations.
- Patients may have anaphylactoid reactions when cysts rupture or leak.

Diagnosis

DIFFERENTIAL DIAGNOSIS
- A typical presentation in a patient who lives in or visited an endemic area strongly suggests the diagnosis of echinococciasis.
- Differential diagnosis should be made between echinococciasis and other diseases that may cause space-occupying lesions, including the following:
  —Tuberculosis
  —Amebic abscess
  —Congenital cysts
  —Malignant diseases

LABORATORY
Serology tests may be helpful.

PATHOLOGIC FINDINGS
- Microscopic examination of excised tissue specimens for identification of the parasite

IMAGING
Imaging tests may show calcification of the external layer of the wall of chronic hydatic cysts.

Echinococcosis

Treatment

MAIN TREATMENT

- There are three main treatment strategies that are used, sometimes in combination:
  — Drug treatment (for *E. granulosus*, albendazole is better than mebendazole)
  — Surgical management (removal of the hydatid cysts)
  — Aspiration of the content of the cyst(s) and administration of a scolicocidal agent in the cyst(s), using a fine needle
- The traditional management of hydatid cyst disease is surgical resection. The use of pharmaceutical agents such as albendazole is recommended prior to and after the operation.
- The recommended dose of albendazole is 400 mg PO every 12 hours. Six 28-day cycles of treatment (interrupted by 14-day off-treatment periods) are recommended.

ALTERNATIVE TREATMENT

Experience with aspiration of contents of cyst(s) using a fine needle has increased in several centers during the last decade. It appears that this approach is safe and effective in experienced hands and offers a good alternative to surgical management, especially if there is only one or few hydatid cysts.

COMPLICATIONS

- Rupture of a hydatid cyst may lead to severe anaphylactoid reactions.
- Hydatid cysts may become infected with bacteria (bacterial superinfection).
- Mass effects due to enlarging hydatid cysts in vital organs may lead to lethal complications.

Follow-Up

- Frequent monitoring of liver and renal function is necessary for patients who receive albendazole or mebendazole.
- Patients may have recurrent disease after treatment of hydatid cyst disease (even after surgical resection due to development of daughter hydatid cysts).

PREVENTION

- Intensive preventive efforts have decreased the incidence of echinococcosis in several countries.
- Countries with high endemicity of echinococciasis until recently (such as Cyprus and Iceland) have accomplished the eradication of this infectious disease due to intensive country-wide efforts of prevention.
- Preventive measures include avoidance of exposure to dog feces, supervision of livestock slaughtering, and safe disposal of infected viscera (preventing dog access to them).

Selected Readings

Falagas ME, Siakavellas E, Sapkas G, et al. Echinococciasis. *Clin Infect Dis* 2000;30:442–443, 567–568.

Filice C, Di Perri G, Strosseli M, et al. Parasitologic findings in percutaneous drainage of human hydatid liver cysts. *J Infect Dis* 1990;161:1290–1295.

Force L, Torres JM, Carrillo A, et al. Evaluation of eight serological tests in the diagnosis of human echinococcosis and follow-up. *Clin Infect Dis* 1992;15:473–480.

Horton RJ. Chemotherapy of *Echinococcus* infection in man with albendazole. *Trans R Soc Trop Med Hyg* 1989;83:97–102.

Saimot AG, Meulemans A, Cremieux AC, et al. Albendazole as a potential treatment for human hydatidosis. *Lancet* 1983;2:652–656.

Wachira TM, Macpherson CN, Gathuma JM. Release and survival of *Echinococcus* eggs in different environments in Turkana, and their possible impact on the incidence of hydatidosis in man and livestock. *J Helminthol* 1991;65:55–61.

Woodtli W, Bircher J, Witassek F, et al. Effect of plasma mebendazole concentrations in the treatment of human echinococcus. *Am J Trop Med Hyg* 1985;34:754–760.

Ehrlichiosis

Basics

DEFINITION
Ehrlichiosis is infection with members of the genus *Ehrlichia*.

ETIOLOGY
- Two pathogens have emerged as etiologic agents of ehrlichiosis in the United States:
  —*Ehrlichia chaffeensis*, which targets mainly macrophages and monocytes, causes human monocytic ehrlichiosis.
  —An *Ehrlichia equi*–like organism causes human granulocytic ehrlichiosis (HGE).
- Recent reports provide evidence suggestive of *Ehrlichia ewingii* infection in humans. The associated disease may be clinically indistinguishable from infection caused by *E. chaffeensis* or the agent of HGE.

EPIDEMIOLOGY
Incidence
- Human monocytic ehrlichiosis (HME) has been documented in more than 400 patients in 30 states by the Centers for Disease Control and Prevention (CDC), as well as in Europe and Africa.
- HGE occurs in North America, mostly Wisconsin and Minnesota, but some cases occur in Massachusetts and Connecticut, and in Western Europe.
- The Lone Star tick (*Amblyomma americanum*) is the major vector for HME, and the white-tailed deer is an important reservoir host of *E. chaffeensis*. Most patients recall tick bites or exposures during the 3 weeks before the onset of illness; usually these events take place in rural areas from April to September, with a peak from May through July.
- Humans acquire HGE from deer ticks (*Ixodes scapularis*) in eastern and central North America and from related ticks in other geographic areas. The agent of HGE and closely related agents infect a variety of wild and domestic animals, including dogs.
- The incidence of HGE peaks in June and July, but the disease occurs throughout the year in conjunction with human exposure to *Ixodes* ticks.

Clinical Manifestations

SYMPTOMS
- After the tick bite inoculation of *E. chaffeensis* and a median incubation period of 9 days, only one-third of persons who seroconvert actually become ill.
  —The clinical signs and symptoms associated with infection due to *E. chaffeensis* include the following:
  —Fever (97%)
  —Headache (81%)
  —Myalgia (68%)
  —Anorexia (66%)
  —Nausea (48%)
  —Vomiting (37%)
  —Rash (6% at onset, 25% during the first week, and 36% overall)
  —Cough (26%)
  —Pharyngitis (26%)
  —Diarrhea (25%)
  —Lymphadenopathy (25%)
  —Abdominal pain (22%)
  —Confusion (20%)
- HGE is clinically similar to the monocytic form of the disease, although rash occurs in fewer than 10% of patients. After a median incubation period of 8 days, patients with HGE usually suffer a flulike illness with the following:
  —Fever (100%)
  —Chills (98%)
  —Malaise (98%)
  —Headache (85%)
  —Nausea (39%)
  —Vomiting (34%)
  —Cough (29%)
  —Confusion (17%)

Diagnosis

DIFFERENTIAL DIAGNOSIS
- Diseases such as endocarditis, other forms of septicemia, vasculitis, and thrombotic thrombocytopenic purpura must be considered.
- Also, other tick-borne infections such as tularemia, babesiosis, Lyme disease, murine typhus, Rocky Mountain spotted fever, and Colorado tick fever may be considered in the differential diagnosis of patients with ehrlichiosis.

LABORATORY
- Serum samples can be obtained during the acute phase of the illness and during convalescence to test for the agent of HGE or *E. chaffeensis*. However, most patients with ehrlichiosis are seronegative for these agents at presentation.
- HME is usually accompanied by leukopenia, thrombocytopenia, and elevated levels of hepatic aminotransferases.
- The CDC case definition for HME requires a clinically compatible history with a minimum antibody titer to *E. chaffeensis* of greater than or equal to 1:64, or a fourfold or greater change in antibody titers from acute and convalescent sera, using indirect fluorescent antibody testing.
- PCR analyses for the organisms associated with HGE and HME (and perhaps *E. ewingii*), if available, would be expected to be positive in untreated patients. However, the use of this modality is still under investigation.
- Culture of the agents of ehrlichiosis is diagnostic, but the process takes several days and the results are reliable only in a few specialized research laboratories.
- The laboratory diagnosis of HGE is more difficult to establish. Serodiagnosis by indirect immunofluorescence assay, with *E. equi*-infected equine neutrophils as

Ehrlichiosis

antigen, is highly sensitive but is useful mainly for retrospective documentation of seroconversion to a titer of 80 or greater during convalescence.
- The sensitivity of the peripheral blood smear as a diagnostic screening tool is unknown, but in one study of patients with HGE, 80% of the patients tested had morulae in the cytoplasm of peripheral blood neutrophils. Clinicians should never discount the diagnosis of HGE in a patient because the peripheral smear does not demonstrate the characteristic morulae in the neutrophils.

Treatment

- Tetracycline drugs such as doxycycline (100 mg twice daily) have been shown to shorten the course of HME. However, no controlled trials of antimicrobial therapy have been conducted.
- The issue of the proper medication for HME in children younger than 9 years is not an easy one. Some institutions use doxycycline (4 mg/kg/d twice daily, with a maximum dose of 100 mg) for the treatment of any patient, regardless of age, with symptomatic HME. If patients are unable to take doxycycline, chloramphenicol (75 mg/kg/d in four divided doses) may be used.
- Although chloramphenicol appears to shorten the course of illness, some patients do not respond to treatment with this agent, and *E. chaffeensis* is resistant to chloramphenicol in cell culture.
- Doxycycline is also an effective therapeutic drug for HGE. Of 35 HGE patients treated with doxycycline, 94% defervesced within 24 to 48 hours. One patient who did not receive doxycycline had the agent of HGE detected by PCR in the blood on day 28 of illness.
- The required duration of administration of doxycycline is not known, but most authorities suggest a 7- to 14-day course.

COMPLICATIONS

- Ehrlichial infections can be severe or even fatal if untreated.
- Over 60% of patients who, at some point, are recognized to have *E. chaffeensis* are hospitalized, 15% of patients have severe infections, and 2% to 3% of patients die.
- Severe illness due to *E. chaffeensis* may lead to the following:
  - Respiratory insufficiency
  - Neurologic involvement (seizures, coma, etc.)
  - Acute renal failure
  - Gastrointestinal hemorrhage
- The natural history of untreated HGE in adults is a 3- to 11-week illness with a possibly fatal outcome.
- Among patients with HGE, elderly patients are more likely to have severe disease, but infections also occur in children. The current mortality rate is estimated to be approximately 5%. So far, 51% of patients have been hospitalized, and 7% have been admitted to an intensive care unit.
- Coinfection with *Borrelia burgdorferi* or *Babesia microti* probably occurs on occasion. It is possible that microbial interactions in this situation lead to more severe disease than infection with a single agent.

Follow-Up

- Persistent ehrlichial infection has been documented after treatment with tetracycline and chloramphenicol.
- Patients with ehrlichiosis usually have a response to treatment within 24 to 48 hours, and the lack of a response should suggest another diagnosis.
- Expert consultation should be obtained before therapy with a drug other than a tetracycline is considered.

PREVENTION

- Ehrlichiosis is prevented by avoidance of tick bite and prompt removal of attached ticks.
- If tick-infested areas cannot be avoided, clothing becomes a protective device. It is preferable to wear light-colored clothing to allow early identification of crawling ticks.
- After returning from tick-infested areas, a thorough body search for attached ticks should be performed, with emphasis on areas containing hair.
- If long-sleeved shirts or long pants are not practical, exposed areas of the skin should be covered with insect repellents containing N, N-diethyl-M-toluamide. This is the most common active agent in insect repellents. Systemic reactions to DEET can occur when concentrations exceeding 35% are used, in patients who repetitively use repellents with lesser concentrations, or in cases of ingestion. Because of these systemic reactions, all DEET-containing compounds should be used with care, and chronic readministration should be avoided.

Selected Readings

Buller RS, Arms M, Hmiel SP, et al. *Ehrlichia ewingii*, a newly recognized agent of human ehrlichiosis. N Engl J Med 1999;341:148–155.

Goodman JL. Ehrlichiosis—ticks, dogs, and doxycycline. N Engl J Med 1999;341:195–197.

van Dobbenburgh A, van Dam AP, Fikrig E. Human granulocytic ehrlichiosis in western Europe. N Engl J Med 1999;340:1214–1216.

Walker D, Raoult D, Brouqui P, et al. Rickettsial diseases. In: Fauci AS, Braunwald E, Isselbacher KJ, et al., eds. *Harrison's principles of internal medicine*, 14th ed. New York: McGraw-Hill, 1998:1045–1052.

Walker DH, Barbour AG, Oliver JH, et al. Emerging bacterial zoonotic and vector-borne diseases. Ecological and epidemiological factors. JAMA 1996;275:463–469.

Encephalitis

Basics

DEFINITION
Encephalitis is inflammation of the brain that is caused by a number of infectious etiologies, including viruses, bacteria, fungi, and protozoa. A wide range of viruses may cause diffuse or localized encephalitis as part of the clinical syndrome. The pathway to the central nervous system (CNS) differs with each organism, but most enter the CNS via the bloodstream.

ETIOLOGY
Viral
- Flaviviridae
  - Japanese encephalitis virus
  - St. Louis encephalitis
  - West Nile virus
  - Central European encephalitis
  - Russian spring-summer encephalitis
  - Murray Valley encephalitis
- Togaviridae
  - Eastern equine encephalitis
  - Western equine encephalitis
  - Venezuelan equine encephalitis
- Bunyaviridae
  - California, La Crosse
  - Rift Valley fever
- Herpesviridae
  - Herpes simplex virus (HSV)
  - Cytomegalovirus (CMV) (in AIDS)
  - Varicella zoster virus (VZV) (in AIDS)
  - Herpes B virus
- Other viruses that are commonly considered
  - Retroviruses (HIV)
  - JC virus
  - Adenovirus
  - Enterovirus(coxsackievirus, echovirus, poliovirus)
  - Influenza
  - Mumps
  - Rabies

Bacterial
- *Listeria*
- *Mycobacterium tuberculosis*
- *Rickettsia*
- *Mycoplasma*
- Syphilis
- Lyme disease
- Whipple's disease
- *Nocardia*

Fungal
- *Cryptococcus*
- Coccidioidomycosis
- *Candida*
- *Aspergillus*
- Protozoa
- Toxoplasmosis
- Malaria

Amoebic
- *Naegleria*

EPIDEMIOLOGY
- Much depends on the specific agent involved.
- Some of the organisms are tick- and mosquito-borne, and thus are seasonal.
- Enteroviral infections tend to occur in the late summer and early fall.
- Encephalitis may be sporadic or part of an outbreak.
- HSV encephalitis is sporadic and occurs in 1 of 250,000 cases annually in the United States.
- West Nile virus: The principal reservoir is in wild birds, such as crows; it is transmitted by mosquitos. The first cases appeared in the United States in 1999 in New York City. In 2000, infected birds and mosquitos were identified in many areas of the northeastern United States.

Clinical Manifestations

- Encephalitis may be acute or chronic.
- Patients often have headache, fevers, and decreased levels of consciousness.
- Seizures are common.
- Because of meningeal inflammation, signs of meningitis may occur, making it hard to distinguish between meningitis and encephalitis.
- Focal signs may occur early, and cranial nerve abnormalities may occur with increased intracranial pressure.
  - Lyme disease is associated with cranial nerve abnormalities.
  - Japanese encephalitis is associated with a movement disorder similar to Parkinson's disease.
  - HSV tends to be located in the temporal lobes; at times, patients have a prodrome of bizarre behavior, with increasing occurrence.
  - *Note:* With all of the CNS events, it is important that systemic signs be sought to help establish a diagnosis. Rashes, when present, are most helpful in diagnosis. Evidence of tick bites or mosquito bites may be lacking.

Diagnosis

LABORATORY
White Blood Cell Count
- The count is often low in viral infections.
- The count is mildly elevated in bacterial infections.
- Large numbers of atypical lymphocytes are seen in Epstein-Barr virus infections.
- Malaria smears and evaluation of WBCs for morulae in *Ehrlichia* should be considered if there is any suspicion that the patient may have malaria or ehrlichiosis.

Encephalitis

Serology

- Diagnosis is made frequently by serology.
- Obtain IgM levels if appropriate.
- Obtain acute and convalescent serum.
- Cerebrospinal PCR evaluation for HSV I and II, as well as CMV, is commercially available.
- Culture, Gram stains, acid-fast bacillus smears, and India ink stains are important.
- West Nile virus can be isolated from blood, cerebrospinal fluid (CSF) tissue, and other body fluids. Antibody is measured in serum; the presence of IgM-specific antibody by ELISA in a single serum sample is diagnostic.
- West Nile virus produces subclinical and mild infection in most persons. Fatalities are seen in 3% to 15% of active cases, usually in the elderly.

Cerebrospinal Fluid Analysis

- CSF analysis is needed when no evidence of a mass lesion is present.
- CSF glucose is often normal in viral infections. Protein is almost always elevated in encephalitis.
- CSF pleocytosis is variable, with usual counts of 10 to 2,000 cells/mm^3 in viral diseases.
  — Cells may be mononuclear or polynuclear.
  — Associated RBCs are present within the CSF with HSV encephalitis.
- Analyze CSF for Venereal Disease Research Laboratory/Rapid Plasmin Reagin (VDRL/RPR) in suspected syphilis.

IMAGING

- CT or MRI can be helpful in determining the location of areas of encephalitis, especially with HSV (temporal lobes).
- Eastern equine encephalitis may produce areas of focal changes in the basal ganglia and thalami.
- Mass lesions may be observed with fungal infections.

DIFFERENTIAL DIAGNOSIS

- Carcinomatous meningitis
- Reye's syndrome
- Toxic metabolic abnormalities
- Drug-induced (recreational along with trimethoprim–sulfamethoxazole, ibuprofen, metronidazole, and others)

Treatment

- Empiric treatment for bacterial and fungal causes should not be done routinely unless the Gram stains reveal organisms or unless other evidence of infection is obtained, such as a positive CNS RPR.
- Acyclovir 10 mg/kg intravenous every 8 hours for 14 to 21 days is used for treatment of HSV encephalitis.
- Ganciclovir and/or foscarnet is used to treat CMV encephalitis.
- Highly active antiviral therapy (HAART) can decrease CSF levels of HIV RNA.
- Other viral causes are treated with supportive therapy.

COMPLICATIONS

Permanent damage is common after some viral encephalitides. This may include cortical blindness, paresis, and seizure disorders.

Follow-Up

Patients require rehabilitation and close follow-up with neurologists. Late onset of seizures may occur.

PREVENTION

- There is no way to prevent HSV encephalitis.
- Avoidance of tick and mosquito bites may limit transmission.
- Vector control in areas where disease is epidemic should be considered.
- Avoidance of swimming in ponds late in the summer may decrease the risk of enteroviral infections.
- A vaccine is available for Japanese encephalitis, and should be given to people who reside in or plan to locate in endemic areas.
- For tourists, prevention of mosquito bites is most likely sufficient to prevent disease.
- Children are vaccinated for measles, mumps and rubella, polio, and varicella.

Selected Readings

Johnson RT. *Viral infections of the nervous system*, 2nd ed. Philadelphia: Lippincott–Raven Publishers, 1998.

McCutchan JA. Cytomegalovirus infections of the nervous system in patients with AIDS. *Clin Infect Dis* 1995;20:747–754.

Whitley, RJ, Kimberlin DW, Roizman B. Herpes simplex viruses. *Clin Infect Dis* 1998;26:541–555.

Endocarditis, Native Valves

Basics

DEFINITION
- Infection of the valves or the endocardium of the heart with bacteria, fungi, or rickettsiae.

ETIOLOGY
- Any valve can become infected, whether it has had previous damage or is normal.
- Infection depends on a number of factors:
  —Integrity of the endocardial surface
  —Flow of blood throughout the heart
  —Virulence of the organism

EPIDEMIOLOGY
- Incidence varies from 1.7 to 3.8 of 100,000 person-years or about 1 per 1,000 admissions per year.
- Approximately 50% of cases occur in patients aged 31 to 60 years.
- Mitral valves are affected most commonly (about 45%), followed by aortic valves (35%). Both mitral and aortic valves are infected concurrently in 35% of cases.
- Commonly, patients have a history of rheumatic heart disease, and the mitral valve is infected in a majority of these patients.
- The pulmonic valve is rarely infected, and the tricuspid valve is infected in 6% of cases.
- Other common heart diseases associated with a risk of endocarditis include the following:
  —Congenital heart disease
  —Bicuspid aortic valve
  —Mitral valve prolapse

Incubation
- Incubation for streptococcal endocarditis is less than 2 weeks.
- Incubation for virulent bacteria is often less than 1 week.

Clinical Manifestations

- Infection can be acute with high fevers and signs of sepsis, or subacute with low-grade fevers and constitutional symptoms over several weeks.
- Fever, chills, and nightsweats are reported in 90% of patients.
- Malaise, back pain, or nonspecific abdominal pains can be noted in acute or subacute cases.
- Splenomegaly is noted in up to 60% of patients with subacute endocarditis.
- Heart failure suggests mitral or aortic regurgitation. A heart murmur is noted in 85% of patients with left-sided disease and in 35% with right-sided disease.
- Cough is often seen with right-sided endocarditis, leading to pneumonitis.
- Clubbing occurs with untreated disease in approximately 50% of patients.
- Petechiae result from microemboli or vasculitis. Janeway lesions are small hemorrhagic macules that present throughout the body, most commonly on the palms and soles.
- Osler nodes are nodules present on the fingers and toes. They are usually less than 15 mm and painful to touch.
- Embolic phenomena occur in 50% of patients. They are seen in the following:
  —Central nervous system, leading to stroke
  —Coronary arteries, leading to myocardial infarcts
  —Lungs in right-heart endocarditis, leading to pulmonary infiltrates and abscesses
  —Kidney, leading to hematuria
  —Spleen, leading to infarction and left upper quadrant pain

Diagnosis

- Multiple positive blood cultures plus an echocardiogram revealing vegetation, a new heart murmur, or embolic phenomena
- In bacterial endocarditis, 90% of the first two blood cultures reveal a positive result.
- Fungal endocarditis has resulted in positive cultures in less than 50% of the cases.
- Culture-negative endocarditis occurs in 18% to 30% of cases in various series.
- Transthoracic echocardiograms are positive in 65% of cases, and transesophageal echocardiograms are positive in 95%.
- Patients often present with anemia and leukocytosis, however, the WBC count may be normal in subacute cases.
- Sedimentation rates are elevated.
- Rheumatoid factor is positive 50% of the time in bacterial endocarditis.
- The urinalysis reveals red blood cells in up to 60% of cases.
- The electrocardiogram, which is useful to follow, may reveal various degrees of SA and AV block.

DIFFERENTIAL DIAGNOSIS
- Atrial myxoma
- Infection of vascular graft or infected aneurysm
- Osteomyelitis

Endocarditis, Native Valves

Treatment

- Treatment depends on the organism present, the sensitivities of that organism, and the need for valvular surgery.
- In general, patients with left-sided disease require 4 to 6 full weeks of antibiotics intravenously.
- For penicillin-sensitive strains of *Streptococcus viridans* and *Streptococcus bovis* (MIC < 0.1 μg/mL of penicillin)
  —Penicillin G 12 to 18 million units i.v. daily in six divided doses, with gentamicin 1 mg/kg i.v. every 8 hours for 2 weeks total
  —Penicillin G 12 to 18 million units i.v. daily, given in six divided doses for 4 weeks
  —Ceftriaxone 2.0 g i.v. daily for 4 weeks
  —For penicillin-allergic patients, use vancomycin 1 g i.v. every 12 hours.
- For *Enterococcus* or *Streptococcus* relatively resistant strains (MIC > 0.5 μg/mL penicillin)
  —Penicillin G 18 to 30 million units i.v. daily, given in six divided doses, plus gentamicin 1 mg/kg every 8 hours for 4 to 6 weeks total
- For *Staphylococcus* that is methicillin-sensitive
  —Nafcillin 2 g i.v. every 4 hours for 4 to 6 weeks, and gentamicin 1.0 mg/kg every 8 hours for 3 to 5 days
- For *Staphylococcus* that is methicillin-resistant, as well as *S. epidermidis*
  —Vancomycin 30 mg/kg i.v. in divided doses for 4 to 6 weeks

COMPLICATIONS

- In addition to emboli and valve failure, patients may develop the following:
  —Osteomyelitis
  —Renal failure
  —Mycotic aneurysms leading to hemorrhage

Follow-Up

Patients should obtain prophylaxis prior to having complicated dental or urologic and gastrointestinal procedures.

PREVENTION

- Antibiotic prophylaxis is needed for patients with the following:
  —Prosthetic valves
  —History of endocarditis
  —Congenital heart disease
  —Mitral valve prolapse with a murmur

Prophylaxis

- For oral surgery or periodontal surgery or tonsillectomy and rigid bronchoscopy
  —Amoxicillin 2 g 1 hour before procedure
- For penicillin-allergic patients, 1 hour before procedure
  —Clindamycin 600 mg
  —Azithromycin 500 mg
  —Clarithromycin 500 mg
- For GU or lower GI tract procedures (controversial)
  —Within 30 minutes of the procedure, ampicillin 2 g i.m. or i.v., plus gentamicin 1.5 mg/kg
  —Six hours after the procedure, amoxicillin 1 g orally or ampicillin 1 g i.v. or i.m
- For penicillin-allergic patients
  —Vancomycin instead of ampicillin
  —No need for the follow-up dose

Selected Readings

Clemens JD, Horwitz RI, Jaffe CC, et al. A controlled evaluation of the risk of bacterial endocarditis in persons with mitral-valve prolapse. *N Engl J Med* 1982;307:776.

Lerner PI. Neurologic complications of infective endocarditis. *Med Clin North Am* 1985;69:385–398.

Moon MR, Stinson EB, Miller DC. Surgical treatment of endocarditis. *Prog Cardiovasc Dis* 1997;40:239–264.

Shapiro SM, Bayer AS. Transesophageal and Doppler echocardiography in the diagnosis and management of infective endocarditis. *Chest* 1991;100:1125–1130.

Tunkel AR, Kaye D. Endocarditis with negative blood cultures. *N Engl J Med* 1992;326:1215–1217.

Watanakunakorn C, Burkert T. Infective endocarditis at a large community teaching hospital, 1980–1990. *Medicine* 1993;72:90.

Endocarditis, Prosthetic Valves

Basics

DEFINITION

Prosthetic valve endocarditis (PVE) is a serious complication of valve replacement surgery, causing high morbidity and mortality. Infection of prosthetic valves accounts for 10% to 20% of all cases of endocarditis. After 10 years, it is thought that 5% of all prosthetic valves will become infected. Infection is harder to detect and eradicate in prosthetic valves than in native valves.

ETIOLOGY

- Infection of the valve may occur at the time of surgery.
- Infection can occur as part of a transient bacteremia or fungemia many years after surgery.
- In contrast to native valve endocarditis, less virulent organisms often cause disease in prosthetic valves. This is in part due to the biofilm that encompasses the prosthesis and sewing ring.
- Bioprosthetic valves are at higher risk of infection than are prosthetic valves.
- PVE that occurs within the first 60 days is termed *early*.
- Early PVE accounts for 37% of cases of PVE.
- Organisms isolated in early PVE include the following:
  - *Staphylococcus epidermidis* or *Staphylococcus aureus* (50% of patients with early PVE)
  - Diphtheroids (10%)
  - Gram-negative organisms (15%)
- This reflects infections obtained at surgery and in the postoperative period.
- Infections that occur after 60 days account for 63% of cases and are termed *late*.
  - *S. epidermidis* and *S. aureus* account for 38% of cases.
  - Streptococci (25%)
  - Diphtheroids are rare.
- *Candida*, along with other fungi, including *Aspergillus*, is more common in PVE than in native valve disease.

EPIDEMIOLOGY

N/A

Clinical Manifestations

- The presentation in many ways is similar to that of native valve endocarditis.
- Fever occurs in almost 100% of patients with PVE.
- Embolization, often to the central nervous system, is present in 40% of patients.
- Splenomegaly, along with petechiae, is commonly encountered.
- Heart failure is present when valvular dysfunction worsens.
- Syncope can occur with valvular obstruction or conduction abnormalities.

Diagnosis

Patients often have a changing murmur or new murmurs. These changes may be hard to detect over a short period of time.

LABORATORY

- Blood cultures are positive for bacteria in 90% of cases.
- Anemia may be caused by chronic disease and by hemolysis due to a paravalvular leak.
- Leukocytosis is common.
- Hematuria due to immune complex-induced glomerulonephritis is seen in over 50% of patients.
- Electrocardiograms reveal conduction abnormalities in patients with intramyocardial abscesses.

Endocarditis, Prosthetic Valves

IMAGING

- Transthoracic echocardiograms (TTEs) frequently cannot resolve vegetations on the valve or intramyocardial abscesses.
- A transesophageal echocardiogram (TEE) is the procedure of choice to evaluate vegetations in PVE.

Treatment

MEDICAL TREATMENT

- *S. epidermidis*
  —Vancomycin 15 mg/kg every 12 hours and rifampin 300 mg orally every 8 hours for 6 weeks, with gentamicin 1 mg/kg every 8 hours for 2 weeks
- *S. aureus*
  —Nafcillin 2 g every 4 hours and rifampin 300 mg orally every 8 hours for 6 weeks, with gentamicin 1 mg/kg every 8 hours for 2 weeks
- Other organisms: depends on sensitivity testing

SURGICAL TREATMENT

- The need for surgery has to be assessed on a daily basis; delay, in order to sterilize the valve, is not warranted. Reasons for surgery include the following:

—Valve dysfunction
—Heart failure
—Multiple emboli
—Persistent fevers with bacteremia
—Fungal infection
—Unstable rocking of the valve
—Intramyocardial abscess with heart block

COMPLICATIONS

Bleeding from mycotic aneurysms occurs if patients are over-anticoagulated. Every effort must be made to avoid this complication while maintaining a therapeutic INR.

Follow-Up

Patients with prosthetic valve endocarditis should be followed closely for signs of valvular leak or obstruction.

PREVENTION

Prophylaxis for dental procedures and urologic and gastrointestinal (GU/GI) instrumentation should be performed. See Section II chapter, "Endocarditis, Native Valves."

Selected Readings

Daniel WG, Mugge A, Martin RP, et al. Improvement in the diagnosis of abscesses associated with endocarditis by transesophageal echocardiography. *N Engl J Med* 1991;324:795–800.

Jault F, Gandjbakeh I, Chastre JC, et al. Prosthetic valve endocarditis with ring abscesses: Surgical management and long term results. *J Thorac Cardiovasc Surg* 1993;105:1106–1113.

Wolf M, Witchitz S, Chastang C, et al. Prosthetic valve endocarditis in the ICU: Prognostic factors of overall survival in a series of 122 cases and consequences for treatment decision. *Chest* 1995;108:688–694.

Endophthalmitis

Basics

DEFINITION

- Endophthalmitis is an inflammatory process involving the ocular cavity and adjacent structures.
- Inflammation involving all ocular tissue layers is termed *panophthalmitis*.

ETIOLOGY

- Infectious endophthalmitis occurs from bacterial, viral, fungal, or parasitic infection of the internal structures of the eye. The most common causes include the following:
  - Bacteria
    - *Acinetobacter* spp
    - *Actinomyces israelii*
    - *Bacillus* spp (usually B. *cereus* and B. *subtilis*)
    - *Clostridium* spp
    - *Corynebacterium* spp
    - *Enterobacter* spp
    - *Enterococcus* spp
    - *Escherichia coli*
    - *Haemophilus influenzae*
    - *Klebsiella* spp
    - *Listeria monocytogenes*
    - *Mycobacteria* spp
    - *Neisseria meningitidis*
    - *Proteus* spp
    - *Propionibacterium acnes*
    - *Pseudomonas aeruginosa*
    - *Salmonella typhimurium*
    - *Serratia marcescens*
    - *Streptococcus* spp
    - *Staphylococcus* spp
    - *Treponema pallidium*
  - Fungi
    - *Aspergillus* spp
    - *Blastomyces dermatitidis*
    - *Candida* spp
    - *Coccidioides immitis*
    - *Fusarium* spp
    - *Histoplasma capsulatum*
    - *Mucor* spp
    - *Penicillium* spp
    - *Rhizopus* spp
    - *Sporothrix schenckii*
  - Viruses
    - Cytomegalovirus
    - Herpes simplex virus
    - Herpes zoster virus
    - Rubella
    - Rubeola
  - Parasites
    - *Taenia solium*
    - *Toxocara canis*
    - *Toxoplasma gondii*
  - Miscellaneous
    - *Pneumocystis carinii*
- Most episodes of endophthalmitis develop from the following:
  - Hematogenous seeding from a remote site, including septic emboli from a diseased heart valve or a dental abscess, that lodges in the retinal circulation
  - Ocular surgery, occasionally months or even years after the operation
  - An occult penetrating foreign body or unrecognized trauma to the globe
- Bacteria such as streptococcal and gram-negative organisms that cause infections with poor visual prognosis are more common after trauma.
- Mixed infections occur frequently after nonsurgical trauma, with an incidence as high as 42% in injuries from a rural environment.

EPIDEMIOLOGY

Incidence

The incidence of endophthalmitis after cataract surgery varies from 0.078% to 0.53%, while the incidence after penetrating trauma is 3.3% to 17%.

Risk Factors

- Any septic focus, localized or systemic, can be the origin of endogenous endophthalmitis.
- Chronically ill, diabetic, or immunosuppressed patients, especially those with a history of indwelling intravenous catheters or positive blood cultures, are at greatest risk for endogenous endophthalmitis.
- Neonates and women in the puerperal period may develop endogenous endophthalmitis.

Clinical Manifestations

SYMPTOMS

- Most patients with endophthalmitis present with ocular pain and injection. However, visual loss is sometimes the only symptom.
- In some instances, a seemingly mild injury may not lead the patient to seek care until the signs and symptoms of infection have developed and infections are revealed weeks after repair of the initial penetrating injury, particularly when the infecting organism is a fungus. In other cases, notably with B. *cereus* infections, the onset of pain and profound visual loss may be rapid.
- Pain with movement of the eye is a prominent feature of panophthalmitis.

SIGNS

- Haziness of vitreous body is essential in the diagnosis.
- Marked swelling, pain, corneal ring infiltrate, fever, and leukocytosis are the usual features of B. *cereus* endophthalmitis.
- White-centered retinal hemorrhages (Roth's spots) are considered pathognomonic for subacute bacterial endocarditis, but they also appear in leukemia, diabetes, and other conditions.

Diagnosis

DIFFERENTIAL DIAGNOSIS

- Other intraocular inflammatory syndromes that can mimic infectious endophthalmitis include the following:
  - Sympathetic ophthalmia
  - Idiopathic uveitis
  - Postoperative sterile inflammation

LABORATORY

- In cases of suspected infectious endophthalmitis, aqueous and vitreous aspiration for microbial culture and smear should be performed.

Endophthalmitis

- Smears should be stained with Gram, Giemsa, and periodic acid-Schiff (PAS) and cultured for aerobic and anaerobic bacteria, mycobacteria, and fungi.

DIAGNOSTIC/TESTING PROCEDURES

Vitreous irrigation material from vitrectomy fluid can be centrifuged and smeared or passed through a filter that can be stained and cultured.

Treatment

MAIN TREATMENT

- Acute bacterial endophthalmitis represents a true ophthalmologic emergency, and therapy should be individualized based on the clinical situation.
  —Postocular surgery (acute): intravitreal amikacin and vancomycin (0.4 mg and 1.0 mg, respectively)
  —Consider periocular injection with tobramycin 40 mg and vancomycin 25 mg or cefazolin 100 mg.
  —Systemic administration of tobramycin and cefazolin
  —Vitrectomy
- Postocular surgery (chronic): vitrectomy and intraocular vancomycin
- Posttraumatic: intravitreal vancomycin and amikacin; also, systemic and intravitreal clindamycin; consider vitrectomy
- Hematogenous spread: third-generation cephalosporin (cefotaxime 2 g every four hours i.v., ceftazidime, or ceftriaxone) and vancomycin 1 g bid; also, intravitreal vancomycin and amikacin. The antibiotic regimen should be adjusted based on culture results.
- Fungal: intravitreal (0.01 mg in 0.1 mL) and intravenous amphotericin B. Also, consider vitrectomy.

- Corticosteroids (systemic prednisone 60 mg PO daily and periocular dexamethasone phosphate 4 mg) are often used to reduce the host immune and antiinflammatory response.

ALTERNATIVE TREATMENT

- Posttraumatic: Systemic vancomycin can be used instead of systemic clindamycin.
- Fungal: Systemic fluconazole for hematogenous endophthalmitis due to *C. albicans* may be less toxic than amphotericin B, but no comparative data are available and resistance of the fungus to fluconazole can occur.

TREATMENT FAILURE

Vitrectomy should be considered, especially if the causative pathogen is virulent or if the interval between onset of symptoms and therapy is prolonged.

COMPLICATIONS

- The visual prognosis for infections after penetrating trauma is worse than that for postoperative cases, in part because the spectrum of bacteria involved is quite different.
- After elective cataract surgery, culture-proven infected eyes achieved visual acuity of 20/40 or better 50% of the time and 20/400 or better 85% of the time, while in recent combined series of posttraumatic endophthalmitis, only 30% of eyes were 20/400 or better.
- The outcome of *B. cereus* endophthalmitis is almost uniformly poor, with loss of all vision and phthisis the usual results.
- The difference in these results probably reflects both the virulence of the infecting organisms in posttraumatic cases and the effects of the initial injury.

Follow-Up

PREVENTION

- Many authorities recommend intravenous, early prophylactic therapy for most cases of penetrating ocular injuries with high risk for infection.
- Both gram-positive and gram-negative coverage should be provided by a combination of antibiotics, such as a combination of vancomycin and ceftazidime or amikacin.
- An intravitreous injection should be considered for maximum protection.
- For trauma limited to the anterior segment, frequent fortified topical antimicrobials, subconjunctival injections at the close of the procedure, and intravenous antimicrobials can produce potentially therapeutic levels of antimicrobials in the anterior chamber.
- Patients with infectious foci and especially those with fungemia due to *Candida* spp should be monitored closely for the development of endophthalmitis.

Selected Readings

Alfonso EC, Flynn HW Jr. Controversies in endophthalmitis prevention. The risk for emerging resistance to vancomycin. *Arch Ophthalmol* 1995;113:1369–1370.

Horton JC. Disorders of the eye. In: Fauci AS, Braunwald E, Isselbacher KJ, et al., eds. *Harrison's principles of internal medicine*, 14th ed. New York: McGraw-Hill, 1998:159–172.

Meredith TA. Posttraumatic endophthalmitis. *Arch Ophthalmol* 1999;117:520–521.

O'Brien TR, Green WR. Endophthalmitis. In: Mandell GL, Bennett JE, Dolin R, eds. *Principles and practice of infectious diseases*, 4th ed. New York: Churchill Livingstone, 1995:1020–1029.

Epidemic Pleurodynia (Bornholm Disease)

Basics

DEFINITION
Epidemic pleurodynia, also known as epidemic myalgia, Bornholm disease (named after the Danish island Bornholm), or devil's grip, is an acute, febrile infectious disease characterized by the abrupt onset of chest or abdominal pain, usually accompanied by fever.

ETIOLOGY
- As its name suggests, the disease often occurs in localized epidemics; it is generally caused by coxsackievirus B.
- Other viruses, such as echoviruses 1, 6, 9, 16, and 19, and coxsackieviruses A4, 6, 9, and 10 have been associated.
- Enteroviral outbreaks involving athletic teams have been reported.

EPIDEMIOLOGY
- Enteroviral infections (coxsackievirus groups A and B, echoviruses, and the newer numbered enteroviruses) are common throughout the late summer and early fall each year in the United States.
- Epidemiologic surveillance suggests that 10 million to 15 million illnesses attributable to nonpolio enteroviruses occur each year.
- Epidemic pleurodynia usually occurs in small or large epidemics, and multiple family members develop symptoms either at the same time or in succession, separated by several days.
- The peak incidence of enteroviral illness coincides with the football and soccer seasons. It has been postulated that close contact either on the playing field or in the locker room facilitates person-to-person transmission, or that water and common containers become contaminated through direct oral contact by infected individuals and serve as a source of virus.
- Intense physical exertion during the incubation period may result in more severe symptomatic infection, making illness among athletes more readily identifiable.

Clinical Manifestations

SYMPTOMS
- Pleurodynia usually has no prodrome and begins with the abrupt onset of fever and spasms of pleuritic chest or upper abdominal pain.
- Fever is usually up to 38.0° to 39.5°C, peaks within an hour after the onset of paroxysms, and subsides when pain resolves.
- Chest pain is more frequent in adults, and abdominal pain is more common in children. Paroxysms of severe, knifelike pain usually last 15 to 30 minutes and are associated with diaphoresis and tachypnea. The involved muscles are tender to palpation, and a pleural rub may be detected.
- Periumbilical pain and pain in the lower abdominal quadrants can occur, especially among children.
- Cases of pain limited to the neck and limbs have been reported.

SIGNS
- Pain can be elicited by pressure on the involved muscles in most cases.
- Swelling of the muscles is seen or felt in some cases.

Diagnosis

DIFFERENTIAL DIAGNOSIS
The differential diagnosis includes pneumonia, pulmonary infarct, myocardial ischemia, herpes zoster, or any cause of acute abdominal pain, particularly acute appendicitis or renal colic (see Section I chapters, "Pleuritic and Chest Pain and Fever" and "Abdominal Pain and Fever").

Epidemic Pleurodynia (Bornholm Disease)

LABORATORY

- The white blood cell count is usually normal.
- Virologic diagnosis can be achieved by isolating group B coxsackievirus from throat washings or feces, or by demonstrating an increase in antibody titers.

IMAGING

Chest radiographs are normal, although, rarely, small pleural effusions can occur.

Treatment

- Treatment includes the administration of nonsteroidal antiinflammatory agents or the application of heat to the affected muscles.
- Opiate analgesics are indicated in severe cases.

COMPLICATIONS

- Symptoms resolve in a few days (usually 4 to 6 days; range, 12 hours to 3 weeks), and recurrences are rare.
- Aseptic meningitis and orchitis can occur (each in fewer than 5% of cases), while pericarditis and pneumonia are even less common.

Follow-Up

PREVENTION

- Specific control measures recommended to avoid outbreaks include the following:
  - Discouraging direct oral contact with common drinking containers
  - Use of disposable cups or individual drinking containers
  - Use of ice packs rather than ice cubes from a team ice chest for injuries
  - Provision of education and information for students, school nurses, and coaching staff

Selected Readings

Ikeda RM, Kondracki SF, Drabkin PD, et al. Pleurodynia among football players at a high school. An outbreak associated with coxsackievirus B1. *JAMA* 1993;270:2205–2206.

Modlin JF. Coxsackieviruses, echoviruses, and newer enteroviruses. In: Mandell GL, Bennett JE, Dolin R, eds. *Principles and practice of infectious diseases*, 4th ed. New York: Churchill Livingstone, 1995:1620–1636.

Pichichero ME, McLinn S, Rotbart HA, et al. Clinical and economic impact of enterovirus illness in private pediatric practice. *Pediatrics* 1998;102:1126–1134.

Epididymitis

Basics

DEFINITION
- Common infection in males transmitted by both sexually transmitted organisms and non-sexually transmitted organisms
- Usually a sexually transmitted disease (STD) in men younger than 35 years and a non-STD in men older than 35 years

ETIOLOGY
- STD: *Chlamydia trachomatis* and/or *Neisseria gonorrhoeae*
- Non STD: uropathogens such as
  —Enterobacteriaceae (mainly *E. coli*)
  —*Pseudomonas aeruginosa*
  —Gram-positive cocci (mainly enterococci)

EPIDEMIOLOGY
Incidence
- One-half million men infected annually in the United States

Risk Factors
- STD: lack of safe-sex practices
- Non STD: surgical manipulation or instrumentation of urinary tract

Clinical Manifestations

SYMPTOMS AND SIGNS
- Fever
- Scrotal pain
- Sometimes urethral discharge and symptoms suggestive of urinary tract infection (50%)
- Frequently preceded by asymptomatic or symptomatic infection of urethra, prostate, bladder, or kidneys
- Inflammation over affected epididymis at onset of infection

Diagnosis

- Sexual history, physical examination, prostate examination, urethra examination, urinalysis, urine culture

DIFFERENTIAL DIAGNOSIS
Noninfectious
- Testicular torsion (causes inflammation over epididymis)
- Testicular cancer
- Tuberculous or fungal epididymitis

LABORATORY
If Sexually Transmitted Disease Suspected
- Urethral smear for white blood cells
- Gram stain
- Culture for *N. gonorrhoeae*
- Test for *C. trachomatis*

Treatment

MAIN TREATMENT
Sexually Transmitted
- Ceftriaxone 250 mg, one dose i.m., followed by doxycycline 100 mg twice per day orally for 10 days

Epididymitis

Non–Sexually Transmitted

- Similar to treatment for acute bacterial prostatitis
  - Mild, no vomiting or nausea
    - Trimethoprim–sulfamethoxazole: one double-strength tablet twice per day orally for 3 to 4 weeks
    - Levofloxacin 500 mg once per day for 3 to 4 weeks
    - Ciprofloxacin 500 mg twice per day orally for 3 to 4 weeks
  - Moderate or severe, with vomiting and/or nausea
    - Hospitalization recommended
    - Parenteral treatment until fever resolves: ampicillin and gentamicin; ciprofloxacin; levofloxacin; then fluoroquinolone orally for 4 weeks

ALTERNATIVE TREATMENT

Sexually Transmitted Disease

- Ofloxacin 300 mg twice per day orally for 10 days

SEX PARTNERS

Evaluate and treat, if indicated.

COMPLICATIONS

N/A

Follow-Up

- High relapse rates, so patients should be followed for cure

PREVENTION

- Safe-sex practices

Selected Readings

Galejs LE. Diagnosis and treatment of the acute scrotum. *Am Fam Physician* 1999;59(4):817–824.

Joly-Guillou ML, Lasry S. Practical recommendations for the drug treatment of bacterial infections of the male genital tract including urethritis, epididymitis and prostatitis. *Drugs* 1999;57(5):743–750.

Paavonen J, Eggert-Kruse W. *Chlamydia trachomatis:* Impact on human reproduction. *Hum Reprod Update* 1999;5(5):433–447.

Steele RW. Prevention and management of sexually transmitted diseases in adolescents. *Adolesc Med* 2000;11(2):315–326.

Epidural Abscess

Basics

DEFINITION
Spinal epidural abscess is most often due to extension of a vertebral osteomyelitis or diskitis.

ETIOLOGY
- *Staphylococcus aureus* causes the majority of cases.
- Other organisms encountered include gram-negative bacteria, streptococcus, and tuberculosis.
- Vertebral osteomyelitis most often occurs following hematogenous spread of bacteria. Vertebral osteomyelitis may also occur
  —After back surgery
  —Post trauma
  —In patients with large decubiti
  —Following spinal or epidural anesthesia
- Epidural abscess is present most often in males.

EPIDEMIOLOGY
- May be seen in intravenous drug users

Clinical Manifestations

- Back pain and fevers are the earliest symptoms.
- Tenderness to palpation over the vertebral body is common.
- At times, swelling and warmth are noted on examination.
- Radicular pain that is unilateral or bilateral is noted over time.
- If an epidural abscess leads to compression of the cord, motor and sensory changes may be noted, which may lead to paralysis.
- Fevers are present in a majority of patients.

Diagnosis

- Leukocytosis and elevated erythrocyte sedimentation rate are common.
- Blood cultures are positive in fewer than 25% of cases.
- Radiographs may show boney destruction consistent with osteomyelitis of the vertebral body.
- CT or MRI defines the extent of the infection in three dimensions and assesses the degree of compression of the cord.
- The lumbar puncture is risky; CT-guided needle aspiration of the lesion is best for diagnosis and is better tolerated.

DIFFERENTIAL DIAGNOSIS
- Tumor
- Guillain-Barré syndrome

Epidural Abscess

Treatment

- Aspiration or placement of a catheter is indicated in many instances when the organism is not known.
- Surgical debridement and laminectomy is performed when there is evidence of cord compromise on the MRI.
- Spinal support
- Antibiotics are given in high dose for 6 to 8 weeks. In some cases, prolonged oral antibiotics are given thereafter.
  —The choice of antibiotics is dictated by the Gram stain and culture and the sensitivities of the organisms.

COMPLICATIONS

- Paralysis may occur, in part due to compression of the cord.
- Spinal instability may require fusion.

Follow-Up

- Patients need adequate pain control, rehabilitation, and close follow-up.
- As in all patients with osteomyelitis, recurrent disease is often possible.

PREVENTION

- There is no way to prevent this rare infection.
- Early intervention with antibiotics for patients with diskitis and vertebral osteomyelitis may reduce the possibility of development of an epidural abscess.

Selected Readings

Baker AS, Ojemann RG, Swartz MN, et al. Spinal epidural abscess. *N Engl J Med* 1975;293:463–468.

Darouiche RO, Hamill RJ, Greenberg SB, et al. Bacterial spinal epidural abscess. Review of 43 cases and literature survey. *Medicine* 1992;71:369–385.

Hlavin ML, Kaminski HJ, Ross JS, et al. Spinal epidural abscess: A ten-year perspective. *Neurosurgery* 1990;27:177–184.

Epiglottitis

Basics

DEFINITION
- Rapidly progressive infection of the epiglottis and adjacent supraglottic structures

ETIOLOGY
- *Haemophilus influenzae* type b is responsible for the majority of pediatric cases (more than 90%) and is frequently isolated from the blood. In adult patients, blood cultures are positive in about 25% of cases.
- Other pathogens isolated from the pharynx of adults with epiglottitis include the following:
  —*Haemophilus parainfluenzae*
  —*Streptococcus pneumoniae*
  —Group A *Streptococcus*
  —*Staphylococcus aureus*

EPIDEMIOLOGY
Incidence and Prevalence
- Epiglottitis is more common among children 2 to 4 years old, but it may also affect older children and adults.
- The incidence has decreased dramatically in countries with widespread use of vaccination against *H. influenzae* type b.

Risk Factors
- Age under 4 years old
- Unvaccinated children
- Immunodeficiency

Clinical Manifestations

SYMPTOMS AND SIGNS
- Symptom onset is usually acute and is preceded by upper respiratory tract symptoms in up to half of the cases.
- Young children usually present within 24 hours of the onset of symptoms with fever, dysphonia, dysphagia, and irritability.
- Respiratory distress, inspiratory stridor, and hoarseness may occur.
- Up to one-third of pediatric patients are in shock, with cyanosis and loss of consciousness on admission.
- The patient prefers to sit leaning forward.
- There is frequently drooling of oral secretions.
- Adolescents and adults may have a less fulminant presentation; sore throat is the most prominent symptom.
- Epiglottis is edematous and erythematous "cherry-red."

Diagnosis

DIFFERENTIAL DIAGNOSIS
- Croup syndrome
  —Usually has a more gradual onset
  —Is more frequently preceded by an upper respiratory tract infection
  —Involves younger children (ages 3 months to 3 years)
  —Has a viral etiology
  —Children with croup do not have prominent drooling or dysphagia and are more likely to lie supine.
- Diphtheria
  —A pseudomembrane is visible in the pharynx.
  —Smear and culture of the membrane demonstrate typical gram-positive rods.
- Allergic laryngeal oedema
  —Patients usually appear less toxic and have no fever.
- Foreign-body aspiration
- Lingual tonsillitis
- Peritonsillar abscess, retropharyngeal abscess

LABORATORY
- Moderate leukocytosis with a left shift
- Positive cultures of blood and epiglottis

IMAGING
- A lateral neck film may show an enlarged epiglottis (the thump sign), ballooning of the hypopharynx, and normal subglottis structures.
- A chest x-ray film may show pneumonia or atelectasis in up to 50% of cases.
- Radiography should not be performed unless physicians who are able to manage acute airway obstruction are present.

DIAGNOSTIC PROCEDURES
- The diagnosis is established by visualizing an edematous "cherry-red" epiglottis.
- The direct examination of the pharynx, using a tongue blade, should not be attempted because of the possibility of laryngospasm and complete airway obstruction.
- The patient should be transferred to an operating room for visualization of the epiglottis with a fiberoptic laryngoscope after all preparations for immediate airway control.

Epiglottitis

Treatment

- Acute epiglottitis constitutes a medical emergency, as airway obstruction may occur suddenly.
- In the event of upper airway obstruction with respiratory distress, an uncuffed endotracheal or nasotracheal tube should be inserted, and the patient must be monitored in an intensive care unit.
- Tracheostomy should be performed if an intact airway cannot be maintained otherwise.
- Observation without intubation of children with epiglottitis is not recommended, because mortality is up to 25% or more in those observed.
- Intravenous antibiotic therapy directed at *H. influenzae* should be given.
  - Cefotaxime 100–200 mg/kg/d in four divided doses
  - Ceftriaxone 50–100 mg/kg/d in one or two divided doses
  - Ampicillin 200 mg/kg/d in four divided doses, plus chloramphenicol 50–100 mg/kg/d in four divided doses
- Duration of therapy is 10 days.
- There are no controlled data to support the use of corticosteroids or epinephrine for the treatment of acute epiglottitis.

COMPLICATIONS

- Complete airway obstruction
- Rarely, *H. influenzae* bacteremia has been associated with metastatic infections such as meningitis and arthritis.
- Iatrogenic complications
  - Aspiration
  - Endotracheal tube dislodgment
  - Tracheal erosion
  - Pneumomediastinum
  - Pneumothorax
  - Pulmonary edema

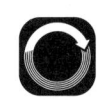

Follow-Up

- Patients with epiglottitis usually improve rapidly, that is, within 12 to 48 hours after starting appropriate antimicrobial therapy.
- Patients can be extubated once they are afebrile, alert, and clinically improved.

PREVENTION

- If the patient with *H. influenzae* epiglottitis has household contacts that include an unvaccinated child under age 4, rifampin prophylaxis given once daily for 4 days in a dose of 20 mg/kg/d (maximum, of 600 mg/d) by mouth is recommended for all members of the household and the patient to eradicate the carriage of *H. influenzae*.
- Immunization against *H. influenzae* type b

Selected Readings

Adams WG, Deaver KA, Cochi SL, et al. Decline of childhood *Haemophilus influenzae* type b (Hib) disease in the Hib vaccine era. *JAMA* 1993;269:221–226.

Crosby E, Reid D. Acute epiglottitis in the adult: Is intubation necessary? *Can J Anaesth* 1991;38:914–918.

Kessler A, Wetmore RF, Marsh RR. Childhood epiglottitis in recent years. *Int J Pediatr Otorhinolaryngol* 1993;25:155–162.

Mayo-Smith MF, Hirsch PJ, Wodzinski SF, et al. Acute epiglottitis in adults: An eight-year experience in the state of Rhode Island. *N Engl J Med* 1986;314:1133–1139.

Sendi K, Crysdale WS. Acute epiglottitis: Decade of change—A 10-year experience with 242 children. *J Otolaryngol* 1987;16:196–202.

Stankiewicz JA, Bowes AK. Group and epiglottitis: A radiologic study. *Laryngoscope* 1985;95:1159–1160.

Walker P, Crysdale WS. Croup, epiglottitis, retropharyngeal abscess, and bacterial tracheitis: Evolving patterns of occurrence and care. *Int Anesth Clin* 1975;30:57–70.

Escherichia coli Infections

Basics

DEFINITION

Escherichia is a genus of gram-negative, facultatively anaerobic, rod-shaped bacteria. *E. coli* is the principal species of the genus. This organism comes in many pathogenic varieties, each with a different mechanism of disease production.

ETIOLOGY

- The most important *E. coli* pathogens are the following:
  — Enterotoxigenic *E. coli*, an important cause of traveler's diarrhea
  — Enteropathogenic or enteroadherent *E. coli*, an important cause of childhood diarrhea, especially in underdeveloped countries and in nursery outbreaks
  — Enteroinvasive *E. coli*, which causes a dysentery-like disease and invades the host cell and provokes a significant inflammatory response
  — Enterohemorrhagic *E. coli*, which causes hemorrhagic colitis and has been associated with the hemolytic–uremic syndrome in children (see Section II chapter, "Hemolytic–Uremic Syndrome")
- In traveler's diarrhea, the heat-labile toxin of enterotoxigenic *E. coli* leads to elevated cyclic monophosphate levels, stimulates chloride secretion, and inhibits sodium chloride absorption. These effects result in net intestinal secretion.
- Enteropathogenic or enteroadherent *E. coli* strains bind to the membranous cells of Peyer's patches and disrupt the overlying mucus layer of the host cell.
- *E. coli* strains lead to urinary tract infections among women that can range from gram-negative septicemia to a cystitis-like illness with mild flank pain. Most of the strains are a unique subgroup of *E. coli* (called uropathogenic strains) that possess specific determinants of virulence that enable them to infect the upper urinary tract of normal, healthy persons. These uropathogenic *E. coli* generally have specific pyelonephritis-associated pili that mediate their attachment to uroepithelial cells.
- Uropathogenic strains of *E. coli* can also cause uncomplicated infection (usually cystitis) in young men. These infections often present with symptoms of cystitis, but in some patients they mimic urethritis, causing urethral discharge and urethral leukocytosis.
- *E. coli* can also be associated with intraabdominal abscesses in any location as well as with cholecystitis and ascending cholangitis.
- In industrialized countries, non-O157 *Shiga*-like toxin-producing *E. coli* strains have been associated with bloody diarrhea and hemolytic–uremic syndrome.
- Infants in their first month of life are predisposed to bacterial meningitis with *E. coli*.
- *E. coli* may also cause the following:
  — Brain abscess
  — Endocarditis
  — Endophthalmitis
  — Osteomyelitis–sinusitis
  — Perinephric abscess
  — Pneumonia
  — Septic arthritis
  — Suppurative thyroiditis

EPIDEMIOLOGY

- *E. coli* is the leading cause of nosocomial bacteremia.
- *E. coli* strains cause 80% of infections in young women with acute uncomplicated cystitis.
- Traveler's diarrhea occurs in individuals from industrialized countries who visit tropical or subtropical regions. In traveler's diarrhea, enterotoxigenic *E. coli* is acquired through the fecal–oral route, usually through consumption of unbottled water or uncooked vegetables.
- The typical acute urinary tract infection occurs in a sexually active female following bacterial colonization of the periurethral region and ascension up the urethra.
- The use of diaphragms and spermicides has been associated with recurrence in some patients with urinary tract infection due to *E. coli*, probably because the spermicide induces colonization of the vagina by *E. coli*.
- Also, susceptibility to urinary tract infection caused by *E. coli* may be genetic, because women with recurrent infections have specific *E. coli*–binding glycolipids that are absent in women who secrete blood-group antigens.
- Among men, risk factors for urinary tract infections due to *E. coli* include the following:
  — Homosexuality (associated with exposure to *E. coli* through anal intercourse)
  — Sexual intercourse with a woman with a sexual partner with vaginal colonization by uropathogens
  — Lack of circumcision (associated with enhanced colonization of the glans and prepuce by *E. coli*)
- Men with HIV infection who have CD4 lymphocyte counts of less than 200 per cubic millimeter may also be at increased risk for urinary infection.

Clinical Manifestations

N/A

Diagnosis

- Any growth of *E. coli* in a normally sterile locale (the bloodstream, cerebrospinal fluid, biliary tract, pleural fluid, etc.) should be assumed to be diagnostic of *E. coli* infection at that site.
- Because *E. coli* is present normally in stool, the diagnosis of *E. coli* gastroenteritis is problematic, but it can be made with techniques that exploit unique properties of specific strains that cause these infections (e.g., sorbitol negativity in EHEC).
- Whether the recovery of *E. coli* from tracheal aspirates in intubated patients indicates colonization or infection must be decided in the context of the patient's clinical state.
- Testing for non-O157 *Shiga*-like toxin-producing *E. coli* strains should be considered in diarrhea without a recognized cause, particularly if the stool has gross blood.

Escherichia coli Infections

Treatment

MAIN TREATMENT

- The mainstay of treatment for localized *E. coli* infections (e.g., abscess) is twofold: antimicrobial therapy and elimination of pus, necrotic tissue, and foreign bodies.
- Traveler's diarrhea is treated with an oral fluoroquinolone (ciprofloxacin 500 mg bid) or trimethoprim–sulfamethoxazole (one double-strength tablet bid) for 3 days. Symptomatic therapy with loperamide can be useful along with the antibiotic.
- Treatment for infection with enteropathogenic or enteroadherent *E. coli* consists of fluid replacement. In severe cases, fluoroquinolones are indicated.
- Uncomplicated cystitis in a healthy woman is treated for 3 days with oral trimethoprim–sulfamethoxazole (one double-strength tablet bid) or a fluoroquinolone (ciprofloxacin 250 mg bid or ofloxacin 200 mg po bid or norfloxacillin 400 mg bid or levofloxacin 250 mg qd) for 3 days. Diabetic or pregnant patients require 7 days of treatment.
- For the pregnant patient with urinary tract infection, the choice of oral agents is limited to amoxicillin, nitrofurantoin, or cefpodoxime. If a pregnant patient develops pyelonephritis, admission to the hospital is indicated.
- The patient with mild uncomplicated pyelonephritis can be treated with oral trimethoprim–sulfamethoxazole or a fluoroquinolone for 10 to 14 days.
- Patients with severe pyelonephritis or other severe infections due to *E. coli* should be given intravenous antibiotics in the hospital. The choices are the following:
    — A fluoroquinolone, such as ciprofloxacin
    — A third-generation cephalosporin, such as ceftriaxone
    — Ampicillin with gentamicin
    — An extended-spectrum penicillin
    — Aztreonam
    — Imipenem/cilastatin
- After acute symptoms resolve, an oral antibiotic should replace the intravenous antibiotic for a total duration of 14 to 21 days.

COMPLICATIONS

- In diarrhea, dehydration can lead to hypovolemia and shock.
- Patients with ischemia of the bowel or other organs (such as patients with diabetes or atherosclerotic vascular disease) are at high risk of developing acute emphysematous cholecystitis, and *E. coli* is a prominent pathogen in this processes.
- Septic shock can complicate *E. coli* infections, especially among patients with poor filtering capacity in the liver (i.e., those with cirrhosis or portosystemic shunts), diminished reticuloendothelial function, or diminished numbers of circulating phagocytic cells.

Follow-Up

- Patients in whom bacteremia with *E. coli* persists despite adequate therapy often have an undrained abscess, most typically intraabdominal.
- Chronic or relapsing urinary tract infections due to *E. coli* are more common among patients with the following:
    — Anatomic defects involving the urinary tract
    — Foreign bodies of the urinary tract
    — Obstruction of the urinary tract
    — Pregnancy
    — Stones

PREVENTION

- Chemoprophylaxis with trimethoprim–sulfamethoxazole, or fluoroquinolones, may be reasonable for the prevention of traveler's diarrhea (especially among certain patient populations, such as for diabetics prone to dehydration, immunocompromised individuals, or persons with underlying inflammatory bowel disease), but because of side effects from the medications and the increasing drug resistance, many authorities do not to recommend chemoprophylaxis for all travelers (see also Section II chapter, "Traveler's Diarrhea").
- Except in selected circumstances (e.g., pregnancy), screening for asymptomatic bacteriuria is unnecessary in adults.

Selected Readings

Eisenstein BI. Enterobacteriaceae. In: Mandell GL, Bennett JE, Dolin R, eds. *Principles and practice of infectious diseases*, 4th ed. New York: Churchill Livingstone, 1995:1964–1980.

Eisenstein BI, Watkins V. Diseases caused by gram-negative enteric bacilli. In: Fauci AS, Braunwald E, Isselbacher KJ, et al., eds. *Harrison's principles of internal medicine*, 14th ed. New York: McGraw-Hill, 1998:936–941.

Hart A, Pham T, Nowicki S, et al. Gestational pyelonephritis-associated *Escherichia coli* isolates represent a nonrandom, closely related population. *Am J Obstet Gynecol* 1996;174:983–989.

Huppertz HI, Rutkowski S, Aleksic S, et al. Acute and chronic diarrhoea and abdominal colic associated with enteroaggregative *Escherichia coli* in young children living in western Europe. *Lancet* 1997;349:1660–1662.

Stamm WE, Hooton TM. Management of urinary tract infections in adults. *N Engl J Med* 1993;329:1328–1334.

Esophagitis, Infective

Basics

DEFINITION
- Infection of the esophagus by a variety of fungi, viruses, bacteria, and parasites

ETIOLOGY
- The most common causes of infectious esophagitis in immunocompromised and immunopotent individuals is one or a combination of the three following organisms: candida, herpes simplex virus (HSV) and cytomegalovirus (CMV).
- Other pathogens that may rarely cause infectious esophagitis are the following:
  - *Aspergillus* species
  - *Histoplasma* species
  - *Blastomyces dermatitidis*
  - Varicella zoster virus
  - Epstein-Barr virus
  - Human papilloma virus
  - *Mycobacterium tuberculosis* and *Mycobacterium avium*
  - Normal oropharyngeal flora (very rarely), such as *Staphylococcus aureus, Staphylococcus epidermidis, Streptococcus viridans,* and *Bacillus* species
  - Acute HIV infection

EPIDEMIOLOGY

Incidence
- Infectious esophagitis is rare in individuals whose immune system is normal but is frequent in immunocompromised patients, in individuals who receive medications that affect the normal esophageal microflora or the immune status, and in the presence of abnormalities that delay the clearance of the esophageal lumen.
- Primary CMV infections are common in preschool children and young adults. However, they cause esophagitis very rarely in immunocompetent persons.

Risk Factors
- Immune defects
- Medications that may alter immune status or esophageal microflora
- Esophageal anatomic abnormalities or motility disorders

Clinical Manifestations

SYMPTOMS AND SIGNS
- Dysphagia, odynophagia, or both are the most frequent complaints.
- Persistent chest pain is also common.
- Other nonspecific clinical manifestations (e.g., weight loss) may occur as a result of these symptoms or as a manifestation of an underlying illness that is responsible for the esophagitis.
- Local complications (e.g., hemorrhage, perforation of the esophagus, or the formation of fistulas) may occur if deep esophageal ulcerations due to infectious esophagitis are present.
- CMV esophagitis may present with systemic symptoms (e.g., fever, nausea, vomiting, or abdominal pain), whereas candida and HSV esophagitis tend to develop oral lesions (e.g., thrush). However, these occasional differences are not distinctive.
- Infectious esophagitis may be asymptomatic. The frequency of asymptomatic esophageal infections is unknown.

Diagnosis

DIFFERENTIAL DIAGNOSIS
- Esophageal cancer (primary or metastatic)
- Systemic illnesses, such as
  - Crohn's disease
  - Sarcoidosis
  - Collagen vascular diseases
- Pill esophagitis, after use of certain antibiotics (e.g., tetracycline, doxycycline, clindamycin, ciprofloxacin, and others), potassium chloride, nonsteroidal antiinflammatory drugs, and quinidine
- Chemotherapy-induced esophagitis (dactinomycin, bleomycin, cytarabine, methotrexate, and other medications)
- Radiation esophagitis or chemoradiation esophagitis (i.e., concomitant radiation with chemotherapeutic drugs)
- Inflammation due to sclerotherapy of esophageal varices
- Oral lesions are commonly encountered in patients with candida and HSV esophagitis, whereas CMV esophagitis is rarely associated with stomatitis.

LABORATORY
- Hematologic profile
- Serologic tests for HSV, CMV, and HIV
- Brush cytology specimens obtained by endoscopy for the diagnosis of candida and HSV esophagitis
- Tissue culture for the diagnosis of HSV and CMV esophagitis. Culture is not routinely recommended for the diagnosis of candida esophagitis. It is reserved for cases with clinical features suggesting the presence of a pathogen resistant to standard antifungal therapy.

PATHOLOGY
Tissue specimens obtained by endoscopy may demonstrate budding yeast cells, hyphae or pseudohyphae in candida esophagitis, multinucleated giant cells and intranuclear inclusion bodies in HSV esophagitis, or cytomegaly of fibroblasts and endothelial cells with intranucleous and cytoplasmic inclusion bodies in CMV esophagitis.

IMAGING
Radiographic examination after a barium swallow shows an irregular, shaggy appearance of the esophageal mucosa in cases of candida esophagitis. Sometimes, the picture is indistinguishable from that seen in cases of HSV and CMV esophagitis.

DIAGNOSTIC PROCEDURES
- Endoscopy and tissue sampling for histologic examination or brush cytology
- The typical endoscopic appearance of candida esophagitis includes white plaques on the mucosa, which often bleed when removed by the endoscope.
- Endoscopy in HSV esophagitis reveals small, demarcated ulcers with a yellowish base. The esophageal mucosa between them may often be normal appearing.

Esophagitis, Infective

- Shallow, elongated ulcerations, surrounded by mucosa that appears to be normal, may be the endoscopic appearance of CMV esophagitis.
- However, the endoscopic features of candida, HSV, or CMV esophagitis may be indistinguishable.

Treatment

MAIN TREATMENT

- The appropriate health care is outpatient, unless the patient's immune status is severely compromised or the infection is very severe. In those cases, hospitalization may be necessary.
- For the treatment of candidal esophagitis, the decision between the use of a topically active, nonabsorbable agent; an orally administered, absorbable agent; or a parenterally administered agent will be made according to the host's immune status and the severity of the infection.
  — In the presence of a mild infection and minimal host immunocompromise, the administration of a topical agent may be sufficient (e.g., oral gel miconazole 10 mL orally qid).
  — The treatment of a moderately severe candidal esophagitis in a substantially immunosuppressed host may require the use of an orally administered absorbable agent (e.g., caps fluconazole 50 mg once daily if the granulocytes are normal and the lymphocytes have no or minimal defects, 100 mg once daily if lymphocyte function is decreased but the granulocytes are normal, and 100 to 200 mg once daily if the granulocyte function is decreased).
  — Severe infections in a severely immunocompromised patient require the use of a parenterally administered agent (e.g., amphotericin B 0.3 mg/kg/d i.v. if the lymphocyte function is decreased but the granulocytes are normal or 0.5 mg/kg/d i.v. if the granulocyte function is decreased).
- HSV esophagitis may require no therapy if the infected individual is immunocompetent.
  — Immunocompromised individuals should be treated with antiviral agents (e.g., acyclovir 5 mg/kg qid i.v. for 7 days, followed by orally administered acyclovir 200 to 400 mg five times daily for at least 1 more week).
  — Prophylactic therapy (acyclovir 200 to 400 mg/d orally or 5 mg/kg bid i.v.) may be indicated if there is high risk for HSV reactivation.
- CMV esophagitis is treated with ganciclovir (5 mg/kg bid for 2 weeks i.v.).
  — Maintenance therapy (5 mg/kg/d for at least 5 days of the week) may be necessary to avoid recurrence of CMV esophagitis in severely immunocompromised persons.
  — In order to prevent CMV infection, CMV seronegative hosts should avoid receiving transplants from seropositive donors. Ganciclovir or CMV immune globulin given as prophylaxis may also be effective in these cases.
  — Concurrent administration of ganciclovir with zidovudine may induce myelosuppression.
- Avoid coadministration of fluconazole and cisapride. Cardiac arrhythmias (possibly lethal) may occur due to elevated blood levels of cisapride, as a result of hepatic cytochrome P450 3A4 isoenzyme inhibition by fluconazole.

ALTERNATIVE TREATMENT

- For the treatment of candida esophagitis, ketoconazole or itraconazole administered orally or fluconazole administered intravenously
- Foscarnet for the treatment of CMV esophagitis resistant to ganciclovir
- If the patient experiences severe odynophagia or the esophagitis is accompanied by oral lesions that make chewing or swallowing impossible, the administration of intravenous fluids may be necessary.

COMPLICATIONS

- Complications are uncommon. If deep esophageal ulcers occur, serious local complications may develop, such as:
  — Massive hemorrhage
  — Perforation of the esophagus
  — Esophagobronchial or esophagomediastinal fistulas

Follow-Up

- The expected course and prognosis depend on the underlying disease and pathogen; if the patient is severely immunosuppressed, prolonged treatment with effective medications is necessary.
- Patients with infectious esophagitis should have a follow-up appointment 2 weeks after resolution of symptoms.

PREVENTION

- Avoidance of risk factors, if possible
- Appropriate antiretroviral treatment to decrease the level of immunosuppression in HIV-infected patients

Selected Readings

Kikendall JW, Friedman AC, Oyewole MA, et al. Pill-induced oesophageal injury. Case reports and review of the medical literature. *Dig Dis Sci* 1983;28:174–182.

Laine L, Bonacini M, Sattler F, et al. Cytomegalovirus and *Candida* esophagitis in patients with AIDS. *J AIDS* 1992;5:605–609.

Laine L, Dretler RH, Conteas CN, et al. Fluconazole compared with ketoconazole for the treatment of *Candida* esophagitis in AIDS. A randomized trial. *Ann Intern Med* 1992;117:655–660.

Levine MS, Macones AJ, Laufer I. *Candida* esophagitis: Accuracy of radiographic diagnosis. *Radiology* 1985;154:581–587.

McBane RD, Gross JB. Herpes esophagitis: Clinical syndrome, endoscopic appearance and diagnosis in 23 patients. *Gastrointest Endosc* 1991;37:600–603.

Tavitian A, Raufman JP, Rosenthal LE. Oral candidiasis as a market for esophageal candidiasis in the acquired immunodeficiency syndrome. *Ann Intern Med* 1986;104:54–55.

Wilcox CM. Esophageal disease in the acquired immunodeficiency syndrome: Etiology, diagnosis, and management. *Am J Med* 1992;92:412–421.

Exanthem Subitum

Basics

DEFINITION
Exanthem subitum is a childhood viral illness caused, in most cases, by human herpesvirus 6B, though it is also caused by human herpesvirus 7. Exanthem subitum is also known as roseola or sixth disease.

ETIOLOGY
- Human herpesvirus 6 is closely related to cytomegalovirus (CMV).
- This virus is implicated in many diseases associated with transplantation in adults, AIDS, chronic fatigue syndrome, and multiple sclerosis in adults.
- The virus persists in a latent state following primary infection.
- It may be found in lymphocytes and monocytes as well as in tissues throughout the body.
- Human herpesvirus 7

EPIDEMIOLOGY
- Infections occur before the age of 3 years, most before the age of 1 year.
- Antibody prevalence is as high as 100% in the U.S. population.
- Antibody titers are high in the newborn, fall until the age of 3 to 9 months, and then rise again.
- Antibody levels may be detectable at high levels until age 60 years.

Clinical Manifestations

PEDIATRIC
- Human herpesvirus 6B causes approximately 10% to 45% of all febrile illness in children.
- Fevers greater than 41°C have been associated with this illness.
- It is a benign illness in children with upper respiratory symptoms and fever.
- A maculopapular rash typically occurs following the febrile period, though disease without a rash may also occur.
- Cervical lymphadenopathy is often present.
- Illness lasts 3 to 5 days.
- Rarely, otitis, gastrointestinal symptoms, respiratory symptoms, and seizures may occur.
- It is a rare cause of encephalitis in nontransplant patients.

ADULT
- Mononucleosis illness
- This may cause upper respiratory illness or pneumonia with hepatitis.
- It is thought that human herpesvirus 6 is associated with lymphomas and leukemia and multiple sclerosis.

TRANSPLANT PATIENTS
- Exanthem subitum must be considered a pathogen in organ transplant patients.
- Human herpesvirus 6 is an important cause of bone marrow suppression and interstitial pneumonitis after bone marrow transplant.

Exanthem Subitum

Diagnosis

DIFFERENTIAL DIAGNOSIS
- CMV
- Viral upper respiratory infection
- Adenovirus
- Hepatitis A, B, and C

LABORATORY
- Leukopenia
- Increased monocytes
- Atypical lymphocytes
- Hepatitis
- Diagnosis is via viral isolation, PCR assay, and serology.
- Rapid shell vial assay is used for transplant patients.

Treatment
- There is no treatment in most cases.
- The disease responds to ganciclovir or foscarnet, but treatment is usually limited to patients who are ill following bone marrow transplantation.

COMPLICATIONS
N/A

Follow-Up

PREVENTION
- At this time, there is no way to prevent initial infection or reactivation with human herpesvirus 6.
- Prophylaxis may be necessary for patients undergoing bone marrow transplantation.

Selected Readings

Campadelli-Fiume G, Mirandola P, Menotti L. Human herpesvirus 6: An emerging pathogen. *Emerg Infect Dis* 1999;5(3):353–366.

Singh N, Carrigan DR. Human herpesvirus-6 in transplantation: An emerging pathogen. *Ann Intern Med* 1996;124:1065–1071.

Filariasis

Basics

DEFINITION
- Filariasis connotes a wide range of tissue-dwelling nematodes within the family Onchocercidae.
- Organisms live within skin and connective tissue, lymphatics, and blood vessels.
- The adult worm may live in the host for over 20 years.

ETIOLOGY
- *Onchocerca volvulus*
  —Enters the human host after a black fly bite
  —Disease seen in South America and Africa
  —Patients have inflammation of the skin and eye, which can lead to blindness. In Africa, the disease is termed *river blindness*.
- *Loa loa*
  —Enters the human host after a tabanid fly bite
  —Worm migration leads to localized swelling, called Calabar swelling.
- *Wuchereria bancrofti*
  —Transmitted from mosquitos
  —The adult worm lives within the lymphatic system.
  —Disease that causes lymphatic destruction and elephantiasis is caused by *W. bancrofti*, *Brugia malayi*, and *Brugia timori*.
- *Mansonella perstans*
  —Transmitted via midges
  —Adult worms live in the peritoneal cavity.
- *Dirofilaria immitis*
  —Dog heartworm
  —Transmitted from dogs to humans via mosquito bites
  —Infection in humans is aborted in the pulmonary parenchyma and may lead to nodules, which can mimic carcinoma. Disease is rare.
  —Infection is worldwide in distribution.

EPIDEMIOLOGY
- *L. loa* is present in West and Central Africa.
- Onchocerciasis is found in Africa and South America. Twenty million people worldwide are infected.
- *O. volvulus*
  —Enters the human host after a black fly bite
  —Disease seen in South America and Africa
- *W. bancrofti*
  —Present worldwide throughout the tropics and transmitted from mosquitos
  —It is estimated that 250 million people are infected with worms that produce lymphatic filaria.
- *M. perstans*
  —Disease found in Africa, Central and South America, and the Caribbean.

Clinical Manifestations

LYMPHATIC FILARIASIS/ WUCHERERIA
- Patients often have recurrent episodes of lymphangitis and lymphadenitis.
- The femoral/inguinal nodes are often affected, and the epididymis and spermatic cord become enlarged.
- Over time, hydroceles develop that may be massive.
- Disease in the lower extremity can lead to elephantiasis.
- Other syndromes associated with lymphatic filariasis include monoarticular arthritis and tropical pulmonary eosinophilia.

ONCHOCERCIASIS
- Skin changes vary from papular rashes to extensive areas of hyper- or hypopigmentation.
- Patients may have eczematoid dermatitis and thickening of the skin. Much pruritus is noted.
- Nodules in the subcutaneous regions reflect areas of inflammation in sites where worms live. They are nontender and may be many centimeters in diameter.
- Onchocerciasis can lead to blindness due to keratitis, optic atrophy, and choroidoretinitis.

LOA LOA
- Adult worms may pass under the conjunctiva or through the skin.
- The worm often takes minutes to transverse vessels in the conjunctiva and then disappears.
- This organism is associated with very little pruritus.
- Calabar swelling is often seen in the wrists and ankles; swelling may last only hours but can be recurrent for years.

Filariasis

Diagnosis

LYMPHATIC FILARIASIS

- Adult worms are infrequently recovered.
- Analysis of blood may reveal the microfilaria.
  - Blood samples are often taken at midnight, when the concentrations of filaria are the highest.
- Serologic diagnosis is available, yet cross-reacting antibodies are common.
- Eosinophilia is often absent.

ONCHOCERCIASIS

- Parasitologic diagnosis is made by obtaining a minute, bloodless skin snip and observing the larvae migrating out of the skin under a microscope.
- Serology is also available but of little use in patients in endemic regions.
- Eosinophilia is present.

LOA LOA

- Diagnosis is clinical.
- Microfilaria can be isolated from the blood. Adult worms can be identified if they are isolated.
  - Blood samples taken at noon have the best yield.
- Serologic diagnosis is not reliable.

DIFFERENTIAL DIAGNOSIS

Lymphatic Filariasis
- Bacterial infection

Onchocerciasis
- *M. streptocerca*
- Scabies
- Leprosy
- Eczema

Loa loa
- Cutaneous larva migrans
- Guinea worm infection

Treatment

LYMPHATIC FILARIASIS/ WUCHERERIA BANCROFTI

- Lymphatic filariasis/*W. bancrofti* can be treated with ivermectin 100 to 400 μg/kg, one time, one dose.
- Children can be treated with both ivermectin 200 to 400 μg/kg and albendazole 400 mg, one dose

Alternative Treatment

- Diethylcarbamazine for 21 days
  - Day 1: 50 mg
  - Day 2: 50 mg tid
  - Day 3: 100 mg tid
  - Days 4 through 21: 2 mg/kg tid

ONCHOCERCIASIS

- Ivermectin 150 μg/kg, one dose, with repeat dose in 3 months and in 6 months
- Adult worms are not killed with medications.
- When eyes are involved, start steroids 1 week prior to therapy.
- Nodules (adult worms) can be removed if palpated.

Alternative Treatment

- Diethylcarbamazine for 21 days
  - Day 1: 50 mg
  - Day 2: 50 mg tid
  - Day 3: 100 mg tid
  - Days 4 through 21: 2 mg/kg tid

LOA LOA

- Ivermectin 200 μg/kg in one dose, or albendazole 200 mg twice a day for 21 days

Alternative Treatment

- Diethylcarbamazine for 21 days
  - Day 1: 50 mg
  - Day 2: 50 mg tid
  - Day 3: 100 mg tid
  - Days 4 through 21: 2 mg/kg tid

COMPLICATIONS

- Use of diethylcarbamazine has been associated with side effects that include headaches and fevers. Some of the side effects may be due to the drug, while others may be related to the release of parasite antigens at the time of parasite death.

Follow-Up

- Treatment is mainly for the microfilarial stage of infection. Adult worms are rarely affected by one dose of medication.
- Repeat therapy is often needed for cure.

PREVENTION

- Vector control needed

Selected Readings

Grove DI. Chemotherapy of the filariases. *Curr Concepts Infect Dis* 1996;9:439–443.

Klion AD, Massougbodji A, Horton J, et al. Albendazole in human loiasis. Results of a doubleblind, placebo-controlled trial. *J Infect Dis* 1993;168:202–206.

Klion AD, Massougbodji A, Sadeler BC, et al. Loiasis in endemic and nonendemic populations: Immunologically mediated differences in clinical presentation. *J Infect Dis* 1991;163:1318–1325.

Food-borne Diseases

Basics

DEFINITION

- Infection arising from consumption of food contaminated with a pathogenic organism, microbial toxin, or chemical

ETIOLOGY

- Bacterial
  - Accounts for 80% of outbreaks in the United States
  - Salmonella (*S. enteritidis* most common cause of food-borne infection in the United States)
  - *Clostridium perfringens*
  - *Staphylococcus aureus*
  - Enterohemorrhagic *E. coli* (0157:H7)
  - *Vibrio* species
  - *Bacillus cereus*
  - *Clostridium botulinum*
  - *Shigella*
- Viral
  - Norwalk virus
  - Hepatitis A
- Parasitic
  - *Giardia lamblia*
  - *Cyclospora cayetanensis*
  - *Cryptosporidium*
  - *Trichinella spiralis*
- Chemical
  - Ciguatoxin
  - Scombrotoxin
  - Shellfish poisoning
  - Heavy metals (especially cadmium)
  - Mushroom (especially *Amanita* species)
  - Monosodium L-glutamate (MSG)

Risk Factors

- Salmonella: meats, poultry
- *B. cereus:* Meats, vegetables, and sauces. Fried rice is implicated in almost all cases of an emetic form of bacterial infection.
- Ciguatoxin: tropical, subtropical regions; barracuda, red snapper, amberjack, grouper
- *C. botulinum:* fish products and home-canned food
- *C. perfringens:* beef, turkey, chicken precooked, then reheated before serving
- Hepatitis A: contaminated seafood, especially shellfish
- *Listeria monocytogenes:* raw and unpasteurized milk, soft cheeses, coleslaw, raw vegetables
- MSG: additive in Chinese cooking; soups contain greatest quantity
- Amatoxins and phallotoxins: poisonous mushrooms
- *S. aureus:* food with high salt content (ham, canned meat) or high sugar content (cream, custard); mode of transmission from food handler to food product

Incubation

- Short incubation (4–8 hours): *S. aureus, C. perfringens, B. cereus,* heavy metal
- Medium incubation (12–48 hours): salmonella
- Long incubation (>72 hours, up to 3 months): hepatitis A, *Listeria*

EPIDEMIOLOGY

N/A

Food-borne Diseases

Clinical Manifestations

SYMPTOMS AND SIGNS

- Diarrhea
- Vomiting
- Cramps

Diagnosis

- History (foods recently consumed), exhibition of clinical symptoms, isolation of organisms specific to each type of infection in stool or serum

LABORATORY

- Blood and stool cultures
- Serum and stool toxin tests

Treatment

Most forms of food-borne disease are treated supportively.

MAIN TREATMENT

- Ciguatoxin: no antidote. Amitriptyline may help alleviate symptoms.
- *C. botulinum:* trivalent equine antitoxin to prevent further paralysis
- *L. monocytogenes:* ampicillin alone or with gentamicin for serious infections
- *Amanita* (mushrooms): thioctic acid partially effective
  — Mushrooms containing muscarine: atropine
  — Mushrooms containing ibotenic acid and muscimol: physostigmine
- Trichinellosis: thiabendazole, mebendazole, albendazole; corticosteroids for severe cases

COMPLICATIONS

N/A

Follow-Up

PREVENTION

- Vaccines for hepatis A: Havrix and Vaqta
- Avoid certain foods
  — Food containing raw or undercooked eggs
  — Unpasteurized dairy products
  — Raw or undercooked meat, poultry, and seafood
  — Soft cheeses
- Avoid cross-contamination in food preparation.

Selected Readings

Appleton H. Control of food-borne viruses. *Br Med Bull* 2000;56(1):172–183.

Jaykus LA. Epidemiology and detection as options for control of viral and parasitic food-borne disease. *Emerg Infect Dis* 1997;3(4):529–539.

Lindsay JA. Chronic sequelae of food-borne disease [see comments]. *Emerg Infect Dis* 1997;3(4):443–452.

Mead PS, Slutsker L, Dietz V, et al. Food-related illness and death in the United States. *Emerg Infect Dis* 1999;5(5):607–625.

Fungal Infections of the Hair, Nails, and Skin

Basics

DEFINITION
Cutaneous fungal infection of the stratum corneum or the nails is very common and is present worldwide. These infections are commonly encountered in clinical practice.

ETIOLOGY
- Dermatophytes are molds. Many are capable of infection of animals as well as humans.
- Infections of the hair are termed *Tinea capitis* (scalp) or *Tinea barbae* (beard). Infections of the skin are termed *Tinea corporis*. The infections are frequently due to *Trichophyton* species and *Microsporum* species.
- *Tinea manuum* occurs on the hand, and *Tinea pedis* occurs between the toes and on the soles of the feet.
- Infection of the nails is referred to as onychomycosis. *Trichophyton* species and *Candida* are often responsible.

EPIDEMIOLOGY
- Dermatophytes are classified as causing disease in animals primarily or humans.
- Zoophilic infections such as *T. verrucosum* (cattle) and *M. canis* (cats and dogs) can cause disease in people.
- *T. corporis* is most common in the tropics.
- Spread of infection is through contact with desquamated skin.
- *T. pedis* is spread through contact within showers or bathroom facilities.

Incidence and Risk Factors
- Children have the highest incidence of *T. capitis*.
- Young adults commonly have *T. pedis*.
- Patients with immunodeficiency often have extensive disease, especially with *T. pedis*.

Clinical Manifestations

TINEA PEDIS *(ATHLETE'S FOOT)*
- Infection occurs in the interdigital space or under the toes.
- Blisters and fissures may occur. Spread of infection to the sole of the foot is common.
- The lesions are pruritic, and maceration may occur as a result of scratching.
- Secondary infection with bacteria may lead to cellulitis.

TINEA CORPORIS *(RINGWORM)*
- Multiple or single round lesions with prominent edges and marked scaling
- Some lesions may contain pustules.
- Some of the lesions may appear nodular, especially on the legs.

TINEA CRURIS *(JOCK ITCH)*
- Present in the groin, often in young men and women, this rash may contain pustules.
- At times, the infection causes itching or burning.

TINEA CAPITIS *(SCALP RINGWORM)*
- This infection is present in children worldwide.
- Infection invades the hair shafts, leading to circular patches of erythema, scaling, and alopecia.
- The lesions are pruritic.

ONYCHOMYCOSIS
- Infection of the nail can be caused by candida and dermatophytes. It is hard to distinguish which organism is leading to disease.
- The nail becomes discolored, and thickening may occur.
- Infection often creeps across the nail from the distal and lateral margins.

Diagnosis

- Diagnosis can be made by microscopic evaluation of scrapings.
- Scrapings can also be cultured on Sabouraud agar.
- A Woods light can pick up infections with Microsporidia, which fluoresces green.

DIFFERENTIAL DIAGNOSIS
- Cutaneous candidal infections can mimic dermatophyte infections.
- Psoriasis
- Contact dermatitis
- Superficial bacterial infections

Fungal Infections of the Hair, Nails, and Skin

Treatment

TINEA CORPORIS, TINEA CRURIS, AND TINEA PEDIS

- Topical therapy with tolnaftate or undecylenic acid. Treatment is for 2 to 4 weeks.
- Oral treatment with ketoconazole 200 mg daily for 4 weeks
- Fluconazole 150 mg orally once a week for 1 to 4 weeks should be considered for refractory cases.
- Terbinafine 250 mg orally daily for 14 days has had excellent results.

TINEA CAPITIS

- Antifungal shampoo such as selenium sulfate for 2 weeks with one of the following:
  —Terbinafine 250 mg orally daily for 2 to 3 weeks
  —Ketoconazole 200 mg daily for 30 days
  —Itraconazole 3 to 5 mg/kg/d for 30 days

ONYCHOMYCOSIS

- Terbinafine 250 mg daily for 6 weeks
- Itraconazole 200 mg daily for 3 months
- Itraconazole 200 mg twice daily for 1 week of each month
  —Fingernail infection is treated for 2 months.
  —Toenail infection is treated for 3 to 4 months.
- Fluconazole 150 to 300 mg once per week
  —Fingernail infection is treated for 3 to 6 months.
  —Toenail infection is treated for 6 to 12 months.

COMPLICATIONS

Bacterial infection can complicate dermatophyte infection, especially on the foot. This is a constant concern in patients with diabetes or peripheral vascular disease.

Follow-Up

Recurrent disease is common; close follow-up after therapy is needed.

PREVENTION

- Wear sandals in communal showers.
- Avoid communal showers if susceptible or being treated for a fungal infection.

Selected Readings

McBride A, Cohen BA. *Tinea pedis* in children. *Am J Dis Child* 1992;146:844.

Walsh TJ. Trichosporonosis. *Infect Dis Clin North Am* 1989;3:43.

Gas Gangrene

Basics

DEFINITION
- Life-threatening infection of muscle and soft tissue caused by *Clostridium*, an anaerobic gram-positive rod

ETIOLOGY
- Necrotizing infection of muscle and surrounding tissues
- Eighty percent of cases are caused by *Clostridium perfringens*. *C. perfringens* produces 12 toxins.
- The other 20% of cases may be caused by *Clostridium septicum* and *Clostridium novyi*.
- Some infections may be due to mixed anaerobic organisms.
- Alpha toxin is responsible for myonecrosis, along with hemolysis and shock.
- Wounds have the proper oxygen tension and nutrients that allow *Clostridium* to germinate and produce pathologic toxins.

EPIDEMIOLOGY
- Trauma accounts for one-half of all cases. Historically, this disease is seen most commonly with wartime injuries.
- Injuries may be major or minor (insect bites, injection sites).
- Other causes include the following:
  - Postoperative abdominal surgery or gastrointestinal surgery
  - Postoperative uterine surgery
  - Spontaneous infection in patients with colonic cancers and polyps, diabetes, and peripheral vascular disease
- In wounds, as many as 40% may be contaminated with potential pathogens, but a fraction of a percentage will become infected.
- The annual number of cases in the United States is about 3,000.
- Clostridia is found in almost all soil samples.
- Patients with gas gangrene have an average age of 35 to 40 years.
- Gas gangrene is two to three times more common in men.

Incubation
Illness typically occurs 1 to 4 days following trauma. At times, incubation may be much longer.

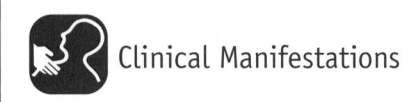

Clinical Manifestations

- Pain is the first symptom of gas gangrene.
- Violaceous skin changes progress to weeping bullae within hours.
- A brownish, foul-smelling discharge runs from the bullae.

Gas Gangrene

- Crepitance may be palpated over the affected area and in areas remote from the origin.
- Patients usually remain conscious despite hypotension.
- Massive hemolysis may lead to profound jaundice and black urine.

Diagnosis

- A Gram stain of discharge from the bullae will show the gram-positive rods (boxcars).
- Surgical debridement reveals pale, necrotic muscle that does not contract with stimulation.
- X-rays of the affected area will show gas within the striated muscle. A CT scan may be needed when gas is deep in the pelvic walls or uterus.

Treatment

- Surgical debridement is the most important life-saving procedure.
- Clindamycin 900 mg i.v. every 8 hours, and penicillin G 4 million units every 6 hours

ALTERNATIVE TREATMENT

- Ceftriaxone 2 g i.v. every 12 hours
- Erythromycin 1 g i.v. every 6 hours

ADDITIONAL TREATMENT

- Hyperbaric oxygen is effective in reducing the toxin production of the organism, but its clinical utility has not been proved.
- *Note*: Arrangement for a chamber should not delay surgical debridement or antibiotics.

COMPLICATIONS

Multisystem failure is common.

Follow-Up

Patients with spontaneous infection, especially with *C. septicum*, should, at some point, be evaluated for colonic polyps, diverticulitis, or malignancy.

PREVENTION

- Irrigation and debridement of wounds and leaving them open when possible reduce the incidence of gas gangrene.
- Rapid surgical debridement may avert the need for radical amputations.

Selected Readings

Caplan ES, Kluge RM. Gas gangrene. Review of 34 cases. *Arch Intern Med* 1976;136:788.

Gorbach SL. Gas gangrene and other clostridial skin and soft tissue infections. In: Gorbach SL, Bartlett JG, Blacklow NR, eds. *Infectious diseases*, 2nd ed. Philadelphia: WB Saunders, 1998:915–922.

Genital Herpes

Basics

DEFINITION
- Sexually transmitted disease manifested as lesions of the herpetic vesicles caused by herpes simplex virus (HSV)

ETIOLOGY
- Caused by HSV-2 in 70% of cases

EPIDEMIOLOGY
Incidence
Approximately 30 million people in the United States have serologic evidence of HSV-2 infection.

Risk Factors
- Sexual intercourse with partner with HSV

Incubation
- Two to 7 days

Clinical Manifestations

SYMPTOMS AND SIGNS
Signs and symptoms during the first episode are more prominent and last longer (up to 3 weeks) than during recurring episodes of genital herpes.

- Multiple vesicles, 1 to 2 mm in diameter, superficial with a serous, erythematous base
- Lymphadenopathy common
- Itching
- Pain
- Dysuria
- Vaginal or urethral discharge
- Fever, headache, malaise, myalgias in approximately 40% of men and 70% of women who seek medical advice
- During primary genital herpetic infection:
  —Secondary yeast infections
  —Aseptic meningitis
  —Extragenital herpetic lesions
  —Sacral autonomic neuropathy

Diagnosis

History and physical examination alone often lead to an inaccurate diagnosis.

DIFFERENTIAL DIAGNOSIS
Infectious
- Syphilis
- Chancroid
- Acute HIV infection
- Mycobacteria (rare)
- Fungi (rare)
- Parasites (rare)
- Lymphogranuloma venereum (rare)
- Granuloma inguinale (rare)
- Donovanosis (rare)

Noninfectious
- Malignancy
- Trauma
- Fixed drug eruption
- Erythema multiforme
- Dermatitis herpetiformis
- Behçet's syndrome

LABORATORY
- Serology culture antigen test for HSV
- Microscopy for antigen detection of HSV

TESTING PROCEDURES
- Gently abrade the lesion with a sterile gauze pad to provoke oozing but not gross bleeding.
- Squeeze the lesion between a gloved thumb and forefinger to increase exudate from lesion.
- Apply the exudate directly onto the microscope slide if used for dark-field and direct immunofluorescence tests.

Treatment

MAIN TREATMENT
- Systemic acyclovir
  —Reduces severity and shortens course of first occurrence.
  —Has no effect on natural history of recurrences
- First occurrence: acyclovir 200 mg PO five times a day for 7 to 10 days

Genital Herpes

- Recurrences
  - Acyclovir 200 mg PO five times a day for 5 days
  - Acyclovir 400 mg PO tid for 5 days
  - Acyclovir 800 mg PO bid for 5 days

ALTERNATIVE TREATMENT

- Valacyclovir for recurrences: 500 mg PO bid for 5 days
- Famciclovir for recurrences: 125 mg PO bid for 5 days

SEX PARTNERS

- Evaluation and counseling, even if asymptomatic

HIV-INFECTED PATIENTS

- Acyclovir 400 mg PO three to five times a day
- Intravenous acyclovir for severe genital herpes
- If no improvement, consider resistance to acyclovir and treat with foscarnet 40 mg/kg i.v. every 8 hours until clinical resolution.
- Valacyclovir 1 g PO bid for 5 days

NEONATES

- Acyclovir is reported safe for the fetus and the mother during all phases of pregnancy.
- Empiric antiviral treatment of neonates delivered through a birth canal infected by HSV has not been studied extensively and is not recommended.

PREGNANCY

Report women who receive acyclovir during pregnancy to the registry maintained by the Burroughs-Wellcome Company in conjunction with the Centers for Disease Control and Prevention: (800) 722-9292, extension 58465.

COMPLICATIONS

- Genital ulcers associated with increased susceptibility and transmission of HIV infection during intercourse
- Pattern of recurrences
- Pregnancy
  - Neonatal HSV infection is usually the result of intrapartum HSV transmission.
  - Neonatal herpes is associated with a 70% mortality rate if untreated.
  - There is an increased risk of spontaneous abortion and prematurity in cases of primary HSV infection.

Follow-Up

- Because recurrence may become frequent, patients should be warned of this possibility.

PREVENTION

- When >5 recurrences occur in a 12-month period, suppressive therapy is recommended:
  - Acyclovir: 400 mg BID, or
  - Famciclovir: 250 mg BID
  - These drugs can be discontinued after 120 days to reassess.

Selected Readings

Ashley RL, Wald A. Genital herpes: Review of the epidemic and potential use of type-specific serology. *Clin Microbiol Rev* 1999;12(1):1–8.

Drake S, Taylor S, Brown D, et al. Improving the care of patients with genital herpes. *BMJ* 2000;321(7261):619–623.

Marques AR, Straus SE. Herpes simplex type 2 infections—An update. *Dis Mon* 2000;46(5):325–359.

Giardiasis

Basics

DEFINITION
- An infection of the upper small bowel with *Giardia lamblia*, which may cause diarrhea.

ETIOLOGY
- A flagellate protozoon, *G. lamblia* (*Giardia intestinalis*), that exists in trophozoite and cyst forms. The infective form is the cyst of the parasite.
- Cysts are infective as soon as passed and remain infective in water for a few months.
- When ingested by a new host, they excyst in the upper gastrointestinal tract and liberate trophozoites, which attach with their suckers to the surface of the duodenal or jejunal mucosa and multiply by binary fission.
- When trophozoites drop off the duodenal and jejunal mucosa, they are carried on with the contents in the gut and encyst.

EPIDEMIOLOGY
- Globally distributed parasitosis
- Commonest where standards of sanitation are low
- Infection is usually sporadic and spreads from person to person directly by the fecal–oral route or indirectly by ingestion of fecally contaminated water or food.
- Epidemics mainly occur where gross *Giardia* cyst contamination of water supplies occurs.
- Epidemics resulting from person-to-person transmission sometimes occur in childcare centers, in institutions for mentally retarded persons, and in male homosexual communities.
- Humans are the principal reservoir of infection, but wild beavers and other animals have also been found to be infected in North America.
- Overland travelers to the Far East are at high risk for infection.

Incubation Period and Natural History
- Infection may be asymptomatic or symptomatic.
- The ratio of asymptomatic to symptomatic cases is high.
- Children usually acquire the infection but exhibit a high degree of tolerance.
- Symptoms develop a few days to several weeks (average, 9 days) after ingestion of cysts.
- Severe infection may develop in immunodeficient hosts.
- Infection may become chronic.

Clinical Manifestations

SYMPTOMS
- The main symptom is diarrhea, usually of subacute onset, although sometimes of acute onset; diarrhea may continue for weeks or months if untreated.
- Stool frequency: usually three to eight bowel motions daily
- Stool: pale, offensive, bulky, with much flatus but no blood or mucus
- Crampy abdominal pain, urgent call to stool; no tenesmus, but perianal soreness may develop
- Bloating, borborygmi, steatorrhea
- Anorexia and possibly vomiting in each stage of symptomatic infection; loss of weight
- Unusual features: urticaria, arthritis, biliary tract disease, gastric infection

SIGNS
- Abdominal distention (typical), flatulence
- Development of anemia is uncommon.

Diagnosis

DIFFERENTIAL DIAGNOSIS
- Secondary disaccharidase deficiency
- Tropical sprue
- Enteropathogenic *E. coli* infection
- Cryptosporidiosis, isosporiasis
- Crohn's ileitis

DIRECT DIAGNOSIS
- Search in a direct saline smear of stool for characteristic cysts.
- Repeat three times for up to 90% success of identifying the cysts versus 50% to 70% on single stool specimen examination.
- Cyst: oval, 8 to 14 μm long, 5 to 10 μm wide; contains four small nuclei and a central refractile axostyle
- The number of cysts found bears no relationship to severity of symptoms.
- Occasionally, trophozoites are found in fresh diarrheal stools. Sometimes, in patients with intense symptoms, no cysts are detected in stool, probably because of high concentrations of trophozoites adhering to mucosa.
- Trophozoite: pear-shaped, 15 μm long, 9 μm wide, 3 μm thick; possesses four pairs of flagella

DUODENAL ASPIRATION
In cases with a high suspicion index for diagnosis, employ the "hairy sting test" (Entero-Test), which may recover trophozoites by duodenal aspiration.

DUODENAL BIOPSY
Intestinal biopsy reveals partial villous atrophy with mild lymphocytic infiltration of the duodenum or jejunum. Trophozoites may be seen on the surface of the bowel.

Giardiasis

INDIRECT DIAGNOSIS

- Serologic methods are emerging as useful diagnostic aids.
- ELISA to detect IgM in serum provides evidence of current infection.
- A polyclonal antigen-capture ELISA can be used to demonstrate submicroscopic infections in faeces.
- An IgA-based ELISA can detect specific antibodies in saliva.

Treatment

MAIN TREATMENT

- Metronidazole (with efficacy up to 80%–95%)
  - In adults (50 kg body weight and above): either 250 to 500 mg (400 mg in the United Kingdom) tid by mouth for 5 days, or 2.0 to 2.5 g by mouth once daily for 3 days
  - Avoid alcohol intake, as it may produce side effects such as headache and flushing.
  - In children, dosage modified: 5 mg/kg tid for 7 days
- Tinidazole (with efficacy up to 90%): not applicable in the United States
  - In adults: A single dose of 2 g is usually effective.

ALTERNATIVE TREATMENT

- Mepacrine/quinacrine
  - In adults (with efficacy up to 90%): 100 mg bid by mouth for 5 to 7 days
  - In children: 2 mg/kg bid for 5 to 7 days
  - Not available in the United States
- Furazolidone (with efficacy up to 80%)
  - *Caution*: Haemolysis in patients with G-6PD deficiency
  - In adults: 100 mg qid by mouth for 5 to 10 days
  - In children: 2 mg/kg daily qid for 5 to 10 days

TREATMENT FAILURE

- A failure rate of about 10% to 20% is expected.
- A repeat course or change to another appropriate drug usually eradicates infection.
- Repeated relapses may be due to infection from another family member or close contact with a person with an asymptomatic infection.
- Treat all suspected cases simultaneously.
- Diarrhea may persist after treatment and may be attributed to secondary lactose intolerance or concomitant tropical sprue.

COMPLICATIONS

- Steatorrhea
- Weight loss
- Hypogammaglobulinemia

Follow-Up

TYPICAL PROGRESSION AND PROGNOSIS

- Monitor symptoms, body weight, and stool examinations.
- Patients with a high degree of tolerance have asymptomatic infection.
- If symptomatic, diarrhea may last for weeks or months and can be self-limiting.
- Patients may have concomitant bacterial infection of the small bowel.

PREVENTION

- Implementation of high standards of environmental sanitation and personal hygiene
- Avoidance of consumption of raw vegetables and tap water in endemic areas
- Boiling destroys cysts rapidly, and appropriate filtering removes them effectively.
- Institution of prevention measures in day care centers, residential communities of children and the mentally handicapped, and homosexual (especially male) communities

Selected Readings

Farthing MJ. Giardiasis. *Gastroenterol Clin North Am* 1996;25(3):493–515.

Vesy CJ, Peterson WL. Review article: The management of giardiasis. *Aliment Pharmacol Ther* 1999;13(7):843–850.

Welch TP. Risk of giardiasis from consumption of wilderness water in North America: A systematic review of epidemiologic data. *Int J Infect Dis* 2000;4(2):100–103.

Gingivitis

Basics

DEFINITION
- Infection of the gingiva that may lead to localized bleeding, systemic fevers, or tooth loss secondary to periodontitis

ETIOLOGY
- A number of organisms are responsible for gingivitis.
  - Streptococci
  - Actinomycetes
  - Spirochetes
  - *Prevotella intermedia*

EPIDEMIOLOGY
Risk Factors
- Poor dental hygiene is an important risk factor for the development of gingivitis.
- There is an increased incidence of disease in immunodeficient states.
- Diabetes and pregnancy are associated with gingivitis.
- Dilantin may be associated with gingival hypertrophy.

Clinical Manifestations

- Bleeding of gums with brushing is the first manifestation.
- Erythema around the dental margin may occur.
- Halitosis may occur.
- With more severe disease, termed *Vincent's angina*, pain, edema, fever, and adenopathy may develop.

Gingivitis

Diagnosis

Gingivitis is a clinical diagnosis.

Treatment

- A combination of debridement of plaque and antibiotics is needed.
- Several oral antibiotics are active against mouth flora. These include the following:
  —Penicillin
  —Metronidazole
  —Clindamycin
  —Tetracycline

COMPLICATIONS

Tooth loss due to periodontal disease is the major complication of severe ulcerative gingivitis.

Follow-Up

Close follow-up is needed with a dental provider.

PREVENTION

Good dental hygiene is needed to prevent disease.

Selected Readings

Chow AW, Roser SM, Brady FA. Orofacial odontogenic infections. *Ann Intern Med* 1978;88:392.

Rams TE, Flynn MJ, Slots J. Subgingival microbial associations in severe human periodontitis. *Clin Infect Dis* 1997;25 [Suppl 2]:S224.

Tanner A, Stillman N. Oral and dental infections with anaerobic bacteria: Clinical features, predominant pathogens and treatment. *Clin Infect Dis* 1993;16 [Suppl 4]:S304.

Granuloma Inguinale (Donovanosis)

Basics

DEFINITION
- Sexually transmitted disease manifested as a single lesion or multiple nodules; also known as donovanosis

ETIOLOGY
- *Calymmatobacterium granulomatis*

EPIDEMIOLOGY
Incidence
- One of the most common STDs in developing countries
- Rare in developed countries

Risk Factors
- Geographic location (endemic in tropics), residence, work, travel

Incubation
- Two to 3 weeks

Clinical Manifestations

SYMPTOMS AND SIGNS
- Nodules on the genitals that slowly enlarge and ulcerate
- Verrucous form likely to occur in the perianal area
- Elongated ulcer with elevated papillary edges
- Ulcer edge is white, on a beefy-red, hypertrophic base

Diagnosis

- Usually based on clinical appearance
- Can identify intracellular "Donovan bodies" from lesion scrapings

DIFFERENTIAL DIAGNOSIS
Infectious
- Genital herpes
- Syphilis
- Chancroid
- Acute HIV infection
- Lymphogranuloma venereum (rare)
- Mycobacteria (rare)
- Fungi (rare)
- Parasites (rare)

Noninfectious
- Malignancy
- Trauma
- Fixed drug eruption
- Erythema multiforme
- Dermatitis herpetiformis
- Behçet's syndrome

Granuloma Inguinale (Donovanosis)

LABORATORY

- Histologic examination of crush or biopsy preparations of the lesion that show typical intracytoplasmic organisms (Donovan bodies)

TESTING PROCEDURES

- Gently abrade the lesion with a sterile gauze pad to provoke oozing but not gross bleeding.
- Squeeze the lesion between a gloved thumb and forefinger to increase exudate from the lesion.
- Apply the exudate directly onto a microscope slide if used for dark-field and direct immunofluorescence tests.

Treatment

MAIN TREATMENT

- Tetracycline: 500 mg PO four times daily for 3 weeks or until clinical resolution
- Trimethoprim–sulfamethoxazole: one double-strength tablet twice daily for 3 weeks

SEX PARTNERS

Follow up with all partners.

COMPLICATIONS

N/A

Follow-Up

PREVENTION

- Use of barrier contraceptives

Selected Readings

Hart CA, Rao SK. Donovanosis. *J Med Microbiol* 1999;48(8):707–709.

Hart G. Donovanosis. *Clin Infect Dis* 1997;25(1):24–30; quiz, 31–32.

Jamkhedkar PP, Hira SK, Shroff HJ, et al. Clinico-epidemiologic features of granuloma inguinale in the era of acquired immune deficiency syndrome. *Sex Transm Dis* 1998;25(4):196–200.

Hantavirus Pulmonary Syndrome

Basics

DEFINITION

- Cardiopulmonary illness with high mortality, identified from a cluster of patients in 1993 in the southwestern United States

ETIOLOGY

- Sin Nombre virus is an RNA virus of the genus *Hantavirus* of the family Bunyaviridae.
- Sin Nombre hantavirus was found to be the etiology of hantavirus pulmonary syndrome; however, many classes have been identified, causing similar symptoms in North and South America.
- Unlike other hantaviruses, the pulmonary type is not transmitted to humans via an arthropod vector.
- The reservoir of this zoonotic infection is the deer mouse.
- Other rodents, such as white-footed mice and cotton rats, have been implicated in causing disease.
- People contract the illness after inhalation of virus-containing aerosols of rodent excreta.
- Person-to-person spread has been seen in rare instances, the result of exposure to infected body fluids.
- Viral infection leads to systemic viremia and a capillary leak syndrome associated with pneumonitis and shock.

EPIDEMIOLOGY

- There have been 250 cases of disease in humans from North and South America from 1993 to the present time.
- The incidence of disease seems to correlate to changes in the deer mouse populations.
- In 1993, at the time the disease was first discovered, the mouse population in the southwestern United States had dramatically increased secondary to increased rainfall that particular year.
- Deer mice (*Peromyscus maniculatus*) inhabit much of the United States.
- There is a low seroprevalence rate in the United States, with higher rates in some parts of rural South America.
- Most cases have been associated with farm work and with sleeping on the ground.
- Indoor invasion of homes by field mice has been implicated for some illness.
- The mean age of patients with the disease is 35 years.

Risk Factors

- Exposure to deer mice or field mice
- Exterminators, farm laborers, sleeping on ground
- Home with field mice infestation

Incubation

- Between 8 and 28 days

Clinical Manifestations

- There is a 2- to 15-day prodrome. Patients note nonspecific viral symptoms of fevers, myalgias, headaches, nausea, and vomiting, along with diarrhea.
- A few patients have only the prodrome.
- Following the prodrome, patients abruptly develop cough and shortness of breath. This progresses to respiratory failure within hours.
- The most common finding on hospital admission is tachypnea.
- Patients develop pulmonary edema and shock during the acute phase of the illness.
- Hemorrhage does not occur.
- Death occurs usually within 1 week of the development of the pneumonia.
- Terminal events include shock and ventricular arrhythmias.

Diagnosis

- Patients often have leukocytosis (with left shift) along with thrombocytopenia.
- Elevated creatine phosphokinase (CPK) consistent with myositis occurs late in the disease course.

Hantavirus Pulmonary Syndrome

- Very mild azotemia with proteinuria occurs early in the course of the disease; however, renal failure is an uncommon complication.
- Chest x-rays reveal interstitial or alveolar infiltrates.
- Serology with Western blots
- PCR analysis of body tissues

DIFFERENTIAL DIAGNOSIS

- Severe bacterial pneumonia including the following:
  - Group A *Streptococcus*
  - Pneumonic plague
  - Atypical pneumonia, including legionella, anthrax, tularemia

Treatment

- Supportive care is paramount.
- Decreased mortality has been noted with extracorporal membrane oxygenation.

COMPLICATIONS

Long-term complications in the patients who have recovered have not been studied.

Follow-Up

- None needed

PREVENTION

- At the present time, no vaccine is available.
- Avoidance of areas inhabited by large numbers of mice is prudent.
- Protecting houses from habitation of field mice may be effective.
- Exterminators and others who deal with large numbers of dead mice should use respirators.
- Respiratory isolation is needed for patients admitted to the hospital with atypical severe pneumonias.

Selected Readings

Duchin JS, Koster FT, Peters CJ, Simpson GL, Tempest B, Ziki SR, Ksiazck TG, Rollin PE, Nichols S, Umland ET. Hantavirus pulmonary syndrome: A clinical description of 17 patients with a newly recognized disease. *N Engl J Med* 1994;330(14):949–955.

Schmaljohn C, Hjelle B. Hantaviruses: A global disease problem. *Emerg Infect Dis* 1997;3(2):95–104.

Helicobacter pylori Infection

Basics

DEFINITION

- Helicobacters are gram-negative, spiral, flagellated bacilli. Most human infections are caused by *Helicobacter pylori*.
- Chronic infection with *H. pylori* has been associated with certain types of upper gastrointestinal pathology and is the foremost cause of peptic ulcer disease, which occurs at some point in the lifetime of about 15% of infected persons in developed countries. It causes gastric and duodenal ulcers and chronic gastritis.

ETIOLOGY

- Humans are the main reservoir of *H. pylori* infection, but the exact route and source of infection are unknown.
- Most *H. pylori*–infected persons do not develop clinical sequelae. That some persons develop overt disease while others do not may be due to bacterial factors, host factors, and environmental factors.
- The individual's age at acquisition of *H. pylori* may influence the pattern of infection in the stomach and the pattern of disease. Thus, infection during early childhood may lead to chronic gastritis, gastric ulcers, and gastric carcinoma, whereas infection later in childhood may lead to antral-predominant gastritis and duodenal ulceration.
- *H. pylori* has an efficient urease that protects it against acid by catalyzing urea to produce ammonia.

EPIDEMIOLOGY

Incidence

- The prevalence of *H. pylori* infection is about 30% in the United States and other developed countries. However, prevalence varies with age: 50% among those over 60 years, and 25% among those 30 to 59 years old. Infection rates in children are 5%.
- In most developing countries, the prevalence of *H. pylori* is 80%, with high rates among children and teen-agers.

Risk Factors

- Spontaneous loss of infection in adulthood is uncommon.
- Risk factors for infection are low socioeconomic status, overcrowding during childhood, and no fixed hot water supply. In adults, the risk rises with the number of children living in the home.
- While oral–oral transmission may occur from parent to child, it does not seem to be a risk factor in young adults.

Clinical Manifestations

- Acute infection with *H. pylori* can cause nausea, upper abdominal pain, vomiting, and burning for 3 to 14 days.
- Chronic infection can be asymptomatic or can cause a heterogenous group of disorders:
  - Duodenal ulceration
  - Gastric ulceration
  - Gastric carcinoma (The relative risk of these adenocarcinomas associated with *H. pylori* infection is about ninefold.)
  - Gastric lymphoma (*H. pylori* is strongly associated with low-grade B-cell mucosa-associated lymphoid tissue [MALT] lymphoma, which is antigen driven and regresses in about half of cases when *H. pylori* infection is eradicated with antimicrobial agents.)
- The prevalence of *H. pylori* is approximately 20% higher among persons with nonulcer dyspepsia than among matched controls.

Diagnosis

DIFFERENTIAL DIAGNOSIS

- A dyspeptic patient should be asked about sinister symptoms (weight loss of 5 kg or more, dysphagia, blood loss from the gut) and about nonsteroidal antiinflammatory drug use. Any sinister symptom mandates endoscopy. Screening for *H. pylori* antibody has been used to avoid endoscopy among patients under 45 years and without a sinister symptom.
- In the absence of nonsteroidal antiinflammatory drug use or acid hypersecretory states such as Zollinger-Ellison syndrome, as many as 90% of patients with duodenal ulcer and 80% of patients with gastric ulcer are infected by *H. pylori*.

LABORATORY

- The commercial urease breath tests show a change in color to indicate infection within a few minutes or up to 1 hour, so that diagnosis can be made with the patient still present. The patient swallows a small amount of labeled urea, and the urease of *H. pylori* rapidly converts the urea to bicarbonate, which is expired as labeled CO_2.
- These rapid urease tests are inexpensive, and a positive breath test within 30 minutes is so specific that additional tests are probably unnecessary. A final reading, after 24 hours, is 90% to 95% specific and sensitive. In a population with a low prevalence of *H. pylori* infection, a negative urease test probably represents a true-negative result, and histology is not cost effective.
- Recent treatment with a proton pump inhibitor, such as omeprazole, or antibacterial drugs usually suppresses *H. pylori* and causes a false-negative breath test, making diagnosis more difficult.
- Serum antibody can be detected in whole blood by individual kits, and the result is available in a few minutes. However, these kits are more expensive, and most are less accurate, than laboratory testing for IgG antibody by enzyme-linked immunosorbent assay. Current reagents are 95% sensitive and specific but are frequently inaccurate in patients over 65.
- Microbiologic culture is expensive, but it is useful to know the antibiotic resistance pattern to guide treatment, particularly after treatment failure.
- Saliva can be collected and tested for antibody but is less sensitive than serum testing.

Helicobacter pylori Infection

DIAGNOSTIC/TESTING PROCEDURES

Invasive diagnosis of *H. pylori* infection is by biopsy specimens obtained at gastroduodenoscopy for a rapid urease test and for histology; microbiologic culture these days is limited to research centres. At endoscopy, jumbo-size biopsy forceps should be used, and for histology, two samples should be taken from the antrum and one from the corpus.

Treatment

MAIN TREATMENT

- *H. pylori* is sensitive *in vitro* to many antibiotics, but only a few are effective clinically.
- *H. pylori* readily becomes resistant to metronidazole, clarithromycin, or other antibiotics when given as monotherapy; therefore standard single therapy should be avoided.
- Recommended regimens for the eradication of *H. pylori* include combinations of one or two antibiotics with ranitidine, a bismuth salt, or a proton pump inhibitor.
- The first choice treatment is the omeprazole–clarithromycin–metronidazole regimen (omeprazole 20 mg, clarithromycin 500 mg, and metronidazole 500 mg twice a day) for at least 7 to 10 days (usually, 10–14 days of therapy is suggested). Studies have demonstrated that this regimen carries an eradication rate of 90% or more and is well tolerated by most patients, resulting in good patient compliance.

ALTERNATIVE TREATMENT

- Bismuth subsalicylate (2 tabs qid)(Pepto Bismol) with tetracycline HCl (500 mg qid) and metronidazole (250 mg tid) for 2 weeks, or
- Bismuth subsalicylate (2 tabs qid) with amoxicillin (500 mg qid) and metronidazole (250 mg tid) for 2 weeks, or
- Omeprazole (20 mg bid) with clarithromycin (500 mg bid) and amoxicillin (1 g bid) for 1 week
- Metronidazole and tetracycline are less expensive than clarithromycin, but they cause more side effects.
- Whether clarithromycin should be given as 250 mg or 500 mg is unclear, as there have been reports of high eradication rates with 250 mg and high eradication values with 7 or 10 days' treatment.
- Lansoprazole, another proton pump inhibitor, has been shown to be just as effective as omeprazole in triple antibiotic therapy.

COMPLICATIONS

Acute infection with *H. pylori* is associated with transient hypochlorhydria. This may be important in communities with poor sanitation and contaminated water supplies, because gut pathogens would survive passage through the stomach.

Follow-Up

- The breath test is the best noninvasive test to check eradication after treatment, but any test for eradication, including endoscopy, must be done at least 1 month after completion of therapy to avoid a false-negative result.
- After eradication of the infection, the antibody titer does not fall until 4 to 6 months later, and acute and convalescent sera must be analyzed together.
- *H. pylori* eradication in nonulcer dyspepsia alleviates symptoms in a low proportion of patients.

PREVENTION

- Testing first-degree relatives of persons with gastric cancer and families in which gastric cancer has occurred in younger members
- In the developed countries, the incidences of *H. pylori* infection and its clinical sequelae are dropping, possibly because of improvements in living standards. However, prevention of infection may be necessary for populations at high risk of gastric cancer. In the United States, these groups include African, Asian, Hispanic, and Native Americans.
- In developing countries, research is underway to prevent and treat *H. pylori* in order to reduce gastric cancer.

Selected Reading

Atherton JC, Blaser MJ. *Helicobacter* infections. In: Fauci AS, Braunwald E, Isselbacher KJ, et al., eds. *Harrison's principles of internal medicine*, 14th ed. New York: McGraw-Hill, 1998:941–943.

Blaser MJ. *Helicobacter pylori* and gastric diseases. *BMJ* 1998;316:1507–1510.

Goodwin CS, Mendall MM, Northfield TC. *Helicobacter pylori* infection. *Lancet* 1997;349:265–269.

Leontiadis GI, Sharma VK, Howden CW. Nongastrointestinal tract associations of *Helicobacter pylori* infection. *Arch Intern Med* 1999;159:925–940.

Peura D. *Helicobacter pylori*: Rational management options. *Am J Med* 1998;105:424–430.

Salcedo JA, Al-Kawas F. Treatment of *Helicobacter pylori* infection. *Arch Intern Med* 1998;158:842–851.

Scheiman JM, Cutler AF. *Helicobacter pylori* and gastric cancer. *Am J Med* 1999;106:222–226.

Hemolytic-Uremic Syndrome

Basics

DEFINITION

- The hemolytic-uremic syndrome (HUS) is defined by the following:
  - Acute renal insufficiency
  - Microangiopathic hemolytic anemia
  - Thrombocytopenia

ETIOLOGY

- HUS can be due to the following:
  - Infectious causes
    - Enterohemorrhagic *Escherichia coli* O157.H7 (EHEC)
    - *Aeromonas enterocolitis*
    - *Campylobacter* spp
    - HIV infection
    - Rotavirus
    - *Shigella* spp
    - *Streptococcus pneumoniae*
    - *Yersinia* spp
  - Sporadic, noninfectious causes
    - Autoimmune diseases (systemic lupus erythematosus, scleroderma, etc.)
    - Autologous stem-cell transplantation
    - Familial
    - Idiopathic
    - Malignancy
    - Medications (mitomycin, cyclosporin, high doses of valacyclovir, etc.)
    - Pregnancy
    - Radiation
- EHEC, most commonly serotype O157:H7 in the United States, is the most common cause of HUS. EHEC produces a *Shiga*-like (vero) cytotoxin. The toxin blocks protein synthesis, leading to cell death. Colonic vascular damage by *Shiga*-like toxin may allow lipopolysaccharides and other inflammatory mediators to gain access to the circulation, thus initiating the HUS.
- Non-O157 *E. coli* organisms that produce Shiga toxin are more difficult to detect than *E. coli* O157 and can cause uncomplicated diarrhea, hemorrhagic colitis, and HUS.
- An association of younger age with HUS might be explained on the basis of increased toxin available per body weight.

EPIDEMIOLOGY

Incidence

- In industrialized countries, the annual incidence of infection with EHEC ranges from 1 to 30 cases per 100,000 people and is highest in young children under 5 years.
- In the United States, EHEC is estimated to cause more than 20,000 infections (total) and as many as 250 deaths each year.
- The rate of EHEC infection follows a seasonal pattern, with a peak incidence from June through September.
- It is estimated that 0.6% to 2.4% of all cases of diarrhea and 15% to 36% of cases of bloody diarrhea or hemorrhagic colitis are associated with EHEC.
- During outbreaks of EHEC infection, about 8% of patients develop HUS.

Risk Factors

- Transmission of the infection is primarily linked to undercooked ground beef, the drinking of contaminated water or unpasteurized milk, and working with cattle.
- Hamburger is a major vehicle, associated with food-borne outbreaks of EHEC infection. Other vehicles include apples, cider, cantaloupe, and contaminated drinking water.
- EHEC can be recovered from the intestines in about 1% of healthy cattle. Cattle may harbor the organisms asymptomatically in the intestinal tract and are an important reservoir for the pathogen.
- Beef can also be contaminated during slaughter, and the process of grinding beef may transfer pathogens from the surface of the meat to the interior of it.
- Water-borne transmission and secondary person-to-person contact can be additional important ways of spread in institutional settings, especially in daycare centers and nursing homes.
- Increased susceptibility to this infection has been described after gastrectomy.

Incubation

The incubation period ranges from 1 to 9 days.

Clinical Manifestations

SYMPTOMS

- Infection with EHEC presents with a wide spectrum of clinical manifestation, including asymptomatic carriage and nonbloody diarrhea. However, bloody diarrhea is the most common symptom and is present in 60% to 90% of cases.
- The infection usually begins with sudden onset of severe abdominal cramps, which are followed within hours by watery diarrhea. Usually within 24 hours after the onset of symptoms, watery diarrhea progresses to grossly bloody stools.
- On presentation, nausea and vomiting may be prominent
- The incidence of fever ranges from none to 32%.
- Bloody diarrhea usually lasts 2 to 4 days, and lasts longer among children.

SIGNS

- Abdominal cramps and diffuse tenderness sometimes accompany infection with EHEC, and may lead to misdiagnosis and even result in unnecessary surgical procedures.
- Oliguria and a marked drop in hematocrit are the first signs of HUS.

Diagnosis

DIFFERENTIAL DIAGNOSIS

Other causes of bloody diarrhea include the following:
- Shigellosis
- Amebiasis
- Campylobacteriosis
- Enteroinvasive *E. coli* infection

- Patients with EHEC infection are usually afebrile, and when fever is present, it is usually mild, unlike that seen with other causes of bloody diarrhea (see also the Section I chapter, "Diarrhea and Fever").
- Other causes are hematochezia hemorrhoids, inflammatory bowel disease, diverticulosis, angiodysplasia, neoplasm, intestinal ischemia
- The differential diagnosis of HUS includes the following:
  - Sepsis with or without disseminated intravascular coagulation (usually due to gram-negative pathogens)
  - Thrombotic thrombocytopenic purpura
  - Dengue
  - Malaria
  - *Hantavirus* infection
- Although skin petechiae and purpura occur frequently with thrombotic thrombocytopenic purpura, they are uncommon with HUS unless there is profound thrombocytopenia.

LABORATORY

- Routine stool cultures do not identify EHEC, and the presence of fecal leukocytes should not dissuade the clinician from considering the diagnosis of EHEC.

Hemolytic-Uremic Syndrome

- Because the rate of recovery of *E. coli* O157:H7 may decline rapidly after the first 4 to 6 days of illness, special stool cultures should be obtained as early in the course of the illness as possible.
- Unlike other *E. coli* serotypes, *E. coli* O157:H7 does not rapidly ferment D-sorbitol. When plated on MacConkey and sorbitol agar, *E. coli* O157:H7 appears sorbitol-negative at 24 hours. These colorless, sorbitol-negative colonies can then be screened for agglutination in O157:H7.
- In HUS, laboratory findings can reveal the following:
  - Severe to moderate anemia associated with red-cell fragmentation and numerous schistocytes on peripheral smear
  - Decreased plasma haptoglobin and an elevated LDH level
  - Negative Coombs' test
  - Thrombocytopenia
  - Elevated creatinine level
  - Hematuria, proteinuria, and granular or hyaline casts

IMAGING

- In patients with EHEC, barium enema studies can show marked thickening of the mucosa and, in some cases, thumbprinting of the colon.
- At endoscopy, the colonic mucosa appears edematous and hyperemic, sometimes with superficial ulcerations.

DIAGNOSTIC PROCEDURES

Renal biopsy is reserved for patients with atypical presentation of HUS.

Treatment

MAIN TREATMENT

- Management is supportive, and no specific treatment for EHEC currently exists.
- Antimicrobial agents have not been shown to modify the course of the illness, and it has been postulated that antibiotics can worsen the clinical course of EHEC infection. Especially, the use of trimethoprim-sulfamethoxazole in EHEC infection has also been questioned, because subinhibitory concentrations of that agent increase the production of *Shiga*-like toxin *in vitro*.
- The antimotility agents are contraindicated because they can lead to bowel stasis and increased toxin absorption.
- Patients with HUS are treated with plasmapheresis, dialysis, and transfusions.
- The efficacy of glucocorticoids and heparin in HUS is uncertain.

ALTERNATIVE TREATMENT

- Fresh-frozen plasma has been given to adults with HUS with some success. A loading dose of 30 to 40 mL/kg, and then a daily dose of 152 to 0 mL/kg, has been recommended. However, a controlled trial in children did not show any benefit.
- If the patient is seen early and is still passing urine, prostacyclin infusion can be tried to inhibit platelet-endothelial interactions and help promote a diuresis, although no controlled study has been done in adults.

COMPLICATIONS

- Infection with EHEC, besides HUS, can lead to hemorrhagic colitis or thrombotic thrombocytopenic purpura.
- HUS can lead to the following:
  - Hypoglycemia
  - Hyponatremia
  - Leukemoid reactions
  - Renal failure (that may require hemodialysis)
  - Rhabdomyolysis
  - Severe anemia (that may require transfusions)
  - Thrombocytopenia

Follow-up

FOLLOW-UP

- Even with advanced therapy, 5% to 20% of patients with HUS die of the acute illness, and the mortality rate is even higher among elderly patients.
- Renal damage progresses slowly over several decades in survivors, an estimated 50% of whom develop significant renal failure and most of whom require long-term dialysis or renal transplantation.

PREVENTION

- The Food and Drug Administration has recommended a minimum internal temperature of 155°F (86.1°C) for cooked hamburgers. Also, patients should be instructed to do the following:
  - Cook ground beef thoroughly, until its interior is no longer pink and the juices run gray.
  - Always use pasteurized milk.
  - Keep food refrigerated or frozen.
  - Thaw frozen food in a refrigerator or microwave.
  - Keep raw meat and poultry separate from other foods.
  - Wash hands carefully with soap before cooking is begun.
  - Wash the working surfaces (including cutting boards), utensils, and hands after touching raw meat or poultry.
  - Keep hot foods hot.
  - Refrigerate leftovers immediately, or discard them.
  - Never taste small bits of raw ground beef during meal preparation.
  - Never place cooked hamburgers back on the unwashed plate that had previously held the raw ground beef.

Selected Readings

Koutkia P, Mylonakis E, Flanigan T. Enterohemorrhagic *Escherichia coli* O157:H7. An emerging pathogen. *Am Fam Physician* 1997;56:853–859.

Neild GH. Hemolytic-uremic syndrome in practice. *Lancet* 1994;343:398–401.

Su C, Brandt LJ. *Escherichia coli* O157:H7 infection in humans. *Ann Intern Med* 1995;123:698–714.

Hepatitis

Basics

DEFINITION
- Hepatitis is inflammation of the liver.
- Fulminant hepatitis is massive hepatic necrosis, usually due to hepatitis B or C.

ETIOLOGY
- Almost all cases of acute viral hepatitis is caused by one of the following viral agents:
  - Hepatitis A virus (HAV)
  - Hepatitis B virus (HBV)
  - Hepatitis C virus (HCV)
  - Hepatitis D virus (HDV)
  - Hepatitis E virus (HEV)
- All these human hepatitis viruses are RNA viruses, except for hepatitis B, which is a DNA virus.
- HDV can either infect a person simultaneously with HBV or superinfect a person already infected with HBV.
- Other viruses can cause hepatitis, such as EOV, CMV, HIV, adenovirus, and enteroviruses.

EPIDEMIOLOGY
- HAV is transmitted almost exclusively by the fecal–oral route. Large outbreaks as well as sporadic cases have been traced to contaminated food and water.
- The major routes of hepatitis B transmission are by blood products and percutaneous exposure.
- HBsAg is infrequent (<0.5%) in normal populations in the United States and western Europe. A prevalence of up to 20% has been found in the Far East and in some tropical countries and in persons with Down's syndrome, leprosy, leukemia, and Hodgkin's disease; in patients on hemodialysis, and in injecting drug users.
- HCV is transmitted by transfusion and other percutaneous routes.
- Some cases of HCV can be due to sexually transmitted infection or perinatal transmission.
- The risk of HCV infection is increased in organ transplant recipients and in patients with HIV.
- HEV is an enterically transmitted virus with epidemiologic features resembling those of HAV. Infection occurs primarily in developing countries.
- HGV is a transmitted by blood transfusion, and can be detected in some patients with acute, chronic, and fulminant hepatitis. Most clinically apparent HGV infections occur in patients coinfected with hepatitis C, but HGV does not alter the severity of hepatitis C.

Incubation Period
- HAV: 15 to 45 days
- HBV: 1 to 6 months
- HCV: 15 to 160 days
- HDV: 1 to 6 months
- HEV: 15 to 60 days

Clinical Manifestations

SYMPTOMS
- The prodromal symptoms of acute viral hepatitis are systemic and include the following:
  - Alterations in olfaction and taste
  - Anorexia
  - Arthralgias
  - Coryza
  - Cough
  - Fatigue
  - Fever (usually low-grade)
  - Headache
  - Malaise
  - Myalgias
  - Nausea and vomiting
- These constitutional symptoms may precede the onset of jaundice by 1 to 2 weeks.
- Symptoms usually diminish with the onset of clinical jaundice.
- A big number of patients with viral hepatitis never become icteric. Hepatitis C occurring after transfusion is more likely to be anicteric.

SIGNS
- In acute viral hepatitis, the liver becomes enlarged and tender and may be associated with right upper quadrant pain and discomfort.
- Splenomegaly and cervical adenopathy are present in 10% to 20% of patients with acute hepatitis.
- The duration of the posticteric phase is variable, ranging from 2 to 12 weeks, and usually is more prolonged in infection with HBV or HCV.

Diagnosis

DIFFERENTIAL DIAGNOSIS
For details on the differential diagnosis and a table reviewing the serologic testing in acute and chronic hepatitis, see the Section I chapter, "Jaundice and Fever."

LABORATORY
- Neutropenia and lymphopenia in acute viral hepatitis are transient and are followed by a relative lymphocytosis.
- Atypical lymphocytes are common during the acute phase.
- Serum aminotransferases increase during the prodromal phase of acute viral hepatitis. Peak levels vary, are usually reached at the time the patient is clinically icteric, and diminish progressively during the recovery phase.
- When jaundice appears, the serum bilirubin typically rises to levels ranging from 85 to 340 mol/L (5 to 20 mg/dL).
- Prolonged prothrombin time (PT) indicates a worse prognosis.
- Hypoglycemia is noted occasionally in patients with severe viral hepatitis.
- Serum alkaline phosphatase may be normal or only mildly elevated.
- A diffuse but mild elevation of the gamma globulin fraction is common during acute viral hepatitis.
- Serologic tests are available with which to establish a diagnosis of hepatitis A, B, C, and D.
- After infection with HBV, HBsAg becomes detectable first. This is followed by the antibody to core antigen (anti-HBc) that usually persists for life. About 3 to 5 months after exposure, HBsAg becomes undetectable, and there is a period of several weeks before the antibody (anti-HBsAg) becomes detectable. During this "window period," testing for IgM anti-HBc can establish the diagnosis.
- The presence of HBeAg during chronic hepatitis B is associated with ongoing viral replication, infectivity, and inflammatory liver injury.
- For HCV infection, the most sensitive indicator (better than anti-HCV) is the presence of HCV RNA with the use of polymerase chain reaction. HCV RNA can be detected within a few days of exposure to HCV.

Hepatitis

DIAGNOSTIC/TESTING PROCEDURES

Liver biopsy is rarely necessary or indicated in acute viral hepatitis, except when there is a question about the diagnosis or when there is clinical evidence suggesting a diagnosis of chronic hepatitis.

Treatment

MAIN TREATMENT

- The treatment of chronic HBV with interferon-alfa is recommended for patients with persistent elevations in serum aminotransferase concentrations; detectable levels of HBsAg, HBeAg, and HBV DNA in serum; chronic hepatitis on liver biopsy; and compensated liver disease. Biopsy of the liver should be performed before therapy to establish the diagnosis, grade the severity of injury, and assess the degree of fibrosis.
- Among patients with chronic HBV infection, interferon-alfa achieves response rates of 30% to 40% within the first year of treatment.
- There are two promising, recent developments for the treatment of chronic hepatitis:
  —Lamivudine has proved beneficial in patients with chronic hepatitis B and is now approved for this indication.
  —The combination of interferon-alfa and ribavirin is a therapy for chronic hepatitis C.
- Patients with chronic viral hepatitis are considered to be at high risk of developing cirrhosis and liver failure. Liver transplantation can be offered to carefully selected patients. Patients with chronic hepatitis C have done as well as any other subset of patients after transplantation, despite the fact that recurrent infection in the donor organ is the rule. In patients with chronic HBV, prophylactic use of hepatitis B immune globulin (HBIG) during and after transplantation increases the success of transplantation.

COMPLICATIONS

- The case fatality rate in HAV and HBV is low (approximately 0.1%) but is increased by advanced age and underlying debilitating disorders.
- In outbreaks of water-borne HEV in India and Asia, the case fatality rate is 1% to 2% and up to 20% in pregnant women.
- The case fatality rate in HBV and HDV coinfection is approximately 5% and in HDV superinfection is approximately 20%.
- Less than 1% of patients with HBV develop fulminant hepatitis, but about 5% to 7% develop chronic carrier states.
- HBV is strongly associated with polyarteritis nodosa.
- Sixty percent to 75% of patients with HCV develop chronic hepatitis, although only 20% develop cirrhosis.
- In acute fulminant hepatitis, patients present with signs and symptoms of encephalopathy that may evolve to deep coma. The liver is small and the PT excessively prolonged. The fatality is greater than 80%. If a donor organ can be located quickly, patients with fulminant hepatitis are candidates for liver transplantation.

Follow-Up

- Carriers of HBsAg have an enhanced risk of hepatocellular carcinoma. The risk of hepatocellular carcinoma is increased as well in patients with chronic HCV infection, almost exclusively in patients with cirrhosis, and usually after three decades of disease.
- No HAV carrier state has been identified after acute HAV, although a few patients experience relapsing hepatitis weeks to months after apparent recovery from the acute episode.

PREVENTION

- Vaccines for HBV (these vaccines are HBsAg) are very effective and widely used. Details are available in Section IV of this book (Drugs and Vaccines).
- Two vaccines made from a strain of HAV attenuated in tissue culture are approved for use and appear to provide adequate protection 4 weeks after a primary inoculation. If travel is more imminent, immune globulin (0.02 mL/kg) should be administered at a different injection site, along with the first dose of vaccine.
- For unvaccinated persons sustaining an exposure to HBV, postexposure prophylaxis with a combination of HBIG and HBV vaccine is recommended.

Selected Readings

Balfour HH Jr. Antiviral drugs. *N Engl J Med* 1999;340:1255–1268.

Dienstag JL, Isselbacher KJ. Acute viral hepatitis. In: Fauci AS, Braunwald E, Isselbacher KJ, et al., eds. *Harrison's principles of internal medicine*, 14th ed. New York: McGraw-Hill, 1998:1677–1692.

Hoofnagle JH, di Bisceglie AM. The treatment of chronic viral hepatitis. *N Engl J Med* 1997;336:347–356.

McCarthy M, Wilkinson ML. Recent advances: Hepatology. *BMJ* 1999;318:1256–1259.

Noskin GA. Prevention, diagnosis, and management of viral hepatitis. A guide for primary care physicians. AMA Advisory Group on Prevention, Diagnosis, and Management of Viral Hepatitis. *Arch Fam Med* 1995;4:923–934.

Herpes Simplex Virus Infections

Basics

DEFINITION

- A group of infections of various organs caused by the herpes simplex virus (HSV)

ETIOLOGY

- There are two types of HSV:
  - HSV type 1
  - HSV type 2
- HSV is a double-stranded, DNA virus that belongs to the herpesviruses group. This group of viruses is an important cause of common infections in humans. The herpesviruses group includes the following viruses:
  - HSV type 1 (the usual cause of herpes labialis and other important infections)
  - HSV type 2 (the usual cause of genital herpes)
  - Varicella zoster virus (VZV)
  - Epstein-Barr virus (EBV)
  - Cytomegalovirus (CMV)
  - Human herpesvirus type 6 (HHV-6)
  - Human herpesvirus type 8 (HHV-8) or Kaposi's sarcoma–associated virus (KSAV)

EPIDEMIOLOGY

Incidence and Prevalence

HSV is the cause of common infections with worldwide distribution, including herpes labialis and genital herpes.

Risk Factors

- Immunosuppression may predispose to severe, systemic herpes simplex infections.
- Neonates are at high risk to develop serious problems if they acquire HSV.
- HSV is also a cause of congenital infection.
- Vaginal delivery in a woman with active genital herpes places the newborn at risk for severe HSV infection.
- Reactivation of HSV, leading to recurrence of herpes labialis or recurrent genital herpes, may be precipitated by several forms of physical or psychological stress, including fever, trauma, stress-provoking situations, and so forth.

Clinical Manifestations

SYMPTOMS AND SIGNS

- Primary infection with HSV-1 is usually mild or subclinical and occurs in early childhood.
- Gingivostomatitis, keratoconjunctivitis, generalized rash, and pharyngotonsillitis may be manifestations of HSV-1 primary infection in a small proportion of children.
- Herpetic whitlow consists of single or multiple vesicular lesions on the distal parts of fingers.
- A significant manifestation of primary HSV infection is meningoencephalitis, which is caused by HSV-1 more commonly than HSV-2.
- A common problem related to HSV is herpetic keratitis.
- Reactivation of HSV-1 from its latent phase usually results in herpes labialis, which is manifested by vesicles on an erythematous base, usually on the lips or elsewhere on the face.
- Genital herpes is usually caused by HSV-2. It is a common infection that may become a recurrent problem.
- HSV-2 has been associated with radiculitis and aseptic meningitis.
- HSV may also cause manifestations from other organs, including diseases such as herpetic esophagitis, hepatitis, skin infection in wrestlers, and pneumonitis.

Diagnosis

DIFFERENTIAL DIAGNOSIS

- Herpes labialis (fever blisters or cold sores) is quite characteristic.
- Similarly, clinical diagnosis without performing any specific test usually suffices in patients with genital herpes.
- Lesions of genital herpes are quite characteristic and should not trouble the clinician. Other causes of genital lesions include syphilis, genital warts, chancroid (*Haemophilus ducreyi* infection), granuloma inguinale, lymphogranuloma inguinale, and neoplasms.
- There are several causes of encephalitis in addition to HSV (reviewed in the Section II chapter, "Encephalitis").

Herpes Simplex Virus Infections

LABORATORY

- Serologic tests may help in the diagnosis of HSV infections.
- PCR for DNA of HSV in cerebrospinal fluid specimens or brain tissue biopsy should be considered early in suspected cases of HSV encephalitis, because antiviral treatment is effective (if started promptly).

PATHOLOGY

A Tzanck preparation of scrapings from the base of HSV lesions commonly demonstrates multinucleated giant cells.

Treatment

MAIN TREATMENT

- Acyclovir has good efficacy against HSV. It should be given in a dose 10 mg/kg i.v. every 8 hours in patients with disseminated herpetic infection or herpetic encephalitis.
- Acyclovir (in smaller doses, e.g., 400 mg PO twice a day) has been also used as a preventive measure in patients with frequent recurrence of genital herpes or severe herpes labialis.

ALTERNATIVE TREATMENT

- HSV may develop resistance to acyclovir.
- Foscarnet may be used in cases of severe infections due to resistance to acyclovir HSV.

COMPLICATIONS

- Disseminated herpetic infection and herpetic encephalitis are potentially fatal diseases.
- Herpetic keratitis may lead to cornea destruction.
- Neonatal herpetic infections are frequently very severe. Serious neurologic and/or eye abnormalities may be the result of the infection in survivors of neonatal HSV infection.

Follow-up

Careful follow-up is necessary after a serious HSV infection, due to the risk of recurrence of HSV and the high probability of residual abnormalities.

PREVENTION

- Patients with herpes labialis should avoid transferring the virus from the facial lesions to the eyes.
- Genital herpes is a sexually transmitted disease. Safe sexual practices are of paramount importance.
- Cesarean section should be performed in women with active genital tract herpetic infection to decrease the probability of HSV infection in the newborn.

Selected Readings

Bryson YJ, Dillon M, Lovett M, et al. Treatment of first episodes of genital herpes simplex virus infection with oral acyclovir. A randomized double-blind controlled trial in normal subjects. *N Engl Med* 1983;308:916.

Corey L, Spear PG. Infections with herpes simplex viruses. *N Engl J Med* 1986;314:686, 749.

Galloway DA, Fenoglio C, Shevchuk M, et al. Detection of herpes simplex RNA in human sensory ganglia. *Virology* 1979;95:265.

McBane RD, Gross JB. Herpes esophagitis: Clinical syndrome, endoscopic appearance, and diagnosis in 23 patients. *Gastrointest Endosc* 1991;37:600.

Rooney JF, Straus SE, Mannix ML, et al. Oral-acyclovir to suppress frequently recurrent herpes labialis. A double-blind, placebo-controlled trial. *Ann Intern Med* 1993;118:268.

Safrin S, Crumpacker C, Chatis P, et al. A controlled trial comparing foscarnet with vidarabine for acyclovir-resistant mucocutaneous herpes simplex in the acquired immunodeficiency syndrome. *N Engl J Med* 1991;325:551.

Straus SE, Croen KD, Sawyer MH, et al. Acyclovir suppression of frequently recurring genital herpes: Efficacy and diminishing need during successive years of treatment. *JAMA* 1988;260:222.

Whitley R, Arvin A, Prober C, et al. Predictors of morbidity and mortality in neonates with herpes simplex virus infections. *N Engl J Med* 1991;324:450.

Whitley RJ, Cobbs CG, Alford CA Jr, et al. Diseases that mimic herpes simplex encephalitis. Diagnosis, presentation, and outcome. *JAMA* 1989;262:234.

Herpes Zoster

Basics

DEFINITION
Herpes zoster (shingles) is a local manifestation on the skin of reactivation of the varicella zoster virus (VZV).

ETIOLOGY
- Primary infection with VZV leads to a subclinical condition or clinically apparent varicella (chickenpox), which is discussed in detail elsewhere in this book.
- The virus remains latent for years after primary infection.
- After a variable period of time (usually many years), basically undetermined factors permit reactivation of VZV, which is manifested by herpes zoster.
- VZV is a DNA virus that belongs to the herpesviruses group.

EPIDEMIOLOGY
Incidence and Prevalence
- VZV affects people worldwide.
- About 90% of people have serologic evidence of past infection by young adulthood.
- Herpes zoster afflicts about 20% of the population overall at some time during their lifetime.
- The incidence of herpes zoster was 4.8 per 1,000 persons in a 7-year study. About 75% of persons who developed herpes zoster were older than 45 years in this study.

Risk Factors
- The elderly are more likely than younger people to develop herpes zoster.
- Immunosuppressed patients, due to medications, neoplasms (especially lymphoproliferative disorders), or infections (e.g., HIV), are predisposed to develop herpes zoster.

Clinical Manifestations

SYMPTOMS AND SIGNS
- Herpes zoster is manifested with vesicles on an erythematous base, with a characteristic distribution of a dermatome (usually unilaterally).
- Severe pain and paresthesia at the area of lesions are common symptoms.
- Thoracic and lumbar dermatomes are most commonly affected.
- However, herpes zoster may affect any dermatome of the body.
- When the first or second branch of the fifth cranial nerve (trigeminal) is affected, herpes zoster may involve the eyelids.
- Herpes zoster ophthalmicus is manifested by keratitis, which may be followed by iridocyclitis and secondary glaucoma.
- The involvement of the maxillary or mandibular branch of the fifth cranial nerve may result in herpes zoster lesions in the mouth.
- Involvement of the geniculate ganglion may lead to Ramsay Hunt syndrome, with pain and vesicular lesions on the external auditory meatus, loss of taste in the anterior two-thirds of the tongue, and ipsilateral fascial palsy.

Diagnosis

DIFFERENTIAL DIAGNOSIS
- The appearance of characteristic herpes zoster skin lesions with a typical dermatomal distribution should suffice for a clinical diagnosis.
- Other viral infections, including herpes simplex virus or coxsackievirus, may very rarely present with lesions with a dermatoma-like distribution.

LABORATORY
Serologic and molecular biology (PCR) tests are available to help establish diagnosis of herpes zoster, but it is emphasized that these tests are not necessary to be performed in clinical practice (because clinical diagnosis usually suffices).

PATHOLOGY
A Tzanck smear of skin lesions (performed by scraping the base of the lesion) may demonstrate multinucleated giant cells, which are more common in herpes simplex virus infection.

Treatment

MAIN TREATMENT
- Acyclovir 800 mg PO 5 times a day (q4h, except a dose that is missed during night sleep) for 7 days is the recommended treatment.
- Acyclovir intravenously (10 mg/kg q8h) is recommended in immunosuppressed patients with severe herpes zoster on multiple dermatomes.

Herpes Zoster

ALTERNATIVE TREATMENT
- Newer antiviral agents with good activity against VZV are now available.
- Valacyclovir 1,000 mg PO q8h or famciclovir 500 mg PO q8h for 7 days may be used to treat patients with herpes zoster.
- It is not clear whether steroid treatment decreases the probability of subsequent postherpetic neuralgia.

COMPLICATIONS
- Herpes zoster in an immunocompromised host may be manifested by a generalized infection with rash distributed very extensively on the skin. In addition, systemic manifestations may appear with pneumonitis, hepatitis, and central nervous system abnormalities.
- Central nervous system involvement, manifested by granulomatous cerebral angiitis, may follow herpes zoster ophthalmicus.
- Secondary bacterial infection may develop on skin lesions due to herpes zoster.

Follow-Up

- A significant proportion of patients develop postherpetic neuralgia, especially the elderly (up to 30%). The management of these patients should start with simple analgesics, such as paracetamol, and proceed to small doses of opiates and/or amitriptyline, if necessary.
- Capsaicin ointments may help patients with postherpetic neuralgia.

PREVENTION
- Use of varicella zoster immunoglobulin (VZIG) is recommended for immunocompromised patients who have no history of chickenpox or herpes zoster and who were substantially exposed to a patient with varicella or herpes zoster. As far as quantification of exposure to a patient with herpes zoster is concerned, intimate contact (e.g., touching or hugging) with a person deemed contagious with herpes zoster is necessary to warrant VZIG administration.
- VZV vaccine in persons with no previous VZV infection prevents chickenpox and herpes zoster.

Selected Readings

Centers for Disease Control and Prevention. Varicella zoster immune globulin for the prevention of chickenpox: Recommendation of the immunization practice advisory committee. *Ann Intern Med* 1984;100:859–865.

Esiri MM, Tomlinson AH. Herpes zoster: Demonstration of virus in trigeminal nerve and ganglion by immunofluorescence and electron microscopy. *J Neurol Sci* 1972;15:35.

Esmann V, Kroon S, Petersblund NA, et al. Prednisolone does not prevent post-herpetic neuralgia. *Lancet* 1987;2:126–129.

Gnann JW, Whitley RJ. Natural history and treatment of varicella-zoster in high risk populations. *J Hosp Infect* 1991;18:317–329.

Huff JC, Bean B, Balfour HH, et al. Therapy of herpes zoster with oral acyclovir. *Am J Med* 1988;85(2A):84–89.

Lawrence R, Gershon AA, Holzman R, et al. The risk of zoster after vaccination in children with leukemia. *N Engl J Med* 1988;318:543–548.

Morton D, Thomson AN. Oral acyclovir treatment of herpes zoster in general practice. *N Z Med J* 1989;109:93–95.

Sheep DH, Dandliker PS, Meyers JD. Treatment of varicella zoster virus infection in severely immunocompromised patients: A randomized comparison of acyclovir and vidarabine. *N Engl J Med* 1986;314:208–212.

Watson PN, Evans RJ. Post-herpetic neuralgia; a review. *Arch Neurol* 1986;43:836–840.

Weibel RE, Neff BJ, Kutter BJ, et al. Live attenuated varicella virus vaccine: Efficacy trial in healthy children. *N Engl J Med* 1984;310:1409–1415.

Histoplasmosis

Basics

DEFINITION
- An inhalation-acquired mycosis mainly affecting the lungs, which was first described in 1905

ETIOLOGY
- The etiologic agent is *Histoplasma capsulatum* (class: Ascomycetes), a dimorphic fungus, with two varieties: var. *capsulatum* and var. *duboisii*. The fungus has mycelial morphology in nature and the yeast form in human body temperature.
- Confirmation of an organism as *H. capsulatum* requires the presence of the typical macroconidia and the conversion of the mold to the yeast.
- *H. capsulatum* usually causes asymptomatic disease but also can be fatal, especially to immunosuppressed persons. It is capable of producing recrudescent disease when the host's cell-mediated immune response is impaired.

EPIDEMIOLOGY

Incidence and Prevalence
- Soil is the natural habitat of *Histoplasma* to a depth of 15 to 20 cm.
- Five hundred thousand individuals become infected annually in the United States, especially within the Ohio and Mississippi River valleys (moisture-holding and acid-containing soil).
- Children under age 1 year and men over age 50 years are more susceptible.
- Even though the skin test with antigens of *H. capsulatum* has the same rate of positivity in males and females (suggesting same rate of asymptomatic acute infection in both sexes), disseminated histoplasmosis is about five times more common in males than in females. Pulmonary histoplasmosis is almost never transmitted from person to person.

Risk Factors
- Living in endemic region: North and Latin America for *H. capsulatum*, and Central Africa for African histoplasmosis; impaired immunologic status; large number of organisms inhaled

Clinical Manifestations

SYMPTOMS AND SIGNS
- The lungs are the mainly involved tissue. There are the following clinical forms:
- Acute primary pulmonary histoplasmosis
  —Ninety percent of cases are asymptomatic. After heavy exposure, patients are likely to develop symptomatic infection. Most symptomatic patients (incubation period, 3-21 days) develop a flulike syndrome that resolves without treatment. Reinfection with the organism simulates an abrupt onset of symptoms (incubation period, <1 week).
  —Fever, chills, headache, anorexia, nonproductive cough, and retrosternal or pleuritic pain may develop. Symptoms last for 2 weeks, then resolve. Fatigability and malaise may persist for months.
  —Hepatosplenomegaly, a transient increase of alkaline phosphatase, erythema nodosum, or erythema multiforme may occur. Rarely, an area of affected lung cavitates.
  —Five percent of patients develop acute pericarditis (bloody fluid), frequently with concurrent pleural effusions; 6% of patients have frank arthritis.
  —In cases of histoplasmosis due to heavy exposure of organisms and/or baseline immunodeficiency state, ARDS, respiratory insufficiency, or obstructive syndromes due to enlarged mediastinal lymph nodes may develop.
- Mediastinal granuloma and fibrosis
  —Extension of infection to paratracheal, hilar, and subcarinal lymph nodes causes nodal enlargement, caseating necrosis, and perilymphadenitis.
  —Resolution of lymphadenitis progresses to extensive fibroplastic proliferation that surrounds caseated nodes.
  —Rarely, progressive fibrosis that invades the mediastinal structures occurs.
  —Large cystic lesions to the mediastinum can cause cough, postobstructive pneumonia, bronchiectasis, and atelectasis. Heavier forms of mediastinal infection may lead to cor pulmonale, respiratory failure, vena cava syndrome, stenosis of esophagus, and/or fistula formation between the esophagus and the respiratory tract.
- Histoplasmoma
  —Large pulmonary lesions that heal to become a residual nodule (1-4 cm), usually in the subpleural regions
- Chronic pulmonary histoplasmosis
  —Occurs usually in men more than 50 years old with COPD
  —Cough, pleuritic pain, night sweats, erythema nodosum or multiforme, sputum production, weight loss, and intermittent hemoptysis are the usual manifestations. Patients may be mildly anemic.
  —Infiltration of the apical and posterior segments of upper lobes in 90% of cases, usually in areas of preexisting emphysema
  —Fifty percent of patients who are not complicated by cavity formation in their lungs progress to healing of the lesions after a progressive fibrosis over a period of 2 to 6 months. Twenty percent will develop cavities.
  —Cavities with thin walls (1-2 mm) will improve spontaneously (one-half of cases); cavities with thick walls (3-4 mm) usually persist and may enlarge.
  —Untreated cases may resolve spontaneously, but they usually progress.
  —Death can be the result (usually due to cor pulmonale, bacterial pneumonia, respiratory failure).
- Progressive disseminated disease
  —Progressive, often lethal illness that occurs in about 1 in 2,000 cases of histoplasmosis in normal adults. The rate is increased in infants and the immunosuppressed (4%-27% in HIV-infected patients). It can develop from pulmonary infection, by exogenous reinfection, or by reactivation.

Histoplasmosis

- It has a broad clinical spectrum: chronic, subacute, and acute forms.
- Acute progressive disseminated histoplasmosis: Fever, weight loss, malaise, cough, dyspnea, hepatosplenomegaly, and cutaneous lesions (erythematous, maculopapular eruptions on the face, trunk, and extremities) are the usual symptoms and signs. HIV patients may present with an acute syndrome, such as septic shock (10%) or meningitis (15%). Only 3% of patients have oropharyngeal ulcers, but 10% have cutaneous lesions.
- Subacute progressive disseminated histoplasmosis: If untreated, it progresses to death in 2 to 24 months. The adrenal glands are vulnerable (80%). Their function should be thoroughly checked in cases of disseminated histoplasmosis, because adrenal insufficiency occurs in 10% of cases.
- Chronic progressive disseminated histoplasmosis: This is an indolent illness that can affect a wide range of sites.
- Diarrhea, weight loss, abdominal pain, polypoid lesions and/or ulcers in the gastrointestinal tract, arthralgias, lytic bone lesions, carpal tunnel syndrome, headache, confusion, cranial nerve dysfunction, anemia, leucopenia, and thrombocytopenia may occur.
- Heart valves can be infected (large vegetations in mitral or aortic valves). These are the only places where hyphae of the organism can be found in pathology specimens.
- The CNS (10%–25%) also can be infected. Patients may have symptoms of chronic meningitis or a cerebral mass lesion.
- Ocular histoplasmosis syndrome: chorioiditis
- One percent to 10% of persons in areas endemic for histoplasmosis have asymptomatic atrophic scars, with 0.2- to 0.7-mm "histospots" located posterior to the equator of the eye, which are presumed to be caused by histoplasmosis. Many of these patients also have typical lung calcifications.
- African histoplasmosis
  - Caused by *H. capsulatum* var. *duboisii*
  - The classic forms of pulmonary infection are not observed.
  - Skin, bones, and soft tissues are usually infected. Arthritis and papular subcutaneous (tender), nodular, psoriasiform, and ulcerated lesions occur. Skin lesions are localized, chronic, and tend to self-heal. Infection of bones (ribs, skull) occurs in 50% of patients. Multiple lesions are often found.

Diagnosis

DIFFERENTIAL DIAGNOSIS

- Acute primary pulmonary histoplasmosis: tuberculosis, sarcoidosis, and infections with *B. dermatides*, *Coccidioides immitis*, *Mycoplasma pneumoniae*, and *Chlamydia pneumoniae*
- Mediastinal granuloma and fibrosis: tuberculosis, tumor
- Histoplasmoma: tumor
- Chronic pulmonary histoplasmosis: tuberculosis, paracoccidioidomycoses, syphilis

LABORATORY

- The mold bears macroconidia (2-5 mm), which is the infectious form of the organism. When inhaled, it is multiplied intracellularly (in the alveolar macrophages) and transforms to the yeast (3×4 mm), which is oval, uninucleate, and has thick walls.
- Hematoxylin and eosin are used to stain biopsy-obtained tissue. Wright-Giemsa is used to stain yeast forms in circulating neutrophils from peripheral blood.
- Skin test: The histoplasmin skin test is used only for epidemiologic studies. A positive result cannot distinguish a past infection from a present one, and a negative result does not rule out active infection. This skin test can augment the titer of serologic tests to significant levels.
- Cerebrospinal fluid (CSF): cells, 10 to 500/mm^3 (mostly neutrophils); protein, greater than 45 mg/dL; glucose, less than 40 mg/dL
- Cultures need 4 to 6 weeks at 30°C. Sputum specimens are positive in 10% to 15% of patients with acute progressive disseminated histoplasmosis, in 60% of patients with chronic pulmonary histoplasmosis or lung cavities, and in 80% to 90% of patients with HIV and progressive disseminated histoplasmosis. CSF specimens are positive in 30% to 60%, and blood and bone marrow in 50% to 90%, depending on the course of the disease. Cultures from the mediastinum are almost always negative.

Histoplasmosis

- Serology: There are tests for complement-fixing (CF) and immunoprecipitating (ID) antibodies (M and H antigens). There is no correlation between level of antibody and severity of illness, especially in the immunosuppressed. Following acute exposure, high levels of antibodies develop within 4 to 6 weeks. CF is most sensitive, and the result becomes positive earlier than with the ID test. No more than 1% patients with a negative CF test will have a positive ID reaction.
- For blood cultures, lysis centrifugation is indicated.
- Specific DNA probes and tests of specific antigens exist in the market. Radioimmunoassay is helpful for detection of *H. capsulatum* polysaccharide antigen in body fluids.

PATHOLOGY

- Well-organized granulomas that contain lymphocytes, epithelioid cells, giant cells, and variable amounts of caseating necrosis. Yeast forms may be sparse.

IMAGING

- Acute primary pulmonary histoplasmosis (x-ray): one or more patchy pulmonary infiltrates. In cases of heavy exposure, soft, nodular infiltrates with irregular outlines, enlarged hilar, or mediastinal lymph nodes, and, rarely, pleural effusions may be seen. Small calcifications of uniform size are sometimes seen in cases of healed histoplasmosis.
- Mediastinal granuloma and fibrosis: mild subcarinal or superior mediastinal widening; calcified debris into bronchi
- Histoplasmoma: coin lesion
- Chronic pulmonary histoplasmosis: nodules (initial phase), infarct-like necrosis (median phase), linear scar formation (final phase); interstitial infiltrates of upper lobes, mediastinal or pulmonary calcifications; if cavities: pleural thickening, hilar retraction, air-fluid levels
- Acute progressive disseminated histoplasmosis: Diffuse pulmonary disease is present in one-half of patients.
- Chronic progressive disseminated histoplasmosis: Chest X-rays often reveal no active disease.
- Subacute progressive disseminated histoplasmosis: diffuse interstitial infiltrates (70%), mediastinal lymphadenopathy (20%); CT: bilateral enlargement of adrenals, with a low attenuation centre
- African histoplasmosis: osteolytic or cystic lesions with new bone formation

Treatment

- Ketoconazole 400 mg/d for 3 to 6 weeks for acute pulmonary histoplasmosis; 400 mg/d for 6 to 12 months for chronic pulmonary histoplasmosis
- Amphotericin B 0.7 to 1.0 mg/kg/d for acute progressive disseminated histoplasmosis. After stabilization, start alternate-day treatment. Long-term suppressive therapy with itraconazole may be needed.
- Amphotericin B 0.5 mg/kg or ketoconazole 400 mg/d for 6 to 12 months for chronic and subacute progressive disseminated histoplasmosis

Histoplasmosis

- Precautions: Amphotericin B can cause significant renal insufficiency and electrolyte abnormalities. Long-term therapy with ketoconazole suppresses steroidogenesis.
- Significant possible interactions: Concomitant use of amphotericin B and other nephrotoxic drugs is dangerous.
- Take surgical measures if vena cava syndrome or other obstructive complications occur.

COMPLICATIONS

The disseminated form of the disease is lethal, not only in immunosuppressed individuals, but also in the healthy, except if early and aggressive treatment is initiated.

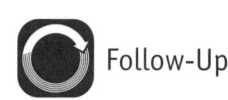

Follow-Up

The status of the infection with use of appropriate antifungal agents should be evaluated every 2 to 3 weeks in patients with chronic pulmonary histoplasmosis.

PREVENTION

An individual is more likely to be exposed to *H. capsulatum* inside caves (soil contaminated from bat droppings), from chicken coops, in bamboo canebrakes, and from decayed wood piles. Avoidance of activity in these areas is advisable for immunosuppressed persons. Decontamination of soil with formalin may prevent exposure.

Selected Readings

Dismukes WE, Bradsher RW Jr, Cloud GC, et al. Itraconazole therapy for blastomycosis and histoplasmosis. *Am J Med* 1992;93:489-497.

Goodwin RA, Loyd JE, des Prez RM. Histoplasmosis in normal hosts. *Medicine* 1981;60:231-266.

Loyd JE, Tillman BF, Atkinson JB, et al. Mediastinal fibrosis complicating histoplasmosis. *Medicine* 1988;67:295-310.

Sharkey-Mathis PK, Velez J, Fetchik R, et al. Histoplasmosis in the acquired immunodeficiency syndrome (AIDS): Treatment with itraconazole and fluconazole. *J AIDS* 1993;6:809-819.

Wheat J, Hafner R, Wulfsohn M, et al. Prevention of relapse of histoplasmosis with itraconazole in patients with the acquired immunodeficiency syndrome. *Ann Intern Med* 1993;118:610-616.

Wheat LJ, Batteiger BE, Sathapatayavongs B. *Histoplasma capsulatum* infections of the central nervous system: A clinical review. *Medicine* 1990;69:244-260.

HIV Infection and AIDS

Basics

DEFINITION

- The term *human immunodeficiency virus (HIV) syndrome* is used to describe the cellular and humoral immunodeficiency and the numerous complications that result from the HIV-1 and HIV-2 infections.
- *Acquired immunodeficiency syndrome* (AIDS) is the spectrum of disorders (HIV-wasting, opportunistic infections, or certain malignancies) resulting from advanced HIV infection. Also, any HIV-infected individual with a CD4+ T-lymphocyte (CD4 cell) count of less than 200/mL has AIDS, regardless of the presence of symptoms or opportunistic infections.

ETIOLOGY

- HIV belongs to the family of human retroviruses and the subfamily of lentiviruses.
- The four recognized human retroviruses belong to two distinct groups:
  —The human T-lymphotropic viruses, HTLV-I and HTLV-II
  —The human immunodeficiency viruses, HIV-1 and HIV-2
- The HIV envelope glycoproteins have a high affinity for the CD4 molecule on the surface of CD4 cells. After HIV binds to CD4, the viral and cellular membranes fuse and the HIV nucleoprotein complex enters the cytoplasm. The RNA viral genome undergoes transcription by the virally encoded reverse transcriptase. The double-stranded viral DNA enters into the nucleus, where integration of the DNA provirus into the host chromosome is catalyzed by integrase (another retroviral enzyme).
- When a CD4 cell with integrated provirus is activated, viral particles are assembled and virions are released from the cell by budding. Productive viral replication is lytic to infected T cells.
- A decrease in function as well as number of CD4 cells is central to the immune dysfunction. Other host cells (such as macrophages, dendritic cells, and Langerhans cells) also are infected by HIV, but these cells do not appear to be lysed by the virus.
- Rapid production and turnover of CD4 cells occur throughout the course of HIV infection. Although a highly dynamic, complex equilibrium between HIV and CD4 cells may be maintained for several years, eventually a decline in circulating CD4 cells occurs in almost all HIV-infected individuals.

EPIDEMIOLOGY

- The most common cause of HIV disease throughout the world is HIV-1, which comprises several subtypes with different geographic distributions. In this chapter, we use the terms *HIV* and *HIV-1* interchangeably.
- Since AIDS was recognized as a distinct disease in 1981, over 50 million individuals worldwide have been infected by HIV-1.
- HIV is transmitted by both homosexual and heterosexual contact, by blood and blood products, and by infected mothers to infants either intrapartum, perinatally, or via breast milk.
- Heterosexual contact has been the dominant mode of HIV-1 transmission, accounting for more than 90% of infections recognized since 1990.
- The virus is present in both semen and cervicovaginal secretions. The concurrent presence of other sexually transmitted diseases, especially those associated with genital ulcerations, strongly facilitates sexual transmission of HIV-1.
- Women, in whom HIV infection is most often acquired via heterosexual sex, now comprise the group in which HIV infection is increasing most rapidly in the United States.
- The risk of HIV transmission following skin puncture from a needle that was contaminated with blood from a patient with HIV infection depends on multiple factors (such as the viral load of the patient, the amount of blood on the needle, etc.) and without antiretroviral therapy is about 0.3%.
- Among injecting drug users, HIV infection occurs through parenteral exposure to infected blood via contaminated drug paraphernalia. The risk of infection depends on the prevalence of HIV infection in the area and increases with the duration of injection drug use and the frequency of needle sharing.
- About 25% of infants born to HIV-1 seropositive mothers who are not receiving antiretroviral therapy are infected by HIV-1.
- Prior to the nationwide implementation of a blood-screening test, infection via transfusion of contaminated blood or blood products accounted for nearly 3% of AIDS cases in the United States.
- Case reports described transmission of HIV from HIV-infected health care workers who performed invasive procedures to patients, but the risk is extremely small.
- HIV can be transmitted by blood and blood products, both among individuals who share contaminated paraphernalia (needles and syringes) for injection drug use and in those who receive transfusions of blood and blood products.
- HIV-2 was originally confined to West Africa, but a number of cases have been identified in Europe, South America, Canada, and the United States.
- HIV-2 is spread through sexual contact and via contaminated blood, but unlike HIV-1, perinatal transmission is limited.

Incubation

- Up to 70% of HIV-infected persons experience a mononucleosis-like syndrome from 2 to 8 weeks after initial infection.
- Acute symptoms last 3 days to 3 weeks and include the following:
  —Arthralgias
  —Fever
  —Headache
  —Lymph node enlargement
  —Maculopapular rash
  —Sore throat
- Ten percent to 20% of patients have neurologic involvement, usually presenting as aseptic meningitis with possible cerebrospinal fluid pleocytosis.
- Progression of disease varies greatly among individuals, and the route of HIV transmission does not influence the rate of progression of immunodeficiency.
- Generalized lymph node enlargement occurs in 35% to 60% of asymptomatic HIV-infected persons, may persist for years, and is not significantly associated with either the rate of progression of immunodeficiency or subsequent development of lymphoma.
- Thrombocytopenia is common during early HIV infection.
- Although HIV-2 causes AIDS, the asymptomatic incubation period after infection with HIV-2 appears to be substantially longer than that following HIV-1 infection.

Clinical Manifestations

- HIV-infection is a protean disease, and clinical manifestations can be due to the HIV or its complications.
- The clinician should view HIV disease as a spectrum ranging from primary infection, with or without the acute syndrome, to the asymptomatic stage, to advanced disease.
- Without antiretroviral therapy, approximately 50% of individuals develop AIDS within 10 years after HIV infection; an additional 30% have milder symptoms related to immunodeficiency, and fewer than 20% are entirely asymptomatic.
- The majority of HIV infected individuals are not diagnosed during the acute retroviral syndrome, are unaware of their infection, and are asymptomatic, with CD4 counts greater than 200 cells/mL.

HIV Infection and AIDS

- Mucocutaneous lesions may be the first manifestations of immune dysfunction, especially recurrent genital herpes simplex virus (HSV) infections, polydermatomal varicella zoster infection (shingles), molluscum contagiosum, and oral hairy leukoplakia (a white, lichenified, plaquelike lesion, most commonly seen on the lateral surfaces of the tongue).
- Fever is common among HIV-infected patients and can be due to the following:
  - *Mycobacterium avium* complex
  - Toxoplasmosis
  - Cytomegalovirus (CMV) infection
  - Tuberculosis
  - *Pneumocystis carinii* infection
  - Salmonellosis
  - Cryptococcosis
  - Histoplasmosis
  - Non-Hodgkin's lymphoma
  - Medications
- HIV-infected individuals often present with endocrine abnormalities that include the following:
  - Adrenal insufficiency
  - CMV adrenalitis
  - Growth failure
  - Hypo- and hyperglycemia
  - Hypocalcemia
  - Hypogonadotrophic hypogonadism
  - Impotence
  - Panhypothyroidism
  - *P. carinii* thyroiditis
  - Syndrome of inappropriate antidiuretic hormone secretion
  - Testicular atrophy
- Cough is a common symptom and can be due to the following:
  - *P. carinii* pneumonia
  - Pulmonary Kaposi's sarcoma
  - Sinus disease (sinusitis occurs in 6%–16% of HIV-infected individuals)
  - Bacterial lung infection
  - Tuberculosis
- Diarrhea is very common in advanced HIV disease, and the etiology includes the following:
  - *Campylobacter* spp
  - *Clostridium difficile*
  - *Cryptosporidium*
  - CMV
  - *Microsporidium* spp
  - *Salmonella enteritidis*
  - *Candida*
  - *Cyclosporidium parvum*
  - *Entamoeba histolytica*
  - *Giardia*
  - HIV
  - *Isospora belli*
  - *M. avium* complex
  - *Shigella* spp
- HIV-infected patients can also develop the following:
  - Cutaneous tumors (due to Kaposi's sarcoma, lymphoma, basal cell carcinoma, squamous cell carcinoma, Bowen's disease, or malignant melanoma)
  - Pruritus (due to dry skin, folliculitis, or scabies)
  - Biliary tract disease (due to *Cryptosporidium parvum*, CMV, or Microsporidia)
  - Pain on swallowing and substernal burning that may indicate *Candida* esophagitis, CMV infection, aphthae, or HSV infection
  - Focal neurologic findings (due to toxoplasmosis, lymphoma, progressive multifocal leukoencephalopathy, cryptococcoma, tuberculoma, or aspergillosis)
  - Headache associated with chronic meningitis (usually due to *Cryptococcus neoformans, Mycobacterium tuberculosis*, coccidioidomycosis, or histoplasmosis)
- The earliest clinical manifestation of HIV infection in women may be the frequent recurrence of *Candida* vaginitis.
- AIDS dementia complex can cause intellectual impairment among persons with a CD4 count less than 50 cells/mL. It is characterized by poor concentration, diminished memory, slowing of thought processes, and motor dysfunction.
- Infection due to nontuberculous mycobacteria (*M. avium-intracellulare* complex, etc.) may cause localized disease, but disseminated disease is much more common. This may present with fever, sweats, weight loss, diarrhea, and anemia, and occurs in 30% to 50% of all patients with AIDS at some stage.

Diagnosis

LABORATORY

- Most centers in the United States use an enzyme-linked immunosorbent assay (ELISA) as the primary screening test for HIV infection.
- If the ELISA test is reactive, the test is repeated in duplicate, and if either or both repeat tests are reactive, the sample is considered positive and a Western Blot (WB) or indirect immunofluorescence assay is done on the same sample for confirmation.
- The WB detects antibodies to specific denatured HIV-1 proteins. The absence of all bands is considered a negative test.
- This protocol for HIV-testing usually has a 3- to 4-week "window period" prior to seroconversion, during which results can be negative or indeterminate.
- Use of p24 antigen as a screening test can reduce the window period. However, most experts suggest the use of plasma viral load (PVL) for patients that may be in the window period. Physicians should keep in mind that PVL is very sensitive and was developed for monitoring the progression of the disease and the effectiveness of antiretroviral therapy, and not for establishing the diagnosis of HIV infection.
- Rapid tests are assays done in 30 minutes or less and are warranted only in certain cases (pregnant women in labor who have not been tested, if the patient is likely not to return for the results, etc.).
- An effective but costly home test is also available. Users perform a finger-stick to obtain a dried-blood specimen on filter paper. The specimen is identified by an anonymous code number and mailed to a laboratory for ELISA. Reactive specimens are confirmed by WB or immunofluorescence assay. The users call a toll-free telephone number to obtain test results, counseling, and referrals.
- The first urine ELISA kits has a relatively low specificity (94.2%).

Treatment

- Once HIV infection is recognized, the physician should discuss with the patient the treatment of HIV infection and appropriate use of laboratory studies.
- It is important that the patient understand the rationale for, and be fully committed to, an effective treatment plan before initiation of antiretroviral therapy.
- The following antiretroviral drugs have been approved by the U.S. Food and Drug Administration. (In parenthesis are the abbreviated names, trade names, and some important side effects.)

ANTIRETROVIRAL DRUGS

- Nucleoside reverse transcriptase inhibitors (NRTIs)
  - Abacavir (Ziagen; severe hypersensitivity reaction, headache, gastrointestinal intolerance, insomnia)
  - Didanosine (ddI, Videx; pancreatitis, peripheral neuropathy, gastrointestinal intolerance)
  - Lamivudine (3TC, Epivir; headache, gastrointestinal intolerance, leukopenia)
  - Stavudine (d4T, Zerit; pancreatitis, peripheral neuropathy, hepatitis)
  - Zalcitabine (ddC, Hivid; pancreatitis, peripheral neuropathy, lactic acidosis)
  - Zidovudine (AZT, Retrovir; bone marrow suppression, myopathy, hepatitis, lactic acidosis)
  - A combination of zidovudine and lamivudine is also commercially available (Combivir).
- Nucleotide reverse transcriptase inhibitor
  - Adefovir/dipivoxil (Preveon; gastrointestinal intolerance, nephrotoxicity)

HIV Infection and AIDS

- Nonnucleoside reverse transcriptase inhibitors (nNRTIs)
  - Delavirdine (Rescriptor; rash, fever, liver abnormalities)
  - Efavirenz (Sustiva; rash, nightmares, dizziness)
  - Nevirapine (Viramune; rash, fever, liver abnormalities; the dose of protease inhibitors needs to be increased when used in combination with nevirapine)
- Protease inhibitors (PIs)
  - Amprenavir (Agenerase; gastrointestinal intolerance, oral/perioral paresthesia, rash)
  - Indinavir (Crixivan; nephrolithiasis, asymptomatic increase of bilirubin, gastrointestinal intolerance)
  - Nelfinavir (Viracept; diarrhea, headache)
  - Ritonavir (Norvir; large increases in plasma concentrations of most benzodiazepines and other drugs metabolized through the P450 system, gastrointestinal intolerance)
  - Saquinavir (Invirase (hard gel), Fortovase (soft gel); gastrointestinal intolerance, must be taken with food)

ANTIRETROVIRAL THERAPY

- The objective of antiretroviral therapy should be to maintain the lowest PVL for as long as possible.
- Monotherapy should not be used with any available antiretroviral drug. Also, therapy with two NRTIs results in viral resistance and is not recommended.
- Three-drug combinations are currently recommended for the initiation of treatment in all patients, although it can result in long-term toxicities.
- The optimal time to initiate therapy for asymptomatic patients is uncertain. Experts suggest those patients with CD4 counts below 350 cells/mL and patients with PVLs greater than 20,000 copies/mL will benefit from effective antiretroviral therapy.

- For patients with CD4 counts between 350 and 500 cells/mL, associated with PVLs less than 10,000 copies/mL, it is not clear whether the potential long-term advantages of treatment outweigh the disadvantages.
- Most experts recommend treatment of patients in whom the acute retroviral syndrome is documented.
- When an effective antiretroviral regimen is initiated in an asymptomatic patient with no previous antiretroviral therapy, the PVL should decrease by 100-fold in 8 weeks and decrease to an undetectable level (<50 copies/mL) within 24 weeks.
- Patients continue to receive clinical and immunologic benefit from antiretroviral therapy despite loss of viral control.

MAIN TREATMENT

- Although each of the recommended regimens can result in durable suppression of PVL, associated with gradual recovery of immunologic function, each regimen has specific advantages and potential toxicities of which the patient must be aware.
- The most widely used combination is two NRTIs (AZT, ddI, 3TC, d4T, or ddC) with a protease inhibitor.
- Zidovudine and stavudine should not be used together because antagonism can occur.
- Didanosine and zalcitabine should not be used together because of additive toxicity.
- Initial data suggest that efavirenz can replace the protease inhibitor.
- Therapeutic studies of patients infected with HIV-2 are lacking.
- A syndrome, which includes the development of "buffalo hump," abnormal fat deposition, systemic dyslipidemias, and glucose intolerance and insulin resistance, has been described as a side effect of aggressive antiretroviral therapy.

ALTERNATIVE TREATMENT

- Nevirapine or delavirdine with two NRTIs (AZT, ddI, 3TC, d4T, or ddC)
- Abacavir with two NRTIs (AZT, ddI, 3TC, d4T, or ddC)
- Hydroxyurea has been used in salvage therapy.

TREATMENT FAILURE

There are currently no data that define the threshold at which a change in therapy should occur. Some experts recommend change as soon as the PVL is above detectable limits on two determinations. Other experts prefer to wait until the viral load again exceeds an arbitrary figure of 10,000 to 20,000 copies/mL.

COMPLICATIONS

- Infections that can occur among HIV-infected individuals with greater than 200 CD4 cells/mL:
  - Herpes zoster involving more than one dermatome
  - *M. tuberculosis* (which may be pulmonary, extrapulmonary, or disseminated)
  - Oral hairy leukoplakia
  - Oropharyngeal candidiasis
  - Recurrent bacterial pneumonia: HIV-infected individuals have a threefold to fourfold increase in incidence of bacterial pneumonias caused by common pulmonary pathogens such as *Streptococcus pneumoniae* and *Haemophilus influenzae*.
- Infections that can occur among HIV-infected individuals with fewer than 200 CD4 cells/mL (the asterisk indicates the infections that usually occur with CD4 counts less than 75 to 100 cells/mL):
  - Aspergillosis* (relatively uncommon)
  - *Candida* esophagitis
  - Infection with *C. neoformans**
  - Enteritis due to *C. parvum* or *I. belli**

HIV Infection and AIDS

—CMV retinitis, colitis or esophagitis*
—Disseminated histoplasmosis or coccidioidomycosis
—Encephalitis due to *Toxoplasma gondii**
—Infection due to nontuberculous mycobacteria (*M. avium-intracellulare* complex, etc.)*
—*P. carinii* pneumonia
- Neoplasms associated with advanced HIV:
—High-grade, B-cell, non-Hodgkin's lymphoma
—Immunoblastic sarcoma
—Invasive carcinoma of the cervix
—Kaposi's sarcoma
—Primary brain lymphoma
—Undifferentiated non-Hodgkin's lymphoma

Follow-Up

- PVL assays should be repeated at 3- to 4-month intervals during therapy.
- Patients with AIDS should receive prophylaxis against *P. carinii, T. gondii, M. avium* complex, and, usually, CMV.
- Prophylaxis is very effective against recurrent HSV-2 infection (acyclovir) and recurrent *Candida* esophagitis (fluconazole), but should generally be reserved for those patients with recurrent symptomatic disease (for details, see relevant chapters for each infection). The current recommendations for prophylaxis can be accessed at www.hivatis.org.
- Immunization against *S. pneumoniae*, flu-vaccine (repeated yearly), and serologic testing for *T. gondii* and syphilis should be performed early in the course of HIV infection.

- Purified protein-derivative testing, in conjunction with chest radiograph, is recommended. Induration of 5 mm or more should be considered positive. Any patient with a positive PPD should be evaluated for the presence of active tuberculosis; if no active disease is present, the patient should receive 1 year of prophylaxis with isoniazid or combination drug therapy for a shorter time period.
- HIV-infected women show an increased prevalence of high-grade squamous intracellular lesions on Papanicolaou (Pap) smear. Women should therefore obtain two Pap smears at a 6-month interval; if the initial two Pap smears are both normal, repeat smears should be done once a year.

PREVENTION

- Adaptation to safer sexual practices has been associated with a decrease in incidence of HIV infection.
- Treatment of HIV-infected women with zidovudine during the third trimester of pregnancy and during delivery, followed by zidovudine treatment of the infant for 6 weeks, decreases maternal–fetal transmission from 25% to 8%. Studies now in progress suggest that administration of combination antiretroviral therapy will further decrease HIV infection in children born to HIV-infected mothers.
- The use of universal blood and body fluid precautions is routinely recommended to protect health care workers. Prompt administration of a combination regimen of indinavir, zidovudine, and lamivudine significantly decreases the likelihood of HIV infection following needle-stick injuries.

Selected Readings

Anonymous. Guidelines for the use of antiretroviral agents in HIV-infected adults and adolescents. Department of Health and Human Services and the Henry J. Kaiser Family Foundation. *Ann Intern Med* 1998;128(12, Pt 2):1079–1100.

Carpenter CC, Fischl MA, Hammer SM, et al. Antiretroviral therapy for HIV infection in 1998: Updated recommendations of the International AIDS Society–USA Panel. *JAMA* 1998;280:78–86.

Centers for Disease Control and Prevention. Update: Provisional recommendations for chemoprophylaxis after occupational exposure to human immunodeficiency virus. *MMWR Morbid Mortal Wkly Rep* 1996;45:468–472.

Chodock R, Mylonakis E, Shemin D, Runarsdottir V, Yodice P, Renzi R, Tashima K, Towe C, Rich JD. Survival of a human immunodeficiency patient with nucleoside-induced lactic acidosis—role of haemodialysis treatment. *Nephrology, Dialysis, Transplantation* 1999;14(10): 2484–2486.

Ho DD, Newman AU, Perelson AS, et al. Rapid turnover of plasma virions and CD4 lymphocytes in HIV-1 infection. *Nature* 1995;362:355–358.

Hofbauer LC. Heufelder AE. Endocrine implications of human immunodeficiency virus infection. *Medicine* 1996;75:262–278.

Mylonakis E, Merriman NA, Rich JD, Flanigan TP, Walters BC, Tashima KT, Mileno MD, van der Horst CM. Use of cerebrospinal fluid shunt for the management of elevated intracranial pressure in a patient with active AIDS-related cryptococcal meningitis. *Diagnostic Microbiology & Infectious Disease* 1999;34(2):111–114.

Mylonakis E, Paliou M, Greenbough TC, Flaningan TP, Letvin NL, Rich JD. Report of a false-positive HIV test result and the potential use of additional tests in establishing HIV serostatus. *Archives of Internal Medicine* 2000;160(15):2386–2388.

Mylonakis E, Paliou M, Lally M, Flanigan TP, Rich JD. Laboratory testing for infection with the human immunodeficiency virus: established and novel approaches. *American Journal of Medicine* 2000;109(7):568–576.

Saag M, Holodniy M, Kuritzkes DR, et al. HIV viral load markers in clinical practice: Recommendations of an International AIDS Society—USA Expert Panel. *Nat Med* 1996;2:625–629.

Infectious Mononucleosis

Basics

DEFINITION

The term *mononucleosis* refers to a common, acute syndrome characterized by fever, lymphadenopathy, exudative pharyngitis, and atypical lymphocytosis.

ETIOLOGY

- The cause of infectious mononucleosis is Epstein-Barr virus (EBV), which belongs to the herpesviruses group.
- A proportion of patients with a syndrome practically identical to infectious mononucleosis have other causative agents (not EBV). The main cause of this infectious mononucleosis–like syndrome is cytomegalovirus (CMV). Other possible causes are toxoplasmosis, drugs, syphilis, and viruses, including HIV and members of the herpesviruses group other than EBV and CMV, such as human herpesvirus type 6 (HHV-6).

EPIDEMIOLOGY

Incidence and Prevalence

- EBV usually causes a subclinical or mild infection, especially in young children.
- If the primary infection with EBV is delayed and occurs during the second half of the second decade or the third decade of life, a clinically apparent syndrome of infectious mononucleosis may occur. This fact is the main cause for the observed major differences in incidence of infectious mononucleosis in various populations.
- Infectious mononucleosis was found to have an annual incidence of about 45 cases per 100,000 persons in a large epidemiologic study in a general population in the United States.
- The syndrome was about 30 times more common in Whites than in Blacks.
- Infectious mononucleosis is diagnosed more commonly among adolescents and young adults (15–25 years old) of higher socioeconomic groups in industrialized countries.
- The incubation period of infectious mononucleosis is highly variable. It is estimated usually to be 30 to 60 days.

Risk Factors

- Humans are the only source of EBV.
- Close personal contact with a person with subclinical EBV infection is common before manifestation of clinical infectious mononucleosis.
- Persons with an inherited, maternally derived, recessive genetic defect may develop a severe, sometimes fatal lymphoproliferative syndrome due to EBV infection. This X-linked lymphoproliferative disorder due to EBV is also known as Duncan's disease and occurs in boys.

Clinical Manifestations

SYMPTOMS AND SIGNS

- EBV has been associated with several clinical syndromes, including the following:
  - Infectious mononucleosis syndrome
  - Burkitt's lymphoma
  - B-cell lymphoma of the central nervous system
  - Posttransplant lymphoproliferative disorder
  - Nasopharyngeal carcinoma
  - Hairy leukoplakia
- Infectious mononucleosis is manifested with a variety of symptoms and signs. The most common presentation is a febrile illness with exudative pharyngitis (sore throat, white or grey exudate covering mainly the tonsils), and lymphadenopathy (mainly in the neck but sometimes also in the axillary and inguinal areas).
- Based on observations from large series of patients with infectious mononucleosis, the following symptoms and signs may be manifested (with indicative proportion of patients who had the various symptoms and signs).
- Symptoms
  - Fever (>90%)
  - Sore throat (82%)
  - Malaise (57%)
  - Headache (51%)
  - Anorexia (21%)
  - Myalgias (20%)
  - Chills (16%)
  - Nausea (12%)
  - Abdominal discomfort (9%)
  - Cough (5%)
  - Vomiting (5%)
  - Arthralgias (2%)
- Signs
  - Lymphadenopathy (94%)
  - Pharyngitis (84%)
  - Splenomegaly (52%)
  - Hepatomegaly (12%)
  - Palatal enanthem (11%)
  - Rash (10%)
  - Jaundice (9%)
- A maculopapular rash appears commonly in patients with mononucleosis who receive a penicillin-type antibiotic (especially ampicillin).

Diagnosis

DIFFERENTIAL DIAGNOSIS

- Patients with atypical lymphocytosis are most likely to have infectious mononucleosis. However other causes include the following:
  - Cytomegalovirus (CMV)
  - Toxoplasmosis
  - Human herpesvirus type 6 (HHV-6)
  - Human immunodeficiency virus (HIV), especially during the acute infection phase
  - Infectious hepatitis
  - Syphilis
  - Measles
  - Mumps
  - Rubella
  - Adenoviral infections
  - Coxsackievirus
  - Drug hypersensitivity reactions
  - Others

LABORATORY

- An important laboratory finding in infectious mononucleosis is the increased number of lymphocytes, including a considerable proportion with atypical morphology (atypical lymphocytes).
- In addition, increased transaminases are found frequently in patients with infectious mononucleosis.
- Thrombocytopenia (usually mild) is also common.
- However, more specific tests are helpful for the diagnosis of infectious mononucleosis, and these are the detection of heterophile antibodies and specific antibodies against EBV.
- Heterophile antibodies may be demonstrable at the onset of the illness or may appear later, during the course of the illness.
- There are several commercial kits for detection of heterophile antibodies. The clinician should become aware of the sensitivity and specificity of the tests performed at the local laboratory.
- Multiple specific serologic tests detect specific antibodies against antigens of EBV. It should be stressed that determination of the presence of EBV-specific antibodies is not indicated for use in every patient to document infectious mononucleosis. Over 90% of patients with infectious mononucleosis will have a positive heterophile antibodies test, which suffices for the diagnosis of an acute EBV infection. In addition, there are only few false-positive results of the heterophile antibodies test if it is performed correctly.

Infectious Mononucleosis

- The specific antibodies most commonly identified in EBV infections are directed against the following EBV antigens:
  - VCA (viral capsid antigen) (IgM antibody)
  - VCA (IgG antibody)
  - Early antigen (anti-D)
  - Early antigen (anti-R)
  - EBNA (Epstein-Barr nuclear antigen)

Treatment

MAIN TREATMENT

- Only symptomatic treatment is usually needed for the majority of patients with clinically apparent infectious mononucleosis.
- Corticosteroids are used in cases of severe infectious mononucleosis with complications such as tonsillar inflammation causing airway obstruction, myocarditis, pericarditis, massive splenomegaly, hemolytic anemia, severe thrombocytopenia, and nervous system abnormalities.
- The preferred dose is prednisone 1 mg/kg/d in a split daily regimen, which is quickly tapered over a period of 7 to 14 days.
- The use of corticosteroids to reduce fever and malaise and improve the feeling of well-being is not recommended in uncomplicated cases of infectious mononucleosis.

ALTERNATIVE TREATMENT

The benefits of specific antiviral treatment, such as with acyclovir, have not been demonstrated for use in patients with infectious mononucleosis.

COMPLICATIONS

- Complications occur rarely in patients with infectious mononucleosis.
- Autoimmune hemolytic anemia (occurs in about 2% of patients)
- Severe thrombocytopenia
- Airway obstruction due to severe tonsillar enlargement
- Neurologic complications (encephalitis, myelitis, Guillain-Barré syndrome, and others)
- Splenic rupture (caution in palpation of spleen during physical examination and avoidance of contact sports are recommended)
- Severe hepatitis
- Myocarditis
- Pericarditis
- Pneumonia
- Lymphoproliferative disorders in susceptible patients (patients who receive immunosuppressive agents, severe immunodeficiency due to HIV, or genetic predisposition, such as individuals with Duncan's syndrome)

Follow-Up

- Follow-up is not necessary for patients with mild infectious mononucleosis who had full recovery.
- Careful follow-up is needed for those with moderate or severe infectious mononucleosis, to promptly detect and appropriately manage potential complications.

PREVENTION

- Patients with a recent history of infectious mononucleosis should not donate blood products.
- Avoid drinking beverages from a common container, to decrease contact with the saliva of an affected person.

Selected Readings

Bender CE. The value of corticosteroids in the treatment mononucleosis. *JAMA* 1967;15:529–531.

Buchwald D, Sullivan JL, Komaroff AL. Frequency of "chronic active Epstein-Barr virus infection" in a general medical practice. *JAMA* 1987;257:2303–2307.

Calender A, Billaud M, Aubry JP, et al. Epstein-Barr virus (EBV) induces expression of B-cell activation markers on in vitro infection of EBV-negative B-lymphoma cells. *Proc Natl Acad Sci U S A* 1987;84:8060–8064.

Fleisher GR, Pasquariello PS, Warren WS, et al. Intrafamilial transmission of Epstein-Barr virus infection among six adult family. *Scand J Infect Dis* 1990;22:363–366.

Ho M, Kaffe R, Miller G, et al. The frequency of Epstein-Barr virus infection and associated lymphoproliferative syndrome after transplantation and its manifestations in children. *Transplantation* 1988;45:719–727.

Horwitz CA, Henle W, Henle G, et al. Heterophile negative infectious mononucleosis and mononucleosis-like illness. Laboratory confirmation of 43 cases. *Am J Med* 1977;63:947–957.

Horwitz CA, Henle W, Henle G, et al. Long-term serological follow-up of patients for Epstein-Barr virus after recovery from infectious mononucleosis. *J Infect Dis* 1985;151:1150–1153.

Peter EM, Gordon LA. Nonsurgical treatment or splenic hemorrhage in an adult with infectious mononucleosis. *Am J Med* 1986;80:123–125.

Sumaya CV, Ench Y. Epstein-Barr virus infection mononucleosis in children. I. Clinical and general laboratory findings. *Pediatrics* 1985;75:1003–1010.

van der Horst C, Joncas H, Aronheim G, et al. Lack of effect of peroral acyclovir for the treatment of infectious mononucleosis. *J Infect Dis* 1991;164:788–792.

Weiss LM, Movahed LA, Warnke RA, et al. Detection of Epstein-Barr virus genomes in Reed-Sternberg cells of Hodgkin's disease. *N Engl J Med* 1989;320:5026.

Influenza

Basics

DEFINITION
Influenza is a zoonotic and emerging respiratory tract virus that can sporadically cause great mortality in a worldwide distribution. The virus leads to damage of the upper or lower respiratory tract.

ETIOLOGY
- Orthomyxoviridae family virus
- Complex lipid-containing envelope with glycoproteins hemagglutinin (HA) and neuraminidase (NA) on the surface
- Internal nucleoproteins determine the type (A, B, C) of the virus.
- HA and NA determine the antigenicity of the virus.
- The genome is negative-stranded RNA.
- It is unique in that the genome is divided into eight separate segments.
- Arrangement of these genomes into the virus leads to a variation that is unique to influenza.
- Antigenic drift, causing mild disease, occurs with mutations of the HA and NA glycoproteins.
- Antigenic shift, often leading to serious disease, occurs with reassortment of the HA and or NA glycoproteins.

EPIDEMIOLOGY
- Worldwide illness occurs in temperate zones during the colder winter months.
- Influenza causes yearly disease and epidemics every 2 to 3 years.
- It causes pandemics with higher mortality every 10 to 20 years.
- Severity of disease is determined by the prevalence of antibodies to the virus in the community.
- The influenza virus is a zoonosis, affecting aquatic birds, chickens, and swine.
- Re-assortment of HA or NA from bird species or swine has the potential for causing disease in humans.
- Bacterial superinfection leads to pneumonia, a major complication of influenza.

Risk Factors
- Risk factors for severe disease include the following:
  - Old age
  - Poor health
  - Lack of antibodies to specific HA and NA proteins on the viral surface

Incubation
- Usually 1 to 2 days

Clinical Manifestations

- Acute onset of fever, cough, myalgias, and headache
- Fevers last 3 to 4 days.
- Sore throat and rhinorrhea may be present.
- Influenza may lead to croup.
- Influenza may lead to pneumonia, which can progress to acute respiratory distress syndrome (ARDS).
- Bacterial superinfection leading to pneumonia often occurs 5 to 7 days after onset of viral symptoms. This is associated with re-emergence of fevers and worsening of cough.
- Myocarditis and pericarditis have been associated with influenza.

Diagnosis

DIFFERENTIAL DIAGNOSIS
- Viral upper respiratory illness
- Respiratory syncytial virus (RSV), adenovirus
- Pneumococcal pneumonia
- Atypical pneumonias such as *Legionella*, *Mycoplasma*

Influenza

LABORATORY

- Cell culture diagnosis from secretions takes 3 to 5 days when available.
- Shell viral rapid assays are available.
- Serology is available for diagnosis.

Treatment

- Rimantadine is used for treatment of type-A influenza. To be most effective, it is started in the first 48 hours of illness, and can be discontinued 24 to 48 hours after symptoms abate; 100 mg orally twice per day.
- Zanamivir is used in treatment of types A and B influenza; two inhalations twice a day for 5 days if given within 48 hours of onset of symptoms.
- Oseltamivir is used in treatment of types A and B influenza; 75 mg orally twice a day for 5 days.

COMPLICATIONS

- Bacterial pneumonia is the most feared complication of influenza, and is associated with the greatest morbidity and mortality.
- Reye's syndrome has been seen in children with influenza who are given salicylates. These drugs should be avoided.

Follow-Up

- None needed

PREVENTION

- Inactivated influenza vaccine is available annually in the fall and should be administered to the following:
  —The elderly
  —Persons with chronic diseases
  —Nursing home patients
  —Children on long-term aspirin therapy
  —Health care workers
- Chemoprophylaxis should be given to the following:
  —Nonimmunized persons residing in nursing facilities
  —Persons with chronic medical or pulmonary conditions
  —Children who are on chronic aspirin therapy
  —Chemoprophylaxis should be given only during the peak period of infection.

Selected Readings

Baker WH, Mullooly JP. Pneumonia and influenza deaths during epidemics: Implications for prevention. *JAMA* 1982;142:84–89.

Douglas RG. Prophylaxis and treatment of influenza. *N Engl J Med* 1990;322:443–450.

Glezen WP, Payne AA, Snyder DN, et al. Mortality and influenza. *J Infect Dis* 1982;146:313–321.

Intraabdominal Abscesses

Basics

DEFINITION

- An intraabdominal abscess is a localized collection of microorganisms and neutrophils in a fibrous capsule associated with tissues, organs, or confined spaces of the abdomen.
- Abscesses may stud the peritoneal cavity; lie within the omentum or mesentery; develop on the surface of viscera, such as liver, spleen, or kidney; or be confined in any abdominal organ. Based on their location, intraabdominal abscesses are divided into the following categories:
  —Intraperitoneal (subphrenic, subhepatic, paracolic, lesser sac, interloop, etc.)
  —Visceral
  —Retroperitoneal

ETIOLOGY

- Intraperitoneal abscesses result from either of the following:
  —Primary or secondary peritonitis
  —Spread of the infection from an adjacent organ
- The liver is the organ most commonly subject to the development of abscesses. Liver abscesses generally arise from the following:
  —Contiguous foci of infection
  —Hematogenous spread
  —Track from other intraabdominal sources
- Splenic abscesses are associated with the following:
  —Bacterial endocarditis
  —Hemoglobinopathy
  —Immunosuppression
  —Injecting drug use
  —Myeloproliferative disease
  —Primary spleen disease
  —Septicemia
  —Trauma
- Perinephric and renal abscesses result from the following:
  —Prior urologic surgery
  —Renal stones
  —Structural abnormalities of the urinary tract
  —Trauma
  —Urinary tract infection
  —Staphylococcal bacteremia
- Some reviews on intraabdominal abscesses also include discussion on pelvic and psoas abscesses. However, in this book these two topics are discussed elsewhere (see Section II chapters, "Pelvic Inflammatory Disease" and "Myositis").

Most Common Pathogens

- Intraperitoneal abscesses
  —*Bacteroides fragilis* (found in 65% of intraabdominal infections overall)
  —Enterobacteriaceae (usually *Escherichia coli*, *Proteus* spp, and *Klebsiella* spp)
  —Anaerobic cocci
  —Enterococci
  —*Staphylococcus aureus*
- Hepatic abscesses
  —Enterobacteriaceae
  —*B. fragilis*
  —Enterococci
  —*Entamoeba histolytica*
  —*Candida* spp
- Splenic abscesses from endocarditis or hematogenous spread
  —Staphylococci (usually *S. aureus*)
  —Streptococci
  —*Candida* spp
- Splenic abscesses from intraabdominal site
  —Enterobacteriaceae
  —Enterococci
  —Streptococci
  —Staphylococci
  —Anaerobes
  —*Salmonella* spp
- Pancreatic abscesses
  —Enterobacteriaceae
  —Enterococci
  —Staphylococci
  —Anaerobes
  —*Candida* spp
- Perinephric abscesses
  —Enterobacteriaceae
  —Staphylococci
  —*Candida* spp

EPIDEMIOLOGY

- Men are two to three times more likely to develop intraabdominal abscesses.
- The highest incidence is in the third to fifth decade.
- Of all intraabdominal abscesses, greater than 70% are not associated with a specific organ.
- In children, appendicitis is the cause of 50% of subphrenic abscesses, while in adults, perihepatic abscesses are usually associated with surgical complications.
- Liver and spleen abscesses due to *Candida* spp are more common among immunosuppressed patients, and are multilocular in more than 90% of cases.
- Bacterial splenic abscesses are unilocular in more than 70% of cases.
- Spleen abscesses due to *Salmonella* spp are more common among patients with sickle cell anemia.
- Splenic and perinephric abscesses are more common among patients with diabetes mellitus.
- Pancreatic abscesses complicate up to 9% of acute pancreatitis cases.

Clinical Manifestations

SYMPTOMS

- Intraabdominal abscesses usually present with fever and abdominal pain. However, the presentation is often nonspecific; therefore, clinical suspicion must be high.
- Patients with liver abscess and particularly those who have associated active biliary tract disease may present with symptoms and signs localized to the right upper quadrant, including pain, guarding, and tenderness. Nonspecific symptoms, such as chills, anorexia, weight loss, nausea, and vomiting, also may develop.
- Fever of unknown origin may be the only presenting manifestation of liver abscess, especially in the elderly.
- Half of patients with splenic abscesses have abdominal pain, and the pain is localized to the left upper quadrant in only half of those.
- Flank and abdominal pain is common in perinephric and renal abscesses. Pain may be referred to the groin or leg. At least 50% of patients are febrile.
- Clinical findings do not distinguish pancreatitis itself from complications such as pancreatic pseudocyst, pancreatic abscess, or intraabdominal collections of pus.

SIGNS

- Only half of patients with liver abscesses have localized signs (right upper quadrant tenderness, hepatomegaly, or jaundice).
- Half of patients with splenic abscesses have clinically significant splenomegaly.
- *Candida* spp may spread to the kidney via the hematogenous route or by ascension from the bladder. The hallmark of the latter route of infection is ureteral obstruction with large fungal balls.

Diagnosis

DIFFERENTIAL DIAGNOSIS

Please see the Section I chapter, "Abdominal Pain and Fever."

LABORATORY

- Amebic serologic testing gives positive results in more than 95% of cases; thus, a negative result helps to exclude this diagnosis.
- Laboratory findings associated with liver abscess include the following:
  —Elevated alkaline phosphatase
  —Leukocytosis
  —Elevated bilirubin

Intraabdominal Abscesses

- —Anemia
- —Elevated aspartate aminotransferase
- —Hypoalbuminemia
- —Bacteremia
- Patients with splenic abscess usually have leukocytosis, and about half of them have positive blood cultures.

IMAGING

- Liver abscess is sometimes suggested by chest radiography, especially if a new elevation of the right hemidiaphragm is seen; other suggestive findings include a right basilar infiltrate and a right pleural effusion.
- Abdominal computerized tomography (CT) has the highest yield in the diagnosis of intraabdominal abscesses.
- Ultrasonography is especially useful for the right upper quadrant and kidneys.
- Gallium- and indium-labeled white blood cell (WBC) scans may be useful in finding an abscess, but, in most cases, these tests must be followed by a CT. Abscesses contiguous with or contained within outpouchings of bowel are particularly difficult to diagnose with scanning procedures.
- In splenic abscesses, chest radiography demonstrates elevation of the left hemidiaphragm and pleural effusion in 70% of patients.

DIAGNOSTIC PROCEDURES

- A diagnostic aspirate of abscess contents should be obtained before the initiation of empiric therapy.
- Some authors have advocated early needle aspiration of pancreatic collections under CT guidance as a mean of distinguishing pancreatic pseudocysts from abscesses.
- On occasion, exploratory laparotomy must be undertaken if an abscess is strongly suspected on clinical grounds, although this procedure has been less commonly used since the advent of CT.

Treatment

MAIN TREATMENT

- The treatment of intraabdominal abscesses involves the establishment of the initial focus of infection, the administration of broad-spectrum antibiotics targeted at organisms involved in the associated infection, and the performance of a drainage procedure.
- For practicing surgeons "in the trenches," the old adage, "Never let the sun set on undrained pus," still applies.
- Factors that favor primary surgical intervention, and not percutaneous drainage, include the following:
  - —An abscess that is inaccessible via the percutaneous route
  - —Associated disease that requires surgery
  - —Lack of a clinical response to percutaneous drainage in 4 to 7 days
  - —Lack of an experienced radiologist or adequate surgical backup
  - —Multilocular or vascular abscess
  - —Large or multiple abscesses
  - —Viscous abscess contents that tend to plug the catheter
- Antimicrobial therapy should be individualized, based on culture and sensitivity results.
- Empiric antibiotic management of intraperitoneal or liver abscesses should be directed against Enterobacteriaceae and *B. fragilis*. Aminoglycosides and second- or third-generation cephalosporins are effective against Enterobacteriaceae, while metronidazole is the most widely used agent against *B. fragilis*.
- The duration of therapy should be individualized based on location, successful drainage, clinical course, and follow-up imaging studies.
- The antibiotic combination should be adjusted when resistant Enterobacteriaceae are the possible culprits.
- If ameba serology is positive, monotherapy with metronidazole may suffice (see the Section II chapter, "Amebiasis").
- Liver abscesses due to *Candida* spp usually require lengthy administration of amphotericin B (500 mg i.v. over 10–14 days), although recent reports have described successful maintenance therapy with fluconazole after an initial course of amphotericin.
- Because of the high mortality rate associated with splenic abscesses, the treatment of choice is splenectomy with adjunctive antibiotics.
- When splenic or perinephric abscess is due to endocarditis or bacteremia, nafcillin, a first-generation cephalosporin, or vancomycin can be used.
- Pancreatic abscess requires early surgical treatment. Imipenem, cefoxitin, ticarcillin–clavulanic acid, piperacillin–tazobactam, and meropenem are the antibiotics used most often.
- Antibiotics for the management of perinephric abscesses associated with urinary tract infection should be directed against Enterobacteriaceae (see chapter "Urethritis and Urethral Discharge").

ALTERNATIVE TREATMENT

- Selected cases, especially those with amebic liver abscess or intraabdominal abscess associated with diverticulitis, can be managed medically but under close combined medical and surgical monitoring.
- Percutaneous drainage has been successful in selected cases of splenic abscess.
- Imipenem and piperacillin–tazobactam are active against *B. fragilis*.

COMPLICATIONS

N/A

Follow-Up

- Always give pneumococcal vaccine to patients who undergo splenectomy.
- If a renal abscess or perinephric abscess is diagnosed, nephrolithiasis should be excluded, especially when a high urinary pH suggests the presence of a urea-splitting organism.
- Close surgical and medical monitoring accompanied by imaging studies is necessary in all cases of intraabdominal abscesses.

PROGNOSIS

- Mortality due to liver abscesses, despite treatment, averages 15%.
- The clinical suspicion for splenic abscess needs to be high, as this condition frequently is fatal if left untreated. Even in the most recently published series, diagnosis was made only at autopsy in 37% of cases.

PREVENTION

- Early and appropriate medical and surgical management of peritonitis, urinary tract infections, and other conditions that predispose to intraabdominal abscesses

Selected Readings

Gorbach SL. Good and laudable pus. *J Clin Invest* 1995;96:2545.

Herman P, Oliveira E, Silva A, et al. Splenic abscess. *Br J Surg* 1995;82:355.

Zalesnik DF, Kasper DL. Intraabdominal infections and abscesses. In: Fauci AS, Braunwald E, Isselbacher KJ, et al., eds. *Harrison's principles of medicine*, 14th ed. New York: McGraw-Hill, 1998:792–796.

Kaposi's Sarcoma

Basics

DEFINITION
Kaposi's sarcoma (KS) is a neoplastic disease that, prior to the AIDS epidemic, was noted to be confined to people from Eastern Europe or those of Mediterranean descent. Since the 1980s, cases have been prevalent in HIV-infected people, this being the most common tumor in this population. KS has also been described in HIV-uninfected individuals and in patients who have had solid-organ transplants and immunosuppressive medications.

ETIOLOGY
- KS is caused by a neoplastic proliferation of spindle cells and other vascular substances.
- Human herpesvirus type 8 (HHV-8) has been isolated from KS lesions, as well as peripheral blood mononuclear cells of affected patients.
- The type-8 virus is sexually transmitted, with viral detection noted in the semen.
- Infection with this virus, in association with profound defects in cell-mediated immunity, leads to a complex mechanism that results in malignant transformation of spindle cells and the development of KS.

EPIDEMIOLOGY
- KS is a rare tumor, first described in 1872.
- It was often described in elderly men of Eastern European or Mediterranean descent, and in patients immunosuppressed due to transplantation.
- In the 1980s, increases in the numbers of homosexual men with KS were noted.
- Between 1981 and 1983, KS was the AIDS-defining illness in 50% of homosexual men in some locales.
- A gradual fall in incidence has been noted over the past 15 years.

Clinical Manifestations

- In elderly men, the disease is often indolent. Lesions are noted mainly on the lower legs.
- In HIV-infected people, the course of KS is quite variable. It appears to be most aggressive with lower CD4 counts. At times, spontaneous remission or regression is noted. This is much more likely after initiation of highly active antiretroviral therapy.
- Patients with AIDS often present with multiple painless, firm, purple skin nodules. In dark-skinned patients, the nodules appear brown or black. Often, the lesions are less than 2 cm, but may increase in size and coalesce with neighboring lesions.
- Lesions can appear anywhere over the entire body, in the conjunctivae, and in the oral cavity. Oral examination may find lesions within the hard palate or gingivae.
- Facial edema or edema of the extremities suggests lymph node involvement. Lymphedema may be massive and lead to recurrent infections and marked morbidity.
- Involvement of the gastrointestinal tract or the lung and airways is common.
- On rare occasions, perforation, bleeding, or obstruction of the gastrointestinal tract may occur; however, these side effects are rare.
- Pulmonary involvement leads to cough and dyspnea. Respiratory failure can occur rapidly in some cases.

Kaposi's Sarcoma

Diagnosis

- Diagnosis is made with histologic examination of biopsy material.
- In the gastrointestinal tract, lesions may be submucosal and less apparent.
- In the respiratory tract, lesions are often endobronchial and appear violaceous. Biopsy of the lesions may lead to bleeding, and the procedure is risky.
- A gallium scan can be useful in determining the nature of the pulmonary involvement. Infections are gallium avid. KS will produce a negative gallium scan.
- Chest x-ray shows a variable pattern in patients with pulmonary involvement. Pleural effusions and hilar adenopathy are frequently seen. Nodular infiltrates are often present; however, a diffuse interstitial infiltrate can be seen in one-third of cases.

Treatment

- There is no evidence that treatment of KS prolongs the life of patients with AIDS.
- Treatment of AIDS, with the initiation of highly active antiretroviral therapy, often leads to remission of disease and accompanying regression of lesions.
- Local treatment of lesions can affect cosmesis or reduce the amount of lymphedema present.
- Injection of small lesions with vinblastine has had good results, as has external beam radiotherapy.
- Small lesions may be treated with liquid nitrogen.
- Systemic therapy with liposomal doxorubicin and daunorubicin, as well as paclitaxel, has had excellent results. Other agents, such as etoposide, vincristine, and bleomycin, are active, and are often used in combination with other drugs.
- Interferon-alfa in high doses has shown a response.
- Steroids have been shown to enhance proliferation of the tumor.

COMPLICATIONS

- Painful and bulky lesions can occur throughout the body.
- Lymph node involvement can lead to marked lymphedema beyond the affected areas.
- Pulmonary involvement can lead to rapid respiratory failure if not treated promptly.

Follow-Up

- Patients should follow up with both infectious disease specialists and oncologists.
- Every effort should be made to continue highly active antiretroviral therapy in patients in remission.

PREVENTION

- It is likely that the HHV-8 is transmitted sexually; therefore, patients should continue to use a barrier method with any sexual activity.
- At present, screening for HHV-8 is not available.

Selected Readings

Biggar RJ, Rabkin CS. The epidemiology of AIDS-related neoplasms. *Hematol Oncol Clin North Am* 1996;10:997.

Gill PS, Akil B, Colletti P, et al. Pulmonary Kaposi's sarcoma: Clinical findings and results of therapy. *Am J Med* 1989;87:57.

Moore PS, Chang Y. Detection of herpesvirus-like DNA sequences in Kaposi's sarcoma in patients with and without HIV infection. *N Engl J Med* 1995;332:1181.

Kawasaki Syndrome

Basics

DEFINITION
- Acute vasculitis in children, which, if untreated, may lead to aneurysms of the coronary arteries

ETIOLOGY
- Disease is due to immune activation; however, an infectious cause has yet to be discovered.
- Possible etiology includes superantigens related to staphylococcal or streptococcal exotoxins.

EPIDEMIOLOGY
- Disease occurs worldwide.
- In Japan, rates of infection in children under the age of 5 years is 90 of 100,000.
- Disease occurs in epidemics, usually in the winter and spring.
- Infection spread among household members is rare.
- Most cases occur between ages 10 and 18 months.

Clinical Manifestations

- Fever for at least 5 days without explanation, often over 40°C
- In addition to fever, four of the following five criteria:
  —Extremity changes, including erythema of palms and soles, induration, and desquamation. Desquamation occurs after 2 weeks of fevers.
  —Polymorphous rash that begins approximately 5 days after fever begins
  —Nonexudative bulbar conjunctivitis
  —Oral cavity changes, including hyperemia, lip edema and erythema, or strawberry tongue
  —Cervical lymphadenopathy

Diagnosis

DIFFERENTIAL DIAGNOSIS
- Viral infections such as adenovirus, cytomegalovirus, Epstein-Barr virus, and influenza
- Group A *Streptococcus* infections, including scarlet fever
- Rocky Mountain spotted fever
- Toxic shock syndrome
- Allergic reactions
- Juvenile rheumatoid arthritis

Kawasaki Syndrome

LABORATORY

- Nonspecific abnormalities
  —Elevated WBC, thrombocytosis
  —Elevated erythrocyte sedimentation rate

IMAGING

- ECGs show tachycardia, along with ST, T, and QT changes.
- Echocardiogram reveals aneurysms in the coronary arteries in 25% of children who are untreated.

Treatment

- It is important to treat as early as possible once the diagnosis is entertained.
- Intravenous immunoglobulin 2 mg/kg in 12 hours as a single infusion: Use before day 10 of illness may reduce the incidence of aneurysm formation.
- Acetylsalicylic acid 80 to 100 mg/kg/d in four divided doses until afebrile, then 3 to 5 mg/kg/d for 6 to 8 weeks
- Antibiotics are not indicated for this syndrome.

COMPLICATIONS

- Cardiac disease with coronary aneurysms occurs in 25% of those untreated or in those treated late in the disease (after 10 days).
- Infarction and sudden death occur most often within 1 year of disease onset.
- One-half of all children with documented aneurysms have regression of the aneurysms over time.
- Recurrent disease has been documented.

Follow-Up

- Children need to have an echocardiogram in 6 to 8 weeks and at 1 year following illness.
- Any evidence of coronary aneurysms should be referred to a pediatric cardiologist.

PREVENTION

There is no way to prevent this syndrome. Patients who recover may have a higher incidence of recurrent disease.

Selected Readings

Melish ME, Hicks RM, Larson EJ. Mucocutaneous lymph node syndrome in the United States. *Am J Dis Child* 1976;130:599–607.

Newburger JW, Takahashi M, Burns JC, et al. The treatment of Kawasaki syndrome with intravenous gamma globulin. *N Engl J Med* 1986;315:341–347.

Rowley AH, Shulman ST. Current therapy for acute Kawasaki syndrome. *J Pediatr* 1991;118:987–991.

Keratitis

Basics

DEFINITION
Keratitis is inflammation of the cornea due to infectious or noninfectious causes.

ETIOLOGY
- Worldwide, the two leading causes of blindness from keratitis are trachoma from chlamydial infection and vitamin A deficiency related to malnutrition. Other infectious causes include the following:
  — Bacteria: *Acinetobacter calcoaceticus, Aeromonas hydrophila, Bacillus* spp, *Bartonella henselae, Borrelia burgdorferi, Brucella* spp, *Clostridium* (*C. perfringens* and *C. tetani*), *Corynebacterium diphtheriae, Enterococcus* spp, *Escherichia coli, Klebsiella pneumoniae, Moraxella* spp, *Morganella morganii, Mycobacterium tuberculosis* and atypica, *Mycobacteria, Neisseria gonorrhoeae, Nocardia* spp, *Pasteurella multocida, Proteus mirabilis, Pseudomonas* spp, *Serratia marcescens, Staphylococcus aureus, Staphylococcus epidermidis, Streptococcus* spp (particularly *S. pneumoniae*), and *Treponema pallidum*
  — Viruses such as adenovirus, cytomegalovirus, Epstein-Barr virus, herpes simplex virus (type 1 rather than type 2), molluscum contagiosum, rubeola, and varicella zoster virus
  — Fungi such as *Aspergillus* spp, *Candida* spp, *Fusarium* spp, and *Penicillium* spp
  — Parasites such as *Acanthamoeba* spp, *Leishmania* spp, *Microsporidia* spp, and *Trypanosoma* spp

EPIDEMIOLOGY

Risk Factors
- A breach in the integrity of the epithelial surface is the most important risk factor.
- In the United States, contact lenses play a major role in corneal infection and ulceration. Additional risk factors for the development of keratitis include the following:
  — Use of homemade saline
  — Use of extended-wear soft contact lenses
  — Wearing of lenses while swimming
  — Inadequate disinfection
- For critically ill patients, the risk factors include the following:
  — Inability to shut the eyes
  — Inadequate blinking
  — Drying associated with epithelial erosions and abrasions
  — Intermittent positive-pressure ventilation
- Infection due to *Nocardia* spp usually follows eye trauma.
- Fungal infection is common in warm, humid climates, especially after penetration of the cornea by plant or vegetable material.
- Keratitis caused by *Acanthamoeba* spp is associated with trauma to the eye and exposure to contaminated water.

Clinical Manifestations

SYMPTOMS
- The most common symptoms are eye pain and the sensation of a foreign body. Other symptoms include the following:
  — Blepharospasm
  — Discharge
  — Photophobia
  — Redness
  — Reflex tearing
  — Tearing
  — Visual loss
- Ocular symptoms due to herpes zoster can occur after zoster eruption in any branch of the trigeminal nerve, but are particularly common when vesicles form on the nose, reflecting nasociliary nerve involvement (Hutchinson's sign).
- *Nocardia* spp cause subacute infection. Nocardial infection involving deeper eye structures is usually a manifestation of dissemination.

SIGNS
- One of the first signs of keratitis is a loss of corneal transparency, best seen with cobalt blue light after installation of fluorescein.
- Severe keratitis inflammation can lead to invasion of the cornea by blood vessels (neovascularization).
- A dendritic pattern of corneal epithelial ulceration (revealed by fluorescein staining) is, when present, characteristic for herpes infection.
- *P. aeruginosa* keratitis usually starts as a small central ulcer that spreads concentrically to involve a large portion of the cornea, sclera, and underlying stroma. The clinical manifestations of *P. aeruginosa* keratitis include the following:
  — Rapidly expanding infiltrate in the bed of an epithelial injury
  — Surrounding epithelial edema
  — An anterior chamber reaction
  — Mucopurulent discharge adherent to the ulcer's surface

Diagnosis

DIFFERENTIAL DIAGNOSIS
- In evaluating the cornea, it is important to differentiate between keratitis and keratoconjunctivitis, which is a more superficial infection.
- Keratitis due to a herpes simplex type can be easily confused with adenoviral conjunctivitis, unless vesicles appear on the periocular skin or conjunctiva.
- For the differentiation between keratitis and the other eye infections, please refer to the Section I chapter, "Red Eye," and the Section II chapter, "Endophthalmitis."

DIAGNOSTIC/TESTING PROCEDURES
- Corneal scrapings are obtained for Gram stain, Giemsa stain, and cultures.
- Slit-lamp examination can show disruption of the corneal epithelium, a cloudy infiltrate or abscess in the stroma, and an inflammatory cellular reaction in the anterior chamber.
- In severe cases of keratitis, pus settles at the bottom of the anterior chamber, giving rise to a hypopyon.
- The irregular polygonal cysts of *Acanthamoeba* may be identified in corneal scrapings or biopsy material, and trophozoites can be grown on special media.

Treatment

MAIN TREATMENT
- If there is clinical suspicion of bacterial keratitis, treatment covering all possible pathogens should be initiated promptly.

Keratitis

- Evaluation by an ophthalmologist should be sought when there is doubt about the diagnosis or what protocol should be followed.

Bacterial Keratitis

- *P. aeruginosa*: tobramycin (14 mg/mL) and piperacillin or ticarcillin eye drops
- Nonpseudomonal: cefazolin and piperacillin or ticarcillin
- Frequency of treatment depends on the clinical situation, but can be up to every 15 to 60 minutes and around the clock for the first 1 to 3 days.
- The duration of treatment is based on clinical response.
- Systemic antibiotic therapy is mainly indicated in cases of severe suppurative keratitis or for infection that involves the sclera. One of the exceptions is Lyme disease, in which keratitis can be a part of the systemic infection and for which parenteral therapy is indicated.

Viral Keratitis

- Herpes keratitis is treated with topical antiviral agents (trifluridine one drop nine times daily for 3 weeks) and cycloplegics. Oral acyclovir has questionable additional benefit.
- Herpes varicella zoster ophthalmicus is treated with antiviral agents (famciclovir 500 mg three times daily PO, or valacyclovir 1 g three times daily PO for 10 days) and cycloplegics. In severe cases, steroids may be added to prevent permanent visual loss from corneal scarring.
- Epidemic keratoconjunctivitis from adenovirus and ocular involvement in infectious mononucleosis usually require only symptomatic care.

Fungal Keratitis

- Natamycin (5%) every 2 to 3 hours

Parasitic Keratitis

Cysts of *Acanthamoeba* are resistant to available drugs, and the results of medical therapy have been disappointing. Some reports have suggested partial responses to propamidine isethionate and neomycin/gramicidin/polymyxin eyedrops. Severe infections usually require keratoplasty.

Symptomatic Therapy

- Cycloplegics should be administered for control of the photophobia and in order to prevent the formation of synechiae.
- The role of topical glucocorticoids is controversial. Steroids are effective in mitigating corneal scarring but must be used with extreme caution because of the danger of corneal melting, prolonging infection, inducing glaucoma, and perforation.

ALTERNATIVE TREATMENT

- Keratitis due to *P. aeruginosa:* ciprofloxacin or ofloxacin (0.3%)
- Nonpseudomonal bacterial keratitis: vancomycin (50 mg/mL) plus ceftazidime (50 mg/mL)
- Herpes keratitis: vidarabine ointment
- Fungal keratitis: topical therapy with amphotericin B (1.5 mg/mL) every 2 to 3 hours. However, this preparation can be toxic to the corneal epithelium.
- *Acanthamoeba* spp: polyhexamethylene biguanide 0.02% or chlorhexidine 0.02%

TREATMENT FAILURE

Severe keratitis (especially due to fungi or *Acanthamoeba* spp) usually requires keratoplasty, corneal transplant, or conjunctival flaps.

COMPLICATIONS

- The inflammation can lead to keratolysis (loss of cornea).
- Corneal ulcer due to *P. aeruginosa* may advance rapidly to involve the entire cornea in 2 days or less, or may evolve subacutely over several days. Complications include corneal perforation, anterior chamber involvement, and endophthalmitis.
- Herpes zoster ophthalmicus produces corneal dendrites, which can be difficult to distinguish from those seen in herpes simplex. Other sequelae include the following:
  —Acute retinal necrosis
  —Anterior uveitis
  —Ocular motor nerve palsies
  —Postherpetic scarring and neuralgia
  —Raised intraocular pressure
  —Stromal keratitis

Follow-Up

Signs of clinical improvement are based on frequent slit-lamp examinations.

PREVENTION

- Contact lenses should not be worn by anyone with an active eye infection.
- Among critically ill patients, frequent inspection of the eye, instillation of sterile artificial tears, and prevention of exposure by maintaining proper closure of the lids at all times are of paramount importance.
- Hospital personnel that care for critically ill patients should avoid the following:
  —Touching ocular surface with tip of ointment tube or drop applicators
  —Using the same ointment tube or drop applicator for both eyes
  —Placing patch or tape over partly open eyes
  —Applying patches on eyes with discharge
  —Suction of respiratory tract secretions across head of patient and without covering patient's eyes
  —Routine eye swabs for culture in comatose patients
  —Leaving contact lenses *in situ*

Selected Readings

Dua HS. Bacterial keratitis in the critically ill and comatose patient. *Lancet* 1998;351:387–388.

Horton JC. Disorders of the eye. In: Fauci AS, Braunwald E, Isselbacher KJ, et al., eds. *Harrison's principles of internal medicine*, 14th ed. New York: McGraw-Hill, 1998:159–172.

Kirwan JF, Potamitis T, El-Kasaby, et al. Microbial keratitis in intensive care. *BMJ* 1997;314:433–434.

O'Brien TR, Green WR. Keratitis. In: Mandell GL, Bennett JE, Dolin R, eds. *Principles and practice of infectious diseases*, 4th ed. New York: Churchill Livingstone, 1995:1010–1020.

Larva Migrans Syndromes

Basics

DEFINITION
- Wide spectrum of syndromes caused by the migrating larvae of helminths through the skin, soft tissues, or the visceral organs of the body

ETIOLOGY
- *Toxocara canis*, a roundworm infection in dogs, may lead to *visceral* larvae migrans or *ocular* larvae migrans in humans via ingestion.
  —The roundworm eggs are deposited in dog feces, become infectious after 3 to 4 weeks, and can infect humans.
  —The eggs hatch in the human stomach and the larvae migrate via mesenteric vessels to the liver. There, the larvae enter the circulation and disseminate throughout the body.
  —Larvae may persist for years in the human host.
  —In the liver and other organs, they cause a granulomatous response, producing nodular lesions.
  —In the eye, subretinal masses may be produced.
- *Ancylostoma braziliense*, a dog and cat hookworm, can cause a *cutaneous* larvae migrans (creeping eruption or "plumbers' itch") in humans.
- Other geohelminths that cause a larvae migrans syndrome include *Ancylostoma duodenale* and *Ancylostoma caninum*.

EPIDEMIOLOGY
- *Toxocara* is widespread in dogs. The infection rate of dogs is as high as 90%.
- Shedding of eggs is most common in puppies.
- Approximately 10% to 30% of playgrounds in the United States are contaminated with *Toxocara*.
- Seropositivity varies from 2% to as high as 54% in children in some communities in the southern United States.
- Visceral larvae migrans generally occurs in preschool-aged children.
- *A. braziliense* is found worldwide in warm climates. In the United States, infections generally are common on the Gulf Coast.

Incubation
- The precise incubation period is not determined. In low-grade infections, the time to development of disease may be years.
- With cutaneous larva migrans, symptoms occur immediately after the larvae penetrate the skin.

Clinical Manifestations

VISCERAL LARVAE MIGRANS
- Most infections are asymptomatic, with larvae arrested in the liver. The degree of symptoms depends on the number of eggs ingested.
- Symptoms, when they occur, include cough, wheezing, and fevers.
- Patients develop hepatomegaly.
- Patients may present with seizures, cardiac dysfunction, or nephrosis.

Ocular Larvae Migrans
- This syndrome causes unilateral eosinophilic inflammatory masses in the posterior chamber of the eye.
- Ocular larvae migrans often occurs by itself and is not associated with visceral disease.

Larva Migrans Syndromes

CUTANEOUS LARVAE MIGRANS

- This is characterized by a papule at the site of entry, with a twisting track within the skin.
- The lesion is very pruritic.

Diagnosis

- The larvae are almost never seen.
- Granulomata are found associated with many eosinophils.
- Patients have leukocytosis and eosinophilia (often greater than 50% of white blood cells).
- Patients have hepatomegaly.
- Cutaneous larva migrans is a clinical diagnosis.

LABORATORY

- Elevated immunoglobulin levels
- Serology (ELISA) using larval antigens has a sensitivity of 90%.

DIFFERENTIAL DIAGNOSIS

Visceral
- Strongyloidiasis
- Schistosomiasis
- *Ascaris*
- *Echinococcus*

Ocular
- Tumor
- Tuberculosis
- Toxoplasmosis

Treatment

VISCERAL
- Diethylcarbamazine 2 to 3 mg/kg orally tid for 10 to 21 days
- Albendazole 400 mg orally bid for 5 days
- Mebendazole 100 to 200 mg orally bid for 5 days
- Add steroids for CNS or cardiac disease.

OCULAR
- Subtenon triamcinolone 40 mg weekly plus prednisone 60 mg every day for 2 weeks

CUTANEOUS
- Ivermectin 150 μg/kg orally one time
- Albendazole 200 mg orally bid for 3 days

COMPLICATIONS

N/A

Follow-Up

- None needed

PREVENTION

- Dogs should be tested and treated for *T. canis*.
- Do not allow dogs to defecate in parks that are frequented by children.
- Handwashing is imperative prior to eating.

Selected Readings

Jones WE, Schantz PM, Foreman K, et al. Human toxocarias in a rural community. *Am J Dis Child* 1980;134:967.

Mok CH. Visceral larva migrans. A discussion based on review of the literature. *Clin Pediatr* 1968;7:565.

Nash TE. Visceral larva migrans and other unusual helminth infections. In: Mandell GL, Bennett JE, Dolin R, eds. *Principles and practice of infectious diseases*, 5th ed. New York: Churchill Livingstone, 1999:2965–2970.

Laryngitis/Laryngotracheobronchitis (Croup)

Basics

DEFINITION

Laryngitis

- Inflammation of the mucosa of larynx

Laryngotracheobronchitis

- Inflammation of the mucosa of the subglottic area of the respiratory tract

ETIOLOGY

Laryngitis

- Viral
  - Influenza virus
  - Rhinovirus
  - Adenovirus
  - Parainfluenza virus
  - Respiratory syncytial virus
  - Coxsackievirus
  - Coronavirus
- Bacterial
  - *Streptococcus pyogenes*
  - *Moraxella catarrhalis*
- Unusual causes
  - Tuberculosis
  - Syphilis
  - Diptheria
  - Candidiasis
  - Histoplasmosis
  - Blastomycosis

Laryngotracheobronchitis

- Several viruses may cause croup.
- Parainfluenza viruses are the major causative agents for all ages (most common, type 1; second most common, type 3; and least common, type 2)
- Influenza viruses are important causes in children older than 5 years of age.
- Respiratory syncytial virus is a frequent cause in the first few months of life.
- Adenoviruses, rhinoviruses, and enteroviruses are less frequent causes.
- *Mycoplasma pneumoniae* may cause croup, mainly in older ages.

EPIDEMIOLOGY

Incidence and Prevalence

- Laryngitis
  - Usually occurs in association with episodes of respiratory tract infections in midwinter.
- Laryngotracheobronchitis
  - Parainfluenza type 1 virus causes outbreaks of infection in the fall, influenza virus types A and B and respiratory syncytial virus in the winter to early spring, and enteroviruses in the summer to early fall.
  - Sporadic cases are commonly associated with parainfluenza type 3 virus and less frequently with adenoviruses, rhinoviruses, and *M. pneumoniae*.
  - Croup is a relatively common infection in young children under 6 years of age.
  - Most cases occur between 3 months and 3 years of age.
  - In several series of cases of croup, boys predominated.

Risk Factors

- Laryngitis
  - Close quarters
  - Occurs in all age groups; more frequent in children
  - Smoking
  - Excess alcohol consumption
  - Immunosuppression
  - Equal occurrence in males and females
- Laryngotracheobronchitis
  - Age (particularly the second year of life)
  - Probably a defect in the regulation of the immune response

Clinical Manifestations

Symptoms and Signs

- Laryngitis
  - Hoarseness
  - Lowering of the normal pitch of voice; occasionally aphonia
  - Symptoms of upper respiratory tract infection
  - Stridor if airway obstruction occurs
  - Examination of the larynx reveals hyperemia, edema, and vascular injection of the vocal cords, and there may be mucosal ulcerations.
- Laryngotracheobronchitis
  - Often, history of acute upper respiratory tract illness
  - Fever (range, 38°C–40°C)
  - Hoarseness
  - A "seal's bark" cough (deepening, not productive, with a striking brassy tone)
  - Inspiratory stridor
  - Tachypnea
  - Often, retractions of the chest wall, usually in the supraclavicular and suprasternal areas
  - In more severe cases, there is stridor on expiration and marked tachypnea and, in auscultation, rales, rhonchi, wheezing, or diminished breath sounds.

Diagnosis

LARYNGITIS

- Help for diagnosis may be offered by the following:
  - Patient's history
  - Clinical findings
- The syndrome of acute viral laryngitis should be distinguished from the following:
  - Bacterial laryngitis
  - A rare cause of laryngitis, such as tuberculosis, syphilis, diptheria, or fungal infections
  - Acute epiglottitis
  - Acute laryngotracheobronchitis
  - Traumatic aphonia
  - Tumors and others noninfectious chronic diseases of the larynx (laryngoscopic examination should be done if hoarseness persists longer than 10–14 days)

LARYNGOTRACHEOBRONCHITIS

- Diagnosis is usually based on the clinical picture.
- Helpful is the anterior–posterior neck x-ray, which shows the characteristic subglottic swelling, the "hourglass" or "steeple" sign.
- The syndrome of croup should be distinguished from the following:
  - Acute epiglottitis: The course is much more rapidly progressive, the patient appears to be more toxic, and there is no history of previous upper respiratory illness. The characteristic cough of croup is absent, and the patient has dysphonia and dysphagia. In croup, the anterior–posterior neck x-ray shows the characteristic subglottic swelling, and, in epiglottitis, the lateral neck x-ray shows an enlarged epiglottis (the thump sign) and normal subglottic structures.
  - Foreign-body aspiration: History is helpful.

Laryngitis/Laryngotracheobronchitis (Croup)

- Allergic reaction: History, other signs of allergy, and no symptoms of infection are helpful.
- Anatomic airway obstruction: Children with a long-standing history of stridor or those (under 3 months of age) with "croup" should be carefully evaluated for anatomic airway obstruction.
- Bacterial tracheitis: dramatic clinical picture with high fever, toxic appearance, stridor, dyspnea, and cough with purulent sputum. It is caused by *S. aureus*, group A β-hemolytic streptococci, and *H. influenzae* type b. The lateral soft-tissue x-ray reveals a normal epiglottis with subglottic narrowing.

LABORATORY

- WBC and differential counts are normal.
- In severe cases, hypoxemia is probably present without or with hypercapnia.

SPECIAL TESTS

For etiologic diagnosis, special serologic or other tests may be used, although they do not have any practical value.

Treatment

LARYNGITIS

- The appropriate health care setting is outpatient.
- Hospitalization is necessary when airway obstruction occurs.
- General measures
  — Inhalation of moistened air
- Medications are not indicated unless bacterial laryngitis is established.

LARYNGOTRACHEOBRONCHITIS

- In mild cases, no specific treatment is needed, as the disease is self-limited. Home care consists of adequate hydration, humidification of air, and fever control.
- In mild to moderate cases, nebulized budesonide (where available) or dexamethasone (oral or intramuscular) in a dose of 0.15 to 0.6 mg/kg results in acute clinical improvement in outpatients, reducing the need for hospitalization. Nebulized racemic epinephrine provides temporary clinical improvement to many children with marked stridor, but such patients should be observed for at least 3 hours because of the possibility of rebound edema and dyspnea. Children requiring two epinephrine treatments should be hospitalized.
- In moderately severe or severe croup, corticosteroid therapy (0.3–0.6 mg/kg dexamethasone or its equivalent every 6 hours for two to four doses) may result in significant clinical improvement and decrease the need for intubation.
- Children with hypoxemia (without hypercapnia) respond to low concentrations of supplemental oxygen. If hypercapnia occurs, mechanical ventilation should be considered. Nasotracheal intubation is the preferred method.
- Antihistamines, decongestants, and antibiotics have no proven efficacy in uncomplicated viral croup.

COMPLICATIONS

Laryngitis

- Airway obstruction

Laryngotracheobronchitis

- Acute complications
  — Acute respiratory failure, often necessitating mechanical ventilation
  — Pneumothorax
  — Noncardiac pulmonary edema
  — Aspiration pneumonia
- Long-term complications (usually after severe croup early in life)
  — Increased frequency of hyperreactivity of the airway
  — Probable altered pulmonary function
  — Occasional occurrence of subglottic stenosis after intubation

Follow-Up

- High fever, significant shortness of breath, and a large amount of respiratory tract secretions may suggest bacterial tracheitis. In this case, antibiotics are needed.
- The diseases are usually self-limited, with a fluctuating course.
- They last about 3 to 4 days, although cough may persist for a longer period.
- In some studies, steroid administration did not shorten the duration of illness, but there was a significant reduction in symptom severity, in the proportion of the hospitalized children, and the required intubation in severe cases of croup.
- Some children have repeated episodes of croup; allergic diathesis or hyperreactivity of the airway may contribute.

PREVENTION

Avoid contact with infected people.

Selected Readings

Denny FW, Murphy TF, Clyde WA Jr, et al. Croup: An 11 year study in a pediatric practice. *Pediatrics* 1983;71:871–876.

Folland DS. Treatment of croup. Sending home an improved child and relieved parents. *Postgrad Med* 1997;101:271–273, 277–278.

Geelhoed GC. Croup. *Pediatr Pulmonol* 1997;23:370–374.

Geelhoed GC, Turner J, Macdonald WBG. Efficacy of a small single dose of oral dexamethasone for outpatient croup: A double-blind placebo-controlled clinical trial. *BMJ* 1996;313:140–142.

Hall CB. Acute laryngotracheobronchitis (croup). In: Mandell GL, Douglas RG, Bennett JE, eds. *Principles and practice of infectious diseases, 4th ed.* New York: Churchill Livingstone, 1995:573–579.

Kaditis AG, Wald ER. Viral croup: Current diagnosis and treatment. *Pediatr Infect Dis J* 1998;17:827–834.

Kairys SW, Olmstead EM, O'Connor GT. Steroid treatment of laryngotracheitis: A meta-analysis of the evidence of randomised trials. *Pediatrics* 1989;83:683–693.

Klassen TP, Feldman ME, Watters LK, et al. Nebulized budesonide for children with mild-to-moderate croup. *N Engl J Med* 1994;331:285–289.

Kristjanson S, Berg-Kelly K, Winso E. Inhalation of racemic adrenaline in the treatment of mild and moderately severe croup. Clinical symptom score and oxygen saturation measurements for evaluation of treatment effects. *Acta Paediatr* 1994;83:1156–1160.

Macdonald WBG, Geelhoed GC. Management of childhood croup [Editorial]. *Thorax* 1997;52:757–759.

Legionnaires' Disease

Basics

DEFINITION

- Legionnaires' disease is the designation for pneumonia caused by bacteria of the genus *Legionella*.
- Pontiac fever is an acute, febrile, self-limited illness that has been serologically linked to *Legionella* species.

ETIOLOGY

- Legionnaires' disease was first recognized during an outbreak of pneumonia involving delegates to the 1976 American Legion convention at a Philadelphia hotel.
- Although 40 different *Legionella* species have been identified, less than half of these have been linked to disease in humans. *Legionella pneumophila* is the most pathogenic, accounting for 90% of the cases of legionellosis, followed by *Legionella micdadei*.
- More than 14 serogroups of *L. pneumophila* have been identified, but serogroup 1 accounts for 80% of the reported cases of legionellosis caused by *L. pneumophila*.
- The natural habitats for *L. pneumophila* are aquatic bodies. Once the organisms enter human-constructed aquatic reservoirs (such as cooling towers or water distribution systems), they can grow and proliferate. Natural bodies of water contain only small numbers of organisms.
- Transmission is due to aerosolization, aspiration, and direct instillation into the lung during respiratory tract manipulations.
- Aspiration is the predominant mode of transmission, but it is unclear whether *Legionella* enters the lung via oropharyngeal colonization or directly from drinking contaminated water.

EPIDEMIOLOGY

- Outbreaks of legionnaires' disease in hotels, cruise ships, and office buildings and sporadic clusters of nosocomial cases have been reported.
- The incidence of *Legionella* as a cause of sporadic community-acquired pneumonia ranges from 2% to 15% of all cases that require hospitalization.

Risk Factors

- Susceptibility is higher among elderly individuals, cigarette smokers, and patients with chronic lung disease or immunosuppression.
- Surgery is a major predisposing factor in nosocomial infection, with transplant recipients at the highest risk.
- The incidence of legionnaires' disease in patients with the acquired immunodeficiency syndrome is low, but is higher than in the general population and the clinical manifestations can be more severe.
- Pontiac fever occurs in epidemics. The high attack rate (above 90%) reflects airborne transmission.

Clinical Manifestations

SYMPTOMS

- The incubation period is 2 to 10 days.
- Patients with legionnaires' disease initially develop nonspecific symptoms, including fever, malaise, myalgias, anorexia, and headache. Later, they develop a broad spectrum of illness, ranging from a mild cough and low-grade fever to stupor, respiratory failure, and multiorgan failure.
- The cough is only slightly productive. Chest pain, occasionally pleuritic, can be prominent.
- Gastrointestinal symptoms are prominent, especially diarrhea, which occurs in 20% to 40% of cases. The stool is watery and not bloody.
- Extrapulmonary legionellosis is rare, but the clinical manifestations are often dramatic. The most common site is the heart, with numerous reports of myocarditis, pericarditis, postcardiotomy syndrome, and prosthetic valve endocarditis. *Legionella* spp have been implicated in cases of sinusitis, cellulitis, pancreatitis, peritonitis, hip-wound infection, and pyelonephritis.
- Pontiac fever is an acute, self-limiting, flulike illness with a 24- to 48-hour incubation period. Malaise, fatigue, and myalgias are the most frequent symptoms. Fever develops in 80% to 90% of cases, and headache in 80%. Other symptoms include arthralgias, nausea, cough, abdominal pain, and diarrhea.

SIGNS

- Patients with legionnaires' disease virtually always have fever. Temperatures in excess of 40.5°C are recorded in 20% of the cases.
- Chest examination reveals rales early in the course, and evidence of consolidation as the disease progresses.
- Abdominal examination may reveal generalized or local tenderness.

Diagnosis

DIFFERENTIAL DIAGNOSIS

- Legionnaires' disease is included in the differential diagnosis of atypical pneumonia, along with infection due to *Chlamydia pneumoniae*, *Chlamydia psittaci*, *Mycoplasma pneumoniae*, *Coxiella burnetii*, and viruses (see Section II chapter, "Pneumonia").
- When compared with other causes of community-acquired pneumonia, patients with legionnaires' pneumonia more frequently
  —Are middle-aged
  —Are male
  —Have failed therapy with betalactamic drugs
  —Have headache, diarrhea, severe hyponatremia, and elevation in serum creatine kinase levels on presentation

LABORATORY

- *Legionella* grows on charcoal-containing medium (buffered-charcoal, yeast-extract agar). Unfortunately, many laboratories either do not culture for *Legionella* or do so inadequately.
- Direct fluorescent antibody staining is a rapid diagnostic test. Its sensitivity is less

Legionnaires' Disease

than that of culture because large numbers of organisms need to be present before they can be readily visualized.
- Usual tissue stains do not reveal the organism.
- The *Legionella* urinary antigen test is a relatively inexpensive, rapid test that detects antigens of *L. pneumophila* in urine. This test has a sensitivity of 70% and a specificity that approaches 100%. Sensitivity can be further improved if the urine is concentrated by ultrafiltration. This test detects only *L. pneumophila* serogroup 1.
- Serologic tests are useful for epidemiologic studies but are less valuable in a specific case, given the requirement for a measurement during convalescence. Antibody screening should include both IgG and IgM, because some patients have only an IgM response.
- Assays based on the polymerase chain reaction have been used to detect *Legionella* in urine samples, bronchoalveolar lavage fluid, and serum.
- In Pontiac fever, modest leukocytosis with a neutrophilic predominance is sometimes detected. The diagnosis is established by antibody seroconversion.
- Hyponatremia is most common in severe cases.

IMAGING

- The chest radiograph cannot be used to distinguish legionnaires' disease from other pneumonias.
- In a few cases of nosocomial disease, fever and respiratory tract symptoms have preceded the appearance of the infiltrate on chest radiography.
- In immunosuppressed patients, especially those receiving corticosteroids, distinctive bilateral nodular opacities may be seen, which may expand and cavitate.
- Pulmonary abscesses can occur in immunosuppressed hosts.

DIAGNOSTIC/TESTING PROCEDURES

Diagnosis is often based on culture and antigen testing (by the method designed for use with urine) of pleural fluid obtained by thoracentesis.

Treatment

MAIN TREATMENT

- Erythromycin (1 g i.v. q6h) has been the drug of choice, but the newer macrolides, especially azithromycin, have superior *in vitro* activity and greater intracellular and lung-tissue penetration. Also, the gastrointestinal intolerance, the requirement for the administration of large volumes of fluid, and ototoxicity related to the 4-g dose of erythromycin have made this drug less attractive.
- Azithromycin (500 mg/d for 5 days) is currently recommended for the treatment of inpatients.
- Quinolones also have good *in vitro* activity and intracellular penetration. Levofloxacin (500 mg/d for 7–10 days) or ciprofloxacin (500 mg q12h for 7–10 days) can be used.
- Parenteral therapy should be given until there is an objective clinical response; most patients become afebrile within 3 days; then, oral therapy can be substituted. The total duration of therapy is 10 to 14 days, but a 21-day course has been recommended for immunosuppressed patients or for those with extensive evidence of disease on chest radiographs.

ALTERNATIVE TREATMENT

- Rifampin is recommended as part of combination therapy with erythromycin for patients who are severely ill.
- Pontiac fever requires only symptom-based treatment, not antimicrobial therapy.

COMPLICATIONS

- With appropriate and timely antibiotic therapy, mortality is low among immunocompetent patients (although in nosocomial infection, the figure has sometimes approached 40% to 50%).
- Higher fatality rates for nosocomial infection are probably due to host-related rather than organism-related factors.

Follow-Up

- Progression of infiltrates on chest radiographs despite appropriate antibiotic therapy is common, and radiographic improvement lags several days behind clinical improvement. Complete clearing of infiltrates on chest radiographs requires one to four months.
- In Pontiac fever, a few patients may experience lassitude for many weeks thereafter.

PREVENTION

- Identify the environmental source and eradicate the organism.
- Disinfection should be considered on the basis of the number of positive culture sites and prior experience with hospital-acquired cases. Numerous methods of disinfection have been tried with variable success. Three methods are now being used: superheating the hot water supply to 70°C to 80°C, with flushing of the distal sites; installing copper–silver ionization units; and hyperchlorinating the water.

Selected Readings

Edelstein PH. Antimicrobial chemotherapy for legionnaires' disease: Time for a change. *Ann Intern Med* 1998;129:328–330.

Lieberman D, Porath A, Schlaeffer F, et al. *Legionella* species community-acquired pneumonia. A review of 56 hospitalized adult patients. *Chest* 1996;109:1243–1249.

Mulazimoglu L, Yu VL. *Legionella* infection. In: Fauci AS, Braunwald E, Isselbacher KJ, et al., eds. *Harrison's principles of internal medicine*, 14th ed. New York: McGraw-Hill, 1998:928–933.

Sopena N, Sabria-Leal M, Pedro-Botet ML, et al. Comparative study of the clinical presentation of *Legionella* pneumonia and other community-acquired pneumonias. *Chest* 1998;113:1195–1200.

Stout JE, Yu VL. Legionellosis. *N Engl J Med* 1997;337:682–687.

Leishmaniasis

Basics

DEFINITION
- *Leishmaniasis* refers to the spectrum of disease caused by the protozoa *Leishmania* and transmitted by a sandfly vector.
- Clinically, leishmaniasis is divided into visceral, cutaneous, and mucosal syndromes.

ETIOLOGY
- *Leishmania* spp have a dimorphic life cycle. In most areas, the *Leishmania* spp are inoculated when the sandfly vector attempts to feed.
- The classic form of old-world cutaneous leishmaniasis (the "oriental sore") occurs throughout tropical and subtropical regions in Asia, China, the Mediterranean, and Africa.
- New-world cutaneous leishmaniasis or American cutaneous leishmaniasis is widespread in Latin America. The causative agents include the following:
  —*L. braziliensis*
  —*L. chagasi*
  —*L. mexicana*
  —*L. braziliensis*
- The incubation period of visceral leishmaniasis varies and depends on the type of the infection, but it can be up to 8 months or more. The incubation period of cutaneous leishmaniasis varies from a few weeks to several months or, in some cases, up to years.

EPIDEMIOLOGY

Incidence
- *Leishmania* infections are among the most common parasitic diseases, with about 10 million infected persons and 400,000 new infections every year.
- In Europe, infections with *L. major* or *L. tropica* are increasingly encountered due to travel and immigration.
- There are two major ongoing epidemics of visceral leishmaniasis (kala-azar), one in Bihar, India, and the other in southern Sudan.
- American cutaneous leishmaniasis is found from Texas to northern Argentina.

Risk Factors
- Children and young adults are the most frequently affected. No animal reservoir has been identified there.
- Leishmaniasis remains an important problem for military personnel operating in endemic regions.
- Visceral leishmaniasis is more common among immunocompromised persons, such as those with HIV infection, or after organ transplantation.

Clinical Manifestations

SYMPTOMS
- "Acute kala-azar" is characterized by the abrupt onset of fever, rigors, malaise, and other nonspecific symptoms as early as 2 weeks after infection.
- American service personnel active in the Gulf War, and infected there by *L. tropica*, developed a chronic viscerotropic disease involving bone marrow and lymph nodes from this normally cutaneous parasite.
- Fever may be intermittent or continuous.
- Sweating with chills accompanies the temperature spikes.
- As time passes, the spleen and liver become enlarged.
- Asymptomatic leishmanial infections have also been documented in persons with HIV.
- Old-world cutaneous leishmaniasis is a local lesion that starts as a papule at the site where promastigotes are inoculated. The papule gradually increases in size, becomes crusted, and finally ulcerates. The ulcer is usually shallow and circular with well-defined, raised, erythematous borders and a bed of granulation tissue. It gradually increases in size and may reach a diameter of 2 cm or more. Satellite lesions that fuse with the original ulcer may be present. There is frequently a serous or seropurulent discharge.
- A wide variety of skin manifestations, ranging from small, dry, crusted lesions to large, deep, mutilating ulcers, are seen in American cutaneous leishmaniasis. In localized cutaneous disease, the initial lesion usually appears 2 to 8 weeks after the sandfly bite as a small, erythematous papule that progresses slowly to form a typical leishmaniotic ulcer: round with raised borders and a granulating base and covered by exudate. The ulcer may persist for months to years.
- Some *Leishmania* spp can persist and lead to mucosal infection.

Leishmaniasis

Diagnosis

DIFFERENTIAL DIAGNOSIS

- The differential diagnosis of cutaneous leishmaniasis includes the following:
  - Fungal infections
  - Lupus vulgaris (skin tuberculosis)
  - Mycobacterial infections of the skin (due to atypical mycobacteria, tuberculosis, or leprosy)
  - Neoplasms
  - Syphilis
- Visceral leishmaniasis can present as organomegaly, fever of unclear etiology, or unexplained chronic anemia, or can mimic other infectious diseases (malaria, typhoid fever, brucellosis, etc.).

LABORATORY

- Anemia, leukopenia, and hypergammaglobulinemia are present in persons with visceral leishmaniasis.
- A definitive diagnosis depends on the demonstration of amastigotes in tissue or isolation of the organism in culture.
- Cultures of bone marrow, liver, spleen, lymph node, and, in some cases, blood may reveal the parasite. Specimens can be inoculated into Novy, McNeal, and Nicolle medium.
- Bone marrow aspiration (Wright- and Giemsa-stained smears) is the most common diagnostic procedure for the diagnosis of visceral leishmaniasis.
- In some areas, liver biopsy and even splenic puncture are routinely performed.
- Enzyme-linked immunosorbent assay (ELISA) and the indirect immunofluorescent antibody assay can be used but are nondiagnostic.
- The leishmanin skin test is useful only in epidemiologic studies.

Treatment

MAIN TREATMENT

- Pentavalent antimonial compounds are most commonly used for the treatment of leishmaniasis. Meglumine antimonate solution contains 85 mg/mL pentavalent antimony, whereas sodium stibogluconate (Pentostam) solution contains 100 mg/mL.
- The dosage is usually 20 mg/kg (i.m. or i.v.) for 3 to 4 weeks.
- Amphotericin B (deoxycholate 0.5 mg/kg given daily, or liposomal formulations) has been used successfully to treat patients who fail to respond or relapse with antimonials.
- In a multicentre study, 20 immunocompetent kala-azar patients treated with liposomal amphotericin B were cured and have not relapsed over a 12- to 24-month follow-up period.
- Pentamidine is a less commonly used alternative.
- Allopurinol monotherapy has no effect on Colombian cutaneous disease primarily caused by *L. braziliensis panamensis* and is therefore unlikely to be effective against cutaneous leishmaniasis in other endemic regions.

COMPLICATIONS

- Mucosal leishmaniasis due to *L. braziliensis* is the only form of American cutaneous leishmaniasis that carries a significant mortality.
- Side effects of pentavalent antimonials include the following:
  - Arthralgias
  - Gastrointestinal symptoms
  - Electrocardiographic changes
  - Headache
  - Pancreatitis

Follow-Up

Cutaneous leishmaniasis can follow the treatment of visceral leishmaniasis.

PREVENTION

Travelers to endemic areas should be educated about the risk of leishmaniasis and the prevention of bites by sandflies.

Selected Readings

Bell SA, Schaller M, Rocken M. Occlusive paromomycin for cutaneous leishmaniasis. *Lancet* 1997;349:29.

Herwaldt BL, Stokes SL, Juranek DD. American cutaneous leishmaniasis in U.S. travelers. *Ann Intern Med* 1993;118:779–784.

Lockwood DN, Pasvol G. Recent advances in tropical medicine. *BMJ* 1994;308:1559–1562.

Magill AJ, Grogl M, Gasser RA Jr, et al. Visceral infection caused by *Leishmania tropica* in veterans of Operation Desert Storm. *N Engl J Med* 1993;328:1383–1387.

Pearson RD, De Queiroz SA. *Leishmania* species: Visceral (kala-azar), cutaneous, and mucosal leishmaniasis. In: Mandell GL, Bennett JE, Dolin R, eds. *Principles and practice of infectious diseases*, 4th ed. New York: Churchill Livingstone, 1995:2428–2442.

Velez I, Agudelo S, Hendrickx E, et al. Inefficacy of allopurinol as monotherapy for Colombian cutaneous leishmaniasis. A randomized, controlled trial. *Ann Intern Med* 1997;126:232–236.

Leprosy

Basics

DEFINITION
- Illness caused by the bacterium *Mycobacterium leprae*.

ETIOLOGY
- *M. leprae* is an acid-fast staining organism that contains a lipid-containing capsule.
- Replication rates are very slow, approaching a 14-day doubling time.
- Two forms of the disease occur: lepromatous leprosy and tuberculoid leprosy.

EPIDEMIOLOGY
- This is a worldwide disease with as many as 6 million people infected. It is endemic in Asia, Africa, and Latin America.
- Most cases in the United States originate in foreign countries.
- Two hundred cases per year are diagnosed in the United States.
- Infection is spread from person to person by nasal secretions.
- It may be transmitted from contaminated soil.
- Leprosy is seen in rural areas in underdeveloped regions of the world.
- Young adults are most often affected.

Incubation
The average incubation period is 5 to 7 years.

Clinical Manifestations

Leprosy affects the peripheral nerves, and many manifestations of disease occur as a result.

FORMS OF DISEASE
- Lepromatous leprosy
  - Organisms produce nodular skin lesions or plaques on the feet and hands, as well as on the ear lobes.
  - Involvement of the nose leads to collapse of the nasal cartilage and a saddle-nose deformity.
  - Upper respiratory disease leads to epistaxis and chronic rhinorrhea.
  - Body hair may be absent in affected areas.
  - Involvement of the peripheral nerves leads to anesthesia of the hands and feet.
- Tuberculoid leprosy
  - Patients with this form of disease often have marked involvement of the peripheral nerves.
  - Hypopigmented skin lesions are also seen in this form of disease.
- Borderline leprosy
  - This type has manifestations of both tuberculoid and lepromatous forms.

Diagnosis

- The diagnosis is usually based on clinical grounds.
- Characteristic skin lesions and peripheral anesthesia are leading clues.
- Finding acid-fast bacilli–positive organisms on biopsy of skin or nerve is necessary for diagnosis however, organisms are infrequently detected in the tuberculoid

Leprosy

lesions. Skin biopsies in patients with this form reveal granulomatous changes with nerve involvement that are consistent with the diagnosis.

DIFFERENTIAL DIAGNOSIS
- Syphilis
- T-cell lymphoma
- Sarcoidosis
- Dermal lupus

Treatment

- Paucibacillary leprosy (tuberculoid type with fewer than five skin lesions without nerve damage)
  - Dapsone 100 mg orally once per day, and rifampin 600 mg orally once every month for 6 months
  - Rifampin 600 mg, ofloxacin 400 mg, and minocycline 100 mg one dose may also be effective.
  - Dapsone 100 mg orally once per day for 5 years
- Multibacillary leprosy (lepromatous or borderline types)
  - Dapsone 100 mg orally once per day and clofazimine 50 mg orally once per day, with rifampin 600 mg orally each month and clofazimine 300 mg orally each month for a 2-year minimum

COMPLICATIONS

Nerve damage, especially to the ulna nerve, can lead to loss of motor function in the hand. Nerve involvement to the peripheral sensory nerves, especially in the hand and foot, can lead to ulceration and infection. Amputation is often needed over time for these extremities.

Follow-Up

Patients should be treated and followed by specialists with experience in treating this illness. The disease takes a long time to regress, there are many treatment factors, and relapse is possible.

PREVENTION

There is no way to effectively prevent infection with leprosy.

Selected Readings

Drutz DJ, Chen TSN, Lu WH. The continuous bacteremia of lepromatous leprosy. *N Engl J Med* 1972;287:159–164.

Nathan CF, Kaplan G, Levis WR, et al. Local and systemic effects of intradermal recombinant interferon-gamma in patients with lepromatous leprosy. *N Engl J Med* 1986;315:6–15.

Waters MF, Rees RJ, Pearson JM, et al. Rifampicin for lepromatous leprosy: Nine years' experience. *BMJ* 1978;1:133–136.

Leptospirosis

Basics

DEFINITION

- An infectious zoonotic disease caused by pathogenic leptospires

ETIOLOGY

- Leptospirosis is caused by one pathogenic leptospire species (*Leptospira interrogans*), which is subdivided into more than 200 serovars.
- More than 20 serovars of *L. interrogans* have been found to cause leptospirosis.
- In the United Kingdom and Oceania, *L. interrogans* serovar *hardjo* seems to be the most common cause of leptospirosis among individuals in close contact with infected livestock.
- In the United States, *L. interrogans* serovars *icterohaemorrhagiae, canicola, autumnalis, australis, bratislava, pomona,* and *hebdomidis* are the most common causes of leptospirosis.

EPIDEMIOLOGY

Incidence and Prevalence

- Leptospirosis is a worldwide infection.
- Most infections are asymptomatic.
- Leptospirosis is an underdiagnosed cause of encephalitis and aseptic meningitis worldwide.
- Serologic evidence for leptospirosis is found in about 10% of cases of meningitis and encephalitis with unclear etiology.

Risk Factors

- Wild and domestic animals are the reservoir for leptospirosis.
- Rats are the main reservoir for *L. interrogans* serovar *icterohemorrhagiae*.
- The main mode of transmission of leptospirosis is via contact of the abraded skin or of mucous membranes with water, vegetation, or soil contaminated with urine of infected animals.
- Subsequently, leptospirosis is a zoonotic disease that mainly affects the following:
  —Farmers
  —Abattoir workers
  —Miners
  —Sewer workers
  —Veterinarians
  —Military troops
  —Bathers
  —Campers
- Leptospirosis is more common in males than females due to epidemiologic reasons related to occupation and preference of recreational activities.
- The incubation period between infection and development of symptoms is usually 1 to 2 weeks (range, 2–25 days).

Clinical Manifestations

SYMPTOMS AND SIGNS

- Fever and chills (fever may be biphasic)
- Headache
- Severe myalgia
- Conjunctival suffusion
- Neck stiffness
- Rash (with palatal enanthem), sometimes hemorrhagic
- Jaundice
- Symptoms from central nervous system disease, including depression, changes in behavior, and confusion
- Symptoms from the respiratory tract, including shortness of breath, cough, and hemoptysis
- Gastrointestinal tract symptoms

Diagnosis

DIFFERENTIAL DIAGNOSIS

- Leptospirosis is an underdiagnosed disease.
- Leptospirosis should come to the mind of the physician as a diagnostic possibility in every febrile patient at risk for the infection due to occupation or recreational activities.
- Cases of leptospirosis are frequently misdiagnosed as a viral infection, including influenza.

LABORATORY

- Serologic tests are helpful in the diagnosis of leptospirosis.
- A problem related to these tests is the fact that IgM antibodies against *Leptospira* may be present for a long time (several months to 1 or 2 years) after an acute leptospirosis infection. Thus, caution is needed in the interpretation of serologic tests.

Leptospirosis

- Culture of *Leptospira* needs special media and requires prolonged intubation.
- *Leptospira* organisms may be seen in the urine of infected patients (using a dark-field microscope).

PATHOLOGY

Leptospira organisms may be seen in tissue biopsy specimens.

Treatment

MAIN TREATMENT

- Penicillin is the drug of choice. The dose may be smaller compared with the dose needed to treat other serious infections. Four to 10 million units of intravenous penicillin G (divided in four to six doses) is sufficient.
- Duration of treatment is 7 days.
- Patients may rarely develop a Jarisch-Herxheimer reaction during treatment.

ALTERNATIVE TREATMENT

- Several other antimicrobial agents also are efficient against leptospirosis.
- Doxycycline 100 mg PO every 12 hours for 7 days may be given in mild cases of leptospirosis.

COMPLICATIONS

- The case fatality rate is 20% for severe (untreated) leptospirosis with liver and kidney dysfunction.
- Main causes of death include the following:
  —Hepatorenal syndrome
  —Adult respiratory distress syndrome
  —Arrhythmias due to myocarditis
  —Vascular dysfunction with severe bleeding
- Recovery of untreated cases may take several months.
- Severe leptospirosis with jaundice is known as Weil's syndrome.
- A leptospirosis syndrome presenting with fever and pretibial rash is known as Fort Bragg fever.

Follow-Up

- Patients with mild leptospirosis syndrome who were treated appropriately and had full recovery need no follow-up.
- Patients with severe leptospirosis should have a follow-up visit about a week after the discontinuation of treatment.

PREVENTION

- Control of the rodent population decreases the incidence of human leptospirosis.
- Exposure to *Leptospira* related to occupation or recreational activities is decreased by wearing protective boots, gloves, and clothing.

Selected Readings

Edwards CN, Nicholson GD, Hassel TA, et al. Penicillin therapy in icteric leptospirosis. *Am J Trop Med Hyg* 1988;39:388–390.

Friedland JS, Warrell DA. The Jarisch-Herxheimer reaction on leptospirosis: Possible pathogenesis and review. *Rev Infect Dis* 1991;13:207–210.

Gochenour WS Jr, Smadel JE, Jackson EB, et al. Leptospiral etiology of Fort Bragg fever. *Public Health Rep* 1952;67:811.

Lai KN, Aarons I, Woodroffe AJ, et al. Renal lesions in leptospirosis. *Aust N Z J Med* 1982;12:276.

Merien F, Amouriaux P, Perolat P, et al. Polymerase chain reaction for detection of Leptospira spp. in clinical samples. *J Clin Microbiol* 1992;30:2219–2224.

O'Neil KM, Rickman LS, Lazarus AA. Pulmonary manifestation of leptospirosis. *Rev Infect Dis* 1991;13:705–709.

Pappas MG, Ballou WR, Gray MR, et al. Rapid serodiagnosis of leptospirosis using the IgM-specific dot-ELISA: Comparison with the microscopic agglutination test. *Am J Trop Med Hyg* 1985;34:346–354.

Takafuji ET, Kirkpatrick JW, Miller RN, et al. An efficacy trial of doxycycline chemoprophylaxis against leptospirosis. *N Engl J Med* 1984;310:497.

Watt G, Tuazon ML, Santiago E, et al. Placedo-controlled trial of intravenous penicillin for severe and late leptospirosis. *Lancet* 1988;1:433–435.

Lice

Basics

DEFINITION
Human pediculosis is a parasitic infectious disease that includes head, body, or pubic lice. Pubic lice infest primarily pubic hairs, and occasionally eyebrows, eyelashes, axillary hair, and the coarse hair on the chests and backs of men. Head and body lice infest scalp hair and other hair on the body, but not pubic hair.

ETIOLOGY
- Pubic or crab lice: *Phthirus pubis*; transmitted via sexual or close body contact
- Body lice: *Pediculus humanus*; transmitted via close body contact
- Head lice: *P. humanus*; transmitted via close body contact

EPIDEMIOLOGY
Incidence
- Head lice: all socioeconomic classes, particularly children of school age
- Body lice: overcrowded populations with poor sanitation
- Pubic/crab lice

Risk Factors
- Children of school age in close contact, infested with head or body lice. Girls are 1.5 times more likely to be infested than are boys; non-Black children are 10 to 30 times more likely to be infested than are Black children.
- Persons living in conditions of poor sanitation
- Sexual contact or close body contact with a person infested with pubic lice

Clinical Manifestations

SYMPTOMS AND SIGNS
- Itching at site of infestation (e.g., scalp, pubic, perineal, and inguinal areas)
- Secondary bacterial infections possible
- An erythematous, maculopapular eruption can be seen on the scalp, the nape of the neck, and the shoulders.

Diagnosis

Diagnosis is based on physical examination. Lice or their nits (eggs) can be observed with the naked eye or with the use of a hand lens.

Lice

Treatment

MAIN TREATMENT

- Permethrin 1% cream rinse applied to affected areas and washed off after 10 minutes
- Lindane 1% shampoo applied to affected areas and washed off after 4 minutes. Lindane is contraindicated for pregnant or lactating women or for children under the age of 2 years.
- Pyrethrins with piperonyl butoxide applied to affected areas and washed off after 10 minutes
- After use of a pediculicide, removal of nits with a fine-tooth comb after drying the hair, using a clean towel
- Soak combs and brushes in a pediculicide for 1 hour or wash in hot water for 20 minutes.
- Eyelashes require application of petroleum jelly two times per day for 10 days.
- Decontaminate clothes and bed linens used within the previous 48 hours by machine washing and drying (using the hot cycle), or dry cleaning.

SEXUAL PARTNERS

- If patients have been sexually active within 1 month of onset of pubic lice symptoms, their partners should be treated.
- When pubic lice are discovered in a child, sexual abuse should be considered.

COMPLICATIONS

Secondary bacterial skin infections may occur.

Follow-Up

- Re-evaluate the patient 1 week after treatment if symptoms persist.
- Retreat the patient if lice or nits are still observed.

PREVENTION

N/A

Selected Readings

Angel TA, Nigro J, Levy ML. Infestations in the pediatric patient. *Pediatr Clin North Am* 2000;47(4):921–935, viii.

Anonymous. Treating head louse infections. *Drug Ther Bull* 1998;36(6):45–46.

Burkhart CG, Burkhart CN, Burkhart KM. An assessment of topical and oral prescription and over-the-counter treatments for head lice. *J Am Acad Dermatol* 1998;38(6 Pt 1): 979–982.

Chosidow O. Scabies and pediculosis. *Lancet* 2000;355(9206):819–826.

Listeriosis

Basics

DEFINITION

- Listeriosis is infection caused by the gram-positive rod *Listeria monocytogenes*. Most common presenting syndromes include the following:
  - Bacteremia and sepsis
  - Chorioamnionitis
  - CNS listeriosis with meningitis or, if there is parenchymal involvement, meningoencephalitis (meningitis with parenchymal involvement), cerebritis, brainstem encephalitis (rhomboencephalitis), and brain or spinal abscess
  - Endocarditis
  - Focal infections, such as skin infection (e.g., a veterinarian or a poultry worker with an ulcerating lesion), endophthalmitis, lymph node infection, septic arthritis, osteomyelitis, liver abscess, hepatitis (usually associated with disseminated infection) or cholecystitis
  - Recurrent spontaneous abortion
  - Transplacental transmission of *L. monocytogenes* can also cause a unique syndrome known as "granulomatosis infantisepticum," characterized by disseminated abscesses and/or granulomas in multiple internal organs, including skin, eyes, liver, spleen, lungs, kidneys, and CNS.
  - Stillbirth

ETIOLOGY

L. monocytogenes is an aerobic or facultatively anaerobic, nonsporulating, intracellular gram-positive bacillus. Identification of serotypes is only of epidemiologic significance.

EPIDEMIOLOGY

- Listeriosis can present as sporadic cases or as outbreaks. It is usually attributed to food-borne transmission of *L. monocytogenes* and is associated with a variety of foods, such as milk, cheese, meat products, and raw vegetables. One percent to 5% of humans are asymptomatic intestinal carriers, providing a reservoir for the pathogen.
- Listeriosis can occur throughout life, even among individuals without predisposing factors. The lack of predisposing factors does not rule out listeriosis.
- At higher risk for the infection are the following:
  - Neonates: *L. monocytogenes* is the third most common cause of neonatal sepsis and meningitis after *Escherichia coli* and group B streptococci.
  - Individuals older than 45 to 50 years and pregnant women: One-third of all listeriosis cases are related to pregnancy. Listeriosis mainly predisposes to non-CNS listeriosis, and it can occur at any time during pregnancy, but more often during the third trimester.

Additional Predisposing Factors

- Hematologic or solid-organ malignancy
- Solid-organ or bone marrow transplantation
- Alcoholism
- Liver disease
- Chemotherapy (especially with fludarabine)
- HIV/AIDS: There is a more than 100-fold increase in incidence among patients with AIDS, but incidence can be reduced by the use of prophylactic trimethoprim-sulfamethoxazole.
- Diabetes mellitus
- Splenectomy
- Autoimmune disorders
- Hemochromatosis

Clinical Manifestations

SYMPTOMS AND SIGNS

Central Nervous System Listeriosis

- Meningitis/meningoencephalitis usually presents with fever (92%), altered sensorium (65%), headache (46%), gastrointestinal symptoms (22%), focal neurologic findings (18%), seizures (5%), and photophobia (3%).
- Up to 15% of patients have symptoms for 5 days or more before hospitalization, and 42% lack meningeal signs on admission.
- Brainstem encephalitis is characterized by asymmetric cranial nerve palsies, cerebellar signs, motor or sensory loss, and impaired consciousness.
- Parenchymal disease without meningeal involvement is uncommon (<5% of all reported cases of CNS listeriosis). It usually presents with fever, abnormal sensorium, headache, and focal neurologic findings. *L. monocytogenes* should be included in the differential diagnosis of brain abscess.

Bacteremia and Sepsis

Primary bacteremia due to *L. monocytogenes* has no distinctive features. Up to one-fourth of the patients have gastrointestinal symptoms (nausea, vomiting, diarrhea, or abdominal pain).

Endocarditis

Listeria is an infrequent cause of (usually subacute) endocarditis, usually involving the left side of the heart. It is more common among patients with preexisting valve lesions. Fever (75%), new or changing murmur (40%), and hepatomegaly or splenomegaly (30%) are the most common findings.

Pregnancy-related Listeriosis

- Most commonly, the mother develops a flulike syndrome, with fever, chills, myalgias, gastrointestinal symptoms, and back pain.
- Neonates in the first 7 days of life usually present with signs of sepsis or pneumonia. Sepsis, CNS infection, and focal infections are the most common syndromes after the first 7 days of life.
- *In utero*–infected neonates that develop granulomatosis infantisepticum might appear very sick, develop cardiopulmonary collapse, or just appear weak.

Focal Infections

Presentation varies with the organ involved.

Diagnosis

DIFFERENTIAL DIAGNOSIS

Central Nervous System Listeriosis

- Meningitis/meningoencephalitis
  - Infection due to *Streptococcus pneumoniae*, *Haemophilus influenzae*, and *Neisseria meningitidis* in adults. *Cryptococcus neoformans* should also be considered in immunocompromised individuals.
  - Metabolic encephalopathy
  - Psychiatric illnesses
- Focal CNS infection (cerebritis/abscess)
  - Brain abscess, tumor, stroke

Bacteremia and Sepsis

- Bacteremia and sepsis are due to a variety of pathogens.

Listeriosis during Pregnancy

- Influenza, congenital syphilis or toxoplasmosis, pyelonephritis, and septic abortion

Listeriosis

Listeriosis in Neonates
- Meningitis due to *E. coli* or group B streptococci
- Bacteremia and sepsis
  —Neonatal sepsis
- Granulomatosis infantisepticum
  —Neonatal sepsis, meningitis, or pneumonia
- Endocarditis and focal infections due to Listeria have no distinctive clinical features and the differential diagnosis includes a variety of possible pathogens (please see respective chapters).

MICROBIOLOGY
- Diagnosis is based on isolation of *Listeria* from a normally sterile site, usually blood, amniotic fluid, or cerebrospinal fluid.
- The organism usually grows within 36 hours on routine culture media, but further identification with biochemical tests is necessary.
- Reports describe cases of autopsy-proven parenchymal CNS listeriosis with sterile blood and cerebrospinal fluid cultures

IMAGING
- Imaging studies are negative in cases of CNS listeriosis without parenchymal CNS involvement.
- In cases of parenchymal CNS involvement, MRI (imaging study of choice) and CT reveal areas of uptake without ring enhancement, involving the brainstem, cerebellum, and cerebral cortex.

SPECIFIC TESTS
- Gram stain of cerebrospinal fluid is negative in two-thirds of cases of meningitis/meningoencephalitis and may be misleading in many of the remaining cases (usually misinterpreted as gram-positive diplococci).
- Cerebrospinal fluid with a high WBC count (>5,000 cells/mm^3) or a high concentration of protein (>200 mg/dL) is uncommon in patients with CNS listeriosis. Also, about half of the patients with meningitis/meningoencephalitis due to *Listeria* have fewer than 75% polymorphonuclear neutrophils in the cerebrospinal fluid.
- However, clinicians should not exclude CNS listeriosis based only on the degree of pleocytosis, the percentage of polymorphonuclear neutrophils, and the concentration of protein or glucose in the cerebrospinal fluid.

Treatment

MAIN TREATMENT
- For severe infections, ampicillin (adult dosage: 200 mg/kg/d i.v. divided in six doses) or penicillin (adult dosage: 300,000 mg/kg/d i.v. divided in six doses) combined with gentamicin (adult dosage: 1–2 mg/kg every 8 hours, adjusted with renal function and followed by levels)
- For pregnant women with mild infection, a lower dose of ampicillin can be used (4–6 g per day in four doses)
- Two to 4 weeks of therapy is probably adequate for bacteremia.
- A minimum of 15 to 21 days (with an aminoglycoside for at least the first 7–10 days) is needed for the therapy of meningitis.
- Longer antibiotic therapy is needed in the presence of localized CNS involvement, for endocarditis, and for severely immunosuppressed patients.
- For neonatal listeriosis, 2 to 3 weeks of antibiotic treatment is needed.

ALTERNATIVE TREATMENT
- Second choice: trimethoprim–sulfamethoxazole (adult dosage: 20 mg/kg/d of the trimethoprim component i.v. in four divided doses)
- Third choice: erythromycin (adult dosage: 60 mg/kg/d i.v. in four doses), chloramphenicol (adult dosage: 60 mg/kg/d i.v. divided in four doses), or tetracycline (adult dosage: 15 mg/kg/d i.v. divided in four doses)

COMPLICATIONS
- Listeriosis during pregnancy can lead to amnionitis, premature labor, recurrent abortion, premature rupture of membranes, and stillbirth.
- Treatment of maternal bacteremia during pregnancy can prevent or limit neonatal infection.
- CNS infection can lead to seizures or severe neurologic compromise (ataxia, personality changes, coma, etc.). Bacteremia might lead to CNS infection.

Follow-Up

TYPICAL PROGRESSION AND PROGNOSIS
- The mortality rate of meningitis/meningoencephalitis is among the highest among all causes of bacterial meningitis (>27%). Mortality is higher among immunocompromised patients and those who develop seizures.
- The mortality rate of cerebritis, CNS abscess, and endocarditis due to *Listeria* is even higher (~50%).
- The exact morbidity and mortality of the pregnancy-associated listeriosis is unclear, but treatment of maternal bacteremia and antibiotic therapy of the newborn can improve outcome.
- Granulomatosis infantisepticum carries the worst prognosis.

PATIENT FOLLOW-UP
- Patients with CNS infection should be monitored for seizures, and those recovering from CNS infection should be monitored for relapse.
- Individuals with listerial bacteremia should be monitored for neurologic findings suggestive of CNS involvement.
- Patients with a history of listerial infection who will undergo aggressive antineoplastic chemotherapy or antirejection treatment should be monitored for relapse, and prophylactic use of antibiotics can be considered.

PREVENTION
- All individuals should cook meat thoroughly, wash vegetables, avoid unpasteurized milk, keep uncooked meat separate from other foods, and wash hands, utensils, and cutting boards after handling uncooked foods.
- Individuals at risk (including pregnant women) should avoid unpasteurized milk and soft cheese and foods from delicatessen counters, and they should cook meat products thoroughly.

Selected Readings

Armstrong RW, Fung PC. Brainstem encephalitis (rhomboencephalitis) due to *Listeria monocytogenes:* Case report and review. *Clin Infect Dis* 1993;16:689–702.

Lorber B. Listeriosis. *Clin Infect Dis* 1997;24:1–9.

Mylonakis E, Hohmann EL, Calderwood SB. Central nervous system infection with *Listeria monocytogenes:* 33 years' experience at a general hospital and review of 776 episodes from the literature. *Medicine (Baltimore)* 1998;77:313–336.

Lung Abscess

Basics

DEFINITION

- A microbial infection of the lung-producing necrosis of pulmonary parenchyma that leads to discrete, walled-off cavities containing purulent material.
- There may be a single abscess, generally >2 cm in diameter, or multiple small abscesses; the latter condition is known as *necrotizing pneumonia*.
- Lung abscess can be classified as acute or chronic, with a dividing line at 4 to 6 weeks. They are also classified as *primary*, occurring in a previously healthy person, or *secondary*, related to an underlying condition such as pulmonary neoplasm, prior surgery in the lung, or an immunocompromising illness. *Putrid* lung abscess refers to the associated foul odor from the sputum and/or breath, related to fermentation by anaerobic bacteria in the lung.
- Lung abscess can also occur secondary to bacteremia (right-sided bacterial endocarditis or jugular vein thrombophlebitis [Lemierre's syndrome]).
- Approximately 80% of lung abscess cases are primary, 60% are putrid, 40% "nonspecific" (no likely pathogen isolated from expectorated sputum), and 40% chronic.

ETIOLOGY

- The usual case of lung abscess is caused by pure anaerobic bacteria (46%) or a mixture of aerobes and anaerobes (43%). Aerobic or facultative bacteria alone account for 11%. The major anaerobic isolates, often in combination, are:
  —Peptostreptococcus
  —Fusobacterium
  —Prevotella
  —Bacteroides
- The major aerobic/facultative bacteria are:
  —Staphylococcus aureus
  —E. coli
  —Klebsiella
  —Pseudomonas aeruginosa
- Rare causes include Legionella, Nocardia, and Actinomyces
- In patients with HIV, Rhodococcus, Salmonella, and Pneumocystis carinii, Cryptococcus and Aspergillus can occur

EPIDEMIOLOGY

- Lung abscess was common in the preantibiotic era but its occurrence has declined 10-fold in recent times.
- Risk factors (present in 80 to 90% of primary lung abscess cases)
  —Conditions that predispose to aspiration, e.g., altered state of consciousness and dysphagia
  —Periodontal infection with pyorrhea or gingivitis

- Incubation period
  —When following a discrete aspiration event, cavitation can develop within 7 to 14 days, although the patient may have only mild symptoms.
  —Some cases, particularly those associated with virulent aerobic/facultative bacteria, can have a short incubation period of 1 to 3 days.

Clinical Manifestations

SYMPTOMS AND SIGNS

- In the more common chronic form, symptoms of fatigue, productive cough (which may be foul-smelling), weight loss, and pleuritic pain can date for weeks to months.
- The sputum is usually purulent

Diagnosis

- Leukocytosis is usually present (15 to 20,000/mm^3)
- Chest radiograph shows a pulmonary infiltrate along with a cavity that may have an air-fluid level, usually confined to a single segment or lobe. CT scan shows

Lung Abscess

cavity formation and may reveal additional cavities as well. The most common sites are those liable to aspiration, e.g., the superior segments of the lower lobes and the posterior segments of the upper lobes.
- One third of patients have coexistent empyema.

DIFFERENTIAL DIAGNOSIS

- Infectious
  —Pneumonia
  —Bronchitis

LABORATORY

- Imaging: Chest x-ray shows pulmonary infiltrate with a cavity.
- Sputum culture
- Gram stain

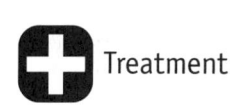

Treatment

MAIN TREATMENT

- Comparative clinical trials have shown that clindamycin is superior to penicillin in treating lung abscess. The initial dose is 750 mg IV three times a day.
- Metronidazole is often used in combination with penicillin, although several studies have shown disappointing results with metronidazole.
- Antibiotic treatment should be started intravenously, but can be switched to the oral route after the fever and toxicity have abated. Duration is usually 3 weeks to several months, based on cavity closure and reduction of the pulmonary infiltrate.
- Surgical drainage is needed in about 10% of cases which are refractory to antibiotics alone. Drainage can be accomplished by a percutaneous needle-guided approach.

ALTERNATIVE TREATMENT

- Alternative therapy (without solid proof of efficacy) is ampicillin/clavulante 4 g/day.

COMPLICATIONS

- Mortality is now 5 to 15%
- Risk factors for a poor prognosis include cavity size >6 cm, persistence of symptoms >8 weeks before diagnosis, elderly and/or debilitated patient, pathogen is aerobic/facultative bacteria, and nosocomial acquisition.
- Obstructed bronchus and/or large abscess can produce failures of medical management, with contiguous involvement of other segments of lung.

Follow-Up

- In the patients with poor prognosis, the chest x-ray should be followed until cavity closure and resolution of the infiltrate to a stable scar.

PREVENTION

N/A

Selected Readings

Hirshberg B, Sklair-Levi M, Nir-Paz R, et al. Factors predicting mortality of patients with lung abscess. *Chest* 1999;115(3):746–750.

Mwandumba HC, Beeching NJ. Pyogenic lung infections: Factors for predicting clinical outcome of lung abscess and thoracic empyema. *Curr Opin Pulmon Med* 2000;6(3):234–239.

Rowe S, Cheadle WG. Complications of nosocomial pneumonia in the surgical patient. *Am J Surg* 2000;179[Suppl 2A]:63S–68S.

Lyme Disease

Basics

DEFINITION

Lyme disease is a multisystemic, tick-borne disease, the infection of which begins at the site of a hard-bodied tick bite, followed by local dissemination of the organism in the skin and subsequent spread by blood or lymph to other skin sites, joints, cerebrospinal fluid, heart, muscle, bone, retina, spleen, liver, and brain. Stages of the disease are classified as acute, localized; subacute, disseminated; and chronic. Stages may overlap.

ETIOLOGY

- Spirochete *Borrelia burgdorferi*
- Restricted to certain members of the *Ixodes* species complex, rarely *Amblyomma americanum*

EPIDEMIOLOGY

Incidence

- United States: 15,000 cases reported annually; over 125,000 cases reported since 1982. However, the disease is greatly underreported.
- Ninety percent of cases arise from ten states (listed by order of most cases): New York, Connecticut, Pennsylvania, New Jersey, Wisconsin, Rhode Island, Maryland, Massachusetts, Minnesota, and Delaware. Rates are highest in the Northeast, followed by the Midwest, then the West.
  —Northeast: *Ixodes dammini/scapularis*
  —Upper Midwest: *I. scapularis*
  —West Coast: *Ixodes pacificus*
  —South: *I. scapularis* and *A. americanum*
- Europe: *Ixodes ricinus*
- Asia: *Ixodes persulcatus*
- Australia

Risk Factors

- Outdoor work or activities in endemic areas

Incubation

- A hard-bodied tick becomes infected in its second developmental stage (the larval stage) with *B. burgdorferi* when it feeds on small mammals or birds.
- Only in the third and fourth developmental stages (nymph and adult) can ticks transmit disease to humans, and only if they are attached for more than 48 hours. Nymphs are the most common source of transmission.

Clinical Manifestations

SYMPTOMS AND SIGNS

Acute, Localized

- Expanding rash, erythema migrans (EM), at site of tick bite 3 days to 1 month later (70%)
- A red macule or papule expands to a larger round or oval patch or erythema, 3 to 68 cm.
  —Frequently, the ring has central clearing with a flat, occasionally raised, intensely erythematous outer border; lesion fades within 1 month.
- Rash can be anywhere on the body, most commonly the groin, thigh, axilla, and popliteal fossa.
- Intermittent symptoms of fever, headache, fatigue, malaise, generalized achiness, migratory musculoskeletal pain, regional or generalized lymphadenopathy, or splenomegaly

Subacute, Disseminated

- Organs
  —Involvement in 70% of untreated patients with EM
  —Liver
  —Spleen
- Musculoskeletal
  —Symptoms develop in 60% of patients with untreated EM.
  —After intermittent episodes of arthralgia or migratory musculoskeletal pain, arthritis develops approximately 6 months after onset of infection.
  —Most patients experience swelling and pain in one or two large joints, especially the knee, lasting several days to a few weeks.
  —Some patients experience pain in the temporomandibular joints, the small joints of the hands and feet, and the periarticular structures, including tendons, bursae, and muscle.
- Neurologic
  —Symptoms are common; approximately 15% of patients with untreated EM develop frank neurologic abnormalities weeks to months after onset of infection.
  —In the United States, it is manifested most commonly as subacute, basilar, lymphocytic meningitis with or without unilateral or bilateral facial palsy or peripheral neuritis.
  —In Europe, it is most commonly manifested as Bannwarth's syndrome, which consists of radiculitis, lymphocytic pleocytosis in cerebrospinal fluid, and sometimes cranial neuritis.
- Cardiac
  —Symptoms develop in 5% of patients with untreated EM 1 week to 7 months after the onset of infection.
  —The most common cardiac manifestations are atrioventricular conduction defects: first-degree, second-degree, Wenckebach, and complete block.
  —Duration is usually brief—a few days to 6 weeks.
- Dermatologic
  —There are secondary annular skin lesions in up to 5% of untreated patients with EM within several days to a few weeks after onset of primary EM.
  —Lesions are smaller than in primary EM, may coalesce, and do not have an indurated center.
- Ocular
  —Follicular conjunctivitis in 10% of patients
- Associated infection
  —Mild hepatitis occurs in 20% of patients.

Chronic

The most common manifestations are musculoskeletal, neurologic, and dermatologic.

- Musculoskeletal
  —Arthritis becomes more persistent, lasting months.
  —Arthritis becomes chronic—at least 1 year of continuing joint inflammation—in 10% of untreated patients.
- Neurologic
  —Subacute encephalopathy, characterized by cognitive defects and disturbances in sleep or mood, occurs months to years after onset of infection in a small percentage of patients.
  —Chronic polyneuropathy (rare)
  —Encephalomyelitis, characterized by cognitive defects, ataxia, spastic paraparesis, and bladder dysfunction (more common in Europe, rare in United States) can occur.
- Dermatologic
  —Acrodermatitis chronica atrophicans: appears on extremities as a doughy, violaceous skin infiltration that gradually becomes indurated, thickened, and hyperpigmented

Lyme Disease

- Borellial lymphocytoma: appears in the dermis, subcutis, or both, as a bluish-red, tumor-like skin infiltration (common in Europe, rare in the United States)
- Cardiac
  - Chronic cardiomyopathy is possible, but evidence suggests that it is rare.

Diagnosis

Diagnosis is based on characteristic clinical symptoms, history of exposure in an endemic area, and laboratory tests. Note the limitations of laboratory testing under the later heading of "Laboratory."

DIFFERENTIAL DIAGNOSIS
Infectious
- Fungal skin infections
- Cellulitis
- Erythema annulare centrifugum
- Guillain-Barré syndrome and sarcoidosis (bilateral facial palsy)
- Insect or spider bites
- Plant dermatitis
- Erysipelas
- Granuloma annulare
- Fibromyalgia (neurologic symptoms)
- Chronic fatigue (neurologic symptoms)

LABORATORY
- Misdiagnosis occurs as a result of misinterpretation, overuse, and suboptimal performance and standardization of laboratory tests for the disease.
- A two-test approach is recommended: sensitive enzyme immunoassay or immunofluorescent assay, followed by a Western immunoblot. Specimens that are negative by enzyme immunoassay or immunofluorescent assay do not need to be confirmed by Western immunoblot, only those that are positive and equivocal.
- *Cautions*
  - Serology tests may have negative results in patients with early Lyme disease; most patients seroconvert within the first 4 weeks after onset of infection.
  - A positive IgM test result late after the onset of Lyme disease does not, by itself, mean that the disease is active.
  - It is not usually possible to culture *B. burgdorferi* from cerebrospinal fluid or joint fluid; amplification of nucleic acid of the organism using the polymerase chain reaction technique has been studied, with promising results.
  - False-positive results for Lyme disease can occur in patients with syphilis, oral infection with other spirochete species, or seronegative spondyloarthropathy due to the low sensitivity and specificity of some tests for Lyme disease.

Treatment

MAIN TREATMENT
- Early disease stage
  - Doxycycline 100 mg twice per day PO for 14 to 21 days
  - Amoxicillin 500 mg three times per day PO for 14 to 21 days
- Lyme arthritis
  - Doxycycline 100 mg twice per day PO for 30 days
  - Amoxicillin 500 mg and probenecid 500 mg three time per day PO for 30 days
  - Ceftriaxone 2 g single dose daily i.v. for 14 to 21 days
  - Penicillin G 20 million units i.v. (divided into four to six doses) for 14 to 21 days
- Lyme neurologic symptoms
  - Facial nerve palsy (without other neurologic manifestations)
    - Doxycycline 100 mg twice per day PO for 30 days
    - Amoxicillin 500 mg three times per day PO for 30 days
  - Other neurologic symptoms
    - Ceftriaxone 2 g single dose daily i.v. for 14 to 21 days
    - Penicillin G 20 million units i.v. (divided into four to six doses) for 14 to 21 days
- Lyme carditis
  - Asymptomatic PR interval prolongation 0.3 second or less
    - Doxycycline 100 mg twice per day PO for 14 to 21 days
    - Amoxicillin 500 mg three times per day PO for 14 to 21 days
  - Symptomatic myocarditis or PR interval prolongation greater than 0.3 second
    - Ceftriaxone 2 g single dose daily i.v. for 14 to 21 days
    - Penicillin G 20 million units (divided into four to six doses) for 14 to 21 days

ALTERNATIVE TREATMENT
- Early Lyme disease
  - Cefuroxime axetil 500 mg twice per day PO for 14 to 21 days
  - Erythromycin 250 mg four times per day PO for 14 to 21 days
  - Azithromycin and clarithromycin being studied as alternatives
- Other neurologic symptoms: less-studied alternatives
  - Doxycycline 100 mg twice per day i.v. or oral
  - Cefotaxime 3 g twice per day i.v.
  - Chloramphenicol 1 g every 6 hours i.v. for 14 to 21 days
- Symptomatic myocarditis or PR interval prolongation greater than 0.3 second
  - Corticosteroids may be helpful if carditis is not responsive to antimicrobial treatment.
  - A pacemaker is only rarely necessary.

COMPLICATIONS
- Arthritis unresponsive to antibiotics, especially patients who are HLA-DR4-positive
- Transplacental transmission of disease has been reported in a few patients (rare).

Follow-Up

PREVENTION
- Avoidance of endemic areas
- Protective clothing, long sleeves and long pants, in endemic areas; light-colored clothing makes dark ticks easier to see.
- Application of tick repellants containing DEET to clothing and exposed skin
- Application of acaricides to clothing; not for use on skin
- Daily and thorough check for ticks attached to skin if in endemic area

Selected Readings

Anonymous. American Academy of Pediatrics Committee on Infectious Diseases. Prevention of Lyme disease. *Pediatrics* 2000;105(1 Pt 1):142–147.

Evans J. Lyme disease. *Curr Opin Rheumatol* 1999;11(4):281–288.

Loewen PS, Marra CA, Marra F. Systematic review of the treatment of early Lyme disease. *Drugs* 1999;57(2):157–173.

Nadelman RB, Wormser GP. Lyme borreliosis. *Lancet* 1998;352(9127):557–565.

Thanassi WT, Schoen RT. The Lyme disease vaccine: Conception, development, and implementation. *Ann Intern Med* 2000;132(8):661–668.

Lymphangitis

Basics

DEFINITION
- Infection within the subcutaneous lymphatic layer of the skin

ETIOLOGY
- Lymphangitis often occurs as part of a localized skin infection, such as an abscess or blister or a paronychia.
- The initial source of infection may be difficult to locate.
- Group A β-hemolytic streptococcus is the most common etiology.
- *Staphylococcus aureus* and *Pasteurella multocida* also cause this disease.

EPIDEMIOLOGY
N/A

Clinical Manifestations

- A red streak develops from the cutaneous source of infection to the regional lymph nodes.
  —The streak is often a few millimeters wide, but, at times, it can be over 1 cm wide.
  —The length depends on the distance to the regional lymph nodes.
- Skin is often tender to palpation over the streak.
- Fever may be present.

Diagnosis

- The organism cannot be cultured from the lymphatic channel.
- Patients often have leukocytosis with a left shift.
- Bacteremia may be present.

Lymphangitis

DIFFERENTIAL DIAGNOSIS
- Superficial phlebitis
- Intravenous line infiltration

Treatment

- Penicillin or a β-lactamase–resistant penicillin should be used.
- Alternatives include a first-generation cephalosporin or vancomycin in severely penicillin-allergic patients.
- Use of a β-lactam/β-lactamase inhibitor such as ampicillin/sulbactam should be used for patients with animal bites that could be infected with *Pasteurella*.

COMPLICATIONS
Bacteremia is a complication of untreated lymphangitis.

Follow-Up

- None specific for this illness

PREVENTION
- Use of appropriate antibiotics early when a skin infection is diagnosed should reduce the incidence of lymphangitis.
- Drainage of abscess and paronychia should be done before lymphangitis occurs.

Selected Readings

Bisno AL, Stevens DL. Streptococcal infections of skin and soft tissues. *N Engl J Med* 1996;334:240.

Lymphogranuloma Venereum

Basics

DEFINITION
Lymphogranuloma venereum (LGV) is a sexually transmitted disease manifested as a lesion at the site of inoculation.

ETIOLOGY
- *Chlamydia trachomatis* serovars L1, L2, L3

EPIDEMIOLOGY
Incidence
- Endemic in Africa, South America, parts of Asia
- Rare in North America, Europe, Australia
- Six to ten times more common in men than in women

Risk Factors
- Geographic location in endemic areas: residence, travel, work
- Inconsistent use of barrier contraceptives

Incubation
- Five to 21 days

Clinical Manifestations

SYMPTOMS AND SIGNS
- Small herpetiform or papular genital lesion (initial stage)
- Cervicitis is the most common initial sign in women.
- Bilateral lymphadenopathy occurs in 30%; it can be extensive.
- If untreated, the lymph nodes can ulcerate and drain.
- In homosexual men and women: anal pruritus, mucus, mucopurulent rectal discharge, rectal pain, tenesmus, fever

Diagnosis

History and physical examination alone often lead to an inaccurate diagnosis.

DIFFERENTIAL DIAGNOSIS
Infectious
- Urethritis
- Mucopurulent cervicitis
- Pelvic inflammatory disease
- Proctitis
- Proctocolitis

Lymphogranuloma Venereum

LABORATORY

- Serologic tests
  - Complement fixation
  - Microimmunofluorescence test
  - Isolation of LGV chlamydial serovars

TESTING PROCEDURES

- Gently abrade the lesion with a sterile gauze pad to provoke oozing, but not gross bleeding.
- Squeeze the lesion between a gloved thumb and forefinger to increase exudate from the lesion.
- Apply the exudate directly onto a microscope slide if used for dark-field and direct immunofluorescence tests.

Treatment

MAIN TREATMENT

- Doxycycline 100 mg PO two times per day for 21 days

- Fluctuant inguinal lymph nodes may require aspiration of incision and drainage through intact skin.

ALTERNATIVE TREATMENT

- Erythromycin 500 mg PO four times per day for 21 days
- Sulfisoxazole 500 mg PO four times per day for 21 days

SEX PARTNERS

- Examination, serologic testing, and presumptive treatment

COMPLICATIONS

- LGV leads to fibrosis of lymph nodes, fistulas, and strictures if untreated.

Follow-Up

PREVENTION

- Safe sex; use of barrier contraceptives

Selected Readings

Kellock DJ, Barlow R, Suvarna SK, et al. Lymphogranuloma venereum: Biopsy, serology, and molecular biology. *Genitourin Med* 1997;73(5):399–401,1997.

Papagrigoriadis S, Rennie JA. Lymphogranuloma venereum as a cause of rectal strictures. *Postgrad Med J* 1998;74(869):168–169.

Malaria

Basics

DEFINITION

- Malaria is a protozoan infection of erythrocytes, transmitted to humans by the bite of an anopheline mosquito.
- Malaria is responsible for as many as 2 million deaths a year. Four strains of protozoa are distributed throughout the tropics.

ETIOLOGY

- Malaria infects 200 to 300 million people per year.
- The four strains are *Plasmodium falciparum*, *Plasmodium vivax*, *Plasmodium malariae*, and *Plasmodium ovale*.
  - *P. falciparum* can invade erythrocytes at all stages of maturation, and is responsible for severe disease with the greatest mortality. It is often drug resistant. Because of the lack of a dormant live stage, *P. falciparum* does not cause relapses.
  - *P. vivax* and *P. ovale* cause acute illness, and they are also responsible for late relapse over 6 to 11 months after acute infection.
  - *P. malariae* infections may persist for decades within the bloodstream, but relapse does not occur, except under rare circumstances, such as trauma or surgery.

EPIDEMIOLOGY

Incidence

- Malaria exists in tropical locations where the anopheline mosquito is present and the pool of infected people is high.
- In parts of the United States, the anopheline mosquito exists; however, malaria is not present, except in rare cases.
- Over 1 million deaths, mainly in children, occur annually in Africa.
- Malaria is so well established in Africa that adaptation with the sickle cell gene, which confers protection, is present in as many as 25% of the population.
- *P. falciparum* exists in tropical locations where mosquitos live year round. In areas where mosquitos do not live year round (dry season), *P. vivax* and *P. ovale* can persist due to the liver hypnozoite stage.
- *P. falciparum* occurs in Africa, Papua New Guinea, Haiti, and east Asia.
- *P. vivax* occurs in Central and South America, India, North Africa, and East Asia.
- *P. ovale* occurs in West Africa.
- *P. malariae* is present worldwide, but it is found mostly in Africa.

Risk Factors

- Immunity plays an important role in the disease that malarial infection causes. Patients with no prior immunity will often have the highest rates of parasitemia and the most complications. Risk of complications also is present in young children with little or no immunity.
- Patients who are asplenic have greater complications.
- Pregnant women have more severe disease.

Incubation

- The time from insect bite to the release of merozoites into the bloodstream varies:
  - *P. falciparum:* between 5 and 15 days
  - *P. vivax:* 13.4 days
  - *P. ovale:* 14.1 days
  - *P. malariae:* 34.7 days

Clinical Manifestations

SYMPTOMS AND SIGNS

- Malaria causes fevers that, at times, are cyclic in nature.
  - In patients with *P. falciparum*, fevers can be continuous, with occasional spikes.
  - Patients with *P. ovale* and *P. vivax* have high fevers every 48 hours. For *P. malariae*, fevers are noted every 72 hours.
- Fevers are associated with rigors, tachycardia, and headaches. After 2 to 6 hours, the patients' fevers will break and sweating occurs.
- In children and people who have no natural immunity, mental status changes, meningismus, seizures, and coma may occur.

Malaria

- Patients may note shortness of breath and cough, which are harbingers of pulmonary edema.
- Renal failure due to hemoglobinuria (blackwater fever) is common in overwhelming *P. falciparum* infection.

Diagnosis

LABORATORY

- Thin and thick smear of blood
- Enzyme-linked immunosorbent assay for a histidine-rich *P. falciparum* antigen
- Assay for parasite lactate dehydrogenase

Other Findings

- Anemia with evidence of hemolysis (elevated LDH and decreased haptoglobin)
- Thrombocytopenia
- Renal insufficiency

DIFFERENTIAL DIAGNOSIS

- Typhoid fever
- Rheumatic fever

Treatment

- Chloroquine-sensitive *P. ovale, malariae, falciparum,* and *vivax*
  —Chloroquine base 600 mg orally, followed by 300 mg orally in 6 hours and 300 mg orally on day 2 and day 3
- Chloroquine-resistant *P. falciparum*
  —Quinine sulfate 650 mg orally every 8 hours for 3 to 7 days, along with doxycycline 100 mg orally twice a day for 7 days, or
  —Quinine sulfate 650 mg orally every 8 hours for 3 to 7 days, followed by pyrimethamine-sulfadoxine 3 tablets orally on the last day of quinine treatment
- For elimination of the hypnozoite stage in *P. ovale* and *P. vivax*
  —Primaquine phosphate base 15.3 mg each day for 14 days
- Exchange transfusion has been used in patients with malaria who have complications and high parasitemia rates.

ALTERNATIVE TREATMENT

- Quinine, followed by clindamycin 900 mg orally tid for 5 days
- Mefloquine 1,250 mg orally as a single dose
- Atovaquone 1,000 mg daily for 3 days and proguanil 400 mg daily for 3 days
- Halofantrine 500 mg every 6 hours for three doses, with repeat three doses given in 1 week

COMPLICATIONS

- Coma due to increased vascular permeability and cerebral edema occur in patients with no immunity who have a high degree of parasitemia.
- Hypoglycemia is multifactorial in etiology. It is due to hepatic glycogen depletion, increased metabolic demands, and hyperinsulinemia.
- Oliguric renal failure can occur with massive hemolysis. This may be due to malaria itself or due to use of quinine in patients with glucose-6 phosphate deficiency.
- Pulmonary edema occurs due to the capillary leak syndrome.

Follow-Up

Signs of malaria may start after a person leaves an endemic region. Travelers should be instructed to seek medical attention if fevers should occur.

PREVENTION

- All travelers should be instructed to use insect repellants with diethyltoluamide (DEET), use mosquito netting, and wear occlusive clothing, especially during the time of day that mosquitos bite.
- Local residents where chloroquine-sensitive *P. malariae* is present
  —Chloroquine base 300 mg once a week
- Local residents where chloroquine-resistant *P. falciparum* is present
  —Mefloquine 250 mg PO once a week
  —Doxycycline 100 mg PO qd
  —Primaquine base 5 mg/kg/d
  —Chloroquine base 300 mg per week and proguanil 200 mg per day
- Drugs should be started 2 weeks before entering an endemic region and continue for 4 weeks after leaving the region.

Selected Readings

Brewster D, Kwiakowski D, White NJ. Neurologic sequelae of cerebral malaria in childhood. *Lancet* 1990;336:1039–1043.

Luxemburger C, Nosten F, ter Kuile F, et al. Mefloquine for drug resistant malaria. *Lancet* 1991;338:1268.

White NJ. The treatment of malaria. *N Engl J Med* 1996;335:800–806.

White NJ, Warrell DA, Chanthavanich P, et al. Severe hypoglycemia and hyperinsulinemia in falciparum malaria. *N Engl J Med* 1983;309:61–66.

Mastitis

Basics

DEFINITION
Mastitis is infection of the breast in nursing mothers.

ETIOLOGY
- Usually, *Staphylococcus aureus* is isolated from the breast.
- On rare occasions, anaerobic streptococci, mycobacteria, nocardia, and other organisms are responsible.

EPIDEMIOLOGY
- Illness occurs in 1% to 3% of nursing mothers.
- Onset occurs within 2 to 3 weeks of delivery of the baby.

Clinical Manifestations

- The spectrum of disease is from a small nodule to a large abscess.
- A plugged duct usually requires moist heat to the affected breast and close observation for signs of infection.
- Mastitis is associated with a red indurated area with occasional streaks. Fevers and chills may occur. Disease is unilateral, often in the upper and outer quadrants.
- Predisposing risk factors include plugged ducts, cracked nipple, engorgement, and changes in feeding patterns.

Diagnosis

- Diagnosis is clinical.
- Incision and drainage is needed if an abscess is present.

DIFFERENTIAL DIAGNOSIS
- Idiopathic granulomatous mastitis
- Carcinoma of the breast

Mastitis

Treatment

- Moist heat is applied to the breast.
- Feeding or pumping should continue every 2 hours.
- Bed rest and avoidance of wearing a constricting bra are recommended.
- Antibiotics such as dicloxacillin or erythromycin are recommended.
- Hospitalized patients should have intravenous antibiotics, and cultures should be obtained to rule out methicillin-resistant staphylococcus.
- Surgery may be required in some patients who have developed mastitis in previously reconstructed breasts. A plastic surgeon should be consulted.

COMPLICATIONS

Mastitis usually resolves with treatment.

Follow-Up

- None specific

PREVENTION

Care should be taken when cracked nipples occur. Breast feeding with the affected breast should be suspended until healing occurs.

Selected Readings

Han BK, Choe YH, Park JM, et al. Granulomatous mastitis: Mammographic and sonographic appearances. *AJR* 1999;173(2):317–320.

O'Hara RJ, Dexter SP, Fox JN. Conservative management of infective mastitis and breast abscesses after ultrasonographic assessment. *Br J Surg* 1996;83(10):1413–1414.

Vogel A, Hutchison BL, Mitchell EA. Mastitis in the first year postpartum. *Birth* 1999;26(4):218–225.

Mastoiditis

Basics

DEFINITION
- Inflammation of the mastoid air cells; classified as acute or chronic, depending on duration of infection

ETIOLOGY
- Infection of the mastoid air cells usually follows middle ear infection.
- In acute mastoiditis, the involved bacteria are similar to those implicated in acute otitis media (usually *Streptococcus pneumoniae, Haemophilus influenzae*, and *Moraxella catarrhalis*).
- In cases of mastoiditis with a prolonged course, *Staphylococcus aureus*, β-hemolytic streptococci, gram-negative bacilli, and anaerobes are frequently involved.
- Tuberculosis and atypical mycobacterial infections are rare causes of chronic mastoiditis.
- Rarely, fungi (mainly *Aspergillus*) can cause mastoiditis in immunosuppressed persons.

EPIDEMIOLOGY

Incidence
- The incidence of mastoiditis has decreased significantly in the antibiotic era because of prompt treatment of otitis media with antimicrobial agents.
- The increasing resistance of microbes to antimicrobial agents during recent years has been associated with increasing rates of mastoiditis.

Risk Factor
- Inadequate treatment of otitis media

Clinical Manifestations

SYMPTOMS AND SIGNS
- Acute otitis media (fever, ear pain, impaired hearing)
- Postauricular pain, tenderness, and swelling over the mastoid bone
- The pinna is often displaced outward and downward.
- Chronic mastoiditis may be manifested by hearing loss, persistent ear discharge, and/or ear pain.

Diagnosis

DIFFERENTIAL DIAGNOSIS
- Postauricular cellulitis
- Postauricular lymphadenopathy
- Parotitis
- Tumors in the mastoid air cells

DIAGNOSTIC STUDIES
- Laboratory studies: usually, increased white blood cell count and erythrocyte sedimentation rate
- Radiography reveals coalescence of the mastoid air cells due to destruction of their bony septa. Also, it may show haziness of the mastoid air cells due to the presence of fluid.
- CT scan is very helpful in evaluating the extension of the disease.
- Cultures of ear discharge should be taken (if the tympanic membrane is not perforated, tympanocentesis should be performed).

Mastoiditis

Treatment

- In acute infection, the antimicrobial drugs of choice are similar to those for acute otitis media.
- Ideally, therapy should be guided by the results of cultures of middle ear fluid. If there is no drainage of middle ear fluid, a myringotomy should be performed.
- Intravenous antimicrobial treatment is preferred for the initial management because mastoiditis is associated with a high probability of complications.
- The recommended duration of treatment is 3 weeks. Oral antibiotics can be used after the initial successful management with intravenous antibiotics.
- Mastoidectomy should be performed when there is evidence of osteomyelitis (by CT scan or MRI), spread to the central nervous system, or failure of medical treatment.
- Surgery is also needed in cases of chronic mastoiditis. The empirical broad-spectrum perioperative antimicrobial therapy should be adjusted on the basis of culture results.

COMPLICATIONS

- Subperiosteal abscess of the temporal bone
- Neck abscess deep to the sternocleidomastoid muscle (Bezold's abscess)
- Cellulitis
- Fascial nerve paralysis
- Intracranial complications (epidural abscess, dural venus thrombophlebitis, meningitis, brain abscess)
- Chronic mastoiditis may cause irreversible hearing loss.

Follow-Up

Follow-up audiograms are needed to check for hearing loss.

PREVENTION

- Early treatment of acute otitis media with effective antibiotics

Selected Readings

Antonelli PJ, Dhanani N, Giannoni CM, et al. Impact of resistant pneumococcus on rates of acute mastoiditis. *Otolaryngol Head Neck Surg* 1999;121:190–194.

Chen D, Lalwani AK, House JW, et al. *Aspergillus* mastoiditis in acquired immunodeficiency syndrome. *Am J Otol* 1999;20:561–567.

Fliss DM, Leiberman A, Dagan R. Acute and chronic mastoiditis in children. *Adv Pediatr Infect Dis* 1997;13:165–185.

Khafif A, Halperin D, Hochman I, et al. Acute mastoiditis: A 10-year review. *Am J Otolaryngol* 1998;19:170–173.

Spiegel JH, Lustig LR, Lee KC, et al. Contemporary presentation and management of a spectrum of mastoid abscesses. *Laryngoscope* 1998;108:822–828.

Swartz JD, Harnsberger HR, Mukherji SK. The temporal bone. *Contemp Diagn Dilem Radiol Clin North Am* 1998;36:819–853.

Wang NE, Burg JM. Mastoiditis: A case-based review. *Pediatr Emerg Care* 1998;14:290–292.

Measles

Basics

DEFINITION
Rubeola virus causes a benign childhood illness that has been controlled since vaccination was initiated. Disease in adults is more severe. In developing countries, measles remains a serious disease, with great morbidity and mortality.

ETIOLOGY
- Enveloped RNA-containing virus of the Paramyxoviridae family

EPIDEMIOLOGY
- Measles occurs worldwide.
- It is spread by respiratory droplets.
- People are most infectious during the catarrhal stage, yet transmission can occur 2 days before obvious symptoms until 4 days after the rash appears.
- Prior to immunization, periodic epidemics occurred every 2 to 5 years, and children ages 5 to 10 years were most affected.
- In developing countries, measles now occurs between the ages of 1 and 5 years.
- Measles worldwide accounts for over 1 million deaths annually.
- Since vaccination, the incidence has dropped in the United States to 1% (around 10,000 cases) of previous years.
- In developed countries, outbreaks have been noted in children over the age of 10 years and in college students.

Risk Factors
- Adolescents who have been immunized only once as a child

Incubation
- Ten to 14 days

Clinical Manifestations

- The initial prodromal phase, with fevers, coryza, cough, and conjunctivitis, lasts several days.
- Patients develop Koplik spots (1-mm spots or grains) along the buccal mucosa during the initial phase.
- Following this, patients develop a red maculopapular and sometimes confluent rash, initially occurring behind the ears and on the forehead, then proceeding down the body to the extremities.
- Patients have high fever during the time the rash is developing. In each location on the body, the rash usually takes 5 days to begin to clear.
- Desquamation of the hands and feet occurs in some cases.
- In adolescents or young adults who had received the live virus vaccination in early childhood but no booster, a mild, atypical infection can occur as immunity has waned. Cough; a mild, evanescent rash; and a pulmonary infiltrate are most common.

COMPLICATIONS
- Bronchitis
- Otitis media
- Bacterial pneumonia
- Death from pneumonia occurs most commonly in infants and small children.
- Acute encephalitis is a rare complication, and occurs typically during the convalescent period.

ADULT MEASLES
- Adult measles carries a very high risk of developing bacterial complications, such as pneumonia, otitis media, and sinusitis.
- Respiratory failure due to measles pneumonia is common in pregnant women and in immunocompromised individuals.

Measles

- The incidence of measles without the characteristic rash in immunocompromised patients is 40%.

ATYPICAL MEASLES

Atypical measles is a term used for patients who get measles but had been immunized with the killed measles vaccine. These patients develop severe illness, with an atypical rash that may be vesicular, hemorrhagic, or pruritic. Patients may have edema of the extremities, hepatitis, and a toxic shock-like syndrome.

Diagnosis

- Diagnosis is made when Koplik spots are identified.
- A serologic diagnosis is often made.
- The virus can be isolated from secretions.
- Leukopenia
- Chest x-rays may show infiltrates if bacterial pneumonia has developed.

Treatment

- Supportive care is needed, as is respiratory isolation.
- Patients should be observed for secondary bacterial complications.

COMPLICATIONS

- Subacute sclerosing panencephalitis (SSPE), a degenerative neurologic disease caused by infection of the brain by a mutated measles virus strain
  —Inflammation, gliosis, and neuronal degeneration occur.
  —The incidence of SSPE is 0.6 to 2.2 cases per 100,000 cases of measles.
  —Increased risk is noted when infection occurs before the age of 4 years.
  —Disease becomes manifest 6 to 8 years after the clinical case of measles (often as children or adolescents).
  —Patients have progressive cognitive dysfunction and incoordination. This progresses to spasms and seizures, and finally stupor and coma. Death takes 1 to 3 years.
- Increased risk of death from pneumonia occurs most commonly in infants and small children.
- Acute encephalitis is a rare complication, occurring during convalescence.

Follow-Up

Following measles, patients have lifelong immunity.

PREVENTION

- Immunization with live virus vaccine
  —Children at the age of 15 months and again at age 11 to 12
  —Patients with HIV who require vaccination should have no problem as long as they are not profoundly immunocompromised.
  —People born in 1957 or prior to 1957
- Passive Immunization
  —Passive immunization with immunoglobulin should be considered for people with deficits of cell-mediated immunity or for people who are not fully immunized.

Selected Readings

Bellini WJ, Rota PA. Genetic diversity of wild-type measles viruses: Implications for global measles elimination programs. *Emerg Infect Dis* 1998;4:29–35.

Griffin DE, Ward BJ, Jauregui E, et al. Immune activation in measles. *N Engl J Med* 1989;320:1667–1672.

Hutchins S, Markowitx L, Atkinson W, et al. Measles outbreaks in the United States 1987–1990. *Pediatr Infect Dis J* 1996;15:31–38.

Mediastinitis

Basics

DEFINITION
Mediastinitis is infection of the mediastinum. This is often a complication of thoracic trauma or surgery, pneumonia, empyema, head and neck infections with inferior spread, or esophageal rupture or surgery.

ETIOLOGY
- Patients with mediastinitis secondary to median sternotomy often have gram-positive organisms such as *Staphylococcus aureus, Staphylococcus epidermidis,* or *Enterococcus.*
- Gram-negative organisms or fungal infections with *Candida* occur less frequently than with gram-positives.
- Patients with mediastinitis secondary to head and neck infections or esophageal perforation often have polymicrobial organisms (anaerobic and aerobic), which include anaerobic streptococci, *Bacteroides, Fusobacterium*, as well as other mouth flora.

EPIDEMIOLOGY
Most cases now are seen in patients who have had heart surgery. The risk of infection after sternotomy is between 0.4% and 5%.

Risk Factors
- Reoperations
- Diabetes
- Obesity
- Lengthy surgical procedures of the thoracic area

Incubation
- The average incubation after a sternotomy is 2 weeks.
- With low-grade pathogens, presentation may be delayed to over 1 year.

Clinical Manifestations

- There is a wide spectrum of presentations, depending on the organism and the location of the infection.
- Redness and drainage are common.
- Sternal click with instability
- Fever with no discernible source
- Increased pain at incision site
- With head and neck infections, the source is often obvious.
  —Patients develop chest pain and sepsis.
  —Hamman's sign is noted (a crunching sound audible over the precordium during systole)
- With esophageal perforation, patients may present with the following:
  —Epigastric or chest pain
  —Fevers
  —Crepitus, especially in the neck or anterior chest wall
  —Hamman's sign

Diagnosis

- Following heart surgery
  —A CT scan in combination with needle aspiration is useful.
  —It is difficult to make diagnosis, in that CT and x-rays are typically abnormal in these postoperative patients.

Mediastinitis

- Following esophageal rupture or head and neck infections
  — An x-ray indicates widening of the mediastinum.
  — Subcutaneous and mediastinal air can be demonstrated.
  — Pleural effusions
- A CT scan is often helpful.
- Patients often exhibit an elevated white blood cell count with shift.

Treatment

- Drainage, debridement
- There is controversy as to whether the wound should remain open or be closed after the initial debridement.
- Antibiotics should be directed at results of culture and Gram stain, and should be administered for a lengthy time.
- Adequate nutrition

COMPLICATIONS

- Sternal osteomyelitis
- Graft destruction
- Infection of hardware such as pacemakers or cardiac prosthetic valves

Follow-Up

Follow closely for evidence of remaining infection.

PREVENTION

- Cefazolin or vancomycin is used as prophylaxis in many cardiovascular procedures, although the benefit is unclear.
- Observe good surgical technique with skin and soft tissues, especially around the sternum.
- Limit the amount of bleeding during operation.
- Limit the use of bone wax.

Selected Readings

Clancy CJ, Mguyen MH, Morris AJ. Candidal mediastinitis: An emerging clinical entity. *Clin Infect Dis* 1997;25:608–613.

Milano CA, Kessler K, et al. Mediastinitis after coronary artery bypass graft surgery. *Circulation* 1995;92:2245–2251.

Rupp ME, Archer GL. Mediastinitis. In: Mandel GL, Bennett JE, Dolin R, eds. *Principals and practice of infectious diseases,* 4th ed. New York: Churchill Livingstone, 1995:813–821.

Meningitis, Acute

Basics

DEFINITION

Acute meningitis is inflammation of the meninges that occurs along with viral and bacterial infections. Acute meningitis typically develops over a period of days and resolves rapidly either by itself, when a viral etiology is implicated, or if treated appropriately when a bacterial etiology is found.

ETIOLOGY

- Viral infections account for most cases.
- Enteroviral infection is the leading cause of aseptic meningitis, especially in the late summer and early fall months.
- Other infections commonly associated with meningitis include the following:
  —HIV (acute retroviral syndrome)
  —Arboviruses
  —Herpesviruses
  —Mumps virus
  —Adenovirus
- Of the bacterial causes of acute meningitis, those that account for most cases are the following:
  —Pneumococcus
  —*Neisseria meningitidis*
  —*Listeria monocytogenes*
  —*Haemophilus influenzae* type B
- *Treponema pallidum* and *Borrelia burgdorferi* invade the CNS and can produce meningitis.
- Group B *Streptococcus* causes disease in neonates.
- Gram-negatives and *Staphylococcus aureus* are encountered on rare occasions.

EPIDEMIOLOGY

- Bacterial meningitis is most frequently seen in children and young adults.
- The three most important pathogens, pneumococcus, meningococcus, and *H. influenzae* are all respiratory pathogens, capable of colonizing the pharynx prior to the development of disease.
- *Pneumococcus* accounts for 40% of community-acquired cases of meningitis.
- There has been a marked decrease in the incidence of meningitis due to *H. influenzae* type B in those countries giving the specific vaccine to children.
- Clusters of meningococcal meningitis occur in young adults spending time in group settings. Meningococcus is the only bacterial pathogen that can lead to epidemics.
- A modest increase in the number of *Listeria* meningitis over the past 10 years most likely can be accounted for by an increase in the numbers of patients who have transplants or are otherwise immunocompromised.

Incidence

- Pneumococcal meningitis: 1.1 case per million
- Meningococcus meningitis: 0.6 case per million
- *H. influenzae* meningitis: 0.2 case per million

Risk Factors

- Unprotected sex would place the patient at risk for viral meningitis due to HIV infection, and at risk for primary syphilis with CNS invasion.
- Bites by the *Ixodes* tick in endemic areas would be a risk factor for Lyme disease.
- Patients who are asplenic have a higher incidence of infections with pneumococcus, meningococcus, and *H. influenzae*.
- Patients with terminal complement deficiency have a higher risk for developing meningococcal meningitis.
- Patients with cerebrospinal fluid (CSF) rhinorrhea, head trauma, otitis media and mastoiditis, and alcoholism have a higher risk of pneumococcal meningitis.

Incubation

Bacterial meningitis generally occurs about 1 to 7 days following the onset of upper respiratory infection.

Clinical Manifestations

VIRAL MENINGITIS

- Fever with headache and nuchal rigidity
- Photophobia
- Nausea and vomiting
- Associated manifestations due to specific viral infections should be sought.
  —Mumps with parotitis or orchitis
  —Herpangina with coxsackievirus A
  —Vesicles on genitalia associated with HSV-2
  —Chickenpox rash with varicella

BACTERIAL MENINGITIS

- Symptoms and signs often differ with respect to the age of the patients.
- Fevers with headache and nuchal rigidity initially
- Rapid progression to confusion, lethargy, and coma
- Cranial nerve abnormalities can be associated with acute bacterial meningitis, especially with Lyme disease.
- Focal neurologic abnormalities can occur with infarction.
- Seizures occur in 30% of cases.
- A skin rash that ranges from petechiae to diffuse ecchymosis would suggest meningococcal disease.
- Pneumonia or otitis media would suggest pneumococcus as the etiology.

Diagnosis

- Lumbar puncture with determination of cell counts and glucose and protein, along with Gram stains are needed for the diagnosis of meningitis.
- Cultures and Gram stains may be positive before CSF pleocytosis occurs.
- Gram stains for bacterial pathogens are positive in the CSF between 50% and 90% of the time.
- CSF polymerase chain reaction, if available, can help with the diagnosis of bacterial and viral (enterovirus) pathogens.

Meningitis, Acute

- In bacterial meningitis, leukocytosis is common. A WBC count less than 5,000/mm³ suggests overwhelming infection.

CEREBROSPINAL FLUID PROFILES

- Bacterial
  - Often show 1,000 to 5,000 WBCs, with 90% or higher polys
  - CSF glucose is often less than 40% of the serum glucose, or less than 40 mg/dL.
  - CSF protein is elevated.
- Viral
  - Generally less than 1,000 WBC cells are seen.
  - Initially, polys are noted; however, over time, lymphocytes predominate.
  - Glucose is normal, except for mumps, in which it can be decreased.
  - CSF protein is often mildly elevated.

DIFFERENTIAL DIAGNOSIS

- Encephalitis
- Meningitis due to drugs such as NSAIDs, carbamazepine, trimethoprim–sulfamethoxazole, and metronidazole
- Brain abscess
- Subarachnoid bleeding
- Cerebral vasculitis

IMAGING

- CT or MRI may show a number of abnormalities, but should not be done prior to the lumbar puncture if no focal abnormalities are noted or the patient is not HIV-positive.
- CT may show cerebral edema, ventriculitis, hydrocephalus, infarcts, or abscess.
- CT may also help with the diagnosis of mastoiditis.

Treatment

COMMUNITY-ACQUIRED BACTERIAL MENINGITIS

- Ceftriaxone 2 g i.v. every 12 hours or cefotaxime 2 g i.v. every 4 to 6 hours
- Many would also start with vancomycin and continue it until penicillin-resistant pneumococcus has been ruled out in the laboratory.
- Dexamethasone 0.4 mg/kg every 12 hours for 2 days should be considered.
- When meningococcus is isolated, treatment with penicillin G or ampicillin is indicated.
- Listeria and gram-negative bacteria
  - Ampicillin 2 g every 4 hours plus ceftazidime 2 g i.v. every 8 hours, along with gentamicin 1 mg/kg every 8 hours
- Meningococcal meningitis is treated for 7 days.
- Pneumococcal meningitis is treated for 10 days.
- Listeria meningitis is treated for 21 days.

COMPLICATIONS

- Late-onset seizures
- Hydrocephalus
- Cognitive abnormalities
- Cranial nerve abnormalities
- Syndrome of inappropriate antidiuretic secretion
- Subdural effusions or subdural empyema
- Cerebral infarcts

Follow-Up

- Patients who survive an episode of meningitis may need rehabilitation and close neurologic follow-up.
- Seizures and hydrocephalus may occur late.

PREVENTION

- Vaccination is available for H. influenzae type B, given in two or three doses beginning at age 2 to 3 months and again at age 6 months. A final dose is given at 12 to 15 months of age.
- Vaccination against meningococcus polysaccharides A, C, W, and Y are available. It should be given to adults and children who are deemed at high risk (military recruits, contacts to index cases, patients going to areas of high incidence, patients with asplenia and terminal complement disorders).
- At times, patients may need vaccination if there is an outbreak in the community.
- College students are now felt to benefit from vaccination.
- A 23-polysaccharide pneumococcal vaccine is available. At this time, it should be given to children and adults with chronic CSF leaks.

Chemoprophylaxis for Meningococcus

- Chemoprophylaxis is given to close contacts of index cases.
- Housemates, daycare contacts, and hospital personnel with close contact with possible respiratory secretions are treated.
- Adults
  - Ciprofloxacin 500 mg orally, one dose
  - Rifampin 600 mg orally every 12 hours for 2 days
  - Ceftriaxone 250 mg intramuscular, one dose
- Children
  - Rifampin 10 mg/kg every 12 hours for 2 days
  - Ceftriaxone 125 mg intramuscular, one dose

Selected Readings

Anderson J, Backer V, Voldsgaard P, et al. Acute meningococcal meningitis: Analysis of features of the disease according to the age of 255 patients. *J Infect Dis* 1987;9:1187–1192.

Connolly KJ, Hammer SM. The acute aseptic meningitis syndrome. *Infect Dis Clin North Am* 1990;4:599–622.

Durand ML, Calderwood SB, Weber DJ, et al. Acute bacterial meningitis in adults. A review of 493 episodes. *N Engl J Med* 1993;328:21–28.

Meningitis, Chronic

Basics

DEFINITION
Chronic meningitis is meningitis that persists for over 4 weeks.

ETIOLOGY
- Tuberculosis is the leading cause of chronic meningeal inflammation; it occurs in 40% of cases of chronic meningitis.
- Atypical mycobacteria, including *Mycobacterium avium* complex, have been rarely associated with chronic meningitis in AIDS patients.
- Other causes of chronic meningitis include syphilis, Lyme disease, and, on occasion, *Listeria*.
- Leptospirosis and relapsing fever are associated with chronic meningitis.
- *Actinomyces* and *Nocardia* may cause focal disease in the brain and are rare causes of chronic meningitis. They usually have a neutrophilic predominance of cerebrospinal fluid (CSF) cells.
- *Cryptococcus neoformans* may produce a chronic meningitis in both immunocompromised and immunocompetent patients. It occurs in 7% of cases of chronic meningitis. It is most often seen in AIDS patients, those who have had transplants, and those on high-dose steroids.
- *Coccidioides immitis* and *Sporotrichosis* produce chronic meningitis, and it is very important to get a good epidemiologic history from patients. With respect to *Coccidioides*, one would need to know whether the patient had been to an endemic area, such as the desert southwestern United States. With respect to *Sporotrichosis*, one would want a history of exposure to the thorns of rose plants.
- As part of disseminated disease syndrome, blastomyces and histoplasmosis can each cause meningitis.
- *Candida* and *Aspergillus* are associated with a neutrophilic predominance of cells in the CSF.
- Parasitic infections may lead to eosinophilic meningitis. *Angiostrongylus cantonensis* is the organism most commonly the cause.
- HIV can lead to a chronic meningitis, especially early in the course of the illness.
- Cytomegalovirus associated with a polyradiculitis at the cauda equina can, at times, have a chronic phase, and the CSF often shows a neutrophilic profile.

EPIDEMIOLOGY
N/A

Clinical Manifestations

- Chronic meningismus
- Headaches
- Fevers
- Nausea
- Vomiting
- Confusion, at times
- Symptoms and signs persist for at least 1 month if untreated.
- Lymphadenopathy
- Vasculitis rashes
- Thrush
- Basilar meningitis with tuberculosis may produce cranial nerve abnormalities, especially a VIth nerve palsy. Choroidal tubercles are, on occasion, seen with tuberculosis meningitis. It is not uncommon that other signs of tuberculosis are present at the same time as meningeal symptoms are noted, such as cough, hemoptysis, fevers, and weight loss.
- *Coccidioides* meningitis often leads to hydrocephalus, and patients may present with headache, confusion progressing to stupor, and coma. Skin nodules can confirm disseminated disease.

Meningitis, Chronic

Diagnosis

A complete physical examination is necessary to help make the diagnosis. Evidence of lymphadenopathy, vasculitic rashes, and thrush should be sought.

DIFFERENTIAL DIAGNOSIS
- Malignancy
- Sarcoidosis
- Granulomatous angiitis
- Behçet's disease
- Lupus
- Chronic parameningeal infection
- Epidermoid cysts
- Idiopathic causes for chronic meningitis occur in a third of patients.

LABORATORY
Tuberculosis Meningitis
- The CSF often shows 100 to 500 cells, with a lymphocytic profile.
- Up to 85% of patients have a decreased glucose in the CSF.
- Acid-fast bacilli from the CSF are positive in 10% to 40% of cases.
- CSF cultures are positive in 38% to 88% of cases.
- Chest x-ray may reveal changes consistent with old tuberculosis or a miliary pattern.
- In one-half of all patients, the chest x-ray is normal.
- Sputum cultures are positive for tuberculosis in 14% to 50% of cases.
- Skin tests for tuberculosis (PPD) may be negative in over 50% of patients with tuberculosis meningitis. In AIDS patients, the percentage is higher.

Cryptococcal Meningitis
- The CSF often shows 40 to 400 cells, with a lymphocytic profile.
- AIDS patients may have fewer than 10 cells.
- CSF glucose is decreased in 55% of patients.
- India-ink evaluation is positive in 50% of patients, and a combination of a positive serum and CSF cryptococcal antigen (greater than 1:8 in the CSF) is diagnostic.
- Cultures are positive.

Coccidioidomycosis
Patients can be diagnosed by growing the fungus from the CSF or by high titers of antibodies in both the CSF and the serum.

Treatment

Treatment depends on the organism isolated. Unless there is a strong concern about the possibility of disseminated tuberculosis, treatment should be delayed until a firm diagnosis is made.

Tuberculosis Meningitis
- Isoniazid, rifampin pyrazinamide, and ethambutol should be used unless known resistance to one or more of these agents is documented.
- Dexamethasone is given in most cases for the first month.
- Serum drug levels of antituberculosis medications should be obtained.

COMPLICATIONS
- Mortality rates for tuberculosis meningitis are up to 30%. Marked morbidity with cranial nerve palsies, seizures, and cerebral infarcts can be permanent.
- Chronic meningitis due to *Coccidioides* can lead to hydrocephalus, which often requires shunt placement.

Follow-Up

Much depends on the etiology of the disease. In some cases (cocci and cryptococcus/AIDS), lifelong treatment is often required.

PREVENTION
There is no way to prevent chronic meningitis.

Selected Readings

Flood J, Weinstock HS, Guroy M, et al. Neurosyphilis during the AIDS epidemic, San Francisco, 1985–1992. *J Infect Dis* 1998;177:931–940.

Swartz M. Chronic meningitis: Many causes to consider. *N Engl J Med* 1987;317:957–959.

Verdon R, Chevret S, Laissy JP, et al. Tuberculosis meningitis in adults: A review of 48 cases. *Clin Infect Dis* 1996;22:982–988.

Mesenteric Adenitis

Basics

DEFINITION
- Inflammation of the mesenteric lymph nodes, leading to abdominal pain, which, on occasion, can mimic appendicitis

ETIOLOGY
- Infection of the colon causes inflammation of the Peyer's patches, which spreads to the regional mesenteric nodes. A few organisms have been associated with adenitis of these nodes.
- *Yersinia enterocolitica* and *Yersinia pseudotuberculosis*, along with group A *Streptococcus* and *Staphylococcus* account for the majority of cases.

EPIDEMIOLOGY
- *Y. enterocolitica* and *Y. pseudotuberculosis* are zoonotic organisms that are infrequently spread to humans. Both can cause mesenteric adenitis, but *Y. enterocolitica* can lead to diarrhea.
- The organism is present in the intestine of many mammals, including pigs, birds, frogs, and crabs.
- *Yersinia* can be present in drinking water.
- Outbreaks of illness have been described from food ingestion, yet the food source is often never identified.
- Household pets have been shown to be able to spread *Yersinia* infections.
- Mesenteric adenitis is frequently seen in children ages 5 to 14 years.

Incubation
It generally takes 2 weeks to begin to develop symptoms after ingestion of tainted meats containing *Yersinia*.

Risk Factors
Eating raw or undercooked pork has led to *Y. enterocolitica* infections and mesenteric adenitis.

Clinical Manifestations

- Fevers and right lower quadrant pain, indistinguishable from appendicitis
- Diarrhea may not be present.
- Patients may have rebound tenderness.
- With *Y. enterocolitica*, a history of previous diarrhea may be given.

Diagnosis

LABORATORY
- Leukocytosis
- Stool reveals fecal leukocytes.
- Stool cultures are frequently positive.
- Serology may be useful to track an outbreak.
- Radiographic studies suggest terminal ileitis in many cases.

Mesenteric Adenitis

DIFFERENTIAL DIAGNOSIS

- Acute appendicitis
- Crohn's disease
- Tuberculosis
- Epstein-Barr virus
- Parvovirus B19

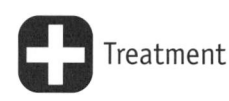

Treatment

- The disease is often self-limited and does not require therapy.
- When treated, sensitivities to medications should be taken into account.
- Trimethoprim-sulfamethoxazole 6 to 12 mg/kg/d divided in 12-hour intervals in children with *Yersinia* infection
- Quinolones in adults with *Yersinia* infection

COMPLICATIONS

- Sepsis with *Yersinia* occurs frequently in patients with iron-overload syndromes.
- Metastatic infection to the spleen, liver, and lung can occur following *Yersinia* sepsis.

Follow-Up

Following treatment, follow-up stool cultures should be obtained.

PREVENTION

- Avoid foods that could have been in contact with *Yersinia* and are not well cooked.
- Avoid contact with animal stool.
- Practice good hygiene in conjunction with household pets.

Selected Readings

Asch MJ, Amoury RA, Touloukian RJ, et al. Suppurative mesenteric lymphadenitis: A report of two cases and review of the literature. *Am J Surg* 1968;115:570–573.

Black RE, Jackson RJ, Tsai T, et al. Epidemic *Yersinia enterocolitica* infection due to contaminated chocolate milk. *N Engl J Med* 1978;298:76–79.

Gutman LT, Ottesen EA, Quan TJ, et al. An inter-familial outbreak of *Yersinia enterocolitica* enteritis. *N Engl J Med* 1973;288:1372–1377.

Mites/Chiggers

Basics

DEFINITION
Mites and chiggers are arthropods with four pairs of legs that can parasitize humans and produce localized skin disease or spread diseases such as typhus or plague. *Sarcoptes scabiei* causes scabies in humans and mange in animals.

ETIOLOGY

Mites That Infest Humans
- *S. scabiei* var. *hominis* causes scabies.
- The mite resides within the skin and lays its eggs.
- Localized inflammation within the burrow, caused by a reaction to the mite, the eggs, and feces, leads to pruritus.
- The mite is not a vector for other infections.
- The life cycle from egg to egg takes less than 2 weeks.

Mites That Infest Animals
- Various species, including *S. scabiei* var. *canis*
- These normally infest dogs but, upon contact with an infected dog, may cause disease in humans.

Chiggers
- These arthropods live in the warm climates; the larval form bites humans.
- Chigger bite leads to intense inflammation and red papules.
- Wheals occur approximately 3 to 6 hours after exposure.
- Chiggers have been known to transmit scrub typhus.

EPIDEMIOLOGY
- Scabies has a worldwide distribution, but is seen most commonly in tropical areas.
- Worldwide estimation of disease is 300 million cases a year.
- Scabies is more common in poorer communities worldwide.
- The organism can be transmitted via fomites or sexual contact with an infected person. The number of organisms on fomites is generally low.
- In patients with a variant called Norwegian scabies, the organisms are abundant and spread is common.
- Secondary household cases can be as high as 38% for all cases of scabies.

Incubation
- Initial infestation may remain silent for 4 to 6 weeks.
- Symptoms often occur rapidly upon subsequent infections.

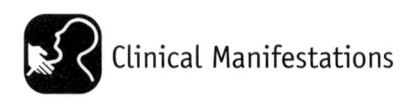

Clinical Manifestations

- Scabies produces linear burrows (3 to 15 mm) and erythematous papular lesions.
  —They may be on the hands or penis initially.
  —Lesions on the hands may be in the web spaces. At times, they can become nodular, especially with Norwegian scabies.
- Norwegian scabies occurs in immunocompromised patients, including AIDS patients.
  —The patient often has widespread nodular, crusty lesions.
  —At times, the lesions are less distinct and resemble psoriasis.
  —The lesions may not be pruritic, leading to confusion and delay in diagnosis. These lesions may become superinfected.

Mites/Chiggers

Diagnosis

- Empiric diagnosis is often made when a patient presents with a pruritic rash.
- Under a magnifying glass, the mites can be visualized.
- The organism or its eggs can be identified in skin scrapings.

Treatment

- Cure rates with permethrin are much higher than with lindane, and the toxicity is much less with permethrin.
- Permethrin 5% cream over the entire body (below chin) for 8 to 10 hours. Repeat in 1 week.
- Lindane 1% lotion over the entire body (below chin) for 8 to 10 hours. Repeat in 1 week.
- Ivermectin 200 μg/kg orally
- Antihistamines to relieve patient's itching

NORWEGIAN SCABIES

- Permethrin or lindane following bathing, repeated in 12 hours. The second dose should be washed off after being on for 12 hours. Repeat in 1 week.
- Alternately, treat with permethrin on the first day and with sulfur 6% in petrolatum on days 2 through 7, repeating the cycle until the condition is clear.
- Lindane is contraindicated in young children and pregnant women due to its neurotoxicity.

COMPLICATIONS

Superinfection may occur with staphylococcal or streptococcal organisms.

Follow-Up

- No follow-up is needed if the patient is fully treated.
- Recurrent disease is common for patients who are not fully treated.

PREVENTION

- Scabies can be prevented in a hospitalized setting by use of contact precautions and frequent, thorough handwashing.
- Norwegian scabies requires persons to be in contact with patients and their clothing and bed linens; wear long-sleeved gowns and shoe covers.
- Laundry workers have been infected; linens should be held in bags for 10 days before laundering.
- Anyone in contact with a patient should be treated empirically, following the regimen for a patient.

Selected Readings

Sargent SJ. Ectoparasites. In: Mayhall CG, ed. *Hospital epidemiology and infection control*. Baltimore: Williams & Wilkins, 1996:465–472.

White GB. Scabies. In: Cook GC, ed. *Manson's tropical disease*, 12th ed. Philadelphia: WB Saunders, 1996:1535–1536.

Mucormycosis

Basics

DEFINITION

- Life-threatening opportunistic fungal infection, mainly involving soft tissues, characterized by extensive vascular occlusion and tissue necrosis, primarily seen in immunosuppressed individuals
- Systems affected: musculoskeletal, central nervous system, respiratory, skin, gastrointestinal, disseminated infection

ETIOLOGY

- Molds belonging to the family Mucorales (genera: *Rhizopus, Rhizomucor, Mucor, Absidia, Cunninghamella, Saksenaea*).
- There is no animal reservoir for Mucorales.
- Mucorales organisms are ubiquitous in nature, and are found in abundance in soil and decomposing organic material.
- Most commonly, inhalation of the spores leads to infection of the lungs and paranasal sinuses; ingestion leads to gastrointestinal infection; traumatic inoculation leads to skin and soft-tissue infections.
- In intravenous drug users, inoculation of the organism occurs via venepuncture and leads to local or distant abscesses formation.
- Mucorales, after inoculation, invades the blood vessels, causing thrombosis, infarction, and tissue necrosis. Adjacent tissue and bone infection follows.
- Dissemination occurs via the haematogenous or lymphatic route.

EPIDEMIOLOGY

Incidence

- There are no good available data for the incidence of mucormycosis.
- Geographic distribution of this infection is worldwide.

Risk Factors

- Uncontrolled diabetes mellitus, particularly patients with ketoacidosis (and other forms of metabolic acidosis)
- Hematologic malignancies (risk increases with neutropenia and prolonged antibiotic use)
- Solid-organ or bone marrow transplantation
- Desferrioxamine therapy for iron and aluminium overload (patients in multiple transfusion programs and in hemodialysis)
- Burns and complicated wounds
- Intravenous drug use
- Protein-energy malnutrition
- Chronic steroid use
- Incidence increasing in HIV infection, mostly related to defective neutrophil numbers and function
- Nosocomial outbreaks in leukemic patients have been described.
- In one outbreak, cutaneous infection cases have been attributed to contaminated dressings.

Clinical Manifestations

SYMPTOMS AND SIGNS

- Symptoms and signs depend on the system affected; clinical course is related to the underlying conditions.
- Rapid onset of fever and tissue necrosis is common to all forms of the disease.
- Rhinocerebral/craniofacial
  —This type is most frequently seen in diabetics and patients with hematologic malignancies.
  —Infection begins in the paranasal sinuses and rapidly spreads to the orbit, face, palate, and/or brain.
  —Unilateral headache, nasal or sinus congestion or pain, and serosanguinous nasal discharge occur.
  —Two-thirds of the patients are comatose by the time of the first clinical examination, due to CNS involvement.
  —Orbital edema, induration, and discoloration
  —Ptosis, proptosis of the eyeball, dilatation and fixation of the pupil, loss of vision, accompanied by drainage of black pus from the eye
  —Violaceous discoloration and/or black necrotic lesion on the hard palate, turbinates; nasal septum or palatal perforation
- Lung
  —Most cases are seen in leukemic patients undergoing intensive chemotherapy.
  —Unexplained fever and progressive development of lung infiltrates, despite broad-spectrum antibiotics
  —Unilateral involvement of one anatomic segment and rapid progress to involve the whole lung
  —Pleural effusion, hemoptysis, and pleuritic chest pain are uncommon.
- Gastrointestinal
  —Most cases occur in malnourished infants and children.
  —Lesions are most commonly found in the stomach, colon, and ileum.
  —Nonspecific symptoms (abdominal pain, haematemesis)
  —Peritonitis (if bowel perforation or infarction occurs)
- Cutaneous
  —Most cases occur in patients with burns, open fractures, and crush injuries or after applying contaminated surgical dressings to the skin.
  —Also at insulin injection sites, catheter insertion sites
  —Fever, persistent swelling, conversion from partial to full-thickness burn, ulceration, induration, tenderness, early separation of eschar, and muscle necrosis
  —Lesions resembling erythema gangrenosum may develop following hematogenous dissemination.
  —They begin as erythematous, indurated, painful lesions that subsequently ulcerate; a black eschar is present.
- Disseminated infection
  —Usually follows pulmonary infection
  —The most common site of spread is the brain, but other sites, such as the spleen, liver, and heart, can be involved.
  —Cerebral infection distinct from the rhinocerebral form results in abscess formation and infarction.
- Unusual focal forms (in intravenous drug users)
  —Endocarditis, osteomyelitis, pyelonephritis

Diagnosis

Differential Diagnosis

- Rhinocerebral/craniofacial
  —Cavernous sinus thrombosis due to extension of staphylococcal face lesions
  —Bacterial orbital cellulitis
  —Rhinocerebral aspergillosis
  —Pseudallescheriasis
  —Rapidly growing orbital tumors
- Lung
  —Gram-negative bacterial pneumonia
  —Aspergillosis
  —Pseudallescheriasis
  —Pulmonary embolism
- Cutaneous
  —Erythema gangrenosum, similar to lesions due to *Pseudomonas aeruginosa* (in leukemic patients)

LABORATORY

- Distinctive clinical appearance: Diagnosis is based on this alone in the majority of cases.

Mucormycosis

- The microbiologic diagnosis is usually made by demonstration of fungal hyphae in biopsy specimens.
- Microscopy: Fungal hyphae (wide, disorganized, with random branching and no septa) can be seen in tissue/fluid KOH preparations. No swabs should be used.
- Cultures are negative in about half of the cases.
- Sources of culture: nasal or sinus tissue, aspirates or biopsies of the lung or other sites
- Mucorales organisms are often contaminants; interpretation of sputum, sinus aspiration material, and bronchial washings culture results should be done with caution.
- Serologic tests are not routinely available.
- Cerebrospinal fluid (CSF) findings are nonspecific. CSF protein may be slightly raised, but glucose is normal. There may be modest mononuclear pleocytosis. CSF cultures are sterile.

PATHOLOGY

- Neutrophil infiltration of tissues, necrosis, thrombosis and haemorrhage, inflammatory vasculitis (arteries and veins)
- Fungal hyphae are present.

IMAGING

- Nonspecific findings
- Plain x-rays: sinus opacification and bone destruction in rhinocerebral/craniofacial disease
- In lung involvement, focal or diffuse infiltrates progressing to consolidation or cavitation
- Unilateral, segmental involvement in the beginning
- Wedge-shaped peripheral lesions, representing haemorrhagic infarction
- CT scans and MRIs: space-occupying lesions and bone destruction findings in rhinocerebral and CNS disease
- Useful in delineating the disease extent and planning surgical intervention

DIAGNOSTIC PROCEDURES

- Stereotactic brain biopsies/skin biopsies/other site biopsies
- Bronchoalveolar lavage

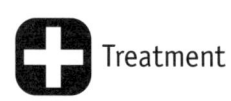

Treatment

MAIN TREATMENT

- Control of underlying conditions
- Surgical debridement of infected tissues should precede any other measure.
- Mucorales organisms are resistant to all antifungals except amphotericin B.
- Full-dose amphotericin should be given from the first day; there is no time for gradual escalation.
- First-line: amphotericin B 1.5 mg/kg i.v. Rifampicin 600 mg bid may exhibit synergism; this can be tested *in vitro*.

ALTERNATIVE TREATMENT

- Second-line: liposomal amphotericin 5 mg/kg/d
- Some cases of cutaneous mucormycosis that responded to surgery only, or to liposomal amphotericin alone, have been reported, but none of these strategies has been studied extensively.
- Adjunctive oxygen therapy has unproved efficacy.

COMPLICATIONS

- Rhinocerebral/craniofacial: cavernous sinus and internal carotid artery thrombosis, brain abscesses
- Lung: If untreated, dissemination follows with brain abscess formation and death within 2 to 3 weeks of onset.
- Gastrointestinal: bowel infarction/perforation, sepsis, gastrointestinal bleed, and hemorrhagic shock, death within weeks
- Cutaneous: extensive local destruction, dissemination with distant abscess formation

Follow-Up

- Monitor hydration status.
- Achieve good control of diabetes mellitus.
- Continue lifelong monitoring for signs of recurrence/residual infection.
- If untreated, rhinocerebral/craniofacial mucormycosis is fatal, usually within a week of onset.
- After appropriate treatment, the survival rate in diabetics with rhinocerebral mucormycosis is 50%.
- The prognosis in other high-risk groups and for other system involvement is very poor.
- Diagnosis of lung and gastrointestinal forms of the disease is usually made postmortem.

PREVENTION

- Oral and trauma hygiene precautions (especially for diabetics and bone marrow transplant/neutropenic patients)
- In neutropenic and bone marrow transplant patients:
  —Primary prophylaxis: Hepa filtered air/laminar air flow is possibly effective, as well as nebulized or intravenous amphotericin B administration.
  —Secondary: Intravenous amphotericin B is possibly effective (1 mg/kg/d is probably enough).
- Emphasis should be given to prevention of diabetic ketoacidosis (good management of diabetes mellitus).
- In comatose diabetic patients, never forget to remove the dentures and examine the palate area.
- Diabetics who have persistence of mental status changes longer than 1 to 2 days after beginning appropriate treatment and resolution of metabolic abnormalities need further exploration, as the probability of mucormycosis is high.

Selected Readings

Boelaert JR, Weruawe PL, Vandepitte JM. Mucormycosis infection in dialysis patients. *Ann Intern Med* 1987;107:782–783.

Christenson JC, Shalit I, Welch DF, et al. Synergistic action of amphotericin B and rifampin against *Rhizopus* species. *Antimicrob Agents Chemother* 1987;31:1775–1778.

Ferstenfeld JE, Cohen SH, Rose HD, et al. Chronic rhinocerebral phycomycosis in association with diabetes. *Postgrad Med J* 1977;53:337–342.

Fisher EW, Toma A, Fisher PH, et al. Rhinocerebral mucormycosis: Use of liposomal amphotericin B. *J Laryngol Otol* 1991;105:575–577.

Munckhof W, Jones R, Tosolini FA, et al. Cure of *Rhizopus* sinusitis in a liver transplant recipient with liposomal amphotericin B. *Clin Infect Dis* 1993;16:183.

Rex JH, Ginsberg AM, Fries LF, et al. *Cunninghamella bertholetiae* infection associated with deferoxamine therapy. *Rev Infect Dis* 1988;10:1187–1194.

Torre Cisneros J, Kusne S, Martin M, et al. Rhinocerebral mucormycosis after liver transplantation. *Transplant Sci* 1992;2:63–64.

Windus DW, Stokes TJ, Julian BA, et al. Fatal *Rhizopus* infections as hemodialysis patients receiving deferoxamine. *Ann Intern Med* 1987;107:678–680.

Mumps

Basics

DEFINITION

Mumps is a benign viral infection of childhood, manifested by swelling of the parotid glands. In adults and, rarely, in children, the disease can cause orchitis, pancreatitis, and aseptic meningitis.

ETIOLOGY

Mumps is an enveloped RNA virus of the family Paramyxoviridae. It is contracted by direct contact with secretions of infected individuals.

EPIDEMIOLOGY

- Mumps is found worldwide and is only present in humans. It is most common in children ages 5 to 9 years.
- In the United States, vaccination programs have reduced the numbers of cases to fewer than 1,000 per year. Of those who become infected, one-third are older than age 15 years.

Incubation

Incubation is from 16 to 18 days.

Clinical Manifestations

- Fever
- Malaise
- Headache
- Painful swelling of the parotid gland develops in the first 2 days.
- Bilateral swelling may occur after another 2 days.
- Resolution of pain, swelling, and fevers occurs within 1 week.
- Meningitis can occur at any time during mumps infection; it is self-limited and resolves in less than 1 week.
- Epididymoorchitis is common in adults with mumps, occurring in as many as 30% of adult patients. Patients present with testicular pain, marked swelling, and high fevers; resolution occurs in less than 1 week.
  —Atrophy of the testes is a complication of severe disease, but sterility is rare, even after bilateral disease.

Diagnosis

- Diagnosis is made on clinical grounds
- Leukopenia may occur.
- Serum amylase and lipase levels are elevated with parotitis.

Mumps

- Serology can be done to confirm the diagnosis.
- Viral isolation from the saliva, cerebrospinal fluid, or urine can be obtained in some laboratories.

DIFFERENTIAL DIAGNOSIS

- Influenza A
- Coxsackievirus
- Parainfluenza 3
- HIV
- Suppurative parotitis

Treatment

- There is no specific treatment of mumps.
- Supportive care and analgesics are recommended.

COMPLICATIONS

- Mumps during pregnancy is associated with congenital malformations, low birth weights, and fetal demise.
- Mumps infection also has been associated with the onset of juvenile diabetes mellitus.
- Low or absent sperm counts

Follow-Up

PREVENTION

- Isolation of suspected cases is warranted.
- Vaccination with attenuated virus at age 12 to 15 months and at 5 to 12 years
- Adults who have not been immunized should be immunized.
- The mumps vaccine is part of the combined measles-mumps-rubella vaccine.

Selected Readings

Candel S. Epididymitis in mumps, including orchitis: Further clinical studies and comments. *Ann Intern Med* 1951;34:20.

Kleiman MB. Mumps virus. In: Lennette EH, ed. *Laboratory diagnosis of viral infections*, 2nd ed. New York: Marcel Dekker, 1992:549.

Levitt LP, Rich TA, Kinde SW, et al. Central nervous system mumps. *Neurology (NY)* 1970;20:829.

Mycotic Aneurysms

Basics

DEFINITION

- An aneurysm that develops in a vessel as part of an infectious process, such as infective endocarditis

ETIOLOGY

- Mycotic aneurysms can form in a number of ways.
  - The most common etiology is from endocarditis, when an infected thrombus lodges in the vasa vasorum and leads to aneurysm formation.
  - Mycotic aneurysms can also form with seeding of the intima during bacteremia. This can be seen in patients with arthrosclerotic plaques.
  - Mycotic aneurysms can also form when a contiguous foci of infection invades a blood vessel. This may occur with infections such as osteomyelitis or deep abscesses.
  - Infection due to direct inoculation during surgery or trauma (intravenous drug abuse) may also lead to aneurysms.
- Any vessel may be affected; however, the sinus of Valsalva and the thoracic aorta are most commonly infected in endocarditis. Aneurysm of the middle cerebral artery has been described in endocarditis.
- Most mycotic aneurysms are caused by *Staphylococcus aureus* or *Salmonella* spp. Fungi such as *Aspergillus* or mucormycosis cause aneurysms due to direct spread from contiguous sites.
- *Candida* spp can cause disease due to fungemia from a distant source.

EPIDEMIOLOGY

- Mycotic aneurysms are very rare, especially when bacteremia is treated rapidly with broad-spectrum antibiotics.
- Two percent to 4% of patients with endocarditis develop intracranial aneurysms.

Clinical Manifestations

- Mycotic aneurysms are often silent until they rupture.
  - Intracranial rupture is associated with headache, meningismus, focal neurologic signs, or coma.
  - Intraabdominal lesions present with peritoneal signs and shock.
  - Peripheral lesions often present with pain and signs of vascular insufficiency.

Diagnosis

- Bacteremia is found in over 50% of cases.
- Leukocytosis is often present.
- CT may suggest blood vessel rupture or aneurysmal dilatation; however angiography is needed for more detail, especially in patients with normal CT scans.
- Transesophageal echocardiography is useful to detect aneurysmal formation at the root of the aorta.

Mycotic Aneurysms

DIFFERENTIAL DIAGNOSIS
- Polyarteritis nodosa
- Congenital aneurysm
- Ruptured viscus

Treatment

- Most patients with intracranial aneurysms have resolution with antibiotics alone.
- Surgery is reserved for those with bleeding intracranial aneurysms or for those with documented enlargement despite adequate antibiotic treatment.
- Infected aortic aneurysms require surgical intervention, as do aneurysms that develop after trauma.
- Antibiotics should be used for at least 6 to 8 weeks when infected aneurysms are detected.

COMPLICATIONS
Rupture, embolization, and vascular insufficiency are the most common complications of mycotic aneurysms.

Follow-Up

Patients who have had mycotic aneurysm treated medically should have serial angiograms or noninvasive imaging procedures to ensure that the aneurysm is getting smaller.

PREVENTION
- There is no way to prevent the development of mycotic aneurysms.
- Initiating antibiotics promptly should decrease the incidence of this disease.

Selected Readings

Cohen OS, O'Brien TF, Schoenbaum SC, et al. The risk of endothelial infections in adults with *Salmonella* bacteremia. *Ann Intern Med* 1978;89:931.

Johnson JR, Ledgerwood AM, Lucas CE. Mycotic aneurysm. New concepts in therapy. *Arch Surg* 1983;118:577.

Morgan MB, Cintron G, Balis JV. Infective "mycotic" aortic root aneurysm following coronary bypass grafting. *Am J Med* 1993;94:550.

Wilson WR, Lie JT, Houser OW, et al. The management of patients with mycotic aneurysm. *Curr Clin Top Infect Dis* 1981;2:151.

Myelitis

Basics

DEFINTION
- Infection of the spinal cord or the adjacent tissues, leading to alteration of cord function

ETIOLOGY
- Inflammation can occur throughout the cross-section of the cord at one or at multiple levels, leading to a focal myelitis or a transverse myelitis.
- Herpesviruses have been implicated in causing transverse myelitis in immunocompromised patients.
- Other causes of transverse myelitis include Lyme borreliosis, schistosomiasis, and leptospirosis.
- Epidural abscess can lead to cord compression, and, thus, transverse myelitis.
- HIV can lead to a diffuse vacuolar myelopathy with myelitis and cord dysfunction.
- HTLV-1 leads to tropical spastic paraparesis, a meningomyelitis.
- Infection of the nerve roots is termed *radiculomyelitis*.
- Infectious agents have various tropisms for compartments within the spinal cord. Poliomyelitis is most commonly found in the anterior horn cells. Similar polio-like illness may occur with coxsackieviruses, echovirus, and enterovirus types 70 and 71.
- Posterior column disease is seen with syphilis, as in tabes dorsalis.
- Dorsal root ganglia are affected in varicella zoster infections. During infection, inflammation of the associated spinal cord segment occurs.

EPIDEMIOLOGY
Much depends on the specific etiology of this diverse group of infections. See individual topics for more detail.

Clinical Manifestations

POLIOMYELITIS
- Patients in the paralytic stage note asymmetric weakness in the arms and legs.
- Examination reveals fasciculations, atrophy, and loss of reflexes—the picture of lower motor neuron involvement.
- Bulbar paralysis may lead to dysphagia and respiratory failure.

TRANSVERSE MYELITIS
- Loss of motor and sensory function
- Much depends on the level of the myelitis.
- Reflexes are initially lost, but then become hyperactive below the lesion.

VARICELLA ZOSTER
- Patients may have inflammation of the dorsal root ganglion.
- Dysesthesias give way to radicular pain in the dermatome.

Myelitis

- Sensory loss is common, but motor impairment occurs in fewer than 5% of patients.

Diagnosis

- Magnetic resonance imaging is used to look for blockage or mass effect.
- Cerebrospinal fluid (CSF) can be obtained and sent for HSV/CMV/VZV polymerase chain reaction, cell counts, and cultures.
- Serology is used to detect possible HIV, enterovirus, syphilis, or borreliosis infections.
- In viral etiologies, CSF glucose is often normal. The protein can be elevated.
- With poliomyelitis, CSF lymphocytosis is noted.
- In herpesvirus infections, polys may predominate.

Treatment

- Treatment of the viral infection likely to be causing the myelitis is necessary.
  —Herpes should be treated with acyclovir.
  —Cytomegalovirus should be treated with ganciclovir or foscarnet.
  —HIV requires highly active antivirals.
- Emergency surgical decompression is indicated when the cord is compromised by epidural abscess.

COMPLICATIONS

- Because of the fragile blood supply to the cord, ischemia and infarction cause irreversible damage to the cord.
- Paralysis is often the outcome with myelitis.

Follow-Up

Patients often require rehabilitation and close follow-up with neurologists.

PREVENTION

Vaccines are available for poliomyelitis, varicella zoster virus, and Lyme disease.

Selected Readings

Lipton HL, Teasdall RD. Acute transverse myelopathy in adults. *Arch Neurol* 1973;28:252.

Whitley RJ, Lakeman F. Herpes simplex virus infections of the central nervous system: Therapeutic and diagnostic considerations. *Clin Infect Dis* 1995;20:414–420.

Myocarditis

Basics

DEFINITION
- Inflammation of the myocardium due to many infectious and noninfectious diseases
- Myocarditis may be due to infection of the heart or due to cross-reacting antibodies to the myocardium.

ETIOLOGY
Viral
- Of the infectious etiologies of myocarditis, coxsackie B virus is the most frequently isolated.
- Other viral etiologies include the following:
  —Coxsackie A virus and echovirus
  —Poliovirus
  —HIV virus
  —Influenza virus
  —Adenovirus
  —Herpesviruses such as cytomegalovirus, Epstein-Barr virus
  —Varicella zoster virus
  —Measles and mumps viruses
  —Rubella virus
  —Rabies virus
  —Dengue and yellow fever viruses

Bacterial
- Bacteria rarely cause myocarditis. When bacteria are a cause, it is due to pericarditis with extension into the myocardium.
- Exceptions include *Borrelia burgdorferi* and *Treponema pallidum*.
- Myocarditis can be seen with rheumatic fever.
- *Corynebacterium diphtheriae* can cause myocarditis via toxin production.
- Other bacteria associated with myocarditis include the following:
  —Gonococci and meningococci
  —Staphylococci and streptococci
  —*Mycoplasma pneumoniae* and *Chlamydia pneumoniae*

Parasitic
- Parasites, including the following, cause myocarditis:
  —*Trypanosoma cruzi*, *Trypanosoma brucei gambiense*, and *Trypanosoma brucei rhodesiense*
  —*Trichinella spiralis*
  —*Toxoplasma gondii*
  —*Echinococcus*

Other
Kawasaki disease causes myocarditis and coronary artery aneurysm; the mechanism is uncertain.

EPIDEMIOLOGY
- The true incidence of myocarditis is not known, because diagnostic evaluations are seldom done and most cases are asymptomatic.
- Up to 5% of all cases of coxsackie B virus are associated with myocarditis.
- Up to 40% of cases of *T. cruzi* are associated with myocarditis.

Risk Factors
HIV infection increases the risk of myocarditis from a wide variety of organisms, including cytomegalovirus, herpes simplex virus, *T. gondii*, and, at times, *Cryptococcus*.

Incubation
Patients develop myocarditis that is symptomatic a few days after a typical viral infection.

Clinical Manifestations

- Patients often have typical upper respiratory tract viral symptoms.
- Over time, fevers, palpitations, shortness of breath, and malaise develop.
- Chest pain, pleuritic in nature, occurs.
- Examination often reveals tachycardia.

Myocarditis

- S3 and signs of failure may develop.
- Arrhythmias

Diagnosis

- Biopsy is needed for diagnosis.
- Echocardiogram shows nonspecific ST/T-wave changes, AV block, or bundle branch blocks.
- Cardiac enzymes may be elevated in a minority of cases.
- Leukocytosis and elevated ESR occur in fewer than 50% of patients.
- Serology with elevated IgM levels and rises in antibodies four times normal can help confirm viral etiologies.

IMAGING

- Echocardiogram may reveal wall motion abnormalities or abnormal thickening of the myocardium.
- In acute myocarditis, the patients have reduced LV function with normal wall thickness.
- CT scan can help define the myocardial wall thickness.
- Gallium- or indium-labeled antimyosin antibodies can detect myocardial inflammation.

DIFFERENTIAL DIAGNOSIS

- Acute myocardial infarction
- Sarcoidosis
- Peripartum cardiomyopathy
- Hyper- and hypothyroidism
- Drugs such as alcohol, cocaine, doxorubicin, and methyldopa
- Antibiotics such as tetracycline and sulfonamides
- Interferon (interleukin-2)
- Rheumatoid disorders such as lupus, rheumatoid arthritis, and scleroderma

Treatment

- Supportive care is very important, as is bed rest.
- Patients should be treated with diuretics and afterload reducers.
- Arrhythmia treatment is important.
- Steroids are not usually indicated.
- Treatment of the specific virus (HIV or herpesviruses) may be beneficial.

COMPLICATIONS

- Sudden cardiac death accounts for 5% to 15% of people with undiagnosed and untreated myocarditis.
- Viral myocarditis leads to up to 20% of all cases of dilated cardiomyopathy.
- Heart failure can be severe, and transplantation may be necessary.

Follow-Up

Patients require close follow-up with a cardiologist and long-term cardiac rehabilitation.

PREVENTION

- None available

Selected Readings

Barbaro G, Di Lorenzo G, Grisorio B, et al. Incidence of dilated cardiomyopathy and detection of HIV in myocardial cells of HIV-positive patients. *N Engl J Med* 1998;339:1093–1099.

Lazar JM, Johnson DH, Cunha BA. Acute myocarditis and acute pericarditis. In: Cunha BA, ed. *Infectious disease in critical care medicine*. New York: Marcel Dekker, 1998:355–375.

Segal LH. Early disseminated Lyme disease: Cardiac manifestations. *Am J Med* 1995;98[Suppl 4A]:258–285.

Myositis

Basics

DEFINITION
- Infection of muscles caused by various types of organisms

ETIOLOGY

Viral
- Viral myositis is associated with the following:
  — HIV and HTLV-1
  — Influenza A virus
  — Adenovirus
  — Coxsackievirus
  — Epstein-Barr virus
  — Cytomegalovirus
  — Herpes simplex virus
  — Parainfluenza virus

Parasitic
- *Trichinella spiralis* can grow within muscle fibers.
- *Toxocara canis* and *Toxocara cati* also enter the muscle compartment as part of visceral larvae migrans syndrome.
- Cysts from *Cysticercus cellulosae* commonly infect muscle tissue, which leads to calcification over time.
- Hydatid disease caused by *Echinococcus granulosus* or *Echinococcus multilocularis* commonly infects muscles. *Toxoplasma gondii* may also encyst within muscles.

Bacterial
- Bacterial myositis is rare. When it occurs, it may be due to local extension from the skin (decubitus ulcer) or from an underlying source (osteomyelitis). On occasion, it may be secondary to hematogenous spread.
- Pyomyositis with *Staphylococcus aureus*, the pathogen in 95% of patients
  — Often seen in tropical areas
  — More recently has been seen in HIV-positive patients
  — Rare causes of pyomyositis include streptococci or coliforms.
- Psoas muscle abscess can be due to extension of a vertebral focus of infection. *S. aureus* and tuberculosis are most commonly implicated.
- Gas gangrene is caused by clostridial infections.
- Group A streptococcal infections can lead to both a fasciitis and a myositis.
- Mixed organisms (aerobic and anaerobic) may, on occasion, cause myositis. Often, the fascia and skin are infected.

Other Organisms
- *Aeromonas hydrophilia*
- *Klebsiella pneumoniae*

EPIDEMIOLOGY
- Pyomyositis is a rare disease in nontropical regions of the world.
- It is often associated with trauma or a foreign body in the muscles or in patients who are intravenous drug users.
- In tropical regions, pyomyositis may account for as many as 4% of hospital admissions.
- Blunt trauma to the muscles may precede development of pyomyositis, presumably due to an area of infarct or hemorrhage.

Risk Factors
- HIV
- Alcoholism

Myositis

- Malignancy
- Residing in a tropical country

Clinical Manifestations

- The onset of symptoms may be insidious.
- Pain associated with fevers may be the only initial symptom or sign.
- Swelling depends on the depth of infection within the muscle.
- Over time, the area becomes indurated and woody, and extreme tenderness is noted on palpation.
- Skin changes may not occur if the infection is within a deep muscle group.
- Sepsis may be a late manifestation.

Diagnosis

- Leukocytosis with a left shift occurs.
- Aldolase levels are often within normal limits.
- Blood cultures may be positive in 5% to 35% of patients.
- A CT or MRI is needed to define the extent of muscles affected.
- Needle aspiration should reveal the organism on Gram stain or culture.
- Bone films should be obtained to rule out infection secondary to extension of osteomyelitis.

DIFFERENTIAL DIAGNOSIS

- Deep vein thrombosis
- Osteomyelitis
- Gas gangrene
- Fasciitis
- Affected muscles over the abdomen may suggest an underlying abdominal process.
- Affected intercostal muscles may suggest ischemic cardiac pain.

Treatment

- A combined medical and surgical approach is needed.
- When an abscess is visualized via CT or ultrasound, it should be drained, preferably by a guided needle aspiration.
- β-Lactamase penicillin (nafcillin 2 g i.v. every 4 hours) or a first-generation cephalosporin (cefazolin 2 g i.v. every 6 hours) is initiated for *S. aureus* infection.

COMPLICATIONS

Infection may develop in the adjacent bone or joints.

Follow-Up

Patients should have physical therapy for joint involvement following medical treatment.

PREVENTION

There is no way to prevent pyomyositis.

Selected Readings

Caplan ES, Kluge RM. Gas gangrene: Review of 34 cases. *Arch Intern Med* 1976;136:788.

Christin L, Sarosi GA. Pyomyositis in North America: Case reports and review. *Clin Infect Dis* 1992;15:668.

Necrotizing Skin and Soft-Tissue Infections

Basics

DEFINITION

Severe infections involving deep fascia and/or muscle compartments: Typically, the necrotizing infections are secondary to an initial break in the skin from trauma or surgery. Depending on the organism causing infection, the disease manifests as necrotizing fasciitis (rare), cellulitis, gangrene, myositis, or pyomyositis.

ETIOLOGY

- Myositis: anaerobic streptococci
- Pyomyositis: *Staphylococcus aureus*, *Streptococcus pneumoniae*
- Gangrene
  - Streptococcal
  - Progressive bacterial synergistic (Meleney's)
  - Clostridial
  - Cellulitis
  - Nonclostridial crepitance
  - Synergistic necrotizing
- Necrotizing fasciitis: *Streptococcus* or *S. aureus*, anaerobic streptococci, mixed infection

EPIDEMIOLOGY

- Synergistic necrotizing cellulitis
  - Seventy-five percent of patients have diabetes.
  - Fifty percent of patients have cardiovascular and/or renal disease.
  - Fifty percent of patients are obese.
- Fournier's gangrene
  - Males age 50 to 60 years, sometimes coexisting disease, frequently no disease
  - Ten percent to 40% mortality rates

Risk Factors

- Trauma or surgical incision, puncture wound, drain site, suture site: myositis and gangrene
- Endemic in tropics, increasingly recognized in temperate climates in patients with HIV or diabetes: pyomyositis
- Perirectal and ischiorectal abscess, perianal disease, surgical incision: cellulitis
- Diabetes: Foot lesions and ulcers associated with necrotizing cellulitis
- Frequent hospitalizations and older age

Incubation

- Six hours to 2 days for streptococcal gangrene
- One to 4 days for progressive bacterial synergistic gangrene and necrotizing fasciitis
- Three to 14 days for cellulitis and vascular gangrene

Clinical Manifestations

SYMPTOMS AND SIGNS

- Severe, constant pain
- Bulbous lesions
- Gas in the soft tissues; putrid odor in the presence of anaerobic bacteria
- Systemic symptoms: fever, renal failure, delirium, leukocytosis
- Rapid disease spread centrally along fascial planes. The course is gradual in cellulitis.
- Skin manifestations vary:
  - Swollen, minimal discoloration: cellulitis
  - Erythematous or gangrenous: synergistic necrotizing cellulitis
  - Erythematous or necrotic: vascular gangrene or streptococcal gangrene
  - Blanched (hard to the touch), erythematous: necrotizing fasciitis

Diagnosis

Diagnosis is based on history and physical examination and observation for common clinical manifestations. Laboratory testing is necessary to confirm the organism of infection.

Necrotizing Skin and Soft-Tissue Infections

DIFFERENTIAL DIAGNOSIS

Clinical presentation and accompanying systemic manifestations distinguish between the superficial skin and soft-tissue infections.

Infectious

- Superficial skin and soft-tissue infection
  - Cellulitis
  - Superficial gangrene
  - Erysipelas

Noninfectious

- Subcutaneous emphysema at site of thoracentesis, chest-tube insertion, or thoracic procedure
- Local emphysema from tracheotomy
- Column of gas along course of an intravenous catheter in the arm or Swan-Ganz catheter (rare)

LABORATORY

- Gram stain of exudate to reveal pathogens
  - Gram-positive cocci in chains suggest *Streptococcus*.
  - Large gram-positive cocci in clumps suggest *S. aureus*.
  - Mixed flora suggest polymicrobial infection.
  - Intravenous drug users often have unusual pathogens from the needles used for injection.
- Deep-tissue culture
- Blood serum cultures
- CT or MRI for revealing exudate along the fascial plane

Treatment

MAIN TREATMENT

- Surgery
  - Debridement
  - Excision
  - Filleting incisions
  - Amputation
- Tissue drainage and colloid therapy
- Antibiotics
  - Mixed infection
    - Imipenem
    - Meropenem
    - Ticarcillin or clavulanate
    - Ampicillin or sulbactam
    - Piperacillin or tazobactam
  - Streptococcal infection
    - Penicillin: Combine with clindamycin for toxic shock or necrotizing fasciitis.
  - *S. aureus* infection
    - Nafcillin
    - Cloxacillin
    - Vancomycin (for resistant strains)

ALTERNATIVE TREATMENT

- Mixed infection
  - Cefotoxin
  - Clindamycin or metronidazole plus aminoglycoside
- *Streptococcus* and *S. aureus* infections
  - Cefazolin
  - Vancomycin

COMPLICATIONS

- Toxic shock
- Loss of muscle or even loss of limb
- Bacteremia, septic shock
- Renal failure

Follow-Up

- At least for 3 months, for recurrence
- Surgical wound care

PREVENTION

- Good initial wound care of traumatic injuries

Selected Readings

Dahm P, Roland FH, Vaslef SN, et al. Outcome analysis in patients with primary necrotizing fasciitis of the male genitalia. *Urology* 2000;56(1):31–35; discussion, 35–36.

Fontes RA Jr, Ogilvie CM, Miclau T. Necrotizing soft-tissue infections. *J Am Acad Orthop Surg* 2000;8(3):151–158.

Meltzer DL, Kabongo M. Necrotizing fasciitis: A diagnostic challenge. *Am Fam Physician* 1997;56(1):145–149.

Urschel JD. Necrotizing soft tissue infections [Review]. *Postgrad Med J* 1999;75(889):645–649.

Neuritis

Basics

DEFINITION

- Infectious neuritis is an inflammation of nerves, caused by a wide variety of organisms and toxins.
- Acute inflammatory demyelinating polyneuritis or the Guillain-Barré syndrome is associated with multiple diverse infections.

ETIOLOGY

- Guillain Barré syndrome is a demyelinating illness involving inflammation of the peripheral nerves.
- The etiology has yet to be resolved, but some cases are associated with the following organisms:
  - *Campylobacter jejuni*
  - Lyme disease
  - Psittacosis
  - *Mycoplasma*
  - Epstein-Barr virus
  - Cytomegalovirus
  - Hepatitis C
  - HIV
- When linked to an infectious etiology, the infection occurs within 1 to 2 months prior to the development of the neuritis.
- Neuritis can be caused by herpesvirus infections.
- Cytomegalovirus can lead to a radicular neuropathy (cauda equina syndrome) in patients with AIDS.
- Herpes simplex and varicella zoster reside within the sensory ganglia and cause neuritis when reactivated.
- HIV can infect peripheral neural tissue and cause severe polyneuropathies.
- Rabies virus can spread into the central nervous system via peripheral nerves.
- Lyme disease is often associated with cranial neuropathy.
- Leprosy leads to neuronal destruction with anesthesia of the skin.
- Trypanosomes have the ability to invade peripheral nerves, leading to neuropathy as well as autonomic dysfunction.
- Toxin produced by *Corynebacterium diphtheriae* may produce injury to Schwann cells and neuronal degeneration, especially of the cranial nerves.
- *Clostridium botulinum* produces a toxin that can lead to ophthalmoplegia along with a descending motor paralysis.
- *Clostridium tetani* produces a toxin that acts at the level of the neuromuscular junction and causes the characteristic muscle spasm.

EPIDEMIOLOGY

Guillain-Barré syndrome occurs in young men and women and is the leading cause of paralysis in this age group. The incidence is 9.5 cases per 10^6 people.

Neuritis

Clinical Manifestations

- Guillain-Barré syndrome starts with weakness of the lower legs, which, over days to weeks, ascends to the entire body, including the respiratory muscles.
- Patients may note mild sensory changes, often paresthesias.
- Autonomic dysfunction also occurs.
- Maximal symptoms occur usually within 1 month.
- Following the paralysis, the patients slowly recover, usually within 1 year of onset.
- One-third of patients are left with mild residual neurologic dysfunction.

Diagnosis

- Diagnosis is often made on clinical grounds.
- Cerebrospinal fluid (CSF) reveals 0 to 200 cells/mm (lymphocytes)
- Elevated CSF protein, which rises in the first month of illness

IMAGING

MRI may show enhancement of the nerve roots.

Treatment

- Treatment includes either plasmapheresis or intravenous immune globulin (0.4 g/kg/d).
- Initiation of these interventions should be done as early as possible.
- Close observation and early intubation are needed with progressive disease.

COMPLICATIONS

- Residual neurologic damage occurs commonly with Guillain-Barré Syndrome.
- Recurrent disease has also been described.

Follow-Up

- Close observation by a neurologist is needed.
- Physical therapy is often required.

PREVENTION

There is no way to prevent either the idiopathic form of Guillain-Barré syndrome or the postinfectious form of the disease.

Selected Reading

Jacobs BC, Schmitz, PIM van der Meche FGA. *Campylobacter jejuni* infection and treatment for Guillain-Barré syndrome [Letter]. *N Engl J Med* 1996;335(3):208–209.

Nocardiosis

Basics

DEFINITION

- Invasive disease associated with *Nocardia* species, first described by Nocard in 1889
- *Nocardia* species belong to higher bacteria—Family: Nocardiaceae; order: Actinomycetales; filamentous growth with true branching; aerobic.
- Localized or disseminated infection
  —Pulmonary disease (transient or subclinical, acute or chronic)
  —Disseminated (hematogenous spread, particularly in the nervous system)
  —Cellulitis, lymphocutaneous syndrome, actinomycetoma
  —Keratitis
- Systems affected: lungs, CNS, heart (endocardium, pericardium), genitourinary (kidneys, prostate, testis, epididymis), thyroid, adrenal, liver, spleen, peritoneum, soft tissues and bones. Dissemination to nearly every organ has been reported.

ETIOLOGY

- Natural soil and dust saprophytes are often found in decaying organic matter.
- *Nocardia* species are neither human nor animal commensals. Other mammals can be infected, too.
- *Nocardia asteroides* is the prominent human pathogen. *N. brasiliensis*, *N. otitidis-caviarum* (*caviae*), *N. farcinica*, *N. nova*, and *N. pseudobrasiliensis* are also associated with human disease.

EPIDEMIOLOGY

Incidence and Prevalence

- The aerosol route is the major portal of entry; the lung is the most common site of infection. The gastrointestinal system is an alternative route, through breaks of mucosa. Traumatic inoculation through the skin or eye occurs rarely.
- Frequent contact with soil or vegetate matter
- No clear evidence for person-to-person transmission
- Approximately 1,000 cases are diagnosed every year in United States (85% pulmonary and/or systematic). Outbreaks are rare.
- Incidence is worldwide but occurs mainly in tropical/subtropical regions (Mexico, Central and South America, Africa, India).
- Predominant age: All ages (even neonates); more common among adults
- Predominant sex: The male–female ratio is 3:1.
- Age-related factors: Infection in childhood may present as cervicofacial syndrome and cause cervical adenitis.

Risk Factors

- Pulmonary alveolar proteinosis
- Malignancy
- AIDS
- Corticosteroid therapy
- Cushing's syndrome
- Organ transplantation
- Chronic granulomatous disease of childhood
- Congenital immunodeficiency diseases
- Every disease/situation that causes deficient cell-mediated immunity
- Can *also* occur in normal hosts

Clinical Manifestations

SYMPTOMS

- Clinical manifestations nonspecific
- Cough is prominent and productive (small amounts of thick, purulent, nonmalodorous sputum).
- Fever, anorexia, weight loss, and malaise are common.
- Dyspnea, pleuritic pain, and hemoptysis are less common.
- Tracheitis and bronchitis are uncommon.
- Remissions over periods of several weeks are frequent.
- Metastatic brain foci may be silent early on. Symptoms and signs depend on location; these are more indolent than abscesses due to other bacteria.
- Meningitis without apparent brain abscess is rare.
- Epididymoorchitis

SIGNS

- Symptoms and signs from abscesses of skin and supporting structures, bone (rarely), muscles, sinuses, kidneys, thyroid, adrenal glands, and so on

Nocardiosis

- Keratoconjunctivitis (traumatic inoculation), endophthalmitis (haematogenous spread)
- Cellulitis (1–3 weeks after breach of skin): pain, swelling, erythema, warmth; firm, not fluctuant, lesions. It may progress to involve underlying tissues. Dissemination is rare.
- Lymphocutaneous syndrome: pyodermatous lesion at site of inoculation, central ulceration, purulent or honey-colored drainage; subcutaneous nodules along local-draining lymphatics
- Actinomycetoma: nodular swelling, typically feet or hands, but also posterior part of neck, upper back, head, and other sites. A fistula appears when the nodule breaks down, and is soon accompanied by others that come and go. There is extensive deformation of affected areas over a period of months to years.

Diagnosis

DIFFERENTIAL DIAGNOSIS

- Tuberculosis
- Bronchogenic carcinoma
- Lung abscess
- Brain tumor
- Brain abscess
- Sarcoidosis
- Actinomycosis
- Fungal disease
- Acute pulmonary infections due to common pathogens
- *Mycobacterium fortuitum* (presenting with postsurgical or skin lesions)
- *Rhodococcus bronchialis* (postsurgical sternotomy infections)
- *Rhodococcus equi* (pulmonary infections)

LABORATORY

- Examination of sputum or pus for crooked, branching, beaded gram-positive filaments. Modified acid-fast or silver stain is needed.
- These organisms grow relatively slowly; culture plates should be held 7 to 10 days. (Sometimes colonies take 2 weeks to appear and 4 weeks to take the characteristic appearance.) Colonies are chalky, raised, pink to orange, and crumbly, with a characteristic odor.
- When there are negative smears, invasive procedures are necessary for diagnosis.
- *Nocardia* species are rarely skin contaminants or respiratory tract saprophytes.
- In immunocompromised patients, a positive sputum culture usually reflects disease. (It is difficult to withhold treatment in these cases.)
- In the immunocompetent, it also usually reflects disease (and not only colonization) when *Nocardia* is detected on Gram stain preparations and multiple positive cultures.
- Routine blood cultures are usually negative. Biphasic culture bottles incubated aerobically for up to 30 days are often positive.
- Disorders that may alter lab results: a high degree of serologic cross-reaction with *Mycobacterium* (including *M. leprae*) and streptomyces species.
- Cerebrospinal fluid or urine specimens should be concentrated and cultured if clinically indicated, but they are rarely positive.
- In actinomycetoma, sulfur granules may be found in the discharge (microscopical examination and culture necessary).
- A serologic diagnosis (hemagglutination, precipitin, complement-fixing antibodies) lacks specificity. Isolation of a 55-KD protein specific for *N. asteroides* is helpful, but is not yet commercially available.
- There are no skin tests for demonstrating delayed cutaneous hypersensitivity.

PATHOLOGY

- Neutrophils and phagocytose organisms limit their growth, but do not kill them efficiently.
- Cell-mediated immunity is important for definite control and elimination of organism.
- Suppurative necrosis and abscess formation are typical.
- Granulation tissue usually surrounds the lesion; extensive fibrosis or encapsulation is uncommon.

Nocardiosis

- Pulmonary lesions: Multiple, confluent abscesses and daughter abscesses are common; peribronchial lymphadenitis may be present. There may be extension to the pleura of chest wall.
- In mycetoma and lymphocutaneous syndromes: Sulfur granules appear (absent in visceral nocardiosis).
- Brain abscesses: any part of brain, usually multiloculated; satellite extensions common

IMAGING

- Chest x-ray: no pathognomonic radiographic picture. Infiltrates vary in size, usually of moderate or greater density. Nodules and cavitation are common. Empyema is evident in one-third of cases. Calcification is rare. Miliary lesions have been recorded.
- CT or MRI of head (with or without contrast material) if brain involvement suspected
- Ultrasound examination of soft tissues (to estimate the presence and size of lesions)

Treatment

- Sulfonamides: the most effective and best-studied drugs. Treatment of choice, even in compromised patients. Sulfadiazine (1.5–2.0 g q6h) or sulfisoxazole
- Sulfamethoxazole–trimethoprim: no good evidence that is more effective; modestly greater risk of hematologic toxicity
- Minocycline: the best-established alternative oral drug for use against all *Nocardia* species (100–200 mg q12h)
- Amikacin: the best-established drug for parenteral use (5.0–7.5 mg/kg q12h)
- Combined therapy: Its value remains unsettled.
  - Imipenem plus cefotaxime
  - Amikacin plus sulfamethoxazole–trimethoprim
  - Imipenem plus sulfamethoxazole–trimethoprim
  - Imipenem plus amikacin
  - Other alternative drugs: ceftriaxone/cefuroxime/cefotaxime/ cefuroxime plus amikacin/amikacin plus amoxicillin/clavulanic acid
- Duration of therapy
  - In the immunocompetent with pulmonary or systemic nocardiosis (outside the CNS) 6–12 months
  - In the immunocompetent with CNS nocardiosis: 12 months. (If all apparent lesions excised, 6 months of therapy may be possible.)
  - In the immunosuppressed, pulmonary or systemic: 12 months
  - In AIDS patients: maybe indefinitely
  - If only soft tissues: 2 months
  - If soft tissues and bone are involved or a slow response of soft lesions: 4 months
  - If unusually extensive soft-tissue lesion or immunosuppressed: longer duration therapy needed
  - In actinomycetoma: 6 to 12 months after clinical cure
  - In keratitis: oral and topical use of sulfonamides until apparent cure and then oral alone for 2 to 4 months
- Aspiration: Transtracheal aspiration should be avoided, because it frequently leads to nocardial cellulitis in tissues around the puncture wound.
- Mortality is increased in patients with acute infection, in those being treated with corticosteroid or antineoplastic agents, in those with Cushing's disease, and in those with dissemination of infection in multiple organs or the CNS.
- There is 15% mortality in otherwise healthy patients with pulmonary nocardiosis.
- There is a higher mortality from pulmonary nocardiosis when there is a serious underlying disease (patients not receiving corticosteroids or cytotoxic agents).
- Dissemination occurs equally in all categories of patients.
- Antinocardial therapy does not influence the rate of appearance of extrapulmonary lesions.
- Death is due to sepsis, brain abscess, and overwhelming pneumonia.

Nocardiosis

SURGICAL MEASURES

Surgical therapy frequently influences the ultimate outcome, although brain abscesses may respond to antimicrobial treatment without surgery.

COMPLICATIONS

- Brain abscesses could drain into ventricles or out into the subarachnoid space.
- Transtracheal aspiration should be avoided, because it frequently leads to nocardial cellulitis in tissues around the puncture wound.
- Mortality is increased in patients
  —With acute infection
  —Being treated with corticosteroid or antineoplastic agents
  —With Cushing's disease
  —With dissemination of infection in multiple organs or the CNS
- Mortality is 15% in otherwise healthy patients with pulmonary nocardiosis.
- There is higher mortality from pulmonary nocardiosis when there is a serious underlying disease (patients not receiving corticosteroids or cytotoxic agents).
- Dissemination occurs equally in all categories of patients.
- Antinocardial therapy does not influence the rate of appearance of extrapulmonary lesions.
- Death is due to sepsis, brain abscess, and overwhelming pneumonia.
- Epidural spinal cord compression from vertebral osteomyelitis
- Pleuropulmonary fistula
- Iliopsoas, ischiorectal, perirectal abscess
- Pericarditis, endocarditis (natural and prosthetic values), aortitis
- Mediastinitis with superior vena cava obstruction
- Empyema
- Obstructive bronchial masses
- Peritonitis (in chronic peritoneal dialysis)
- Septic arthritis and bursitis
- Diffuse organ abscesses

Follow-Up

- All patients with cutaneous nocardiosis should initially be evaluated for disseminated disease. Cutaneous lesions are not always due to inoculation: Occasionally, disseminated disease results in secondary seeding of the skin.
- Investigate any evidence of complication or recurrence until several months after apparent cure, because there is a tendency for relapse or appearance of metastatic abscesses during or after effective therapy (at least 6 months after therapy has ended).
- If there is a poor response or development of a new pulmonary or extrapulmonary lesion, investigate for a second pathogen (*Pneumocystis carinii, Aspergillus, Cryptococcus, M. tuberculosis*)
- Any child with nocardiosis and no known cause of immunosuppression should undergo tests to determine the adequacy of the phagocytic respiratory burst.

PREVENTION

- Avoidance of direct contact with soil or vegetable matter (patients with immunosuppression)

Selected Readings

Smego RA Jr, Gallis HA. The clinical spectrum of *Nocardia brasiliensis* infection in the United States. *Rev Infect Dis* 1984;6:164–180.

Smego RA, Moeller MG, Gallis HA. Trimethoprim–sulfamethoxazole therapy for *Nocardia* infections. *Arch Intern Med* 1983;143:711–718.

Stropes L, Bartlett M, White A. Case report: Multiple recurrences of nocardial pneumonia. *Am J Med Sci* 1980;280:119–122.

Wallance RJ Jr, Steele L, Sumter G, et al. Antimicrobial susceptibility patterns of *Nocardia asteroides*. *Antimicrob Agents Chemother* 1988;32:1776–1779.

Wallance RJ, Septimus EJ, Williams TW, et al. Use of trimethoprim–sulfamethoxazole for treatment of infections due to *Nocardia*. *Rev Infect Dis* 1982;4:315–325.

Nontyphoidal *Salmonella* Infections

Basics

DEFINITION
Salmonella spp are responsible for diarrhea, along with sepsis and, occasionally, metastatic infection in humans.

ETIOLOGY
- Gram-negative rod in the Enterobacteriaceae family
- The organism is found in the gastrointestinal tract of many species of mammals, birds, reptiles, amphibians, and insects. Some, but not all, species cause disease in humans.
- *Salmonella typhi* is present only in humans, with no animal reservoir.
- Nontyphoidal *Salmonella* spp have the ability to live within macrophages.
- Infection of the small and large intestines occurs.

EPIDEMIOLOGY
- Disease is found worldwide.
- Up to 3.7 million cases occur each year in the United States.
- Disease is most common in undeveloped tropical regions of the world.
- Most cases in humans occur by eating contaminated meat or eggs.
- Nosocomial spread has been documented
- Pet animals, especially reptiles, have been implicated in some cases of disease in humans.
- Following symptomatic infection, patients often remain culture-positive for over 1 month.
- Long-term carriers occur in 0.2% to 0.6% of those infected.

Incubation
- Six to 48 hours

Clinical Manifestations

- Fevers and diarrhea are the most common manifestations of *Salmonella* infections.
- Infection is usually self-limited. Fevers resolve after 2 to 3 days, and diarrhea resolves in the first week.
- Dysentery or cholera-like symptoms are uncommon in salmonellosis.
- Bacteremia occurs up to 4% of cases in healthy people with gastroenteritis.
- In elderly patients or young children, bacteremia is more common.
- Patients with HIV have a 100× increased risk of bacteremia.
- Metastatic spread of infection to vascular grafts, bone, heart valves, joints, kidney, and liver or spleen has been well documented in bacteremic patients.
- Osteomyelitis has been described in patients with sickle cell anemia and *Salmonella* bacteremia

Diagnosis

- Stool and blood cultures should identify the organism.
- Leukocytosis is common.

DIFFERENTIAL DIAGNOSIS
- *E. coli* strains
- *Campylobacter*
- *Yersinia*
- *Shigella*
- *Clostridium difficile*

Treatment

- No antibiotics should be used for uncomplicated cases of *Salmonella* gastroenteritis.

Nontyphoidal *Salmonella* Infections

- Patients at risk of bacteremia (the elderly, the young, the immunocompromised, those with vascular grafts or prosthetic valves) should be treated with oral or intravenous ciprofloxacin until afebrile.
- Severe diarrhea can be treated with ciprofloxacin 500 mg orally twice per day for 3 to 5 days.
- Alternatives include trimethoprim–sulfamethoxazole (double-strength) orally twice per day for 3 to 5 days.
- Patients with simple bacteremia should be treated with ciprofloxacin 400 mg i.v. twice per day for 14 days.
- Alternatives include ceftriaxone 2 g i.v. daily for 14 days.
- Endovascular infection, seen with high-grade bacteremia, should be treated for at least 6 weeks. Patients with unresectable foci may require suppressive antibiotics for life.
- Patients with HIV have recurrent *Salmonella* bacteremia and require long-term suppressive ciprofloxacin.

COMPLICATIONS

- Metastatic infections throughout the body can occur following gastroenteritis with sepsis.
- Vascular grafts or infection of aneurysms often requires surgery for eradication.

Follow-Up

Infected health care workers or food handlers should take great precaution to avoid direct contact with patients or food. Often, negative stool cultures are required prior to their going back to full-time employment.

PREVENTION

- Outbreaks of infection should be reported to state authorities for investigation.
- Meat and poultry should be washed prior to cooking, and be well cooked.
- Eggs should be well cooked.
- Pets such as reptiles should be avoided in families with young children or immunocompromised individuals.
- Good handwashing is always important after contact with pets.

Selected Readings

Herikastad H, et al. Emerging quinolone-resistant *Salmonella* in the United States. *Emerg Infect Dis* 1997;3:371–372.

Lewin CS. Treatment of multiresistant *Salmonella* infection. *Lancet* 1991;337:47.

Mishu B, et al. Outbreaks of *Salmonella enteritidis* infections in the United States, 1985–1991. *J Infect Dis* 1994;169:547–552.

Wang JH, et al. Mycotic aneurysm due to non-typhi *Salmonella*: Report of 16 cases. *Clin Infect Dis* 1996;23:743–747.

Odontogenic Infections

Basics

DEFINITION
Odontogenic infections are those originating within the mouth, associated with the teeth and surrounding structures. These infections can range from small apical abscesses to large soft-tissue infections extending to the neck and beyond. Infections may occur within the gums (gingivitis), the alveolar bone and supporting structures (periodontitis), and the enamel and dentin of the tooth itself (caries).

ETIOLOGY
- Determining the cause of the large array of infections associated with teeth requires understanding of the oral flora, the normal anatomy, and host factors.
- The flora of the oral cavity includes the following:
  - *Streptococcus*
  - *Peptostreptococcus*
  - *Bacteroides*
  - *Fusobacterium*
  - *Actinomyces*
  - *Spirochetes*
  - Many other species
- *Streptococcus mutans* is associated with the development of caries.
- Anaerobes are associated with periodontal infections.
- Gingivitis is associated with *Prevotella intermedia* and other anaerobic gram-negative rods.

EPIDEMIOLOGY
- Pertubation of the colonizing microflora can lead to the development of disease within the mouth.
- Diet, especially concentrated sugars, plays a role in establishment of certain organisms within the mouth.
- Patients with poor oral hygiene in general have higher colony counts of mouth flora.
- Hospitalized patients have higher numbers of gram-negative facultative rods (e.g. *E. coli*, *Klebsiella*).
- Disorders of salivation are associated with greater numbers of organisms.
- Disorders of cell-mediated immunity, deficiency of IgA, and reduction in neutrophils are all risk factors for the development of oral infections.

Risk Factors
- Pregnancy
- Diabetes
- Immunodeficiency

Clinical Manifestations

- Periapical abscess and pulpitis occur when bacteria enter the tooth through caries.
- Patients complain initially of hot and cold sensitivity of the tooth; this may develop into a throbbing sensation that is worsened with eating.
- Eventually, the tooth will generate continuous pain.

GINGIVITIS
- Inflammation of the gums may lead to bad breath and bleeding after brushing.
- The gums are hyperemic.
- In the worst cases, termed *Vincent's disease* or *trench mouth*, fevers may occur.
- The gingival surface becomes necrotic.

PERIODONTITIS
- Periodontal disease is often associated with localized pain along with hot and cold sensitivity.
- Gingivitis may be present. Loss of the supporting structure may lead to motion of the tooth, and pressure on the tooth leads to formation of pus around the tooth.

Diagnosis

Infections of the gingiva are easily identified clinically.

IMAGING
- Radiographs should detect bone loss, areas of abscess formation, and loss of dentin and enamel.

Odontogenic Infections

- With deep extension of infection, CT or MRI scanning is most helpful.

LABORATORY

Cultures generally reveal mixed infections, and thus are not useful.

Treatment

- All abscesses need to be drained. There are many intraoral routes for drainage.
- At times, the crown of the tooth needs to be removed or the tooth extracted.
- Clindamycin 300 mg orally every 6 hours is the drug of choice for most minor odontogenic infections.
- Amoxicillin–clavulanate 250 to 500 mg orally every 8 hours is an alternative to clindamycin.
- Erythromycin 250 to 500 mg orally every 6 hours can be used in patients who are allergic to β-lactams or clindamycin.
- Deep neck infections should be treated with intravenous penicillin G and metronidazole, or a combination β-lactam/β-lactamase inhibitor, clindamycin, or a carbapenem.

COMPLICATIONS

- Simple odontogenic infections
  —Endocarditis
  —Infections of prosthesis
  —Deep face/neck infections
  —Brain abscesses
- Deep space infections
  —Fevers
  —Marked swelling
  —Induration of the affected area
- Submandibular/sublingual space infections
  —Ludwig's angina, a bilateral infection that causes elevation of the tongue and floor of the mouth
  —The airway may become occluded rapidly.
  —Patients need hospitalization.
- Pharyngeal space infections
  —Lateral pharyngeal space infections are rarely caused by an odontogenic source.
  —Patients have trismus and swelling of the lateral pharyngeal wall.
  —Airway occlusion may occur, and hospitalization is necessary.
- Buccal and parotid space infections
  —Massive swelling over the side of the face.
  —Trismus is not commonly encountered.
- Intracranial spread
  —Dreaded complications of cavernous sinus thrombosis and suppurative jugular thrombophlebitis may have an odontogenic source.
- Osteomyelitis
  —Osteomyelitis of the jaw can occasionally occur and lead to great morbidity.
  —The infection may be chronic and require months of antibiotics and extensive oral surgery for cure.

Follow-Up

- Frequent periodontal scaling can avert plaque formation and periodontitis.
- Frequent follow-up with a dentist, at least every 6 months, is mandatory.

PREVENTION

- Good oral hygiene is needed to prevent plaque build-up.
- Fluoride promotes remineralization of the teeth and can prevent caries.
- Chlorhexidine can reduce the amount of plaque formation and prevent disease.

Selected Readings

Bloomquist IK, Bayer A. Life-threatening deep facial space infections of the head and neck. *Infect Dis Clin North Am* 1988;2:237.

Chow AW, Roser SM, Brady FA. Orofacial odontogenic infections. *Ann Intern Med* 1978;88:392.

Tanner A, Stillman N. Oral and dental infections with anaerobic bacteria: Clinical features, predominant pathogens and treatment. *Clin Infect Dis* 1993;16[Suppl 4]:S304.

Orchitis

Basics

DEFINITION
Orchitis is infection of the testicle(s), most often caused by the mumps virus. Other viral infections, as well as bacterial, mycobacterial, or fungal infections, may be the cause.

ETIOLOGY
- The most common cause of orchitis in unimmunized older children and adults is mumps.
- HIV often infects the testes, without symptoms.
- Bacterial orchitis occurs via spread of infection from the epididymis. Enteric pathogens are often isolated; however, *Pseudomonas* and *Staphylococcus* are, on occasion, isolated.
- Gonorrhea leads to an epididymis orchitis infection if untreated.
- Tuberculosis orchitis has been well described, most likely secondary to hematogenous spread.
- Systemic fungal infections such as histoplasmosis, blastomycosis, or coccidioidomycosis can produce chronic orchitis.
- Disseminated toxoplasmosis in AIDS patients may infect the testes, leading to a low-grade orchitis.

EPIDEMIOLOGY
- Orchitis is a rare disease, and it is most often seen in cases of mumps.
- Mumps orchitis is rare before puberty but is seen in 20% to 30% of mumps patients after puberty.

Incubation
In mumps infection, orchitis follows the onset of symptomatic parotiditis by a few days.

Clinical Manifestations

- Patients with symptomatic mumps infection may note unilateral or bilateral testicular swelling and tenderness. The disease is unilateral in two-thirds of cases.
- Mild disease lasts 4 to 5 days.
- Severe diseases can last as long as 1 week.
- Pyogenic orchitis leads to the following:
  —Fevers
  —Swelling
  —Severe pain in the testes
  —Possible formation of abscess
  —Possibility that entire scrotum may become edematous and hard

Diagnosis

- The diagnosis is often clinical.
- Urethral cultures are taken to rule out gonorrhea.
- Midstream urine cultures should be obtained.
- It may be hard to differentiate orchitis from epididymitis when severe inflammation is present.
- A CT scan may reveal edema and abscess

Orchitis

DIFFERENTIAL DIAGNOSIS

- Torsion
- Infarction
- Tumor with necrosis
- Trauma
- Gonorrhea
- Epididymitis

Treatment

- Mumps orchitis can be treated symptomatically with elevation of the scrotum and bed rest.
- Gonorrhea should be treated with ceftriaxone, followed by doxycycline 100 mg orally 2 times per day for 10 days.
- Alternative treatment includes ofloxacin 300 mg postprandial twice per day for 10 days.
- Pyogenic orchitis due to coliforms should be treated with β-lactam/β-lactamase inhibitor or a third-generation cephalosporin or ciprofloxacin. Duration of treatment should be 7 to 10 days.

COMPLICATIONS

- Testicular infarction or damage leading to sterility is a dreaded complication of orchitis, but it is rare.
- Abscess formation can occur with pyogenic infection.

Follow-Up

Close observation for the development of a scrotal or testicular abscess is needed in the recovery period.

PREVENTION

- Vaccination for mumps should be universal, with two doses given in childhood. The first dose is given at age 12 to 15 months and the second dose at age 5 to 12 years.
- Vaccination should be considered for adults who have no history of childhood vaccination.
- Early treatment of epididymitis may decrease the chances of testicular involvement.

Selected Readings

Beard CM, Benson RC, Kelalis PP, et al. The incidence and outcome of mumps orchitis in Rochester Minn. Mayo Clinic, 1935–1974. *Mayo Clin Proc* 1977;52:3.

Candel S. Epididymitis in mumps, including orchitis: Further clinical studies and comments. *Ann Intern Med* 1951;34:20.

Osteomyelitis

Basics

DEFINITION
Osteomyelitis is an infection of bone, usually bacterial and rarely fungal in nature.

ETIOLOGY
Infection can occur via the following:

- Hematogenous spread
  - In adults, hematogenous spread to bone often occurs with *Staphylococcus aureus*.
  - *Mycobacterium tuberculosis* may be isolated, often in the thoracic spine. It spreads from the intervertebral disks to involve bone above and below the disk and is the result of hematogenous spread in most instances.
- Direct inoculation during trauma or surgery
- Spread from contiguous sites, such as joints or soft-tissue infections
  - Infection contiguous to a prosthetic device may lead to persistent infection despite adequate antibiotic therapy.
- Infection is often subacute in nature.
- All areas of the bone, including the cortex, medullary cavity, and periosteum can be affected. Necrotic bone is termed the *sequestrum*.
- Osteomyelitis in children often is present in the metaphysis of long bones.
- *Pseudomonas* is often isolated in osteomyelitis in intravenous drug users and in diabetics with foot infections.
- *Pseudomonas* can inoculate bone when a sharp object, such as a nail, penetrates a wet sneaker.
- *Staphylococcus epidermidis* can infect bone contiguous to an infected prosthetic device, such as a rod or total knee replacement.
- Enterobacteriaceae can cause vertebral osteomyelitis. It is often spread from Batson's plexus in patients with bladder or prostate infections. These organisms also may be present in the bones of the foot in patients with diabetes or vascular insufficiency.
- Atypical mycobacterial infection with *M. avium-intracellulare* is seen within the bone marrow of patients with AIDS. Cases with bony destruction are seen during a reconstitution syndrome in patients starting highly active antiretroviral therapy.
- Fungal osteomyelitis is seen with coccidioidomycosis and blastomycosis.
- Infections with *Candida* are seen in patients with chronic indwelling catheters and in intravenous drug users.

EPIDEMIOLOGY
Refer to the specific infection.

Risk Factors

- Although *S. aureus* is more common, patients with sickle cell anemia account for most of the bone infections with *Salmonella*.
- Diabetics have increased risk for osteomyelitis caused by *S. aureus*. Diabetic foot ulcers predispose to bone infections.
- Intravenous drug users
- Patients with peripheral vascular disease or peripheral neuropathy

Clinical Manifestations

- There is a wide range of clinical presentations in patients with osteomyelitis.
- Much depends on the acuity of the infection, the location of the involved bones, and the organism isolated.
- In general, patients present with fever and pain over the affected bone.
- Swelling may be present.
- When the infection is chronic, sinus drainage may occur.
- Overlying cellulitis is common. Recurrent cellulitis should alert the clinician to the possibility of an underlying osteomyelitis.

Diagnosis

The diagnosis of osteomyelitis should be considered in any patient who presents with bone pain or swelling that is not associated with trauma.

DIFFERENTIAL DIAGNOSIS

- Tumors of the bone

Osteomyelitis

LABORATORY

- The organism responsible for osteomyelitis can be recovered via positive blood cultures in 40% of cases of acute osteomyelitis.
- Sinus tract cultures, if positive for *S. aureus*, may be accurate; however, other organisms found in the tract may not reflect the infection in the bone, especially when overlying cellulitis is present.
- Bone biopsy while the patient is not on antibiotics is the only reliable way to recover the organism causing osteomyelitis.
- An elevated erythrocyte sedimentation rate (ESR) is helpful in making the diagnosis and in following treatment of the disease.

IMAGING

- X-rays are important in making the diagnosis; however, the radiographs may be normal in the early stages of illness.
- CT scans may reveal subtle cortical changes and soft-tissue changes before they are seen on plain x-rays.
- MRI is useful for evaluation of the spine in suspected osteomyelitis.
- Radionuclide scanning is the best means of making an early diagnosis. The entire body can be scanned and occult sites of metastatic infection can be detected.

Treatment

- Long-term antibiotic therapy can work only if necrotic tissue and bone are surgically debrided.
- In early disease, it is not always necessary to debride.
- At times, revascularization is necessary for adequate treatment.
- Foreign bodies, if infected, should be removed, if possible.
- *S. aureus* should be treated with oxacillin or nafcillin for 6 weeks.
- Susceptible gram-negative rods and *Pseudomonas* should be treated with ciprofloxacin.
- Coagulase-negative *Staphylococcus* should be treated with vancomycin and rifampin.
- Diabetic foot osteomyelitis should be treated with a β-lactam/β-lactamase combination, or a carbapenem or a combination such as ciprofloxacin and metronidazole.

COMPLICATIONS

- Bony destruction may lead to loss of function of the bone or limb.
- Vertebral osteomyelitis may produce an epidural abscess and cord compression and myelitis. Spread to the paravertebral area may lead to a psoas abscess.
- Osteomyelitis of the base of the skull may lead to cranial neuropathies.

Follow-Up

- Osteomyelitis may recur, and close follow-up is always needed.
- Follow-up x-rays may not indicate whether the infection is eradicated. Bone is often in the process of remodeling, and the findings on x-ray may be hard to evaluate.
- Following ESRs every month for the first 2 months and then every 4 months is suggested for the first year following treatment.

PREVENTION

- Diabetic patients with neuropathy should always be made aware of the risk of developing ulcers on their feet.
- Every effort should be made to provide a sterile operating room environment for patients receiving prosthetic joints.

Selected Readings

Gathe J Jr, Harris R, Garland B, et al. Candida osteomyelitis. Report of 5 cases and a review of the literature. *Am J Med* 1987;82:927–937.

Lew DP, Waldvogel FA. Current concepts of osteomyelitis. *N Engl J Med* 1997;336:999–1007.

Lew DP, Waldvogel FA. Quinolones and osteomyelitis: State-of-the-art. *Drugs* 1995;49[Suppl 2]:100–111.

Otitis Externa

Basics

DEFINITION
- Infection of the external auditory canal; subdivided into four categories:
  - Acute localized otitis externa
  - Acute diffuse otitis externa (swimmer's ear)
  - Chronic otitis externa
  - Invasive ("malignant") otitis externa

ETIOLOGY
- Acute localized otitis externa: pustule or furuncle associated with hair follicles; usually due to *Staphylococcus aureus*
- Acute diffuse otitis externa (swimmer's ear): occurs mostly in hot, humid weather and may be due to a decrease in canal acidity. The most common pathogens are *Pseudomonas aeruginosa*, other gram-negative bacilli, *S. aureus*, and fungi (e.g., *Aspergillus* spp).
- Chronic otitis externa: due to irritation of the external auditory canal from drainage of a chronic middle-ear infection. Rare causes include tuberculosis, syphilis, yaws, and leprosy.
- Invasive ("malignant") otitis externa: severe, necrotizing infection that slowly invades from the squamous epithelium of the ear canal into adjacent soft tissues, blood vessels, cartilage, and bone. *P. aeruginosa* is the pathogen involved in more than 95% of cases; in the remaining cases, the pathogens include *Staphylococcus epidermidis, Aspergillus, Fusobacterium,* and *Actinomyces*.

EPIDEMIOLOGY

Incidence
- All forms of otitis externa (except the invasive form) are common.
- Exact data for the incidence of the disease are not available.

Risk Factors
- Hot, humid weather; water exposure; and mechanical trauma are risk factors for acute diffuse otitis externa.
- Diabetic, elderly, immunocompromised, and debilitated patients are at particular risk for invasive ("malignant") otitis externa.

Clinical Manifestations

SYMPTOMS AND SIGNS
- Acute localized otitis externa
  - Presentation of pustule or furuncle
- Acute diffuse otitis externa (swimmer's ear)
  - Otalgia, pruritus
  - Manipulation of the auricle often elicits pain.
  - Often purulent discharge
  - Erythema and edema of the ear canal skin
  - Erythematous tympanic membrane. In contrast to acute otitis media, however, it moves normally with pneumatic otoscopy.
- Chronic otitis externa: causes pruritus rather than ear pain and is associated with chronic suppurative otitis media
- Invasive ("malignant") otitis externa
  - Severe pain and tenderness from the tissues around the ear
  - Drainage of pus from the canal
  - Edematous canal with granulation tissue, usually in the posterior wall
  - Permanent facial paralysis is frequent (cranial nerves VI, IX, X, XI, or XII also may be affected).
  - Fever is rare and of low grade.

Diagnosis

- Otoscopy is essential.
- In invasive ("malignant") otitis externa:
  - Laboratory studies usually reveal a normal WBC but an increased erythrocyte sedimentation rate.

Otitis Externa

— CT, MRI, and radionuclide medicine scanning are helpful for defining the extent of bone and soft-tissue involvement.
— Cultures of discharge from the external canal are unreliable. A deep-tissue specimen should be obtained for culture and pathologic examination.
— Diagnostic tests for underlying disease should be performed.

Treatment

MAIN TREATMENT

- Acute localized otitis externa
  — Otic drops containing antibiotics with antistaphylococcal action are usually effective.
  — Antibiotics by mouth (e.g., dicloxacillin 500 mg q6h or amoxicillin/clavulanic acid 500/125 mg q8h for 7 days if local antibiotic treatment is not effective)
- Acute diffuse otitis externa (swimmer's ear)
  — Protection of the ear from additional moisture and avoidance of further mechanical injury by scratching
  — Gentle removal of debris and cleaning with mixture of alcohol and acetic acid
  — Otic drops containing a mixture of antibiotic and corticosteroid in an acid vehicle (e.g., neomycin–polymyxin and hydrocortisone) are very effective.
- Chronic otitis externa: Treatment for chronic otitis media will also treat this condition.
- Invasive ("malignant") otitis externa
  — Intravenous antibiotic treatment active against *P. aeruginosa* should be used for 6 to 8 weeks. Use one of the following:
    — Imipenem 0.5 g q6h
    — Meropenem 1 g q8h
    — Ciprofloxacin 400 mg q12h
    — Ceftazidime 2 g q8h
    — Cefepime 2 g q12h
    — Piperacillin 4 to 6 g q4–6h plus an antipseudomonal aminoglycoside antibiotic
    — Ticarcillin 3 g q4h plus an antipseudomonal aminoglycoside antibiotic
  — In early cases, oral ciprofloxacin alone (750 mg q12h) may follow the initial 2 weeks of intravenous therapy if cultures reveal a *P. aeruginosa* strain sensitive to this drug.
  — Cleansing of the canal and removing of the devitalized tissue
  — Surgical debridement of the infected bone is reserved for cases of deterioration despite medical therapy.

COMPLICATIONS

In invasive ("malignant") otitis externa, the infection may spread to the temporal bone, sigmoid sinus, jugular bulb, base of the scull, cranial nerves, meninges, and brain.

Follow-Up

- Otoscopy in a follow-up appointment

PREVENTION

Good management of diabetes mellitus may decrease the risk of invasive otitis externa.

Selected Readings

Doroghazi RM, Nadol JB, Hyslop NE, et al. Invasive external otitis. *Am J Med* 1981;71:603–613.

Johnson MP, Ramphal R. Malignant external otitis: Report on therapy with ceftazidime and review of therapy and prognosis. *Rev Infect Dis* 1990;12:173–180.

Phillips P, Bryce G, Shepherd J. Invasive external otitis caused by *Aspergillus*. *Rev Infect Dis* 1990;12:277–281.

Rapoport Y, Shalit I, Redianu C, et al. Oral ofloxacin therapy for invasive external otitis. *Ann Otol Rhinol Laryngol* 1991;100:632–637.

Otitis Media

Basics

DEFINITION
- Inflammation of the mucosa of periosteum of the middle ear
- Acute otitis media: presence of fluid in the middle ear, with signs or symptoms of acute illness
- Recurrent acute otitis media: three or more episodes in 6 months, four or more in 1 year, or two or more episodes in the first year of life
- Otitis media with effusion or serous otitis media: persistence of middle-ear fluid for several months without other signs of infection
- Chronic suppurative otitis media: chronic purulent drainage from the affected ear through perforated tympanic membrane with or without cholesteatoma

ETIOLOGY
- Anatomic or physiologic dysfunction of the eustachian tube appears to play a critical role in the development of otitis media. This dysfunction results in fluid collection in the middle ear and mastoid cavities, providing a culture medium for any bacterium present. Viral upper respiratory infections, which can cause congestion of the mucosa of the eustachian tube, often precede episodes of acute otitis media.
- Acute otitis media
  - In children (nonneonates)
    - *Streptococcus pneumoniae*: 35%; the most common types in order of decreasing frequency are 19, 23, 6, 14, 3, and 18.
    - *Haemophilus influenzae*: approximately 25%; about 90% of *H. influenzae* infections are due to nontypable strains; bacteremia or meningitis may accompany infections due to type b *H. influenzae*.
    - *Moraxella catarrhalis*: approximately 15% (90% of *M. catarrhalis* strains produce beta-lactamases)
    - Group A streptococci: 12%
    - *Staphylococcus aureus*: 12%
    - Sterile (no pathogen grown in cultures of middle ear fluid): up to 25% to 30% in some studies
  - In neonates: Group B streptococci and gram-negative bacilli are important causes. Also, in this age group, *Chlamydia trachomatis* infection may be a pathogen in cases of acute otitis media.
  - In adults: *H. influenza* (26%) and *S. pneumoniae* (21%) are the most common pathogens.
- Recurrent acute otitis media
  - Most cases are due to the same pathogens that cause acute otitis media. Most cases of early recurrence (75%) are not due to relapse (of the same strain) but to new infections due to organisms different from those that caused the initial episode.
- Otitis media with effusion
  - Eustachian tube dysfunction is important for pathogenesis.
  - Cultures of middle-ear fluid are frequently negative.
- Chronic suppurative otitis media
  - Aerobic cultures of draining fluid reveal a high percentage of *S. aureus*, *P. aeruginosa*, and enteric gram-negative bacilli (*Klebsiella, Escherichia coli, Proteus*)
  - Anaerobes, including *Prevotella, Fusobacterium, Porphyromonas*, and some *Bacteroides* species, are found in 50% of cases, usually in mixed culture with aerobes.
  - Tuberculous otitis media is a rare cause of chronic suppurative otitis media. It is characterized by a tympanic membrane with multiple perforations, extensive granulation tissue, and severe hearing loss.

EPIDEMIOLOGY

Incidence and Prevalence
- More than two-thirds of children under age 3 have at least one episode of acute otitis media and one-third have three or more; the prevalence among adults is only 0.25%.
- Predominant age: The peak incidence is at ages 6 to 24 months (with a second smaller peak between 5 and 6 years, the time of school entrance); incidence declines after age 6 years, and is infrequent in adults.
- Predominant sex: Acute otitis media occurs more often in males than in females.

Risk Factors
- Anatomic changes (cleft palate, cleft uvula)
- Alteration of normal physiologic defenses (patulous eustachian tube)
- Congenital or acquired immunologic deficiencies
- Daycare
- Passive smoking
- Family history
- Being young age at the time of the first episode is a risk factor of recurrent middle ear infections.
- Breastfeeding for 3 or 4 months is associated with decreased risk for acute otitis media in the first year of life.

Clinical Manifestations

SYMPTOMS AND SIGNS
- Acute otitis media
  - Earache
  - Fever (may be absent)
  - Decreased hearing
  - Ear drainage if eardrum is perforated
  - Vertigo, nystagmus, and tinnitus may occur.
  - Decreased eardrum mobility (as observed by pneumatic otoscopy)
  - The eardrum is usually red, opaque, and bulging. Redness is an early sign of acute otitis media, but erythema alone is not diagnostic of middle ear infection.
- Acute otitis media in infants
  - May cause no symptoms or cause septic profile
  - Often irritability, anorexia, nausea, vomiting, and diarrhea
  - Eardrum as above
- Otitis media with effusion
  - Usually asymptomatic
  - Associated with an approximate 25-dB hearing loss of the affected ear
  - Sense of fullness in the affected ear
  - Vertigo or tinnitus may occur.
  - The eardrum is often dull but not bulging, is hypomobile, and occasionally is accompanied by air bubbles in the middle ear.
- Chronic suppurative otitis media is divided into two groups: with or without cholesteatoma.
  - Chronic purulent drainage from the affected ear
  - Hearing loss
  - Perforation of the tympanic membrane
  - May be accompanied by mucosal changes, such as polypoid degeneration and granulation tissue, and osseous changes, such as osteitis and sclerosis

Diagnosis

DIFFERENTIAL DIAGNOSIS
- Earache with a normal otoscopic examination may be caused by referred pain from the jaw or teeth.
- In an adult with persistent unilateral serous otitis media, nasopharyngeal carcinoma must be excluded.

SPECIAL TESTS
- Tympanometry, acoustic reflex measurement, or acoustic reflectometry: to document the presence of middle ear fluid

Otitis Media

- Hearing testing in patients with otitis media with effusion or chronic suppurative otitis media
- In patients with chronic suppurative otitis media, a CT scan should be used to rule out a surgically treatable nidus of infection, such as an infected cholesteatoma or mastoid sequestrum.

DIAGNOSTIC PROCEDURES

- Tympanocentesis to define the microbiology (cause of infection) should be considered in the following:
  — The patient who is critically ill at the onset
  — The patient who has not responded to initial antimicrobial therapy in 48 to 72 hours and is toxic
  — The patient with altered host defenses, including the newborn infant

Treatment

MAIN TREATMENT

Acute Otitis Media: Antimicrobial Chemotherapy

- In children (nonneonates) and adults
  — Drug of choice: amoxicillin 40 mg/kg/d divided q8h or 1 g tid in adults for 10 days
  — Alternative drugs are indicated for the following cases: patients with penicillin allergy, persistent symptoms after 48 to 72 hours of amoxicillin treatment, and in immunocompromised hosts
    — Amoxicillin–clavulanate: 40 mg/kg/d for amoxicillin component divided q8h or 625 mg tid in adults for 10 days
    — Cefaclor: 40 mg/kg/d divided q8h or 500 mg tid in adults for 10 days
    — Cefuroxime axetil: 30 mg/kg/d divided q12h or 250 mg bid in adults for 10 days
    — Cefprozil: 30 mg/kg/d divided q12h or 500 mg bid in adults for 10 days
    — Loracarbef: 30 mg/kg/d divided q12h or 400 mg bid in adults for 10 days
    — Cefixime: 8 mg/kg/d divided q12h or 200 mg bid in adults for 10 days
    — Cefpodoxime proxetil: 10 mg/kg/d divided q12h or 100 mg bid in adults for 10 days
    — Ceftibuten: 9 mg/kg/d qd or 400 mg qd in adults for 10 days
    — Ceftriaxone: 50 mg/kg i.m. single dose
    — Clarithromycin: 15 mg/kg/d divided q12h or 250 mg bid in adults for 10 days
    — Azithromycin: 10 mg/kg qd on day 1 and then 5 mg/kg qd on days 2 to 5; in adults, 500 mg qd on day 1 and then 250 mg qd on days 2 to 5
    — Trimethoprim-sulfamethoxazole (TMP/SMX): 8 mg TMP/kg/d divided q12h or 160 mg TMP/800 mg SMX bid in adults for 10 days
    — Erythromycin–sulfisoxazole: 40 mg/kg/d for erythromycin component divided q6h
- In neonates: Initially, intravenous antimicrobial chemotherapy is needed (ampicillin plus cephalosporin of third generation)

Recurrent Acute Otitis Media

- Chemoprophylaxis for 3 to 6 months or during winter and spring
  — Amoxicillin: 20 mg/kg qd or 250 mg qd in adults, or
  — Sulfisoxazole: 75 mg/kg qd or 500 mg qd in adults
- Immunoprophylaxis: pneumonococcal vaccines (more effective in children over the age of 2 years)
- Referral for surgery if more than two or three acute otitis media recurrences while on chemoprophylaxis

Otitis Media with Effusion

- Antihistamines and decongestants (usually are ineffective)
- Some suggest a short course of oral antibiotics or steroids, or even a combination of the two, but they are probably of little lasting benefit.
- Referral for surgery if the patient has the following: more than 4 to 6 months of bilateral otitis media with effusion, more than 6 months of unilateral otitis media with effusion, and/or hearing loss greater than 25 dB.

Chronic Suppurative Otitis Media

- Surgical drainage of infected areas of the middle ear, followed by a prolonged course of topical antibiotic drops
- Surgical management of cholesteatoma
- In exacerbations of chronic suppurative otitis media: culture of the drainage and, by mouth, antimicrobial chemotherapy based on antibiogram

APPROPRIATE HEALTH CARE

- Outpatient except when surgery is indicated

SURGICAL MEASURES

Otitis media with effusion, recurrent acute otitis media: Surgical management of the persistent effusion of the middle ear includes the use of myringotomy, adenoidectomy, and the placement of tympanostomy tubes (when surgery is indicated).

COMPLICATIONS

- Acute and chronic mastoiditis
- Labyrinthitis
- Facial nerve paralysis
- Petrous apicitis, Gradenigo's syndrome
- Otogenic skull base osteomyelitis
- Sigmoid sinus thrombosis
- CNS infection (meningitis, epidural abscess, subdural abscess, intraparenchymal brain abscess)
- Hearing loss

Follow-Up

- Follow-up is not necessary if symptoms of acute otitis media clearly disappear with appropriate treatment.
- Appropriate antimicrobial treatment of patients with acute otitis media decreases the probability of recurrence.

PREVENTION

- Vaccination against Pneumococci and *Haemophilis* influenzae
- Breastfeeding is associated with decreased incidence of acute otitis media in infants.

Selected Readings

Celin S, Bluestone C, Stephenson J, et al. Bacteriology of acute otitis media in adults. *JAMA* 1991;266:2249–2252.

Chonmaitree T, Howie VM, Truant AL. Presence of respiratory viruses in middle ear fluids and nasal wash specimens of children with acute otitis media. *Pediatrics* 1986;77:698702.

Fria TH, Cantekin EI, Eichler JA. Hearing acuity of children with effusion. *Arch Otolaryngol* 1985;111:10–16.

Henderson FW, Collier AM, Sanyal MA, et al. A longitudinal study of respiratory viruses and bacteria in the etiology of acute otitis media with effusion. *N Engl J Med* 1982;306:1377.

Kaleida PH, Casselbrant ML, Rocjette HE, et al. Amoxicillin or myringotomy or both for acute otitis media: Results of a randomized clinical trial. *Pediatrics* 1991;87:466–474.

Klein JO, Bluestone CD. Acute otitis media: Management of pediatric infectious diseases in office practice. *Pediatr Infect Dis* 1982;1:66–73.

Teele DW, Klein JO, Rosner B. Epidemiology of otitis media during the first seven years of life in children in greater Boston: A prospective, cohort study. *J Infect Dis* 1989;160:83–94.

Parvovirus Infections

Basics

DEFINITION

- Parvovirus infections are a group of diseases caused by parvovirus B19.
- Parvovirus B19 has been associated with erythema infectiosum (fifth disease), transient aplastic crisis in chronic hemolytic anemia patients, chronic anemia in immunocompromised (including HIV-infected) patients, and fetal infection (hydrops fetalis and fetal death).
- Parvovirus B19 is responsible for the most transient aplastic anemia episodes in patients with chronic hemolytic disorders (i.e., 80%–92% of transient pure red-cell aplasia crises in sickle cell disease).

ETIOLOGY

- Parvovirus B19 is a small, nonenveloped, single-stranded DNA virus, the only human-specific member of the family Parvoviridae. It has been named after the code number of the human serum where it was discovered in the early 1970s.
- It is resistant to ether, chloroform, acid (up to pH 3.0), and heat (up to 60°C).

EPIDEMIOLOGY

- Global distribution: Humans are the principal infection reservoir.
- Seroprevalence rates rise rapidly between the ages of 5 to 18, and reach 30% to 60% in adults.
- Erythema infectiosum is a childhood illness and occurs in outbreaks in schools, mostly during late winter and early spring, but it can affect any age. Secondary attack rates rise up to 50%.
- Although there is no sex predominance for most manifestations of parvovirus infection, arthritis most commonly affects women.
- Failure to clear parvovirus B19 viremia seems to be a common causative factor for chronic anemia (not related to antiretroviral agents) in HIV-positive patients. Parvovirus B19–related chronic anemia has been described in other forms of congenital and acquired immunodeficiency states.
- Transmission may occur via the respiratory route and close person-to-person contact. The virus is present in oral and/or respiratory secretions.
- Parenteral transmission via blood and blood products has also been documented. Risk by single blood donation is 1:50,000, but this increases with the use of concentrated coagulation factors.
- Vertical transmission also occurs and may lead to hydrops fetalis and fetal death.
- Nosocomial and laboratory transmission has been documented.
- Viremic patients with aplastic crises are highly infective for other patients belonging to the high-risk groups.

High-Risk Groups

- Seronegative pregnant women
- Patients with chronic hemolytic anemias (thalassemia, sickle cell disease, etc.)
- HIV-positive individuals
- Patients with other forms of cell-mediated immunity suppression

Incubation Period and Natural History

- Infection may be asymptomatic or symptomatic.
- Incubation lasts about a week and is followed by viremia of 1 week's duration. During the viremic period, the virus can be detected in oral and/or respiratory secretions.
- About the tenth day, pure red-cell aplasia in bone marrow has been established, due to infection and lysis of the red-cell precursors.
- Rash appears after resolution of viremia (more than 2 weeks after challenge) and lasts for 2 to 3 days. Joint involvement may persist several days after the rash resolution. Both phenomena seem to be immune-mediated reactions.
- IgM–parvovirus B19 complexes can be detected on about day 10, and IgG about 1 week later.
- Resolution of anemia and recovery from viremia correlate with virus-specific IgM and IgG antibodies. The latter may persist lifelong.
- Failure to form a proper antibody response results in chronic infection in the immunocompromised patient.
- Failure to effectively overcome the pure red-cell aplasia in hemolytic anemia patients results in transient aplastic crisis.
- Infection of the fetus may lead to severe anemia, resulting in cardiac failure, hydrops fetalis, and endometrial death.

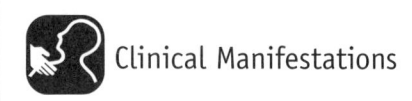

Clinical Manifestations

SYMPTOMS

- The appearance of the rash is preceded by mild symptoms (fever, malaise, myalgias, headache, pruritus).
- There may be sore throat and respiratory and abdominal symptoms.
- Joint symptoms (stiffness, pain) begin about 1 day after rash resolution, mostly affecting women. Hands, knees, and wrists are usually involved. Peripheral polyarthropathy is symmetric and improves in about 2 weeks.
- Symptoms of severe anemia predominate in aplastic crises and in hemolytic anemia patients.

SIGNS

- Erythema infectiosum appears about the tenth day of illness, presenting as a fine, reticular, maculopapular, bright-red facial rash (slapped cheek). It spares the region around the mouth, but may involve the extremities and, less often, the trunk, the palms, and the soles. It usually resolves within 1 week but can recur for several weeks after exposure to heat, cold, exercise, or stress.
- Swelling of the affected joints and fluid formation can be present.
- Signs of severe anemia predominate in aplastic crises and in hemolytic anemia patients. Rash may be absent.

Parvovirus Infections

Diagnosis

DIFFERENTIAL DIAGNOSIS

- Rubella
- Scarlet fever
- Facial erysipelas
- Roseola
- Infectious mononucleosis
- Echovirus infection
- Toxic shock syndrome
- Rickettsioses
- Meningococcemia
- Lyme disease
- Vasculitic disease
- Allergic and drug reactions

LABORATORY

- Diagnosis of erythema infectiosum in children is clinical.
- Diagnosis of parvovirus B19 infection is important during pregnancy, especially because, when hydrops fetalis develops, maternal IgM is no longer present. Maternal α-fetoprotein, ultrasound of the fetus to detect hydrops, amniotic fluid, and cord blood PCR are used.
- Detection of viral IgM (RIA, ELISA) can be achieved within 3 days of onset of symptoms of viremia. The IgM level decreases after 1 month but remains detectable by 2 to 3 months.
- A fourfold or larger increase of viral IgG (RIA, ELISA) between acute phase and convalescent serum samples confirms the diagnosis.
- Also useful are detection of parvovirus B19 antigen by RIA or ELISA and detection of parvovirus B19 DNA by hybridization or PCR in respiratory secretions, bone marrow, spleen, amniotic fluid, fetal organs, serum, and tissue specimens.
- Parvovirus B19–related aplastic episodes in the setting of hemolytic anemia are suspected when the degree of anemia is high (Hg <2 g/dL below baseline, reticulocytes <0.2%), and bone marrow is hypoplastic, with characteristic giant pronormoblasts present.
- Antibodies might be of no help in immunocompromised individuals, as the titer's rise might be transient or absent.

Treatment

MAIN TREATMENT

- Parvovirus B19 infection in the nonimmunocompromised is self-limited and does not need specific treatment.
- Symptomatic relief with antiinflammatory drugs may be necessary in cases of arthritis.
- Transient aplastic crisis and chronic anemia
  - —Supportive blood transfusions
  - —Intravenous immunoglobulin (IVIG) infusions
  - —Decreasing the amount of immunosuppressive drugs (i.e., cyclosporine) in the immunocompromised might be of benefit.
  - —Counseling parents in the case of infection during pregnancy. Therapeutic abortion is not indicated. Intrauterine transfusions may be necessary in the case of hydrops fetalis.

TREATMENT FAILURE

Recurrence of aplastic anemia and chronic anemia responds to retreatment with IVIG.

COMPLICATIONS

- There are no major complications in nonimmunocompromised.
- Erythema infectiosum and related arthritis are benign, self-limited conditions.
- In the case of infection during pregnancy, risk of fetal infection is 33%, and overall risk of hydrops fetalis and fetal death is 9%.
- Transient aplastic episodes in hemolytic anemia patients may be fatal if not readily managed.
- Chronic anemia in immunocompromised patients has a high recurrence rate but responds to IVIG retreatment.

Follow-Up

- Complete blood count, reticulocytes in hemolytic anemia and immunocompromised (including HIV-positive) patients
- Maternal α-fetoprotein, ultrasound of the fetus to detect hydrops, in the case of maternal infection during pregnancy

PREVENTION

- Prevention by vaccine is not available.
- As the patients are infectious before the appearance of any signs and symptoms, prevention by exclusion from school or the workplace is of no help. Exclusion should be individualized (i.e., exclusion of a high-risk individual during an outbreak).
- Handwashing in the case of direct contact
- Separation of patients admitted from those in high-risk groups (including seronegative pregnant hospital workers)
- When treating viremic patients, hospital staff should wear gowns, gloves, and masks to avoid hospital outbreaks.
- The future use of recombinant coagulation factors will diminish the transfusion-associated risk of infection.

Selected Readings

Brown KE, Young NS. The simian parvoviruses. *Rev Med Virol* 1997;7(4):211–218.

Frickhofen N, Abkowitz JL, Safford M, et al. Persistent B19 parvovirus infection in patients infected with human immunodeficiency virus type 1 (HIV-1): A treatable cause of anemia in AIDS. *Ann Intern Med* 1990;113:926–933.

Gillespie SM, Canter ML, Asch S, et al. Occupational risk of human parvovirus B19 infection for school and daycare personnel during an outbreak of erythema infectiosum. *JAMA* 1990;263:2061–2065.

Kurtzman G, Frickhofen N, Kimball J, et al. Pure red-cell aplasia of 10 years' duration due to persistent parvovirus B19 infection and its cure with immunoglobulin therapy. *N Engl J Med* 1989;321:519–523.

Trapani S, Ermini M, Falcini F. Human parvovirus B19 infection: Its relationship with systemic lupus erythematosus. *Semin Arthritis Rheum* 1999;28(5):319–325.

Pelvic Inflammatory Disease

Basics

DEFINITION

Pelvic inflammatory disease covers a spectrum of inflammatory disorders of the upper female genital tract, manifesting with lower abdominal or pelvic pain, increased or changed vaginal discharge, dyspareunia, dysuria, metrorrhagia, or menorrhagia. Disorders include the following:

- Endometritis
- Salpingitis
- Parametritis
- Oophoritis
- Tuboovarian abscess
- Pelvic peritonitis

ETIOLOGY

- Common organisms (50% of cases), either alone or in combination
  —*Neisseria gonorrhoeae*
  —*Chlamydia trachomatis*
  —Anaerobes, such as *Bacteroides* and *Peptostreptococcus*
- Other organisms frequently isolated from inflamed tissue, but that may not be involved in pathogenesis
  —*Gardnerella vaginalis*
  —Enteric gram-negative rods, such as *E. coli*
  —Streptococci, mainly *Streptococcus agalactiae* (group B *Streptococcus*)
  —*Mycoplasma hominis*
- Rarely, actinomycosis in women with an intrauterine device (IUD)
- In developing countries, *Mycobacterium tuberculosis* is a common cause.

EPIDEMIOLOGY

Incidence and Prevalence

- Over 1 million cases reported annually in United States
- Adolescent girls most prevalent

Risk Factors

- Multiple sex partners
- Unprotected sexual intercourse
- IUDs, typically older models; not associated with newer versions unless the woman is exposed to sexually transmitted diseases (STDs)

Clinical Manifestations

SYMPTOMS AND SIGNS

- Lower abdominal or pelvic pain, usually dull, bilateral, and subacute at onset
- Increased or changed vaginal discharge
- Metrorrhagia
- Menorrhagia
- Dyspareunia
- Dysuria
- Adnexal tenderness or swelling
- Cervical motion tenderness
- Elevated temperature
- Mucopurulent cervicitis

LESS COMMON SYMPTOMS AND SIGNS

- Nausea and vomiting
- Pleuritic or right upper quadrant pain, caused by perihepatitis of Fitz-Hugh and Curtis syndrome
- Symptoms of proctitis

Diagnosis

DIFFERENTIAL DIAGNOSIS

- Acute appendicitis
- Ectopic pregnancy
- Endometriosis
- Ovarian tumor
- Fibroids
- Mesenteric lymphadenitis
- Urinary tract infection
- Ruptured ovarian cyst
- Corpus luteum bleeding

LABORATORY

- Complete blood cell count (CBC)
- Pregnancy test
- Erythrocyte sedimentation rate
- C-reactive protein
- Gram stain of cervical discharge
- Gonococcal culture
- Testing of endocervical mucus specimens for chlamydia

IMAGING

- If there is diagnostic uncertainty
  —Ultrasound or CT examination of the pelvis
  —Laparoscopy when noninvasive tests are inconclusive

Treatment

MAIN TREATMENT

- Hospitalization if no clear improvement within 72 hours of initiation of drug therapy

Pelvic Inflammatory Disease

- Drug therapy: outpatient
  - Cefoxitin 2 g i.m. plus probenecid 1 g orally (PO) in a single concurrent dose
  - Ceftriaxone 250 mg i.m. or other parenteral third-generation cephalosporin, for example, ceftizoxime or cefotaxime, plus doxycycline 100 mg orally twice daily for 14 days
  - Ofloxacin 400 mg orally twice daily for 14 days plus clindamycin 450 mg four times daily or metronidazole 500 mg twice daily for 14 days
- Drug therapy: inpatient
  - Cefoxitin 2 g i.v. every 6 hours
  - Cefotetan 2 g i.v. every 12 hours plus doxycycline 100 mg i.v. or orally every 12 hours. *Continue at least 48 hours after the patient demonstrates substantial clinical improvement.*
  - Clindamycin 900 mg i.v. every 8 hours plus gentamicin 2 mg/kg i.v. or i.m. as a loading dose, then gentamicin 1.5 mg/kg every 8 hours. The maintenance dose should be adjusted for renal dysfunction. *Continue at least 48 hours after the patient demonstrates substantial clinical improvement*, after which, doxycycline 100 mg orally twice daily or clindamycin 450 mg orally four times daily should be continued for a total of 14 days.
- Sex partners
  - Evaluate and treat for the likelihood of asymptomatic or symptomatic gonococcal and/or chlamydial infection. There is a high risk of reinfection of the patient if a partner is left untreated.
  - Empiric treatment for both gonococcal and chlamydial infection, regardless of microbiologic test results

ALTERNATE TREATMENT

- Ampicillin/sulbactam plus doxycycline
- Ofloxacin plus clindamycin or metronidazole

TREATMENT FAILURE

- Hospitalize the patient if the following applies:
  - Diagnosis is uncertain and surgical emergencies such as appendicitis and ectopic pregnancy cannot be excluded.
  - Severe illness or nausea and vomiting preclude outpatient management.
  - The patient is pregnant.
  - The patient has HIV infection.
  - A pelvic abscess is suspected.
  - Clinical follow-up within 72 hours if starting antibiotics cannot be arranged.
  - The patient is an adolescent (due to the likelihood of noncompliance with therapy and follow-up in this population).
  - The patient is unable to follow or tolerate an outpatient regimen.
  - The patient does not respond clinically to outpatient therapy.

COMPLICATIONS

- Infertility may occur in 11% of women after one episode of pelvic inflammatory disease, in 23% after two episodes, and in 54% after three episodes.
- Ectopic pregnancy occurs seven to ten times more frequently after pelvic inflammatory disease.
- The syndrome of chronic abdominal pain attributed to pelvic adhesions may occur, mainly in infertile women with a history of multiple episodes of pelvic inflammatory disease.
- Death occurs in about 6 per 100,000, usually caused by a ruptured tuboovarian abscess, with generalized peritonitis.

Follow-Up

- Seventy-two hours after initiation of drug therapy, the patient should show clear, marked improvement.
- Three to 5 days from initiation of therapy for hospitalized patients, substantial clinical improvement should be evidenced by defervescence and reduction in abdominal, uterine, adnexal, and cervical motion tenderness.
- Seven to 10 days after completing drug therapy, all patients should have microbiologic examination.

PREVENTION

- General recommendations for avoiding STDs
  - Safe-sex practices
    - Use condoms.
    - Limit the number of sex partners.
    - Treat infected partners.
  - Do not give IUDs to women with multiple sex partners who are at risk of acquiring an STD.

Selected Readings

Jackson SL, Soper DE. Pelvic inflammatory disease in the postmenopausal woman. *Infect Dis Obstet Gynecol* 1999;7(5):248–252.

Munday PE. Clinical aspects of pelvic inflammatory disease. *Hum Reprod* 1997;12[Suppl 11]:121–126.

Paavonen J. Pelvic inflammatory disease. From diagnosis to prevention. *Dermatol Clin* 1998;16(4):747–756, xii.

Steele RW. Prevention and management of sexually transmitted diseases in adolescents. *Adolesc Med* 2000;11(2):315–326.

Pericarditis

Basics

DEFINITION
Pericarditis is inflammation of the pericardium, and is caused by a wide assortment of infections, including viral, bacterial, fungal, and protozoal etiologies. Noninfectious etiologies also are common and must be ruled out.

ETIOLOGY
- Most cases of idiopathic pericarditis are never fully diagnosed, and thus are attributed to viral causes.
- Viral
  —Coxsackievirus A and B are the most common infections, leading to pericarditis and myocarditis.
  —Herpesviruses (Epstein-Barr virus, varicella zoster virus, herpes simplex virus, and cytomegalovirus)
  —Hepatitis B virus
  —Adenovirus
  —Mumps
  —Echovirus
  —Influenza
- Bacterial
  —Contiguous pulmonary processes such as pneumonia or empyema, caused by tuberculosis, *Pneumococcus*, *Staphylococcus*, and gram-negative organisms such as *Klebsiella*, *Legionella*, and *Haemophilus influenzae*
  —Part of a generalized infection of the mediastinum in patients who have had a median sternotomy as part of cardiac surgery
  —Nosocomial organisms, such as *Staphylococcus aureus*, or gram-negative organisms are often discovered.
- Fungal
  —Histoplasmosis
  —*Coccidiodes immitis*
  —*Candida*
  —All are seen as part of a disseminated syndrome.
- Protozoal
  —Disseminated toxoplasmosis
  —Spread of *Entamoeba histolytica* can occur from involvement of the liver, usually the left lobe, with extension through the diaphragm.

EPIDEMIOLOGY
N/A

Clinical Manifestations

- Retrosternal chest pain and fever are common. Patients get relief from the pain by sitting forward.
- Associated viral symptoms, such as upper respiratory tract infections in winter or the rash of chicken pox
- In bacterial pericarditis, chest pain occurs in only one-third of patients with disease.
- Fevers
- Tachypnea and unexplained tachycardia; can lead to early tamponade
- Physical examination may reveal a pulsus paradoxus, along with decreased pulse pressure.
- A three-component friction rub or decreased heart sounds may be noted.

Diagnosis

- Enteroviral isolation of the throat or stool should be attempted for cases in young healthy people who develop pericarditis.

Pericarditis

- An ECG often shows ST elevation in multiple leads, along with PR depression.
  - An ECG is the best diagnostic method.
  - Hemodynamic consequences can be seen.
  - An ECG shows evidence of constrictive pericarditis as is seen in cases of tuberculosis.
- T-wave inversions occur late.
- Tamponade can be diagnosed via ECG or via catheterization of the right heart or pulmonary artery.
- Electrical alternans and low voltage are seen with large pericardial effusions.
- Computed tomography scans can distinguish pulmonary processes and assess the thickness of the pericardium.
- Pericardiocentesis or surgical pericardial biopsy can help establish the diagnosis while relieving tamponade (window procedure).
- Serum should always be stored for acute and convalescent serology studies.

DIFFERENTIAL DIAGNOSIS

- Uremia
- Collagen–vascular diseases
- Postmyocardial infarct
- Sarcoidosis
- Postradiation

Treatment

- Nonsteroidal antiinflammatory medications are used to treat pain.
- Steroids are not given for most causes. Exceptions are constrictive pericarditis with tuberculosis, for which the use of steroids is recommended.
- Bed rest is considered a mainstay of therapy.
- Close observation is necessary to rule out tamponade.
- Pericardiotomy is often required in purulent pericarditis or when tamponade has occurred.
- Antiviral agents are used when the viral diagnosis is evident.
  - Cytomegalovirus can be treated with ganciclovir 5 mg/kg/d.
  - Herpes simplex virus can be treated with acyclovir 5 mg/kg q8h.
  - Influenza can be treated with rimantadine 100 mg PO bid.
- Purulent pericarditis needs to be treated with appropriate antibiotics for at least 4 to 6 weeks.

COMPLICATIONS

N/A

Follow-Up

Patients should have follow-up echocardiograms in order to rule out late fluid reaccumulation and tamponade.

PREVENTION

- There is no way to prevent idiopathic pericarditis.
- Early diagnosis and treatment may prevent the need for surgery.

Selected Readings

Park S, Bayer AS. Purulent pericarditis. *Curr Clin Top Infect Dis* 1992;12:56-82.

Rubin RH, Moellering RC. Clinical, microbiological and therapeutic aspects of purulent pericarditis. *Am J Med* 1975;59:68–78.

See D, Tilles J. Pericarditis and myocarditis. In: Gorbach SL, Bartlett, Blacklow. *Infectious diseases*, 2nd ed. Philadelphia: WB Saunders, 1998:683–690.

Peritonitis

Basics

DEFINITION

Peritonitis is inflammation of the peritoneum, usually due to an infectious etiology. Peritonitis is classified as one of the following:

- Primary (bacterial infection not associated with an intraabdominal source)
- Secondary (infection secondary to inflammation or perforation of a gastrointestinal or genitourinary source)
- Tertiary (diffuse peritonitis, without a well-defined focus of infection)
- Related to peritoneal dialysis

ETIOLOGY

Primary Peritonitis or Spontaneous Bacterial Peritonitis

- This occurs on rare occasions in healthy young children. More commonly, it occurs in children with the nephrotic syndrome. Often, the etiology is not known, but respiratory tract pathogens, including *Pneumococcus*, have commonly been isolated.
- Most cases of spontaneous peritonitis occur in adult patients with advanced cirrhosis and ascites.
- It is believed that the source of the infection is most likely the bloodstream, but transmural spread of bacteria across the bowel wall, lymphatics, or the fallopian tubes has been suggested as well.
- In most cases, underlying cirrhosis leads to bypass of the reticuloendothelial system (liver and spleen).
- Infections with gram-negative enteric organisms, such as *E. coli* and *Klebsiella*, account for 70% of cases.
- Infections with gram-positive organisms, including *Streptococcus* species along with the *Pneumococcus*, account for 25% of cases.
- *Staphylococcus aureus* accounts for only 2% to 4% of cases.
- Isolation rates of anaerobes are low.
- Tuberculosis peritonitis occurs infrequently in developed countries.

Secondary Peritonitis

- Intraabdominal source of infection
  —Includes diverticular abscess, ruptured appendicitis, cholecystitis, and penetrating abdominal trauma
- Multiple aerobic and anaerobic organisms are isolated, derived from the bowel flora.
  —*Candida* may be isolated from perforations of the stomach and small bowel.
  —*Enterococcus* is isolated in as many as 20% of intraabdominal infections; however, eradication has been noted despite antibiotic regimes not specific for the organism.
  —*Pseudomonas aeruginosa* can be isolated in 20% of cases in some hospitals, despite its not being a usual colonizer of the intestine.

Tertiary Peritonitis

- *Candida, Pseudomonas, Enterococcus*
- Fifty percent mortality, prolonged course
- Multiple-organ failure

EPIDEMIOLOGY

Incidence

- Spontaneous bacterial peritonitis
  —Occurs in 25% of patients with cirrhosis of the liver
  —The most frequent infectious complication in patients with ascites
- Peritoneal dialysis infections
  —Occur an average of once a year in patients undergoing chronic peritoneal dialysis

Risk Factors

- Severe liver disease with ascitic fluid albumin less than 1 g/dL
- Shock
- Gastrointestinal bleed
- Urinary tract infection
- Intestinal overgrowth
- Patients with the following:
  —Nephrotic syndrome
  —Severe heart failure
  —Acute hepatitis
  —Metastatic carcinoma
  —Systemic lupus erythematosus

Clinical Manifestations

SPONTANEOUS BACTERIAL PERITONITIS

- Onset may be subclinical, with nothing more than a decompensation in fluid balance, low-grade fever, or mild encephalopathy.
- Fevers occur in 50% to 80% of patients.
- Abdominal pain occurs in 60% of patients.
- Increased encephalopathy is noted in 50%, and this may be the only sign of infection.
- Diarrhea occurs in 33% of patients.
- Hypothermia occurs in 17% of patients.
- *Note*: Ten percent of patients have no symptoms and signs.

SECONDARY PERITONITIS

- Symptoms are related to inflammation of the peritoneum adjacent to the organ affected.

Peritonitis

- Patients present with abdominal rebound tenderness, which becomes diffuse and boardlike if the infection spreads.
- Fevers and hypotension are often present.
- Some pelvic infections may be occult and present with fevers and colonic irritation leading to diarrhea.

TERTIARY PERITONITIS

- Same as in secondary peritonitis
- Chronic peritoneal drainage of purulent, culture-positive exudate
- Hypotension, renal failure

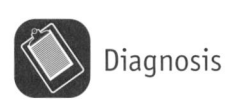

Diagnosis

DIFFERENTIAL DIAGNOSIS

- Peritoneal CA
- Pancreatitis

LABORATORY

- Ascitic fluid with greater than 250 polys/mm^3
- Ascitic protein less than 3.5 g/L
- Ascitic fluid pH less than 7.35 and lactate greater than 25 mg/dL
- Positive blood cultures in 75% of patients with spontaneous bacterial peritonitis
- On rare occasion, patients will not have time following infection to mount a WBC response in the ascitic fluid. Cultures may be positive, with few WBCs present.
- Peritoneal fluid should be inoculated directly into blood culture bottles.
- Tuberculosis must be considered when routine cultures are negative. Peritoneal biopsy is often necessary to make this diagnosis.

IMAGING

- X-rays often help with the diagnosis of secondary peritonitis. Air under the diaphragm suggests disruption of the bowel or stomach wall.
- CT scans are needed to help diagnose the etiology of secondary peritonitis.

Treatment

SPONTANEOUS BACTERIAL PERITONITIS

- Aminoglycosides should be avoided.
- Initial empiric treatment with cefotaxime 2 g i.v. every 8 hours
- A β-lactam/β-lactamase inhibitor or carbapenem should be considered.
- Treatment should be administered for 10 days to 3 weeks.

SECONDARY PERITONITIS

- A combined medical–surgical approach is beneficial.
- Antibiotics should be directed against aerobes and anaerobes. Examples of regimens include the "gold standard" of gentamicin and clindamycin, second- or third-generation cephalosporins or quinolones with metronidazole, β-lactam/β-lactamase inhibitors, or carbapenems.

TERTIARY PERITONITIS

- Various drainage procedures have been used.
- Systemic antibiotics are used only for high fever and hypotension; local instillation of antibiotics is not effective.

COMPLICATIONS

Patients with cirrhosis are in precarious balance; often, decompensation due to peritonitis is fatal.

Follow-Up

Follow-up paracentesis should be performed to make sure the leukocyte counts in the ascitic fluid are falling. This should be done in 48 hours after the initial paracentesis, or sooner if the patient has not responded.

PREVENTION

Use of trimethoprim-sulfamethoxazole, double-stranded, every day for 5 days per week has been shown to reduce the rate of peritonitis in patients with end-stage liver disease.

Selected Readings

Johnson CC, Baldesarre J, Levison ME. Peritonitis: Update on pathophysiology, clinical manifestations, and management. *Clin Infect Dis* 1997;24:1035-1047.

Peterson PK, Matzke GR, Keane WF. Current concepts in the management of peritonitis in continuous ambulatory peritoneal dialysis patients. *Rev Infect Dis* 1987;9:604-612.

Such J, Runyon BA. Spontaneous bacterial peritonitis. *Clin Infect Dis* 1998;27:669-676.

Pertussis

Basics

DEFINITION

Infection due to *Bordetella pertussis* and *Bordetella parapertussis* is responsible for whooping cough.

ETIOLOGY

- *B. pertussis* is a small gram-negative coccobacillary organism.
- A number of toxins are produced, including a tracheal cytotoxin and a pertussis toxin.

EPIDEMIOLOGY

- Pertussis is worldwide in distribution.
- Incidence peaks every 3 to 4 years.
- It is estimated that the rate of infection is 176 cases per 100,000 person-years.
- It accounts for 600,000 deaths a year worldwide.
- With lower rates of immunization in developed countries, pertussis is now much more common.
- Transmission is from aerosol, and attack rates are very high.
- Carrier states are rare; most people infected are symptomatic.
- Prior to vaccination, the disease was seen in children between the ages of 1 and 5 years.
- Since vaccination, disease is now seen more commonly in adults and in infants who do no have passive immunity. These adults are now the reservoir for infection.

INCUBATION

Incubation is between days and weeks.

Clinical Manifestations

- In many studies, the incidence of pertussis causing prolonged cough after what was presumed to be a viral infection is between 12% and 32%.
- The initial phase of the illness is the catarrhal phase.
  —This lasts less than 2 weeks.
  —It is associated with rhinorrhea, fevers, and conjunctivitis and is no different from other upper respiratory infections obtained.
- The next phase is the paroxysmal phase.
  —Gradually, the patient develops a dry cough with episodes of coughing fits.
  —It lasts as long as 2 to 4 weeks.
- Over the next 1 to 2 weeks, the patient enters the convalescent phase, wherein the episodes of coughing decrease and the patient returns to normal.
- The whoop, which is not seen in all children, is associated with a paroxysm of coughing, followed by cyanosis and then by vomiting.
- Infants without the benefit of passive antibodies have the most severe disease.

Diagnosis

- Culture of the organism via sputum or nasopharyngeal swab is positive within the first 2 weeks of illness. Cultures become negative after 5 days of antibiotic therapy.
- Serology can be used to make the diagnosis of presumed disease if there is a rise of the IgG or IgA titers.
- Diagnosis can be made with a single high antibody titer to pertussis toxin.

Pertussis

LABORATORY
Lymphocytosis may be marked at the onset of the paroxysmal phase.

IMAGING
Chest x-ray may reveal pneumonia in 20% of severe cases.

DIFFERENTIAL DIAGNOSIS
- Pneumonia, bacterial or viral
- Bronchitis and asthma
- Foreign-body aspiration in an infant
- Gastroesophageal reflux in infants

Treatment

- Supportive care is needed, especially in infants under the age of 1 year.
- Antibiotics do not reduce the duration of coughing if given initially in the paroxysmal phase.
- Adults: erythromycin 500 mg orally four times per day for 14 days, or trimethoprim-sulfamethoxazole (TMP-SMX), double-stranded, orally twice per day for 14 days

COMPLICATIONS
- Major complications include secondary bacterial respiratory infections.
- Coughing may lead to intracranial hemorrhage.
- Seizures may occur in children and, less frequently, in adults.
- Barotrauma from coughing may cause pneumothorax.

Follow-Up

PREVENTION
- Standard immunization
- Pertussis acellular or whole-cell vaccine is given in conjunction with diphtheria and tetanus at ages 2, 4, 6, and 15 to 18 months and at ages 4 to 6 years.
- Consideration is being given to adding the acellular vaccine to tetanus and diphtheria for administration to adults.
- Antibiotic prophylaxis of household contacts is needed, and should be started as soon as possible after the diagnosis is made.
- Erythromycin or TMP-SMX should be used for a full 14 days.

Selected Readings

Cherry JD. Pertussis in adults. *Ann Intern Med* 1998;128: 64–66.

Nenning ME, Shinefield HR, Edwards KM, et al. Prevalence and incidence of adult pertussis in an urban population. *JAMA* 1996;275:1672–1674.

Orenstein WA. Pertussis in adults: Epidemiology, signs, symptoms, and implications for vaccination. *Clin Infect Dis* 1999;28[Suppl 2]:S147–S150.

Pharyngitis/Tonsillitis

Basics

DEFINITION
- Inflammation of the mucosa of the pharynx and tonsils

ETIOLOGY
- Several different groups of microorganisms can be the cause of the pharyngitis.
- Viral: rhinovirus, coronavirus, adenovirus (types 3, 4, 7, 14, 21), herpes simplex virus (types 1, 2), parainfluenza virus (types 1–4), influenza virus (types A and B), coxsackievirus A (types 2, 4, 5, 6, 8, 9, 10, 21), coxsackievirus B (types 1–5), echovirus, enterovirus 71, Epstein-Barr virus, cytomegalovirus, human immunodeficiency virus, human herpesvirus 6 (HHV-6), and others
- Bacterial: group A β-hemolytic *Streptococcus*; groups C, G, and B β-hemolytic *Streptococcus*; *Neisseria gonorrhoeae*; *Haemophilus influenzae* type b; *Corynebacterium diphtheriae* (diphtheria); *Corynebacterium ulcerans*; *Arcanobacterium haemolyticum* (*Corynebacterium haemolyticum*); *Yersinia enterocolitica*; *Treponema pallidum*; and mixed anaerobic infection
- Chlamydial: *Chlamydia pneumoniae* (strain TWAR)
- Mycoplasmal: *Mycoplasma pneumoniae*, *Mycoplasma hominis* (type 1)
- In approximately 30% of patients with pharyngitis, the cause is unknown.

EPIDEMIOLOGY

Incidence and Prevalence
- Most cases occur during the colder months of the year, with peak rates in late winter and early spring.
- It occurs in all age groups. Streptococcal pharyngitis is more frequent in children 5 to 10 years old (~15% of all cases).
- Incidence is equal in males and females.

Risk Factors
- Age (the young are more susceptible)
- Close quarters, such as in new military recruits
- Fatigue
- Smoking
- Excess alcohol consumption
- Oral sex (mainly for cases of gonococcal pharyngitis)
- Diabetes mellitus
- Recent illness
- Immunosuppression

Clinical Manifestations

SYMPTOMS AND SIGNS
- Streptococcal pharyngitis
  —The severity of illness varies greatly.
  —Fever (>39°C in severe cases)
  —Pharyngeal pain, odynophagia
  —Headache, chills, malaise, and anorexia may occur.
  —Pharyngeal erythema, enlarged tonsils, and exudate that covers the posterior pharynx and tonsillar area
  —Edema of the uvula and soft palate petechiae
  —Cervical adenopathy
  —Absence of cough, hoarseness, or lower respiratory symptoms
  —In scarlet fever (strains of *Streptococcus pyogenes*, which produce erythrogenic toxin), there is a characteristic erythematous rash (punctate erythematous macules with reddened flexor creases and circumoral pallor) that involves the face and skin folds and is followed by desquamation. The tongue is red, and the papillae are enlarged (strawberry tongue).

Pharyngitis/Tonsillitis

- In cases of pharyngitis due to strains of group C or G β-hemolytic streptococci, the symptoms and signs are similar to those due to *S. pyogenes* (may be less severe).
- Pharyngitis in patients with influenza
  —Sore throat
  —Fever
  —Myalgia, headache, malaise
  —Coryzal symptoms, hoarseness, possible cough
  —Edema and erythema of the pharyngeal mucosa
  —Pharyngeal exudates and adenopathy usually not present
- Pharyngoconjunctival fever (adenoviral pharyngitis)
  —Sore throat
  —Fever
  —Myalgia, headache, malaise
  —Pharyngeal erythema and exudate may be present, mimicking streptococcal pharyngitis.
  —In one-third to one-half of cases, there is also conjunctivitis.
- Acute herpetic pharyngitis (due to herpes simplex virus, primary infection)
  —Vesicles and shallow ulcers of the palate are characteristic.
  —Often, there is an associated gingivostomatitis.
- Herpangina (caused by coxsackievirus A)
  —It is characterized by the presence of small vesicles (diameter, 1–2 mm) on the soft palate, uvula, and anterior tonsillar pillars. After rupture of these lesions, small white ulcers are present.
  —In some cases, there is abdominal pain mimicking acute appendicitis.
- Infectious mononucleosis (due to Epstein-Barr virus)
  —Exudative tonsillitis or pharyngitis occurs in approximately one-half of the cases (often membranous).
  —It is associated with fever, cervical or generalized adenopathy, persistent fatigue, and, often, splenomegaly.
- HIV infection
  —Febrile pharyngitis (hyperemia; often mucosal ulcerations, but not exudate) associated with myalgia, arthralgia, adenopathy, and, often, maculopapular rash is a feature of primary infection with HIV.
- Pharyngitis associated with the "common cold"
  —It is characterised by soreness or irritation of the pharynx.
  —Mild edema and erythema may be present.
  —Fever is unusual (except in children).
  —Symptoms of acute upper respiratory illness are always present.
- Infection with *Corynebacterium diphtheriae*
  —This still occurs in unvaccinated populations.
  —The characteristic tonsillar or pharyngeal membrane is gray and firmly adherent to the mucosa.
- Infection with *C. haemolyticum*
  —It is clinically mimicking streptococcal pharyngitis.
  —It affects mainly children and young adults and is associated with a diffuse, erythematous, maculopapular skin rash on the extremities and trunk.
- Vincent's angina
  —It is a mixed infection due to aerobic and anaerobic bacteria.
  —The most often isolated microorganism is *Fusobacterium necrophorum*.
  —It is characterized by a purulent exudate and a foul odor to the breath. It may be complicated with peritonsillar abscess and jugular vein septic phlebitis (Lemierre's disease)
- Gonococcal pharyngitis: *N. gonorrhoeae* may be a cause of mild pharyngitis.
- Yersinial pharyngitis: *Y. enterocolitica* may be a cause of exudative pharyngitis.
- Chlamydial pharyngitis: *C. pneumoniae* (strain TWAR) may cause pharyngitis as a separate illness or in association with pneumonia or bronchitis.
- Mycoplasmal pharyngitis: *M. pneumoniae* may cause mild pharyngitis without distinguishing clinical features.

Pharyngitis/Tonsillitis

Diagnosis

- The primary objectives in the diagnosis of infectious pharyngitis are the following:
  —To distinguish infectious pharyngitis from noninfectious pharyngitis, which may be associated with conditions such as systemic lupus erythematosus, Behçet's syndrome, Kawasaki syndrome, pemphigus, bullous pemphigoid, drug reactions, agranulocytosis, chemical irritation, and neoplasms
  —To detect cases due to *S. pyogenes*
  —To identify the occasional case due to an unusual or rare cause for which treatment is available.
- Specifically, help for an etiologic diagnosis may come from the following:
  —Patient's history
  —Epidemiologic factors
  —Patient's age

CLINICAL

- Presence of pharyngeal exudate: group A β-hemolytic *Streptococcus*; groups C and G β-hemolytic *Streptococcus*; *C. diphtheriae*; *C. haemolyticum*; *Y. enterocolitica*; anaerobic infection; adenovirus; herpes simplex virus; Epstein-Barr virus
- The presence of small vesicles or ulcers suggests herpes simplex virus infection or herpangina.
- The presence of membranous exudate suggests diphtheria, Vincent's angina, or Epstein-Barr virus. If it is pseudomembrane and firmly adhered, it suggests diphtheria.
- The presence of petechiae of the soft palate suggests group A β-hemolytic *Streptococcus* or Epstein-Barr virus.
- The presence of skin rash suggests infection with S. pyogenes, *C. (Arcanobacterium) haemolyticum*, HIV, and Epstein-Barr virus.
- The presence of conjunctivitis suggests infection with adenovirus and some types of enterovirus.
- Helpful also may be the presence of adenopathy (regional or generalized), splenomegaly, or other extrapharyngeal features.

LABORATORY

- Leukocytosis suggests infection with bacteria.
- Special tests are helpful for an etiologic diagnosis.
- Group A β-hemolytic *Streptococcus*: blood agar throat culture from swab, antigen agglutination test from throat swab, serologic tests (ASO titer) (rarely helpful)
- *N. gonorrhea*: may be detected on Thayer-Martin media from throat swab
- Vincent's angina: a crystal violet–stained smear of the pharyngeal exudate
- Diphtheria: throat culture using Loeffler's medium
- Primary HIV infection: detection of HIV antigen in serum or HIV RNA
- Epstein-Barr virus: Monospot test or specific serologic test
- Specific serologic tests are available for other etiologic agents.

Treatment

- Appropriate health care is usually outpatient. Hospitalization is necessary with some types of pharyngitis that are associated with systemic illness or have serious complications.
- General measures
  —Saltwater gargles
  —Acetaminophen
- Streptococcal pharyngitis: The primary aim of treatment is the eradication of the microbe and prevention of acute rheumatic fever. (Initiation of treatment within 1 week of the onset of streptococcal pharyngitis will prevent acute rheumatic fever.)

Pharyngitis/Tonsillitis

- Drug of choice
  - Penicillin V 50,000 IU/kg/d divided q6h in children or 500,000 IU qid in adults for 10 days, or
  - Benzathine penicillin G 25,000 IU/kg i.m. to a maximum of 1.2 million IU as a single dose or 1.2 million IU i.m. in adults
  - In patients who are allergic to penicillin: erythromycin 40 mg/kg/d divided q6h or 500 mg q8h in adults for 10 days
- Alternative drugs: first-generation cephalosporins, newer macrolides
- Recurrent pharyngitis associated with the documented presence of *S. pyogenes.* in the pharynx and failure of the first-choice treatment: amoxicillin–clavulanate, ampicillin-sulbactam, or clindamycin
- Asymptomatic carrier: no treatment required except in well-documented epidemics of streptococcal infection and high-risk situations such as
  - Occurence of rheumatic fever or nephritis in a population such as military recruits or school
  - Cases of streptococcal infection in families with a member who suffers from rheumatic fever or acute streptococcal toxic shock syndrome
- *C. diphtheriae*: antitoxin plus erythromycin 40 mg/kg/d (divided in four doses) i.v., or erythromycin 500 mg PO 26 h for 7 to 14 days. Strict isolation is necessary until at least 24 hours after initiation of appropriate treatment and two samples of pharyngeal secretions cultures are negative.
- Vincent's angina: penicillin G 4 million IU q4h i.v.
- Gonococci: ceftriaxone 250 mg i.m. as a single dose

- *A. haemolyticum*: Susceptibility to antibiotics varies; frequently nonsensitive to penicillin or other β-lactams. Doxycycline, vancomycin, or fluoroquinolones may be needed.
- Viral: Antiviral agents are not indicated, except for herpes simplex virus 1 or 2 infection (acyclovir 200 mg five times per day for 10 days) and HIV infection.

COMPLICATIONS

- *S. pyogenes* pharyngitis
  - Suppurative complications, which include sinusitis, otitis media, mastoiditis, peritonsillar abscess, retropharyngeal abscess, bacteremia, and pneumonia
  - Nonsuppurative complications, which include acute rheumatic fever, acute poststreptococcal glomerulonephritis, toxic shock syndrome, and scarlet fever
- Jugular vein septic phlebitis (Lemierre's disease) is a complication of Vincent's angina and is usually due to *F. necrophorum*.

Follow-Up

- Not necessary in appropriately managed cases with full recovery

PREVENTION

- Avoid contact with infected people. Patients are presumed to be noninfectious after 24 hours of antibiotic coverage.
- Tonsillectomy reduces the incidence of throat infections in children who were severely affected with recurrent pharyngitis.
- Secondary prophylaxis for rheumatic fever is recommended.

Selected Readings

Cohen D, Ferne M, Rouach T, et al. Food-borne outbreak of group G streptococcal sore throat in an Israeli military base. *Epidemiol Infect* 1987;99:249–255.

Hayden GF, Murphy TF, Hendley JO. Non-group A streptococci in the pharynx. Pathogens or innocent bystanders? *Am J Dis Child* 1989;143:794–797.

Kessler HA, Blaauw B, Spear J, et al. Diagnosis of human immunodeficiency virus infection in seronegative homosexuals presenting with an acute viral syndrome. *JAMA* 1987;258:1196–1199.

Krober MS, Bass JW, Michels GN. Streptococcal pharyngitis. Placebo-controlled double-blind evaluation of clinical response to penicillin therapy. *JAMA* 1985;253:1271.

McMillan JA, Sandstrom C, Weiner LB, et al. Viral and bacterial organisms associated with acute pharyngitis in a school-aged population. *J Pediatr* 1986;109:747–752.

Miller RA, Brancato F, Holmes KK. *Corynebacterium haemolyticum* as a cause of pharyngitis and scarlatiniform rash in young adults. *Ann Intern Med* 1986;105:867–872.

Paradise JL, Bluestone CD, Bachman RZ, et al. Efficacy of tonsillectomy for recurrent throat infection in severely affected children. Results of parallel randomized and nonrandomized clinical trials. *N Engl J Med* 1984;310:674.

Pilonidal Abscess

Basics

DEFINITION
- Chronic infection located in a pilonidal cyst in the area between the buttocks.

ETIOLOGY
- It is unclear as to whether this is an acquired problem or is part of a congenital defect.
- Often, hair follicles are found within the sinus. Growth of hair may be the mechanism of disease.

EPIDEMIOLOGY
- The peak incidence of disease is between ages 16 and 20 years.
- Males predominate 3:1 over females.
- It is estimated that there are 40,000 to 70,000 cases of infected pilonidal abscess in the United States per year.

Clinical Manifestations

- Patients often complain of pain in the buttocks area.
- Swelling and signs of drainage present when the infection is chronic.
- Symptoms may wax and wane for weeks.
- In acute infections, an abscess forms, with edema, erythema, and warmth.
- A large pilonidal abscess may be associated with sepsis and shock.

Diagnosis

- Physical examination, looking for an abscess or fistula, is needed to make the diagnosis.

Pilonidal Abscess

- The fistula may be small, and signs of inflammation may be minimal.

DIFFERENTIAL DIAGNOSIS

- Crohn's disease
- Foreign body
- Radiation proctitis
- Necrotizing fasciitis or Fournier's gangrene
- Herpes simplex virus

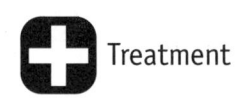

Treatment

- Surgical incision is needed for drainage of the abscess.
- Definitive surgical treatment includes excision of the cavity, sinus tract, and removal of any infected tissue.
- The wound is left to heal by secondary intent.
- Antibiotic therapy, when used in conjunction with surgery, should be directed to bowel flora.

COMPLICATIONS

Patients may be prone to recurrent disease.

Follow-Up

Proctoscopy is no longer recommended for evaluation of this disease.

PREVENTION

There is no way to prevent pilonidal abscess, but good perineal hygiene may decrease the incidence of disease.

Selected Readings

Surrell JA. Pilonidal disease. *Surg Clin North Am* 1994;74(6):1309–1315.

Plague

Basics

DEFINITION
Plague is a zoonotic infection caused by *Yersinia pestis*. Of great historical significance, this organism caused the "Black Death" in the Middle Ages. The disease may be bubonic (lymph node involvement), pneumonic, septicemic, or meningeal.

ETIOLOGY
Y. pestis, a gram-negative coccobacillus, is in the Enterobacteriaceae family.

EPIDEMIOLOGY
- Plague is a zoonotic disease found worldwide.
- Most cases occur in poor, developing countries.
- Epidemic urban disease is associated with poor sanitation and squalid living conditions.
- Animal reservoirs include rodents, prairie dogs, squirrels, and domestic cats.
- Flea vectors spread disease to humans; however, direct contact with infected animals may spread disease.
- Pneumonic plague can be spread from person to person by respiratory droplets or from cats that have either plague pneumonia or submandibular abscesses.

Incubation
Following exposure, incubation is generally between 2 and 8 days.

Clinical Manifestations

BUBONIC PLAGUE
- Illness begins with fevers, chills, and headache.
- After 24 hours, patients note the onset of buboes, or painful, massively enlarged lymph nodes. Usually, they occur near areas of inoculation, such as the axilla (arm) or inguinal area (leg).
- Small pustules or papules may be present in the area of the flea bite in 25% of patients.
- Patients progress to multisystem disease.
  - Sepsis
  - Hypotension
  - Disseminated intravascular coagulation (DIC)
  - Encephalitis
  - Diarrhea
- Pneumonia occurs in 20% of patients with bubonic disease.

PNEUMONIC PLAGUE
Pulmonary infiltrates can occur as part of the septicemic complication of bubonic plague or as a primary site of inoculation of the organism. Unless diagnosed early, progression to respiratory failure may occur.

SEPTICEMIC PLAGUE
Septicemic is the term for most severe forms of plague, originally the bubonic form. Mortality rates are as high as 50%. In 10% of cases, buboes are not present.

MENINGITIC PLAGUE
Pyogenic meningitis is a rare complication, caused by seeding of the CNS at the time of bacteremia.

Diagnosis

DIFFERENTIAL DIAGNOSIS
- Incarcerated inguinal hernia
- Chancroid and lymphogranuloma venereum

Plague

- Streptococcal skin infection
- Tularemia
- Atypical pneumonia
- Hantavirus

LABORATORY

- Leukocytosis is most commonly seen.
- DIC may develop.
- Aspiration of the bubo should reveal bipolar, staining coccobacilli organisms.
- Blood and sputum cultures should be obtained and should reveal the organism.
- Cultures are done in broth and MacConkey agar.
- Direct fluorescent antibody stains are available.
- Serology is available.

IMAGING

- Chest x-rays reveal either patchy pneumonia or lobar pneumonia that progresses to cavitation.
- Acute respiratory distress syndrome with diffuse opacity can be present.

Treatment

- Gentamicin 2 mg/kg i.v., followed by 1.7 mg/kg every 8 hours i.v.
- Streptomycin 1 g i.v. or i.m. every 12 hours

ALTERNATIVES

- Doxycycline 100 mg oral or i.v. every 12 hours
- Chloramphenicol 500 mg oral or i.v. every 6 hours should be used if meningitis is present.
- Contacts of patients with respiratory disease should be treated prophylactically with doxycycline.
- Contacts of patients with buboes should be treated only if they develop an unexplained febrile illness.

COMPLICATIONS

Infection of buboes with *Staphylococcus aureus* may occur at any time, and may need surgical drainage.

Follow-Up

- No specific recommendations

PREVENTION

- In endemic areas, household pets need to be screened for fleas.
- Rodent control is necessary, especially in populated areas.
- Sanitation measures should be taken.
- Vaccine is available to people at high risk in endemic areas.

Selected Readings

Crook LD, Tempest B. Plague: A clinical review of 27 cases. *Arch Intern Med* 1992;152:1253–1256.

Kaufmann AF, Boyce JM, Martone WJ. Trends in human plague in the United States. *J Infect Dis* 1980;141:522–524.

Pneumocystis carinii Infection

Basics

DEFINITION
Pneumocystis carinii is an opportunistic pathogen, the natural habitat of which is the lung. The organism is an important cause of pneumonia in the compromised host.

ETIOLOGY
- *P. carinii* has a worldwide distribution.
- Recent studies favor the taxonomy of *P. carinii* in the fungal kingdom.

EPIDEMIOLOGY
Incidence
- The frequency of *P. carinii* infection among HIV-infected patients far exceeds that among other immunocompromised hosts.
- In 1992, *P. carinii* pneumonia accounted for 42% of all AIDS-indicator diseases. However, with the advent of the highly effective antiretroviral therapy, the incidence of *P. carinii* pneumonia in this population is declining.
- In recent years, the diagnosis of *P. carinii* pneumonia has increasingly been reported among non–HIV-infected individuals not receiving prophylaxis.
- Extrapulmonary *P. carinii* infection is involved in fewer than 3% of cases.

Risk Factors
- *P. carinii* pneumonia occurs in the following hosts:
  - Premature, malnourished infants
  - Children with primary immunodeficiency disease
  - Patients receiving corticosteroids or other immunosuppressive therapy
  - Patients with autoimmune diseases and a lymphocyte count of less than $0.4 \times 10^9/L$
  - Severely immunosuppressed patients with hematologic or other malignancies, organ transplantation, and so forth.
  - HIV-infected individuals
- Administration of aerosolized pentamidine is a risk factor for extrapulmonary *P. carinii* infection in HIV-infected patients.

Incubation Period
- Serologic surveys indicate that most healthy children have been exposed to the organism.
- On the basis of animal studies, the incubation period is thought to be 4 to 8 weeks.

Clinical Manifestations

SYMPTOMS
- The clinical picture is quite variable. Patients with *P. carinii* pneumonia usually develop the following:
  - Dyspnea (that is exacerbated with exercise)
  - Fever
  - Nonproductive cough.
- Symptoms in non–HIV-infected patients often begin after the glucocorticoid dose has been tapered, and typically last 1 to 2 weeks.
- HIV-infected patients are usually ill for several weeks or longer and have relatively subtle manifestations.
- The most common sites of extrapulmonary involvement are the following:
  - Lymph nodes (in up to 50% of cases)
  - Spleen
  - Liver
  - Bone marrow
- Less common sites of extrapulmonary involvement are the gastrointestinal and genitourinary tracts, adrenal and thyroid glands, heart, pancreas, eyes, ears, and skin.
- Clinical manifestations of extrapulmonary involvement range from incidental findings at autopsy to specific organ involvement.

SIGNS
- Physical findings of *P. carinii* pneumonia include the following:
  - Tachypnea
  - Tachycardia
  - Cyanosis
- Lung auscultation is usually unremarkable.

Diagnosis

DIFFERENTIAL DIAGNOSIS
- The differential diagnosis of *P. carinii* pneumonia is very broad and includes infectious diseases, such as the following:
  - Atypical pneumonia (due to *Mycoplasma* or *Chlamydia* spp, etc.)
  - Atypical presentation of pneumococcal or fungal pneumonia
  - Legionnaires' disease
  - Tuberculosis
  - Viral pneumonia
- Also, *P. carinii* pneumonia can mimic noninfectious diseases, such as congestive heart disease, Kaposi's sarcoma or lymphoma involving the lungs, and pulmonary embolism.

LABORATORY
- There is no reliable way to cultivate the organism *in vitro*.
- A definitive diagnosis is made by histopathologic staining. Stains include reagents such as methenamine silver, toluidine blue, and cresyl echt violet, which selectively stain the wall of *P. carinii* cysts, and reagents such as Wright-Giemsa, which stain the nuclei of all developmental stages.
- Immunofluorescence with monoclonal antibodies is more sensitive than traditional staining.
- The yield from different diagnostic procedures is higher in HIV-infected patients than in non–HIV-infected patients, probably because of the higher organism burden.
- Elevated serum concentrations of lactate dehydrogenase have been reported but are not specific to *P. carinii* infection.
- The white blood cell count is variable.
- Exercise-induced oxygen saturation is probably the most sensitive and specific noninvasive test for diagnosis of *P. carinii* pneumonia.
- Arterial blood gases usually demonstrate hypoxia, an increased alveolar-arterial oxygen gradient ($PAO_2–PaO_2$), and respiratory alkalosis.
- There also may be changes in the oxygen saturation with pulmonary function test values (diffusing capacity) and increased uptake with nuclear imaging techniques (gallium scan).

IMAGING
- The classic findings on chest radiography consist of bilateral diffuse infiltrates involving the perihilar regions. Atypical manifestations also have been reported.
- Early in the course of pneumocystosis, the chest radiograph may be normal.
- Patients who receive aerosolized pentamidine have an increased frequency of upper lobe infiltrates and pneumothorax.

Pneumocystis carinii Infection

DIAGNOSTIC/TESTING PROCEDURES

- Fiberoptic bronchoscopy with bronchoalveolar lavage remains the mainstay of *P. carinii* diagnosis.
- Sputum induction is a simple, noninvasive technique, but its sensitivity has varied at different institutions.
- Transbronchial biopsy and open lung biopsy, which are the most invasive procedures, are reserved for situations in which a diagnosis cannot be made by lavage.

Treatment

MAIN TREATMENT

- Trimethoprim–sulfamethoxazole is the drug of choice for all forms of *P. carinii* infection. It is administered orally or intravenously at a dosage of 15 to 20 mg of trimethoprim/kg/d in three or four divide doses.
- Several studies have shown that the administration of glucocorticoids to HIV-infected patients with moderate to severe pneumocystosis (a PO_2 of 70 mmHg or a PAO_2–PaO_2 of 35 mmHg) can improve the rate of survival. The recommended regimen is 40 mg of prednisone PO twice daily, with tapering to a dose of 20 mg/d over a 3-week period.
- The use of steroids as adjunctive therapy in non-AIDS patients remains to be evaluated.
- Ten percent to 45% HIV-infected patients experience serious adverse reactions, including fever, rash, neutropenia, thrombocytopenia, hepatitis, and hyperkalemia.
- Treatment of *P. carinii* pneumonia should be continued for 14 days in non–HIV-infected patients, and for 21 days in persons with AIDS.
- Clinicians should wait for a few days before concluding that therapy has failed.
- Other important measures include the maintenance of oxygenation, nutrition, and electrolyte balance.
- Treatment for the extrapulmonary forms of pneumocystosis is the same as that for pneumonia.

ALTERNATIVE TREATMENT

- The other major drug used to treat *P. carinii* pneumonia is pentamidine isethionate. Pentamidine is given as a single dose of 4 mg/kg/d by slow intravenous infusion. Its principal adverse effects are hypotension, cardiac arrhythmia, pancreatitis, dysglycemia, azotemia, electrolyte changes, and neutropenia.
- Other alternative treatments are clindamycin given intravenously (600 mg four times daily) or by mouth (300–450 mg four times daily) and primaquine by mouth (15 mg daily). Primaquine should be avoided in patients with glucose-6-phosphate dehydrogenase deficiency.
- Trimethoprim plus dapsone and atovaquone are less toxic oral regimens that are used in mild to moderate *P. carinii* pneumonia.

COMPLICATIONS

- In the typical case of untreated *P. carinii* pneumonia, progressive respiratory compromise leads to death.
- Therapy is most effective when instituted early in the course of the disease, before there is extensive alveolar damage.
- Concurrent pulmonary infections complicate management, but the presence of cytomegalovirus usually does not affect the outcome of *P. carinii* pneumonia.

Follow-Up

- Patients should be followed for
  - Close monitoring of the oxygenation
  - The response to treatment
  - The development of antibiotic-related side effects
  - The occurrence of pneumothorax or other complications

PREVENTION

- Primary prophylaxis is indicated for HIV-infected patients at high risk of developing pneumocystosis—that is, those who have CD4+ cell counts of, ora history of, persistent fever or opportunistic infections.
- Guidelines for the administration of primary prophylaxis to other immunocompromised hosts are less clear. Currently, in most centers, prophylaxis is given to patients in known risk groups, such as bone marrow transplant recipients and children with acute lymphoblastic leukemia.
- Secondary prophylaxis is indicated for all patients who have recovered from *P. carinii* pneumonia.
- The prophylactic regimen of choice is one double-strength tablet of trimethoprim–sulfamethoxazole (160 mg of trimethoprim) per day. Alternative regimens include the following:
  - Trimethoprim–sulfamethoxazole at a reduced dose or frequency
  - Dapsone (50 mg daily), pyrimethamine (50 mg once per week), and folinic acid (25 mg once per week)
  - Dapsone (100 mg daily)
  - Nebulized pentamidine (300 mg once per month via a Respirgard II nebulizer)

Selected Readings

Furrer H, Egger M, Opravil M, et al. Discontinuation of primary prophylaxis against *Pneumocystis carinii* pneumonia in HIV-1-infected adults treated with combination antiretroviral therapy. Swiss HIV Cohort Study. *N Engl J Med* 1999;340:1301–1306.

Miller RF, Mitchell DM. AIDS and the lung: Update 1995. 1. *Pneumocystis carinii* pneumonia. *Thorax* 1995;50:191–200.

Sepkowitz KA, Brown AE, Armstrong D. *Pneumocystis carinii* pneumonia without acquired immunodeficiency syndrome. More patients, same risk. *Arch Intern Med* 1995;155:1125–1128.

Weltzer PD. *Pneumocystis carinii* infection. In: Fauci AS, Braunwald E, Isselbacher KJ, et al., eds. *Harrison's principles of internal medicine,* 14th edition. New York, McGraw-Hill, 1998:1161–1163.

Pneumonia

Basics

DEFINITION

- Pneumonia is a lower respiratory tract infection. Inflammation of the lung is classified as the following:
  - *Community acquired (CAP)*: acquired in community setting
  - *Nursing home*: acquired in nursing home setting
  - *Nosocomial*: acquired in the hospital setting, not incubating at time of admission
  - *Compromised host*: patient with major defect in normal host defenses
  - *Aspiration*: abnormal entry of fluids or particulate material in lower airways from the upper airways or stomach

ETIOLOGY

Community-acquired Pneumonia

- *Streptococcus pneumoniae* (30%–50%)
- *Mycoplasma pneumoniae* (15%): common in patients with "walking pneumonia"
- *Haemophilus influenzae* (10%–15%)
- *Chlamydia pneumoniae* (5%–10%)
- *Staphylococcus aureus* (2%–5%): more common with influenza
- Miscellaneous bacteria (rare): *Moraxella catarrhalis, Neisseria meningitidis, Staphylococcus pyogenes*

Nosocomial

- Gram-negative bacilli (50%–70%): *Pseudomonas aeruginosa*, Enterobacteriaceae
- Anaerobic bacteria (10%–20%): usually in combination with gram-negative bacteria
- *S. aureus* (15%–30%)
- Viral (10%–20%): primarily respiratory syncytial virus in pediatric patients and cytomegalovirus in the compromised patient
- *Legionella* (4%): may be found in epidemics associated with contaminated water supply
- *Mycobacterium tuberculosis* (less than 1%): rare, but important to recognize and be aware of

Compromised Host

- Splenectomy and hypogammaglobulinemia
  - *S. pneumoniae*
  - *H. influenzae*
  - *N. meningitidis*
- Neutropenia
  - Gram-negative bacilli
  - *Aspergillus*
- Cell-mediated immunity defects
  - Parasitic infection: *Pneumocystis carinii*
  - Fungal infections: *Histoplasma capsulatum, Coccidioides immitis, Blastomyces dermatitidis*
  - Mycobacteria: *M. tuberculosis, M. avium, M. kansasii*, etc.
  - Bacteria: *Nocardia, S pneumoniae, H. influenzae, S. aureus, P. aeruginosa, Legionella*
  - Viruses: cytomegalovirus, herpesvirus 6, herpes simplex virus, adenovirus

EPIDEMIOLOGY

Incidence

- Four million patients with pneumonia annually in the United States
- CAP: 10 to 15 per 1,000 annually in the United States; highest in winter months
- Nosocomial: 0.4% to 0.7% of hospitalized patients
- Compromised host: epidemics possible, resulting from contaminate air supplies
- *Note:* Pneumonia is the major cause of death from infectious disease.
- About 40% of *Streptococcus* pneumococcus strains are currently resistant to penicillin, and many are also resistant to macrolides and tetracyclines, and some to cephalosporins as well.

Risk Factors

- Hospital or nursing home setting, especially the ICU
- Immunocompromised patients
- Age greater than 65 years
- Associated underlying disease

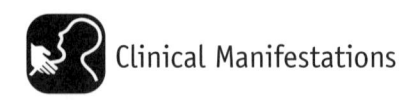

Clinical Manifestations

SYMPTOMS AND SIGNS

- Fever with respiratory symptoms: cough, sputum, pleurisy, dyspnea (80%)
- Crackles heard upon auscultatory examination (80%)
- Physical findings of consolidation (30%)
- Pulmonary infiltrate evident on chest x-ray

DIFFERENTIAL DIAGNOSIS

Infectious

- Bronchitis
- Lung abscess
- Empyema

Pneumonia

Noninfectious
- Lung cancer
- Lymphoma
- Sarcoidosis

LABORATORY

- Imaging: chest x-ray indicating infiltrates
- Computed tomography more sensitive than x-ray for detecting infiltrates
- Culture specimens uncontaminated by upper airway secretions
- Expectorated sputum

Treatment

- The first decision is whether to hospitalize.
- Indications for hospitalization
  - Age greater than 65 years
  - Coexisting disease
  - Respiratory rate greater than 30 per minute
  - Systolic pressure less than 90 mm Hg or diastolic pressure less than 60 mm Hg
  - Fever greater than 38.3°C
  - Altered mental status
  - White blood cell count less than 4,000/dL or greater than 30,000/dL
  - Hematocrit less than 30%
  - Alveolar PO$_2$ less than 60 mm Hg on room air
  - Renal failure
  - Chest x-ray indicating multiple lobe involvement, rapid spread, or pleural effusion
- *S. pneumoniae*
  - Penicillin G intravenous
  - Amoxicillin
  - Vancomycin (for penicillin-resistant strains)
  - Cephalosporin (e.g., third-generation, such as ceftriaxone or cefotaxime; may be a better choice for penicillin-resistant strains).
  - Macrolide (e.g., erythromycin, azithromycin, or clarithromycin)
  - Moxifloxacin and gatifloxacin
- *H. influenzae*
  - Cephalosporin, trimethoprim–sulfamethoxazole
- *C. pneumoniae* or *M. pneumoniae*
  - Doxycycline
  - Erythromycin, azithromycin, or clarithromycin
  - Quinolones such as ciprofloxacin, moxifloxacin, or gatifloxacin
- *S. aureus*
  - Nafcillin or oxacillin plus rifampin or gentamicin
  - Vancomycin plus rifampin or gentamicin
- *Legionella*
  - Erythromycin plus rifampin
  - Quinolone

COMPLICATIONS

- Failure to respond to treatment as a result of the following:
  - Disease too far advanced or treatment delayed too long
  - Wrong diagnosis
  - Inadequate dose of antibiotic
  - Compromised or debilitated host
  - Resistant pathogen
- Empyema
- Lung abscess

Follow-Up

- Pneumococcal pneumonia
  - Fever resolves in a mean of 3 to 5 days.
  - Blood cultures are negative in bacteremic patients by day 2.
  - Chest x-ray should show resolution in a mean of 3 weeks for young, previously healthy adults, and in 13 weeks for patients older than 65 years or in compromised patients with associated disease.
- Legionella
  - Fever resolves in a mean of 5 days.
  - Chest x-ray should show resolution of infiltrates in a mean of 11 weeks.

PREVENTION

- Pneumococcal vaccine

Selected Readings

Bartlett JG, Dowell SF, Mandell LA, et al. Practice guidelines for the management of community-acquired pneumonia in adults. *Clin Infect Dis* 2000;31:347–382.

Fine MJ, Smith MA, Carson CA, et al. Prognosis and outcome of patients with community-acquired pneumonia. A meta-analysis. *JAMA* 1996;275:134.

Marrie, TJ. Pneumococcal pneumonia: Epidemiology and clinical features. *Semin Respir Infect* 1999;14:227.

Poliomyelitis

Basics

DEFINITION

- Poliovirus is an enterovirus, a small RNA virus that affects the central nervous system.
- This virus has no animal reservoir.

ETIOLOGY

- Poliovirus is transmitted by the fecal–oral route and through respiratory secretions.
- It is most often spread through contaminated water, such as ponds or lakes.
- The virus infects intestinal cells. From there it spreads and replicates in local lymphatics, causing a minor viremia. The infection either ends at this stage or spreads throughout the body, a major viremia.
- The virus causes destruction of anterior horn cells and motor nuclei in the spinal cord, pons, and medulla. This leads to motor weakness or paralysis of the axial skeleton or the cranial nerves or brainstem.

EPIDEMIOLOGY

- Infection before the year 1900 occurred in very young children, and immunity developed without much paralytic disease. By the 1950s, children were being exposed at a later age, and paralysis was much more common.
- Inactivated vaccine was used in 1955; oral vaccine was introduced in 1962.
- Because of the worldwide effort to vaccinate children and adults, polio has been eliminated from most developed countries. No transmission of polio occurs in the American continent.
- Polio still exist in Asia, Africa, and the Middle East. An effort is underway to eradicate this disease entirely.

Clinical Manifestations

Most cases of polio (95%) have no symptoms.

MINOR ILLNESS

- Abortive polio (4%–8%) infection is classified as "minor illness."
- The first phase of illness resembles a nonspecific upper respiratory tract illness, with sore throat and low-grade fevers.
- There may be abdominal pains and diarrhea.
- Three to 10 days after the onset of the mild viral symptoms, central nervous system manifestations begin.
- At times, headache and signs of meningeal inflammation occur, but paralysis does not develop.
- Symptoms of headache and meningismus last 1 to 3 days.

MAJOR ILLNESS

- Paralytic polio (<1%) infection is classified as "major illness."
- Two to 5 days following the "minor illness stage," the patient notices the rapid onset of localized muscle pains. Fasciculations are visible. Fevers return, and signs of meningitis and the rapid (2 to 3 days) onset of asymmetric flaccid paralysis occur. Reflexes are lost.
- Leg weakness is more common than arm weakness, and proximal muscles are more affected than distal groups.
- Bulbar disease leads to problems with swallowing, speech, and, at times, breathing.
- Cranial nerves IX and X are frequently involved.

INCUBATION

The incubation period from exposure to the onset of paralysis is 11 to 17 days.

Diagnosis

- Cerebrospinal fluid pleocytosis occurs.
- Viral isolation is needed to determine whether the virus is vaccine-related or wild-type.

Poliomyelitis

- Cultures should be obtained from stool, throat swabs, and the central nervous system.
- Central nervous system cultures are often negative.
- Serology is also available for diagnosis.

DIFFERENTIAL DIAGNOSIS

- Guillain-Barré syndrome
- Other enteroviral infections
- Epidural mass lesion
- Neuropathy
- Stroke
- Tick paralysis
- Transverse myelitis

Treatment

- There is no specific antiviral therapy for poliovirus.
- Patients require supportive treatment and, at times, intubation.

COMPLICATIONS

- Patients may note progression of symptoms up to 35 years after the initial event.
- Weakness often occurs in areas most affected by the initial episode of disease.

Follow-Up

PREVENTION

- Two vaccines are available: attenuated oral polio vaccine (OPV) and inactivated polio vaccine (IPV).
- To eliminate the risk of vaccine-associated paralytic polio (VAPP), an all-IPV schedule is now recommended for routine childhood polio vaccination in the United States. All children should receive four doses of IPV at 2 months, 4 months, 6 to 18 months, and 4 to 6 years. OPV (if available) may be used only for the following special circumstances:
  —Mass vaccination campaigns to control outbreaks of paralytic polio
  —Unvaccinated children who will be traveling in less than 4 weeks to areas where polio is endemic or epidemic
  —Children of parents who do not accept the recommended number of vaccine injections: These children may receive OPV only for the third or fourth dose, or both; in this situation, health care professionals should administer OPV only after discussing the risk for VAPP with parents or caregivers.
  —During the transition to an all-IPV schedule, recommendations for the use of remaining OPV supplies in physicians' offices and clinics have been issued by the American Academy of Pediatrics (see *Pediatrics*, December 1999).

Selected Readings

Centers for Disease Control and Prevention. Paralytic Poliomyelitis—United States, 1980–1994. *MMWR Morbid Mortal Wkly Rep* 1997;46:79–83.

Dalakas MC, Elder G, Hallet M, et al. A long-term follow-up study of patients with post-poliomyelitis neuromuscular syndrome. *N Engl J Med* 1986;314:959–963.

Strebel PM, Sutter RW, Cochi SL, et al. Epidemiology of poliomyelitis in the United States one decade after the last reported case of indigenous wild virus–associated disease. *Clin Infect Dis* 1992;14:568–579.

Progressive Multifocal Leukoencephalopathy

Basics

DEFINITION

- Rare, subacute demyelinating disease of the brain white matter, caused either by primary infection or reactivation of JC virus (JCV).
- First identified as a clinical entity in 1958, it is primarily seen in patients with AIDS or other forms of cell-mediated immunity suppression, and is mainly characterized by rapidly deteriorating focal neurologic deficits, with a usually fatal outcome.
- Progressive multifocal leukoencephalopathy (PML) is an AIDS-defining disease in patients with HIV infection, according to the Centers for Disease Control and Prevention (CDC) case surveillance definition.

ETIOLOGY

- JC virus (JCV)
- Rare cases have been attributed to simian virus 40 (SV40). Both JCV and SV40 are DNA viruses, belonging to the family Papovaviridae, genus *Polyomavirus*.
- The third known human polyomavirus, BK virus (BKV), does not cause PML.
- Demyelination occurs as a result of the direct infection of CNS oligodendrocytes (myelin-producing cells) by JCV and the subsequent cytopathic effect, which leads to decreased myelin production.

EPIDEMIOLOGY

Incidence

- Incidence in the United States has increased since the AIDS epidemic.
- Reported deaths due to PML in pre-HIV era: 1.5 in 10 million persons in 1974
- Reported deaths due to PML in 1987: 6.1 in 10 million persons
- One percent to 4% of HIV-positive persons will develop PML if left untreated. In 1992, 2% of HIV-related deaths were due to PML.
- JCV seroprevalence in adults in the United States and Europe is about 60% to 80%. A very small proportion of those show evidence of active viral replication, against about 33% among HIV-infected individuals.
- Antibody-based studies show that primary JCV infection occurs during childhood (10–14 years).
- Asymptomatic JCV and BKV viruria has been described in immunosuppressed patients, pregnant women, and the elderly.

Risk Factors

- AIDS, mainly late disease (CD4 count $<100/mm^3$): More than 60% of cases of PML occur in this setting.
- Rare case reports of other forms of congenital or acquired immunosuppression (organ transplant recipients are at increased risk if seropositive for JCV donor), patients with hematologic malignancies, and patients in chronic steroid use (including patients with systemic lupus erythematosus, rheumatoid arthritis, or sarcoidosis)
- Fewer than 5% of overall cases develop in the absence of any identifiable immunodeficiency.

Incubation Period: Natural History

- Incubation period and the mode of transmission are not known. Primary infection has been documented in renal transplant recipients from a seropositive donor.
- Demyelination results in rapid deterioration (over weeks) with multiple focal neurologic deficits, without signs of increased intracranial pressure. The disease is fatal.

Clinical Manifestations

SYMPTOMS AND SIGNS

- No constitutional symptoms, such as fever.
- At presentation: hemiparesis (42%), visual field deficits (32%–45%), typically homonymous hemianopia, cognitive impairment (36%), aphasia (17%), ataxia (21%), and/or cranial nerve deficits (13%), sensory deficits (9%), seizures (accounts for 1% of seizures in HIV-positive patients), dementia, confusion, personality changes
- Late in the course: severe neurologic deficits (cortical blindness, quadriparesis, profound dementia, and coma; motor weakness in 75%)
- The clinical presentation can be much more impressive than the imaging and/or pathology findings.
- Clinical presentation in HIV-positive patients is similar to that in HIV-negative patients.

Diagnosis

DIFFERENTIAL DIAGNOSIS

- HIV encephalopathy and leukoencephalomyelopathy
- Other opportunistic infections (cytomegalovirus, neurosyphilis, cryptococcosis, tuberculous meningitis, toxoplasmosis) and malignancies (primary CNS lymphoma, Kaposi's sarcoma) associated with HIV infection
- Acute multiple sclerosis
- Acute hemorrhagic leukoencephalitis
- Herpes simplex virus meningoencephalitis
- Multifocal varicella zoster virus leukoencephalitis

Progressive Multifocal Leukoencephalopathy

- Postinfectious or vaccinal immune-mediated encephalomyelitis
- Cyclosporin toxicity (encephalopathy, seizures) in transplant recipients

LABORATORY

- Diagnosis is made by detection of JCV antigen or genomic DNA in brain tissue by immunocytochemistry, *in situ* hybridization, or PCR amplification, in association with the characteristic pathologic changes. Detection is not diagnostic unless accompanied by pathologic changes.
- JCV grows slowly in culture (over weeks to months), and susceptible cells are not readily available.
- Serum and cerebrospinal fluid (CSF) antibodies are not helpful.
- CSF-nonspecific pleocytosis, increased IgG, and monoclonal bands have been described.
- Detection of virus in CSF by PCR needs further evaluation.

PATHOLOGY

- Stereotactic brain biopsy is necessary to confirm the diagnosis.
- Multifocal areas of demyelination, varying greatly in size, scattered throughout the CNS, with minimal inflammation
- Typical changes in oligodendrocytes and astrocytes
- Cerebral hemispheres, cerebellum, and brainstem may all be involved. Spinal cord involvement is rare.
- Electron microscopy shows polyomavirus inclusions into enlarged nuclei of oligodendrocytes.

ELECTROENCEPHALOGRAPHY

- Focal or diffuse slowing. Sometimes, abnormalities precede CT changes.

IMAGING

- CT scan: hypodense, nonenhancing subcortical white matter lesions without edema or mass effect; usually periventricularly, in the centrum semiovale, in the parietal–occipital region, and in the cerebellum
- MRI scan: more sensitive than CT scan; shows multiple, asymmetric subcortical white matter lesions, with high signal on T2-weighted images

Treatment

MAIN TREATMENT

- If the patient is HIV-positive, aggressive antiretroviral treatment to reverse immunosuppression is begun.
- Supervised drug administration may be necessary in patients with dementia.
- There is no available specific treatment for PML.
- Intravenous or intrathecal cytarabine (cytosine arabinoside) and cidofovir are under clinical evaluation, but the evidence is conflicting.
- High doses of zidovudine, interferons alpha and beta, and 5-iodo-2'-deoxyuridine have been reported to be of some benefit.

COMPLICATIONS

Death occurs within about 6 months of the diagnosis, but spontaneous fluctuations over a period of 2 to 3 years have been described in HIV-positive patients, except if immunosuppression improves with aggressive management of HIV infection.

Follow-Up

- Frequent clinical follow-up to check for recurrence of illness
- HIV infection monitoring

PREVENTION

- Proper antiretroviral treatment to avoid severe immunosuppression

Selected Readings

Berger JR, Pall L, Lanska D, et al. Progressive multifocal leukoencephalopathy in patients with HIV infection. *J Neurovirol* 1998;4(1):59–68.

Huang SS, Skolasky RL, Dal Pan GJ, et al. Survival prolongation in HIV-associated progressive multifocal leukoencephalopathy treated with alpha-interferon: An observational study. *J Neurovirol* 1998;4(3):324–332.

Re D, Bamborschke S, Feiden W, et al. Progressive multifocal leukoencephalopathy after autologous bone marrow transplantation and alpha-interferon immunotherapy. *Bone Marrow Transplant* 1999;23(3):295–298.

Weber T, Major EO. Progressive multifocal leukoencephalopathy: Molecular biology, pathogenesis and clinical impact. *Intervirology* 1997;40(2-3):98–111.

Prostatitis

Basics

DEFINITION
- The term *prostatitis* encompasses several infectious and noninfectious processes, including the following:
  - Acute bacterial prostatitis
  - Chronic bacterial prostatitis
  - Nonbacterial prostatitis
  - Prostatodynia (prostatosis)
  - Granulomatous prostatitis

ETIOLOGY
- Acute bacterial prostatitis: caused by the usual uropathogens, mainly
  - *Escherichia coli*
  - Other Enterobacteriaceae
  - *Pseudomonas aeruginosa*
  - Enterococci
- Chronic bacterial prostatitis: usually caused by the same uropathogens
- Nonbacterial prostatitis (also known as the prostatitis syndrome)
  - Uncertain etiology
  - Some cases caused by *Chlamydia* or *Mycoplasma* species
- Prostatodynia (prostatosis): symptoms similar to those of nonbacterial prostatitis without evidence of an inflammatory response in prostatic secretions
  - Uncertain etiology
  - In some cases, a voiding dysfunction is found by urodynamic testing, caused by dyssynergy between bladder detrusor and internal sphincter muscles.
- Granulomatous prostatitis: a rare condition caused by the following:
  - Tuberculosis
  - Atypical mycobacteria
  - Fungi, mainly cryptococcosis, blastomycosis, coccidioidomycosis, or histoplasmosis
  - The prostate can be the focus of persistent cryptococcosis in patients with AIDS.

EPIDEMIOLOGY
- Prostatitis should be considered in every man with symptoms and/or signs consistent with urinary tract infection.

Clinical Manifestations

SYMPTOMS AND SIGNS
ACUTE BACTERIAL PROSTATITIS
- May cause the following:
  - Perineal, pelvic, or lower back pain
  - Urinary frequency
  - Dysuria or urgency
  - Systemic symptoms such as fever with chills
- A rectal examination, which should be done gently to avoid precipitating bacteremia, reveals an enlarged, tender prostate.

CHRONIC BACTERIAL PROSTATITIS
- Can be the cause of persistence of bacteria in the urinary tract and leads to recurrent urinary tract infections (UTIs)
- Patients are usually asymptomatic in the periods between recurrent UTIs, although they sometimes complain of symptoms similar to those reported in nonbacterial prostatitis and prostatodynia.

NONBACTERIAL PROSTATITIS AND PROSTATODYNIA
- May cause various pelvic and genitourinary symptoms
  - Perineal, pelvic, lower back, scrotal, or inguinal pain or vague discomfort is common and may be continuous or spasmodic.
  - Urinary frequency, dysuria, dribbling, hesitancy, urgency, or ejaculatory complaints are sometimes present.

Diagnosis

PATHOPHYSIOLOGY
- Bacterial prostatitis is associated with secretory dysfunction of the prostate.
- Prostatic secretions have an increased pH, which influences the local pharmacokinetic properties of several antibiotics.
- There is a reduced level of prostatic antibacterial factor, a zinc-containing polypeptide with antimicrobial properties found in prostatic secretions.

ACUTE BACTERIAL PROSTATITIS
- Prostate involvement should be considered in any man with symptoms suggestive of a UTI.
- A tender prostate supports the diagnosis.
- Specimens for urinalysis, urine culture, blood urea nitrogen, and creatinine should be taken before initiation of antimicrobial treatment.

CHRONIC BACTERIAL PROSTATITIS/NONBACTERIAL PROSTATITIS/PROSTATODYNIA
- These three syndromes cause similar symptoms, except that chronic bacterial prostatitis leads to recurrent UTIs.
- The differential diagnosis is based on the interpretation of segmented urine cultures.
  - For the appropriate collection of segmented urine cultures, the patient retracts the foreskin and cleans the glans penis.
  - The first 10 mL of voided urine is the urethral specimen and is labeled VB1 (voided bladder 1).
  - A midstream urine specimen is labeled VB2 (attention should be paid not to empty the bladder fully).
  - While the patient maintains foreskin retraction, the physician massages the prostate with continuous strokes for collection of the expressed prostatic secretions.
  - If there is no fluid, the patient milks the penis from the base toward the tip.
  - Finally, the first 10 mL of voided urine after the prostate massage is collected and labeled VB3. This specimen represents a mixture of prostatic secretions and urine.
- If the bladder urine (VB2) is sterile or has less than 10^3 CFU/mL, the diagnosis of bacterial prostatitis is indicated by higher colony counts of bacteria from the expressed prostatic secretions or the urine after the prostate massage (VB3) than from the urethral specimen (VB1), preferably by at least tenfold.

Prostatitis

- If the bladder urine (VB2) has more than 10^3 CFU/mL, a prostatic infection may be masked by a coexistent bladder infection. In this case, a 3-day regimen should be given with an antibiotic that will treat the bladder infection but will not penetrate well into the prostate (e.g., oral ampicillin 500 mg four times daily or oral nitrofurantoin 100 mg three times daily). The segmented urine cultures test should then be repeated.
- In the absence of urethral, bladder, and kidney infections, 10 or more white blood cells per high-power microscopic field of the expressed prostatic secretions or the urine after the prostate massage (VB3) is indicative of prostatic inflammation.
- Elderly men with symptoms of chronic prostatitis without evidence of infection should have urine cytology, a bladder ultrasound examination, and, if necessary, cystoscopy to exclude the possibility of bladder cancer.

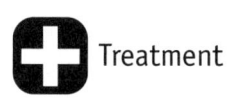

Treatment

ACUTE BACTERIAL PROSTATITIS

- Severity of illness and the presence of nausea or vomiting dictate the route of treatment.
- Mild illness, no nausea or vomiting
  - Trimethoprim–sulfamethoxazole (TMP-SMX), one double-strength tablet twice daily, orally, or
  - A fluoroquinolone (e.g., levofloxacin 500 mg once daily or ciprofloxacin 500 mg twice daily, orally)
  - Drugs are given for 3 to 4 weeks.
- Moderate or severe illness
  - Parenteral treatment (ampicillin and gentamicin, or ciprofloxacin, levofloxacin, or TMP-SMX) until fever resolves; then oral TMP-SMX or a fluoroquinolone for a total of 4 weeks
  - Adjunctive treatment includes stool softeners, analgesics, and antipyretics.
  - Transurethral catheterization should be avoided.
  - Acute urinary retention is managed by suprapubic catheterization.
  - Bacteremia and prostatic abscess may complicate acute bacterial prostatitis.
- Persistence of the pathogen would prompt retreatment for a 12-week course.

CHRONIC BACTERIAL PROSTATITIS

- Because many antimicrobial drugs do not penetrate well into the prostate that is not acutely inflamed, selection of an antibiotic based only on the segmented urine cultures results is not appropriate.
- The preferred regimens for penetration into the prostate are oral TMP-SMX, one double-strength tablet (160 mg TMP, 800 mg SMX) twice daily for 6 weeks or an oral fluoroquinolone (e.g., levofloxacin 500 mg once daily, or ciprofloxacin 500 mg twice daily for 4 weeks).
- About one-third of patients with chronic bacterial prostatitis have a complete response, one-third have a partial response, and one-third have no response to this regimen.
- For patients in the latter two categories, a 12-week course with the same or an alternative antibiotic is given. Infected prostatic calculi can cause bacterial persistence in the prostate despite appropriate, prolonged therapy.
- When a cure is not achieved, continuous antimicrobial treatment with oral TMP-SMX, one single-strength tablet daily, is given for suppression of prostatic infection and prevention of recurrent UTIs.
- In elderly men with considerable morbidity because of frequent recurrent UTIs despite suppressive antimicrobial treatment, transurethral, or even total, prostatic resection should be considered.

NONBACTERIAL PROSTATITIS

- There is no good therapy for this syndrome because the etiology is uncertain.
- A 2-week trial course of an antibiotic for the possibility of *Chlamydia* or *Mycoplasma* infection is reasonable.
- The preferred agent is oral doxycycline 100 mg twice daily or an oral macrolide (erythromycin 500 mg four times daily)
- If there is no clear improvement, additional antimicrobial treatment should not be given; if there is improvement, continue treatment for 2 to 4 more weeks.
- Reassurance about the benign nature of the illness and nonspecific therapy (hot sitz baths, antiinflammatory agents such as ibuprofen) are helpful.
- Prostatic massage, oral zinc, and vitamins have unproved efficacy. Sexual activity is encouraged.

PROSTATODYNIA

- Patients with urodynamic dysfunction may benefit from therapy with an alpha-blocker (e.g., prazosin or terazosin).
- Some patients with prostatodynia seem to have tension myalgia of the pelvic floor.
- Diathermy, special exercises, and diazepam have been helpful in these patients.

COMPLICATIONS

- Prostatic abscess and septicemia may complicate acute bacterial prostatitis.

Follow-Up

A follow-up culture of urine should be performed 14 days after completing therapy in cases of acute bacterial prostatitis.

PREVENTION

- Effective management of acute prostatitis cases will decrease incidence of recurrent prostatitis or chronic bacterial prostatitis.

Selected Readings

Domingue GJ Sr, Hellstrom WJ. Prostatitis. *Clin Microbiol Rev* 1998;11(4):604–613.

Lipsky BA. Prostatitis and urinary tract infection in men: What's new; what's true? *Am J Med* 1999;106(3):327–334.

Nickel JC. Prostatitis: Myths and realities. *Urology* 1998;51(3):326–362.

Thin RN. Diagnosis of chronic prostatitis: Overview and update. *Int J STD AIDS* 1997;8(8):475–481.

Pseudomonas Infections/Melioidosis/Glanders

Basics

DEFINITION
- Members of the genus *Pseudomonas* are motile, gram-negative, aerobic bacteria.
- Infections caused by *Burkholderia pseudomallei* constitute a broad spectrum of disease processes called melioidosis.
- Glanders is infection due to *Burkholderia mallei*.

ETIOLOGY
- *Pseudomonas aeruginosa* is the most common human pathogen in this group. Also, this group includes the following:
  —*Brevundimonas diminuta*
  —*Brevundimonas vesicularis*
  —*Burkholderia cepacia* (formerly *Pseudomonas cepacia*), which has been reported to cause bacteremia, burn-wound infections, chronic infections of the respiratory tract in patients with cystic fibrosis, endocarditis, meningitis, peritonitis, pneumonia, surgical wound infections, and urinary tract infections (UTIs)
  —*B. mallei* (formerly *Pseudomonas mallei*)
  —*Burkholderia pickettii*
  —*B. pseudomallei* (formerly *Pseudomonas pseudomallei*)
  —*Comamonas acidovorans*
  —*Pseudomonas fluorescens* (mainly associated with infections related to the administration of contaminated stored blood products)
  —*Pseudomonas pseudoalcaligenes*
  —*Pseudomonas putida*
  —*Pseudomonas stutzeri*
  —*Stenotrophomonas maltophilia* (formerly *Xanthomonas maltophilia*), which has been associated with pneumonia, bacteremia, cholangitis, endocarditis, meningitis, peritonitis, UTI, and wound infection

EPIDEMIOLOGY

Incidence
- *P. aeruginosa* is one of the most common causes of complicated and nosocomial infections of the urinary tract.
- *B. pseudomallei* and the infections it causes are found mainly in the tropics and are endemic in Southeast Asia. Person-to-person transmission is rare.
- Glanders is a disease of equine animals that is occasionally transmitted to humans.

Risk Factors
- Most *P. aeruginosa* infections are hospital acquired. Risk factors for *P. aeruginosa* infection include the following:
  —Bypass of the normal barriers (e.g., endotracheal intubation, urinary bladder catheterization)
  —Immune compromise
  —Disruption of the normal bacterial flora by broad-spectrum antibiotic therapy
- Risk factors for central nervous system infections include the following:
  —Cancer of the head and neck
  —Central nervous system tumors
  —Cerebrospinal fluid leaks
  —Indwelling hardware
  —Lumbar puncture
  —Neurosurgical procedures
  —*P. aeruginosa* bacteremia
  —Parameningeal infection
  —Penetrating head trauma
  —Spinal anesthesia
- Patients with cystic fibrosis can develop a chronic infection of the lower respiratory tract with *P. aeruginosa*.
- Vertebral osteomyelitis is associated with complicated UTI, genitourinary instrumentation, and intravenous drug abuse.
- UTIs may be chronic or recurrent and usually result from the following:
  —Instrumentation
  —Obstruction
  —*P. aeruginosa* bacteremia
  —Stones or other persistent foci
  —Surgery
  —Urinary tract catheterization
- *P. aeruginosa* causes necrotizing enterocolitis in infants and a similar disease in neutropenic patients.
- External otitis usually affects the external auditory canal, particularly under moist conditions ("swimmer's ear"). Occasionally, *P. aeruginosa* leads to "malignant external otitis," an invasive process that is typically slow but destructive and is more common among diabetics and immunocompromised individuals.
- *P. aeruginosa* infections of the symphysis pubis are associated with pelvic surgery and intravenous drug use.
- *B. cepacia* endocarditis is usually related to injection drug use.

Clinical Manifestations

SYMPTOMS
- Pneumonia due to *P. aeruginosa* is an acute, life-threatening infection.
- Among patients with early cystic fibrosis, *P. aeruginosa* usually causes mild recurrent upper respiratory symptoms. As cystic fibrosis advances, episodes of pneumonia develop and can lead to chronic productive cough, generalized weakness, growth retardation, respiratory compromise, weight loss, and wheezing.
- The clinical features of bacteremia, meningitis, and UTIs due to *P. aeruginosa* are usually indistinguishable from those of other bacterial infections.
- *P. aeruginosa* causes bacterial keratitis or corneal ulcer and endophthalmitis. Corneal ulcer due to *P. aeruginosa* may advance rapidly to involve the entire cornea. The clinical manifestations of *P. aeruginosa* keratitis are described in the Section II chapter, "Keratitis."
- Patients with *P. aeruginosa* infections of the symphysis pubis present with pain. Fever is variable, and the duration of symptoms before diagnosis ranges from days to months.
- Otalgia and otorrhea are common presenting symptoms of malignant external otitis.
- Manifestations of glanders are determined by the route of infection:
  —Chronic suppurative infection presents as multiple abscesses.
  —Mucous membrane infection results in the production of a mucopurulent discharge involving the eye, nose, or lips, with the subsequent development of granulomatous ulcers.
  —Pulmonary and systemic infection can present with fever, myalgia, headache, pleuritic chest pain, and diarrhea.
- Melioidosis most often involves the lungs and presents with fever, productive cough, and marked tachypnea. It can also cause acute or chronic suppurative infections involving the skin or internal organs.

SIGNS
- Pathognomonic skin lesions termed *ecthyma gangrenosum* develop in

Pseudomonas Infections/Melioidosis/Glanders

- a relatively small minority of patients with *P. aeruginosa* bacteremia. The lesions begin as small hemorrhagic vesicles surrounded by a rim of erythema and undergo central necrosis with subsequent ulceration.
- *P. aeruginosa* causes diffuse pruritic maculopapular and vesiculopustular rashes associated with exposure to contaminated hot tubs, spas, whirlpools, and swimming pools.
- In external otitis due to *P. aeruginosa*, there is a purulent discharge, and pain is elicited by pulling on the pinna.
- Physical examination in cases of malignant external otitis almost always reveals abnormalities of the external auditory canal, including swelling, erythema, purulent discharge, debris, and granulation tissue in the canal wall.
- In glanders, lymphadenopathy and splenomegaly may be documented.

Diagnosis

DIFFERENTIAL DIAGNOSIS

- The diagnosis of melioidosis should be entertained when a febrile patient who has been in an endemic area presents with an acute lower respiratory tract infection or exhibits unusual skin lesions.
- The diagnosis of glanders may be suggested by the clinical picture and a history of close contact with equines.

LABORATORY

- A positive culture is usually required for the discrimination of *P. aeruginosa* from most other infections due to gram-negative pathogens.
- In malignant external otitis, peripheral leukocytosis is infrequent, while the erythrocyte sedimentation rate usually is markedly elevated and cerebrospinal fluid occasionally exhibits pleocytosis and an elevation in the protein level.

IMAGING

- In malignant external otitis, computed tomography and magnetic resonance imaging typically reveal bony erosions and new bone formation.
- In melioidosis, chest roentgenograms typically reveal upper lobe consolidation or thin-walled cavities. Progressive upper lobe disease can mimic tuberculosis.

Treatment

MAIN TREATMENT

- Most types of *P. aeruginosa* disease are treated with one or, usually, two antibiotics to which the infecting organism is sensitive (usually a combination of an aminoglycoside or a quinolone and a β-lactam).
- Antibiotics with antipseudomonal activity include the following:
  - Aminoglycosides (gentamicin, tobramycin, etc.)
  - Carbapenems
  - Certain extended-spectrum penicillins (e.g., ticarcillin, piperacillin)
  - Certain third-generation cephalosporins (e.g., ceftazidime, cefoperazone)
  - Fluoroquinolones (e.g., ciprofloxacin)
  - Monobactams
- Malignant external otitis is treated with ciprofloxacin.
- Trimethoprim–sulfamethoxazole (TMP-SMX) and chloramphenicol have been used successfully in the treatment of *B. cepacia* infections.
- TMP-SMX is often useful for the treatment of infections due to drug-resistant strains of *S. maltophilia*.
- Severe melioidosis: TMP (8 mg/kg/d), SMX (40 mg/kg/d), and ceftazidime (120 mg/kg/d). Parenteral therapy is given for 2 weeks, followed by oral treatment for 6 months.
- Sulfadiazine (100 mg/kg/d) has proved effective against glanders. Antibiotics are administered for at least 30 days in uncomplicated infections, and longer in complicated cases.

TREATMENT FAILURE

- Alternative agents for *S. maltophilia* include ticarcillin–clavulanate, ciprofloxacin, and minocycline or doxycycline.
- Ciprofloxacin and ampicillin–sulbactam may be considered as alternative agents for use against sensitive strains of *B. cepacia*.
- Cefotaxime, imipenem, and amoxicillin–clavulanate are possible alternatives in melioidosis and glanders.
- In melioidosis and glanders, abscesses may require surgical drainage.

COMPLICATIONS

- UTIs exhibit a propensity for persistence, chronicity, resistance to antibiotic therapy, and recurrence.
- Complications of *P. aeruginosa* keratitis include corneal perforation, anterior chamber involvement, and endophthalmitis.
- All forms of melioidosis are subject to possible early or late relapse.
- In malignant external otitis, advancing osteomyelitis can involve the cranial nerves and the cavernous sinus, or, in rare cases, can lead to central nervous system infection.

Follow-Up

Prevention
N/A

Selected Readings

Pollack M. Infections due to *Pseudomonas* species and related organisms. In: Fauci AS, Braunwald E, Isselbacher KJ, et al., eds. *Harrison's principles of medicine*, 14th ed. New York: McGraw-Hill, 1998:943–950.

Sanford JP. *Pseudomonas* species (including melioidosis and glanders). In: Mandell GL, Bennett JE, Dolin R, eds. *Principles and practice of infectious diseases*, 4th ed. 1995:2003–2009.

Wilson R, Dowling RB. Lung infections. 3. *Pseudomonas aeruginosa* and other related species. *Thorax* 1998;53:213–219.

Psittacosis

Basics

DEFINITION

- Psittacosis is primarily an infectious disease of birds that is caused by *Chlamydia psittaci*. Transmission of infection from birds to humans results in a febrile illness characterized by pneumonitis and systemic manifestations. Inapparent infections or mild influenza-like illnesses also may occur.
- The name of the disease is derived from the Greek word for "parrot," *psittakos*. Because almost any bird may be a vector, some observers have recommended changing the name to *ornithosis*.

ETIOLOGY

- Psittacosis is a multisystem infection with a predilection for the lungs, causing an atypical pneumonia.
- In psittacosis, chlamydial organisms can be seen as inclusion bodies, less than 1 μm in diameter, in the cytoplasm of pneumonocytes and inflammatory cells in alveoli from patients with pneumonia, in smears of lung tissue, and in tissue culture. The organisms are demonstrated well with a Giemsa stain. The respiratory epithelium of the bronchi and bronchioles usually remains intact.

EPIDEMIOLOGY

Incidence

- *C. psittaci* is estimated to cause 0.5% to 1.5% of cases of community-acquired pneumonia.
- Almost any avian species can harbor *C. psittaci*. Psittacine birds (parrots, parakeets, and budgerigars) are most commonly infected, but human cases have been traced to contact with pigeons, ducks, turkeys, chickens, and many other birds.
- The agent is present in nasal secretions, excreta, tissues, and feathers of infected birds.

Risk Factors

Psittacosis is an occupational disease of pet shop owners, poultry workers, pigeon fanciers, taxidermists, veterinarians, workers at poultry-processing plants, and zoo attendants.

Clinical Manifestations

SYMPTOMS

- The clinical manifestations and course of psittacosis are extremely variable.
- After an incubation period of 7 to 14 days or longer, the disease may start abruptly with shaking chills and fever, with temperatures ranging as high as 40.5°C (105°F). Less commonly, the onset is gradual, with fever increasing over a 3- to 4-day period.
- Diffuse, severe headache is almost always a prominent symptom.
- Many patients present with a dry, hacking cough that is usually nonproductive, but small amounts of mucoid or bloody sputum may be raised as the disease progresses.
- Chest pain, pleurisy with effusion, and a friction rub may all occur, but are rare. Symptoms of upper respiratory tract infection are usually not prominent.
- Photophobia and epistaxis can be present.
- Patients often report generalized myalgia, and spasm and stiffness of the muscles of the back and neck may lead to an erroneous diagnosis of meningitis.
- Lethargy, mental depression, agitation, insomnia, and disorientation have been prominent features of the illness in some epidemics.
- Gastrointestinal problems such as abdominal pain, nausea, vomiting, and diarrhea are noted in some cases.
- A pink, blanching maculopapular rash is seen in 1% of patients.

SIGNS

- Most patients have a normal or slightly increased respiratory rate.
- The initial examination may reveal fine sibilant rales, or clinical evidence of pneumonia may be completely lacking. Rales usually become audible and more numerous as the illness progresses.
- The pulse rate is slow in relation to the fever.
- The reported incidence of splenomegaly ranges from 10% to 70%.
- Nontender hepatic enlargement also occurs, but jaundice is rare.

Diagnosis

DIFFERENTIAL DIAGNOSIS

- The pulmonary diseases that may be confused with psittacosis include the following:
  - Carcinoma of the lung with bronchial obstruction
  - *Chlamydia pneumoniae* pneumonia
  - Coccidioidomycosis
  - Common bacterial pneumonias
  - *Coxiella burnetii* pneumonia
  - *Legionella pneumophila* pneumonia
  - *Mycoplasma* pneumonia
  - Q fever
  - Viral pneumonia (influenza A and B viruses, respiratory syncytial virus, adenovirus, and parainfluenza)
- Because culture of *C. psittaci* is difficult (and hazardous for lab workers), the key to the diagnosis is an appropriate history of exposure. Exposures have ranged from mouth-to-beak contact to passage through a room where infected birds were present.
- In some studies, up to 25% of patients with psittacosis report no exposure to birds. Such patients may, in fact, not have psittacosis because of serologic cross-reactivity between its agent and the more recently discovered pathogen *C. pneumoniae*, which has no particular relation to birds.

Psittacosis

LABORATORY

- The white blood cell count is normal or moderately decreased in the acute phase of the disease but may rise in convalescence.
- The erythrocyte sedimentation rate frequently is not elevated.
- Transient proteinuria is common.
- The cerebrospinal fluid sometimes contains a few mononuclear cells but is otherwise normal.
- The results of liver function tests are generally normal or mildly elevated.
- The most commonly used diagnostic method is a test for complement-fixing antibody. Both an acute-phase and a convalescent-phase specimen should always be tested. A confirmed case of psittacosis is defined as one in which the culture is positive or the antibody levels increase by a factor of 4, to a titer of at least 1:32. A single titer of 1:32 can be the basis of a presumptive diagnosis in a patient with an illness compatible with psittacosis.
- Acute infections with *C. trachomatis* or *C. pneumoniae* can also produce titer rises in the complement-fixing antibody test. However, these species have different major outer-membrane proteins that are the principal antigens in more sensitive tests, which can be used to differentiate among them.

IMAGING

- Pneumonia, when present, is generally more extensive on radiography than would be expected from clinical signs.
- As with other forms of atypical pneumonia, no diagnostic patterns are recognized on chest radiographs, but they may show pneumonic lesions, which are usually patchy in appearance but can be hazy, diffuse, homogeneous, atelectatic, wedge-shaped, nodular, or miliary.

Treatment

MAIN TREATMENT

The tetracyclines (tetracycline 500 mg PO qid or doxycycline 100 mg PO bid for 10–21 days) are consistently effective in the treatment of psittacosis. Defervescence and alleviation of symptoms usually take place within 24 to 48 hours after the institution of therapy with 2 g daily in four divided doses. To avoid relapse, treatment should probably be continued for at least 7 to 14 days after defervescence.

ALTERNATIVE TREATMENT

Erythromycin can be used in patients who are allergic to or intolerant of tetracyclines.

TREATMENT FAILURE

In severe cases, hospitalization and pulmonary intensive care may be indicated.

COMPLICATIONS

- Relapses occur but are rare.
- Occasional patients develop culture-negative endocarditis. Pericarditis and myocarditis have been reported.
- Pancarditis, hepatitis, anemia, arthritis, meningoencephalitis, skin lesions, and, rarely, interstitial nephritis, glomerulonephritis, and acute renal failure are seen.
- Thrombophlebitis is not unusual during convalescence and may cause pulmonary infarction, which is a late complication and may be fatal.

Follow-Up

- In untreated cases of psittacosis, sustained or mildly remittent fever persists for 10 days to 3 weeks, or occasionally for as long as 3 months.
- If psittacosis is untreated, the fatality rate is up to 20%. With treatment, it drops to less than 1%.
- The response to therapy is usually prompt. In one series of 135 patients, 92% were afebrile 48 hours after starting treatment.

PREVENTION

- Cases in the United States have declined with the introduction of tetracycline-laced bird feed and the requirement of a 30-day quarantine period for imported birds.
- Infected birds should be treated with tetracycline, chlortetracycline, or doxycycline for at least 45 consecutive days.

Selected Readings

Anonymous. Case records of the Massachusetts General Hospital. Weekly clinicopathological exercises. Case 16-1998. Pneumonia and the acute respiratory distress syndrome in a 24-year-old man. *N Engl J Med* 1998;338:1527–1535.

Chang KP, Veitch PC. Fever, haematuria, proteinuria, and a parrot. *Lancet* 1997;350:1674.

Cotton MM, Partridge MR. Infection with feline *Chlamydia psittaci*. *Thorax* 1998;53:75–76.

Johnson SR, Pavord ID. Grand Rounds—City Hospital, Nottingham. A complicated case of community acquired pneumonia. *BMJ* 1996;312:899–901.

Williams J, Tallis G, Dalton C, et al. Community outbreak of psittacosis in a rural Australian town. *Lancet* 1998;351:1697–1699.

Pyelonephritis

Basics

DEFINITION
Pyelonephritis is an "upper" urinary tract infection (UTI), causing inflammation of the renal parenchyma, calyces, and pelvis. It is classified as acute uncomplicated, chronic ascending, or xanthogranulomatous. Chronic pyelonephritis is characterized macroscopically by uneven scarring of kidney and microscopically by chronic inflammatory changes, mainly in the renal interstitium and tubules of one or both kidneys.

ETIOLOGY
- Chronic
  —Infectious or noninfectious causes
- Acute uncomplicated
  —Bacterial infection, typically *Escherichia coli* (90%)
  —*Proteus* (4%)
  —*Klebsiella* (4%)
  —Mixed (5%)

EPIDEMIOLOGY
Incidence
- Seven million cases of UTIs overall in the United States annually
- UTIs are more prevalent in the following:
  —Younger than 3 months, boys more than girls
  —Girls ages 1 to 15 years: 4.0% and 0.5% for girls and boys, respectively
  —Women ages 16 to 35 years: 20% and 0.5% for women and men, respectively

Risk Factors
- Pregnancy
- Obstruction (prostate enlargement or inflammation; urethral obstruction)
- Stone formations
- Sexual intercourse (young women)

Clinical Manifestations

SYMPTOMS AND SIGNS
- Systemic (headache, nausea, vomiting, malaise, fever, chills)
- Unilateral or bilateral flank pain and/or tenderness
- Low back pain
- Abdominal pain
- Symptoms of "lower" UTI either concurrent or 1 to 2 days preceding symptoms of upper UTI
- Elderly: paucity of symptoms
- Children: usually present with nonspecific symptoms for all UTIs

Diagnosis

- History, physical examination, urinalysis, pretreatment urine culture, blood urea nitrogen, and/or creatinine
- Imaging for patients with slow or no improvement, recurrent episodes, or atypical features (e.g., colicky pain and/or persistent hematuria)

DIFFERENTIAL DIAGNOSIS
- Cystitis
- Urethritis
- Vaginitis
- Appendicitis
- Pelvic inflammatory disease

NONINFECTIOUS
- Tumor in bladder or kidney

LABORATORY
- Urine culture
- Imaging: Use if symptoms persist longer than 72 hours with appropriate treatment.

Pyelonephritis

— A plain x-ray of kidneys, ureter, and bladder may locate radiopaque calculi and soft-tissue masses and detect gas in the kidney(s) in cases of emphysematous pyelonephritis.
— Ultrasonography is the preferred initial method in recurrent or atypical pyelonephritis.
— Computed tomography is used if further clarification of renal anatomy is required, such as in intrarenal and/or perinephric abscess.

Treatment

MAIN TREATMENT
Acute Uncomplicated
- Trimethoprim–sulfamethoxazole (TMP-SMX) 160 to 800 mg orally every 12 hours for 10 to 14 days
- Norfloxacin 400 mg every 12 hours orally for 10 to 14 days
- Ciprofloxacin 500 mg every 12 hours orally for 10 to 14 days
- Amoxicillin 500 mg every 8 hours orally for 10 to 14 days
- Cefpodoxime 200 mg 12 hours orally for 10 to 14 days

Severe Illness or Possible Urosepsis
- Hospitalization recommended
- TMP-SMX 160 to 800 mg every 12 hours parenterally
- Ciprofloxacin 200 to 400 mg every 12 hours parenterally
- Levofloxacin 250 to 500 mg once per day parenterally
- Gentamicin 1 mg/kg every 8 hours parenterally
- Ceftriaxone 1 to 2 g once per day
- Ampicillin 1 g every 6 hours
- Imipenem/cilastatin 250 to 500 mg every 6 to 8 hours
- Ticarcillin/clavulanic acid 3.2 g every 8 hours
- Aztreonam 1 g every 8 to 12 hours

Outpatient after Fever Resolves
- Follow oral regimen for 14 days; dosages as under "Acute Uncomplicated"
  — TMP-SMX
  — Norfloxacin
  — Ciprofloxacin
  — Levofloxacin

COMPLICATIONS
- Bacteremia, septic shock
- Renal abscess
- Perinephric abscess

Follow-Up

- Posttreatment urine culture

PREVENTION
N/A

Selected Readings

Roberts JA. Management of pyelonephritis and upper urinary tract infections. *Urol Clin North Am* 1999;26(4):753–763.

Weir M, Brien J. Adolescent urinary tract infections. *Adolesc Med* 2000;11(2):293–313.

Q Fever

Basics

DEFINITION

Q fever, a rickettsiosis (Q for *query*, because the cause was unknown when the infection was first described in 1935), is an acute and occasionally chronic infection caused by *Coxiella burnetii*.

ETIOLOGY

- *C. burnetii* displays an antigenic-phase variation that is unique among the rickettsiae.
- *C. burnetii* exists in antigenic phase I in nature, but it changes to phase II after continuous passage in tissue culture. The transition from phase I to phase II occurs when one or more carbohydrate components are deleted from the lipopolysaccharide moiety.
- In acute Q fever, antibodies to *C. burnetii* phase II antigen dominate the immune response, whereas in chronic Q fever, phase I antigen levels become elevated.
- The ability of *C. burnetii* to form spores allows it to survive in harsh environments. Indeed, it can survive for more than 40 months in skim milk at room temperature and is readily recovered from soil up to 1 month after contamination.

EPIDEMIOLOGY

Incidence

- Q fever is a zoonosis. The primary reservoirs of *C. burnetii* are cattle, sheep, and goats, but many other species, including rodents and cats, can be infected.
- The infection in animals is usually not clinically apparent, but *C. burnetii* may be excreted in milk, urine, feces, and amniotic fluid.
- *C. burnetii* is mostly contracted by inhaling infected aerosols; it has an incubation period of around 3 weeks.
- The organism is particularly infectious (one to ten organisms is sufficient to infect humans) and is usually transmitted following contact with parturient ewes or cows, in which the organism is endemic in certain areas.
- In some series, up to 80% of the cases occurred between February and May.
- A high ratio of male to female patients (up to 1.0:3.5) has been noted.
- Reports of both sporadic cases and epidemics have been published.
- Infections due to *C. burnetii* occur in most countries. In the United States, about 3% of the cases of community-acquired pneumonia are due to *C. burnetii*, and Western Europe studies showed the presence of antibodies reactive with *C. burnetii* in 48.7% of the population.

Risk Factors

- Persons at risk for Q fever include abattoir workers, veterinarians, and others who come into contact with infected animals.
- The primary manifestation of acute Q fever differs from place to place, probably reflecting differences in the route of infection. In Nova Scotia (Canada), it is pneumonia, while in Marseille (France), it is granulomatous hepatitis. In the Basque country of Spain, both pneumonia and granulomatous hepatitis occur.
- Endocarditis due to *C. burnetii* usually occurs in patients with previous valvular heart disease, immunosuppression, or chronic renal insufficiency.

Clinical Manifestations

SYMPTOMS

- Acute *C. burnetii* infection causes a variety of clinical syndromes, the most common of which are a self-limited febrile illness, a flulike syndrome, and a mild-to-moderate atypical pneumonia.
- Other symptoms include chills, sweats, nausea, vomiting, and diarrhea, which occur in 5% to 20% of patients.
- Unlike other rickettsial diseases, Q fever is not usually associated with a rash, but a nonspecific skin rash may be evident in some patients.
- Headache is the most common neurologic manifestation of *C. burnetii* infection.
- Uncommon manifestations of acute Q fever include the following:
  - Epididymitis
  - Erythema nodosum
  - Extrapyramidal neurologic disease
  - Guillain-Barré syndrome
  - Hemolytic anemia
  - Inappropriate secretion of antidiuretic hormone
  - Mediastinal lymphadenopathy
  - Mesenteric panniculitis
  - Optic neuritis
  - Orchitis
  - Pancreatitis
  - Priapism
- Years after the initial infection with *C. burnetii*, chronic Q fever can occur in the form of endocarditis, usually involving abnormal or prosthetic cardiac valves. Fever is absent or, if present, is of low grade.
- Other manifestations of chronic Q fever include the following:
  - Hepatitis
  - Infection among immunocompromised hosts
  - Infection during pregnancy
  - Infection of aneurysms
  - Infection of vascular prostheses
  - Meningoencephalitis
  - Myocarditis
  - Osteomyelitis
  - Pericarditis
  - Prolonged fever
- Meningoencephalitis and abnormal cerebrospinal fluid findings are much less frequent in Q fever than in other rickettsial diseases.

SIGNS

- Hyperthermia is the main clinical feature in acute Q fever, with temperatures that can reach 40°C in up to 60% of the patients with pneumonia.

Q Fever

- The dissociation between pulse rate and temperature is found in one-third to one-half with Q fever.
- Hepatomegaly and splenomegaly can occur in certain cases.

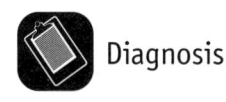

Diagnosis

DIFFERENTIAL DIAGNOSIS

- The differential diagnosis of *C. burnetii* pneumonia includes all other possible causes of atypical pneumonia, and *C. burnetii* should be considered in cases of culture-negative endocarditis (see also Section II chapter, "Pneumonia" and both chapters on endocarditis).
- Hepatitis due to *C. burnetii* can present as fever of unknown origin.

LABORATORY

- *C. burnetii* can be isolated from buffy-coat blood samples or tissue specimens by a shell-vial technique, but most clinical laboratories are not permitted to attempt the isolation of *C. burnetii*, because it is considered highly infectious.
- PCR can be used to amplify *C. burnetii* DNA from tissue or biopsy specimens. This technique also can be used on paraffin-embedded tissues.
- Serology is the most commonly used diagnostic tool. Three techniques are available:
  - Complement fixation
  - Indirect immunofluorescence (method of choice)
  - Enzyme-linked immunosorbent assay
- A fourfold rise in titer between acute- and convalescent-phase samples is seen in acute Q fever.
- Positive rheumatoid factor, high erythrocyte sedimentation rate, high C-reactive protein level, and/or increased gamma globulin concentrations suggest this diagnosis.

- The white blood cell count is usually normal, but monocytosis can occur with acute Q fever. Thrombocytopenia is present in about 25% of patients.
- Altered liver function, consisting more frequently in elevated alkaline phosphatase (70% of the cases) rather than transaminase, is found.

IMAGING

Despite the absence of specific radiologic findings, several features of *C. burnetii* pneumonia have been described, such as increased reticular markings and multiple round lesions or alveolar opacities, with a preferential topography in the lower lobes and frequent bilateral involvement.

Treatment

MAIN TREATMENT

- Treatment of acute Q fever with doxycycline (100 mg twice daily for 14 days) is usually successful.
- Doxycycline (100 mg twice daily) with hydroxychloroquine (200 mg tid) is becoming the treatment of choice in *C. burnetii* endocarditis.
- The optimal duration of antibiotic therapy for chronic Q fever remains undetermined, but a minimum of 3 to 4 years of treatment is usually recommended. Therapy should be discontinued only if the phase I IgA antibody titer is less than or equal to 1:50 and the phase I IgG titer is less than or equal to 1:200.

ALTERNATIVE TREATMENT

- The combination of rifampin (300 mg qd) and doxycycline (100 mg bid) has been used with success for the treatment of chronic Q fever.
- Quinolones are also effective and can be used in the treatment of chronic Q fever, instead of rifampin.

COMPLICATIONS

Mortality due to *C. burnetii* endocarditis is up to 25% to 60%, and relapse is common.

Follow-Up

- Most acute Q fever infections resolve spontaneously.
- Chest radiographs return to normal in 80% of the patients within the first month.

PREVENTION

- Consumption of only pasteurized milk
- Aborted material from goats and sheep should be destroyed, and affected dams isolated.

Selected Readings

Anonymous. Case records of the Massachusetts General Hospital. Weekly clinicopathological exercises. Case 38-1996. An 18-year-old man with severe headache, pleocytosis, and ataxia. *N Engl J Med* 1996;335:1829–1834.

Ayres JG, Flint N, Smith EG, et al. Postinfection fatigue syndrome following Q fever. *Q J Med* 1998;91:105–123.

Caron F, Meurice JC, Ingrand P, et al. Acute Q fever pneumonia: A review of 80 hospitalized patients. *Chest* 1998;114:808–813.

Walker D, Raoult D, Brouqui P, et al. Rickettsia, mycoplasma, and chlamydia. In: Fauci AS, Braunwald E, Isselbacher KJ, et al, eds. *Harrison's principles of internal medicine*, 14th ed. New York: McGraw-Hill, 1998:1045–1064.

Rabies

Basics

DEFINITION
Rabies virus is a rodlike virus in the family Rhabdoviridae. Rabies virus causes infection with a 100% mortality rate in humans.

ETIOLOGY
- Rabies virus is an enveloped virus with an RNA genome.
- Rabies virus is a zoonosis that infects many species of mammals.
- There is antigenic variation between various strains of rabies virus; this helps in the identification of the source of infection.
- Rabies virus incubates for a variable length of time within the muscles prior to entering into the peripheral nerves. It travels within the peripheral nerves between 12 and 24 mm/d until it reaches either the brain or the spinal cord. From this point, the virus replicates in the spinal ganglia.
- Encephalitis occurs after the virus enters the brain and is spread throughout the entire body via the peripheral nerves.

EPIDEMIOLOGY
- Incidence of disease in humans is proportional to the disease in domestic animals.
- Infected dogs represent the highest risk group for transmission to humans.
- Cats are less likely to be infected and transmit disease, as are farm animals.
- In the wild, bats are the most likely vector for transmission to humans.
- Other animals that can be infected include wolves, foxes, skunks, and raccoons.
- Small rodents or birds are rarely infected.
- Rabies is not present in England, Australia, and the Antarctic.
- The majority of cases occur in underdeveloped countries.
- In some parts of India, China, and the Middle East, rates as high as 3 in 100,000 are noted.
- Children have the greatest risk of exposure to the virus.
- In the United States, a few cases of rabies are reported each year.
- Most rabies from dog exposure takes place in either the southeastern United States close to Mexico, or in patients who were exposed to dogs in foreign countries.
- Bat rabies predominates in people who have not traveled.
- Raccoon rabies, which has caused extensive animal disease in the northeastern United States, does not account for much disease in humans. Infected skunks are a threat, however.

Incubation
The average incubation is 20 to 90 days, with cases occurring as early as 4 days and as late as 19 years following exposure.

Risk Factors
- People who work with animals
- Hunters
- Laboratory workers
- Cases have been transmitted within caves, most likely from aerosolized bat excreta.

Clinical Manifestations

PRODROME
- Patients may note paresthesias at the site of the initial bite.
- Constitutional symptoms and signs, such as malaise and fevers, nausea, vomiting, and sore throat, may occur.
- The prodrome lasts 2 to 10 days.

ACUTE NEUROLOGIC PERIOD
- Patients have encephalitis at this stage.
- Hyperactivity, agitation, biting, and hallucinations occur.
- Patients may also have hyperthermia, hypertension, and spasms of the pharynx and larynx.
- Hydrophobia occurs, as does exacerbation of symptoms with any tactile stimuli.
- The symptoms can wax and wane, and, between episodes of agitation, the patients are cooperative.
- On occasion, patients will have progressive confusion and clouding of consciousness, which progresses rapidly to coma. The patients complain of headache. Paralysis may occur at this stage.
- The acute neurologic stage lasts less than 1 week and progresses to coma and death.
- Death is due to a number of factors, including myocarditis and arrhythmias or intractable seizures. Respiratory failure and vascular collapse are infrequent.

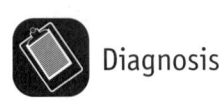

Diagnosis

DIFFERENTIAL DIAGNOSIS
- Encephalitis of multiple causes
- Toxin or substance abuse
- Tetanus
- Guillain-Barré syndrome
- Polio

Rabies

LABORATORY

- A serologic diagnosis with the rapid fluorescent focus inhibition test can give results in 48 hours.
- Viral cultures are often positive but do not help in the diagnosis because of the length of time these cultures take to develop.
- The white blood cell count is only mildly elevated.
- Cerebrospinal fluid evaluation reveals fewer than 100 cells, with a monocytic predominance, a normal glucose, and protein.
- Biopsy is taken from the nape of the neck. Fluorescent antibody tests should reveal the organisms in 50% of cases by the first week of illness.
- Corneal impressions may be positive for virus.
- Biopsy of the brain should reveal Negri bodies or intracytoplasmic inclusions.
- Every effort should be made to capture the animal, in order to test its central nervous system for virus.

IMAGING

Computed tomography and magnetic resonance imaging are normal.

Treatment

- There is no useful therapy to prevent death in patients with clinical rabies.
- Treatment is supportive at best, and strict isolation is needed in order to prevent secondary cases.

COMPLICATIONS

N/A

Follow-Up

It is mandatory that people who are at high risk of infection be checked for antibody titers frequently, at least once every 2 years.

PREVENTION

Prophylaxis

- Determination as to who does and does not need prophylaxis should be made on an individual basis.
- People at high risk may want to be immunized prior to any potential exposure.
- Public health measures taken to decrease the risk of disease in domestic animals has had great success in developed countries. Travelers should be alerted to the risks when traveling into less-developed areas.

Postexposure

- Rabies is transmitted through the saliva. Usually, animals will be sick or become sick within 10 days of an attack. Duration of illness in the dog is 3 days; in the cat, it is 5 days.
- Wild dogs, skunks, raccoons, foxes, and bats have the highest risk of infection.
- Bites from potentially rabid bats often go unnoticed; anyone who has, while sleeping, possibly been exposed to a bat should be treated as if they have been bitten.
- Whenever possible, the animal should be recovered and either quarantined or killed and sent to the laboratory for examination.
- The wound must be scrubbed with soap as soon as possible after the bite.
- Vaccination should be given as soon as possible for a high-risk bite, but it can be delayed for a few days while awaiting results from the laboratory in low-risk situations.
- Passive antibody administration with human rabies immune globulin, at a dose of 20 IU/kg, should be given. One-half of the dose should be administrated around the wound, and the other half given intramuscularly in the thigh or upper outer buttocks.
- Vaccination should be given in 1-mL doses on days 0, 3, 7, 14, and 28. Vaccination should be administered in the deltoid area only.
- In people who have high-risk professions or are traveling into high risk locations where animal contact is possible, pre-exposure vaccination is indicated. In this case, vaccine (1 ml intramuscular) should be given at day 0, 7, and 21 or 28. Antibody titers should be determined at least every 2 years. There should be neutralization at the 1:5 level via the rapid fluorescent focus inhibition test.
- For people with a high-risk exposure who have been fully immunized prior to the exposure, vaccine boosters on days 0 and 3 are adequate.

Selected Readings

Anderson LJ, Nicholson KG, Tauxe RV, et al. Human rabies in the United States. 1960–1979: Epidemiology, diagnosis, and prevention. *Ann Intern Med* 1984;100:728–735.

Centers for Disease Control. Extension of raccoon rabies epizootic–United States, 1992. *MMWR Morbid Mortal Wkly Rep* 1992;41:661–664.

Human rabies—Virginia. 1998. *MMWR Morbid Mortal Wkly Rep* 1999;48:95–97.

Relapsing Fever

Basics

DEFINITION
- A spirochetal infection manifested with fever that lasts few days and subsequent recurrence(s) of fever after short period(s) with normal temperature

ETIOLOGY
- The pathogenic spirochetes causing relapsing fever are transmitted to humans by arthropods.
- The human body louse (*Pediculus humanus corporis*) transmits *Borrelia recurrentis* to humans, causing epidemic relapsing fever.
- Several species of ticks transmit the many species of *Borrelia* to humans, causing endemic relapsing fever.

EPIDEMIOLOGY

Incidence and Prevalence

- The incidence of relapsing fever due to *B. recurrentis* (louse-borne epidemic relapsing fever) depends on socioeconomic and ecologic factors.
- Louse-borne relapsing fever usually occurs in epidemics related to catastrophic events, such as war, serious weather-related events, or famine because of easy dissemination of lice between humans due to overcrowding.
- There are a few areas of the world (highlands of Central and East Africa and the South America Andes) where louse-borne relapsing fever is still endemic.
- The incidence of tick-borne relapsing fever is mainly influenced by environmental and social factors, which determine the probability of tick bites of humans.
- A large outbreak of tick-borne relapsing fever in the Western Hemisphere occurred in 1973 in Arizona and affected 62 campers.
- Tick-borne relapsing fever has a worldwide distribution but is especially endemic in tropical Africa.
- The incubation period of relapsing fever is usually 8 days (range, 5–15 days).

Risk Factors

- Overcrowding is a major risk factor for louse-borne relapsing fever.
- Recreational activities in areas where tick bites are more likely to occur increase the probability of tick-borne relapsing fever in humans.

Clinical Manifestations

SYMPTOMS
- Acute onset of fever, accompanied by a combination of the following symptoms:
  - Chills
  - Rigors
  - Headache
  - Malaise
  - Arthralgias
  - Diffuse myalgias
  - Lethargy
  - Cough
  - Jaundice
  - Photophobia
- A petechial, macular, and/or papular rash may appear.
- Manifestations from the heart and/or the central nervous system may also complicate relapsing fever.
- The febrile episode terminates abruptly in 3 to 6 days.
- After 7 to 9 days with no fever, the patient has recurrence of the symptoms (relapsing fever).
- The number of relapses of fever is usually one to two in louse-borne relapsing fever, while multiple relapses of fever are common in tick-borne relapsing fever.

SIGNS
- Common signs may include the following:
  - Conjunctival infection and edema
  - Hepatomegaly
  - Splenomegaly
  - Diffuse abdominal tenderness
  - Abnormal respiratory sounds (rales and rhonchi)
  - Lymphadenopathy

Diagnosis

DIFFERENTIAL DIAGNOSIS
The possibility of a coexisting epidemic of typhus should be entertained in cases of epidemic louse-borne relapsing fever.

Relapsing Fever

LABORATORY

- Demonstration of *Borrelia* in the peripheral blood of a febrile patient is the definitive test for the diagnosis of relapsing fever.
- Thick and thin smears of peripheral blood stained with Giemsa or Wright should be carefully checked.
- Dark-field microscopy of peripheral blood may also prove the presence of *Borrelia*.
- Serology tests may be of help, but results should be interpreted with caution due to their limited sensitivity and specificity.

Treatment

MAIN TREATMENT

- A single dose of 0.5 g tetracycline PO is the recommended treatment for louse-borne relapsing fever.
- A tetracycline regimen of longer duration (0.5 g every 6 hours PO for 7 days) is the recommended treatment for tick-borne relapsing fever.

ALTERNATIVE TREATMENT

- Erythromycin (instead of tetracycline) is the best alternative for both louse-borne and tick-borne relapsing fever.
- The dosage and duration of treatment with erythromycin is similar with the tetracycline regimen described above.

COMPICATIONS

- The case-fatality rates for untreated relapsing fever are 4% to 40% for louse-borne relapsing fever and 2% to 5% for tick-borne relapsing fever.
- Liver damage, arrhythmias due to myocarditis, and cerebral hemorrhage are the main causes of death.

Follow-Up

Careful follow-up is necessary for patients with relapsing fever, due to the high probability of recurrence of the syndrome.

PREVENTION

- Control of lice and ticks

Selected Readings

Barbour AG. Antigenic variation of a relapsing fever *Borrelia* species. *Annu Rev Microbiol* 1990;44:155–171.

Burgdorfer W. The enlarging spectrum of tick-borne spirochetoses: R.R. Paker Memorial Address. *Rev Infect Dis* 1986;8:932–940.

Butler T. Relapsing fever: New lessons about antibiotic action. *Ann Intern Med* 1985;102:397.

Horton JM, Blaser MJ. The spectrum of relapsing fever in the Rocky Mountains. *Arch Intern Med* 1985;145:871–875.

Le CT. Tick-borne relapsing fever in children. *Pediatrics* 1980;66:963–966.

Negussie Y, Remick DG, DeForge LE, et al. Detection of plasma tumor necrosis factor, interleukins 6 and 8 during the Jarisch-Herxheimer reaction of relapsing fever. *J Exp Med* 1992;175:1207–1212.

Perine PL, Teklu B. Antibiotic treatment of louse-borne relapsing fever in Ethiopia: A report of 377 cases. *Am J Trop Med Hyg* 1983;32:1096–1100.

Scioto CG, Lauer BA, White WL, et al. Detection of *Borrelia* in acridine orange-stained blood smears by fluorescence microscopy. *Arch Pathol Lab Med* 1983;107:384–386.

Respiratory Syncytial Virus Infection

Basics

DEFINITION
- Contagious viral infection that causes lower respiratory tract infections in children and adults, and is particularly severe in infants and children with congenital heart disease, in immunocompromised adults, and in the elderly.

ETIOLOGY
- Paramyxoviridae
- Enveloped RNA virus
- Natural infection in only humans and chimpanzees

EPIDEMIOLOGY
- Worldwide distribution
- In the United States, outbreaks peak in the winter and spring months.
- Immunity to the virus is not established; therefore, children as well as adults can have recurrent disease.

Children
- Almost all children are infected in the first years of life.
- Infection is via respiratory secretions and via fomites.
- Respiratory syncytial virus (RSV) causes pneumonia and bronchiolitis in children.
- The virus is commonly isolated in daycare settings.
- Children below the age of 6 months, who should normally have maternal antibodies, are affected with severe disease. Pneumonia and severe bronchiolitis may occur in 30% to 71% of these patients.

Risk Factors
- Children with the following:
  —Compromised immune systems
  —Cystic fibrosis
  —Congenital heart disease

Incubation
The incubation period is 5 days.

Clinical Manifestations

- Initially, children and adults have an upper respiratory-like infection, with coryza and sore throat.
- Children may have high fevers.
- Symptoms are similar to those of a common cold, but worse.
- Over time, children may develop a deepening cough, with spasms (bronchiolitis) and wheezing.
- Hoarseness is not common.
- Croup may occur in 10% of cases, but is usually mild.
- Tachypnea with retractions of the respiratory muscles occurs in infants and small children.
- Otitis media may be present.
- Elderly adults commonly develop bronchopneumonia as a complication of RSV.

Diagnosis

- Nasal washings can be sent for viral culture.
- The shell-vial test may take up to 40 hours for detection, and routine cell culture evaluation takes less than 5 days on average.
- Many rapid tests are available for screening of respiratory secretions; they take several hours to complete.
  —Indirect immunofluorescence assays
  —ELISA
  —Enzyme immunoassays

Respiratory Syncytial Virus Infection

—Serologic diagnosis is available for community-screening purposes.

DIFFERENTIAL DIAGNOSIS

- Rhinovirus
- Influenza virus
- Parainfluenza virus
- Childhood asthma

IMAGING

- Chest x-rays for children, to watch for the following:
  —Consolidation
  —Interstitial infiltrates
  —Hyperaeration

Treatment

- Ribavirin, via small-particle aerosol for 12 to 20 hours a day, is beneficial. The dosage is 1.1 g/d.
- Supportive care
- Bronchodilators if reactive airways present

COMPLICATIONS

- In very young children, sudden infant death syndrome has been associated with RSV. Apnea associated with infection appears to contribute to this.
- Development of asthma is possibly connected to recurrent RSV infections in childhood.
- Bacterial pneumonia or otitis is a complication of infection.
- Myocarditis has been associated with RSV.
- Rare cases of myelitis or encephalitis have occurred during RSV infection.
- Children and adults with heart disease (congenital) or immunosuppression are at particular risk with RSV. Interstitial pneumonitis is common.
- In adults with bone marrow transplants, mortality rates of 50% are seen with untreated RSV.

Follow-Up

- None required unless bronchospasm develops on a recurrent or permanent basis

PREVENTION

- The nosocomial infection rate is high.
- Strict isolation is needed when patients are admitted to the hospital.
- There should be consideration in high-risk children (immunocompromised, cystic fibrosis, congenital heart disease) for intravenous immunoglobulin given monthly.

Selected Readings

Hall CB, Walsh EE, Schnabel KC, et al. Occurrence of groups A and B of respiratory syncytial virus over 15 years: Associated epidemiologic and clinical characteristics in hospitalized and ambulatory children. *J Infect Dis* 1990;162:1283–1290.

Henderson FW, Collier AM, Clyde WA, et al. Respiratory syncytial virus infections, reinfections and immunity. A prospective, longitudinal study in young children. *N Engl J Med* 1979;300:530–534.

Jackson GG, Muldoon RL. Viruses causing common respiratory infections in man. III. Respiratory syncytial virus and coronaviruses. *J Infect Dis* 1973;128:674–692.

Smith DW, Frankel LR, Mathers LH, et al. A controlled trial of aerosolized ribavirin in infants receiving mechanical ventilation for severe respiratory syncytial virus infection. *N Engl J Med* 1991;325:24–29.

Rheumatic Fever

Basics

DEFINITION
Rheumatic fever is a clinical syndrome that occurs following group A streptococcal pharyngitis. A constellation of signs and symptoms is associated with this illness, and they range from arthritis and atypical fleeting rashes to pancarditis with cardiac valve dysfunction.

ETIOLOGY
- Group A streptococcal pharyngitis initiates rheumatic fever.
- Specific strains have been associated with this disease.
- Pathogenesis is related to antibodies that cross-react between streptococcal antigens and heart valves exists.
- Patients with rheumatic fever have inflammatory lesions in connective tissue and Aschoff nodules in the myocardium. This is a pancarditis involving all parts of the heart.

EPIDEMIOLOGY
- Rheumatic fever is a worldwide disease.
- It accounts for 40% of the heart disease in developing countries.
- Rheumatic fever is a disease of childhood, usually affecting children ages 6 to 15 years.
- One-third of cases occur after a subacute or asymptomatic case of group A streptococcal pharyngitis.
- The attack rate following untreated cases of streptococcal pharyngitis ranges from 0.4% to 3.0%.
- Rates in the United States have dropped secondary to antibiotic use.
- The estimated incidence within the United States is 0.5 per 100,000.
- Epidemics of disease reflect the specific strain of *Streptococcus* present in the community.

Risk Factors
- Overcrowding
- History of rheumatic fever

Incubation
- One to 5 weeks, with an average of 19 days

Clinical Manifestations

MAJOR MANIFESTATIONS
- Polyarthritis in 75%
- Carditis in 50%
- Chorea in 15%
- Subcutaneous nodules in fewer than 10%
- Erythema marginatum in fewer than 10%

Polyarthritis
- Rheumatic fever often begins with fevers and polyarthritis.
- It involves the knees, ankles, elbows, and wrists. Most children have multiple joints involved. They may have arthralgias or frank arthritis.
- Symptoms resolve within 1 month.

Carditis
- Pancarditis may be silent.
- On occasion, patients present with congestive heart failure.
- Most acute valvular disease presents with mitral regurgitation and, to a lesser extent, aortic regurgitation.

Chorea
- *Chorea* is defined as irregular, purposeless movement of the muscles.
- It may occur at all times of the day, and it includes the face and extremities.
- Chorea is often present, along with carditis and arthritis.

Subcutaneous Nodules
- Painless nodules appear over tendons, often near the joints.
- They may be as large as 2 cm.
- They occur often in conjunction with carditis.

Erythema Marginatum
- These irregular areas of erythema may be macular and are often present on the trunk and extremities.
- The rash is evanescent and may be hard to detect.

MINOR MANIFESTATIONS
- Fever
- Arthralgias without frank arthritis

Rheumatic Fever

- Laboratory evidence that can constitute minor criteria includes a prolonged PR interval or elevated, acute-phase reactants such as an elevated erythrocyte sedimentation rate or C-reactive protein.
- The symptoms, if untreated, last an average of 3 months.

Diagnosis

- This is a clinical diagnosis, and there are many diseases with which it may be confused. This is especially true if the rheumatic fever is chronic or recurrent, in which case, manifestations may be less obvious.
- Clinical diagnosis is made with two major criteria, or one major criteria and two minor criteria.

LABORATORY

- Evidence of a recent streptococcal infection needs to be determined.
- A positive throat culture or a serum ASO titer of greater than 200 Todd units/mL is necessary.
- Other serologic tests that should be elevated following a significant streptococcal infection include an antihyaluronidase antibody or anti-DNAseB.
- Should all serology be negative, the diagnosis needs to be questioned.

DIFFERENTIAL DIAGNOSIS

- Primary rheumatologic illness, such as juvenile rheumatoid arthritis and lupus
- Infections such as Lyme disease, gonococcal arthritis, and endocarditis
- Viral diseases such as rubella and coxsackievirus A or B
- Other illnesses, such as drug reactions, sickle cell crisis, sarcoidosis, inflammatory bowel disease, and leukemia

Treatment

- Treatment with salicylates is necessary.
- Steroids are used if inflammation cannot be reduced with salicylates alone.
- Steroids are used when carditis leads to congestive heart failure.
- Aspirin is often given in high doses for 8 weeks. Start with 90 to 100 mg/kg/d. When used in conjunction with steroids, aspirin should be continued for 4 weeks after steroids are finished (usually steroids are given over a 1-month period).

COMPLICATIONS

- Complications include refractory heart failure or valve dysfunction, leading to cardiac failure.
- In addition, patients may develop endocarditis secondary to the damaged valves.

Follow-Up

Patients who have had rheumatic fever need close follow-up with the pediatrician and possibly the pediatric cardiologist.

PREVENTION

- For streptococcal pharyngitis, penicillin treatment for 10 days prevents rheumatic fever. Penicillin can be given up to 9 days following the start of sore throat.
- Patients with a history of rheumatic fever have a good chance of developing recurrent disease.
- Many possible regimes are available, including benzathine penicillin G, to be given intramuscularly every month. Alternatives also include sulfadiazine orally, penicillin VK orally, or erythromycin orally.
- Patients with valvular disease require antibiotic prophylaxis for dental procedures.

Selected Readings

Bisno AL. Group A streptococcal infections and acute rheumatic fever. *N Engl J Med* 1991;325:783–793.

Dajani AS, Ayoub E, Bierman FZ, et al. Guidelines for the diagnosis of rheumatic fever: Jones criteria, updated 1992. *Circulation* 1993;87:302–307.

Wallace MR, Garst PD, Papadimos TJ, et al. The return of acute rheumatic fever in young adults. *JAMA* 1989;262:2557–2561.

Rocky Mountain Spotted Fever

Basics

DEFINITION

Rocky Mountain spotted fever (RMSF) is an acute, often fatal infection caused by *Rickettsia rickettsii*, a small, pleomorphic, obligate intracellular parasite that survives only briefly outside a host.

ETIOLOGY

- RMSF has been documented in 48 U.S. states and in Canada, Mexico, Costa Rica, Panama, Colombia, and Brazil.
- It is transmitted by the following:
  —*Dermacentor variabilis*, the American dog tick, in the eastern two-thirds of the United States and California
  —*Dermacentor andersoni*, the Rocky Mountain wood tick, in the western United States
  —*Rhipicephalus sanguineus* in Mexico
  —*Amblyomma cajennense* in Mexico and Central and South America
- The rickettsiae are released from the salivary glands of feeding adult ticks during their 6 to 10 hours of attachment.
- A tick bite is recalled by approximately 50% of patients.
- *R.rickettsii* is more invasive than other rickettsiae, routinely spreading to infect vascular smooth-muscle cells.
- Although occlusive thrombosis and ischemic necrosis are often cited as the pathologic basis for tissue and organ injury in RMSF, it is, in fact, increased vascular permeability, with resulting edema, hypovolemia, and ischemia, that is responsible.
- The incubation period ranges from 3 to 12 days (usually about 7 days).

EPIDEMIOLOGY

Incidence

- Between 600 and 1,200 cases are reported annually in the United States.
- Most infections are acquired in the south Atlantic coastal and the western and south central states.
- The disease typically occurs during spring in the western states and during summer in the eastern states.

Risk Factors

- Most infections arise from exposure in rural or suburban environments, but rare urban foci exist.
- Children, in particular those 5 to 9 years old, outdoor recreationalists, and farmers appear to be at higher risk.
- Other reported risk factors include exposure to dogs, residence in a wooded area, and male gender.

Clinical Manifestations

SYMPTOMS

- Illness begins abruptly with the following:
  —Fever (in virtually all patients)
  —Malaise (95%)
  —Severe frontal headache (90%)
  —Myalgias (80%)
  —Vomiting (60%)
- Other symptoms include abdominal pain, diarrhea, headache, myalgia, and anorexia.

SIGNS

- The typical rash, which begins 1 to 15 days after the onset of illness, first appears as macules on the wrists and ankles and subsequently spreads to involve the trunk, face, palms, and soles. These cutaneous lesions often develop papular, petechial, or purpuric features.
- At the time of initial presentation, the classic triad—fever, rash, and history of exposure to ticks—is found in only 60% to 70% of confirmed cases.
- Involvement of the palms and soles, often considered diagnostically important, usually occurs relatively late in the course (after day 5 in 43% of cases), and does not occur at all in many cases.
- The absence of a rash does not exclude the diagnosis, because 10% of patients never develop a rash; this type of manifestation is called Rocky Mountain "spotless" fever.
- Encephalitis due to vascular injury, presenting as confusion or lethargy, is apparent in 25% of cases. Numerous other neurologic abnormalities have been seen, including cranial nerve palsies, hearing loss, severe vertigo, nystagmus, dysarthria, aphasia, unilateral corticospinal signs, ankle clonus, extensor toe signs, hyperreflexia, spasticity, fasciculations, athetosis, neurogenic bladder, hemiplegia, paraplegia, and complete paralysis.
- Respiratory failure, renal dysfunction, hypotension, dysrhythmias, hepatosplenomegaly, myocarditis, lymphadenopathy, and hepatic injury can develop.
- Ocular involvement includes conjunctivitis in 30% of cases and retinal vein engorgement, flame hemorrhages, arterial occlusion, and papilledema.

Diagnosis

DIFFERENTIAL DIAGNOSIS

- Early in the illness, when medical attention usually is first sought, RMSF is difficult to distinguish from many self-limiting viral illnesses, as well as leptospirosis, typhoid fever, gram-negative or gram-positive bacterial sepsis, and other rickettsial diseases.
- Central nervous system infection, including bacterial and viral meningoencephalitis, should be considered in the presence of seizures, coma, and neurologic signs.
- The presence of cough, pulmonary signs, and chest roentgenographic opacities leads to consideration of bronchitis or pneumonia.
- Many other illnesses considered in the differential diagnosis are associated with a rash, including rubeola, rubella, meningococcemia, disseminated gonococcal infection, secondary syphilis, toxic shock syndrome, drug hypersensitivity, idiopathic thrombocytopenic purpura, thrombotic thrombocytopenic purpura, Kawasaki syndrome, and immune complex vasculitis.

Rocky Mountain Spotted Fever

- Clinical and epidemiologic considerations are more important than a laboratory diagnosis early in the illness.

LABORATORY

- Findings include a normal white blood cell count, with increased numbers of immature myeloid cells and increased plasma concentrations of proteins of the acute-phase response.
- Hyponatremia is reported in 50% of cases.
- Skeletal muscle injury, clinically manifested as myositis, has been documented in several individual cases by marked elevations in serum creatine kinase levels or histopathologic evidence of vascular injury in skeletal muscle and multifocal rhabdomyonecrosis.
- Meningoencephalitis results in cerebrospinal fluid pleocytosis in about one-third of cases. The protein concentration in cerebrospinal fluid may be increased, but the glucose concentration is usually normal.
- An elevated serum bilirubin concentration and frank jaundice are sometimes found and are probably consequences of both hemolysis and hepatocyte injury.
- Serologic tests are usually negative at the time of presentation. The most common laboratory test for confirmation of the diagnosis is the indirect immunofluorescence assay. Between 7 and 10 days after the onset of illness, a diagnostic titer of 64 is usually detectable. Latex agglutination and a solid-state enzyme immunoassay are also available commercially. Latex agglutination usually yields a diagnostic titer of 128 at 1 week after onset.
- The historically significant, but insensitive and nonspecific, Weil-Felix *Proteus vulgaris* OX-19 and OX-2 agglutination tests are unreliable and should not be used.

IMAGING

Imaging studies in cases of encephalopathy associated with RMSF have been limited. The computed tomography scan usually shows only generalized cerebral edema. Magnetic resonance imaging has showed increased signal intensity in an apparent perivascular-space distribution on T2-weighted images.

DIAGNOSTIC/TESTING PROCEDURES

The only specific test currently available to diagnose RMSF in its early stages is a direct immunofluorescent examination of skin biopsy samples for *R. rickettsii* antigen. The test is available from the Centers for Disease Control and Prevention (CDC) but is impractical and not widely used.

Treatment

MAIN TREATMENT

- Doxycycline is the drug of choice for the treatment of adults with RMSF and is administered orally (or, in the presence of coma or vomiting, intravenously) at a dosage of 200 mg/d in two divided doses.
- Therapy should be continued for 5 to 7 days and for at least 48 hours after the resolution of fever.

ALTERNATIVE TREATMENT

Other regimens include oral tetracycline (25–50 mg/kg/d) in four divided doses, or chloramphenicol (50–75 mg/kg/d) in four divided doses.

TREATMENT FAILURE

- The most seriously ill patients are managed in intensive care units, with careful supportive care.
- In the most severe cases, shock results in acute tubular necrosis–induced renal failure, which may require hemodialysis.

COMPLICATIONS

- In the pre-antibiotic era, the mortality rate was 20% to 25%; it still runs around 5%, primarily because of delayed diagnosis and treatment.
- The case–fatality ratio is higher for males than for females and increases with each decade of life above age 20.
- Sometimes, full-blown thrombotic thrombocytopenic purpura develops, or, more commonly, disseminated intravascular coagulation.
- Bleeding is a potentially life-threatening effect of severe vascular damage. Blood is detected in the stools or vomitus of 10% of patients, and death has followed massive upper gastrointestinal hemorrhage.

Follow-Up

Although survivors of RMSF usually return to their previous state of health, patients who have been severely ill may sustain permanent sequelae, including neurologic deficits, and may need to have gangrenous extremities amputated.

PREVENTION

Avoidance of tick bites is the only available preventive approach. When exposure to ticks is possible, use of tick repellents and inspection of the skin and clothing several times daily and before going to bed are effective.

Selected Readings

Anonymous. Case records of the Massachusetts General Hospital. Weekly clinicopathological exercises. Case 32-1997. A 43-year-old woman with rapidly changing pulmonary infiltrates and markedly increased intracranial pressure. *N Engl J Med* 1997;337:1149–1156.

Conlon PJ, Procop GW, Fowler V, et al. Predictors of prognosis and risk of acute renal failure in patients with Rocky Mountain spotted fever. *Am J Med* 1996;101:621–626.

Drage LA. Life-threatening rashes: Dermatologic signs of four infectious diseases. *Mayo Clin Proc* 1999;74:68–72.

Spach DH, Liles WC, Campbell GL, et al. Tick-borne diseases in the United States. *N Engl J Med* 1993;329:936–947.

Walker D, Raoult D, Brouqui P, et al. *Rickettsia, Mycoplasma*, and *Chlamydia*. In: Fauci AS, Braunwald E, Isselbacher KJ, et al., eds. *Harrison's principles of internal medicine*, 14th ed. New York: McGraw-Hill, 1998:1045–1052.

Roundworms, Intestinal

Basics

DEFINITION
Only a few roundworms are clinically important in humans; however, many people worldwide are infected. It is estimated that there are 1 billion cases of ascariasis worldwide. Intestinal nematodes are transmitted to humans through the soil.

ETIOLOGY

Trichuriasis, or Whipworm
- The habitat is the cecum and ascending colon. Ingested eggs hatch in the intestine, and larvae penetrate the intestinal villus. From there, they move along the bowel to the cecum.
- The worm lies embedded in the intestinal villi, with a life span of 1 year.
- Contact with mature eggs occurs in contaminated soil.

Enterobiasis, or Pinworm
- A small worm with a lifespan of 11 to 35 days
- The adult lives in the terminal ileum and cecum and migrates to the perineal area to lay eggs during the night.
- Pruritus leads to scratching and reinfection.

Ascariasis
- *Ascaris lumbricoides*
- The worm can be up to 35 cm in length and lives in the small intestine.
- Eggs pass into the soil and becomes infectious in 3 to 12 weeks.
- After ingestion, the rhabditiform larvae penetrate the small bowel, migrate via the bloodstream to the lungs, and break out into the alveoli. There they are swallowed and begin to develop into adults within the small intestine. Adults live about 1 year.

Hookworm
- *Necator americanus* and *Ancylostoma duodenale*
- Hookworms are small worms about 1 cm in length. The larvae enter the patient via the skin. Larvae pass into the bloodstream and enter the lungs, where they penetrate the alveoli. The larvae are then swallowed and hook onto the mucosa of the small intestine. Adults can live for decades.

Strongyloidiasis
- *Strongyloides stercoralis*
- This tiny (2.2-mm) worm lives in the upper small intestine.
- Larvae pass into the stool and are deposited in the soil, where they can either develop into infectious filariform larvae or become adult free-living worms.
- Infection occurs either via skin contact with infected soil or via autoinfection when the larvae penetrate the bowel wall. Infection can enter the bloodstream to the lungs, through the alveoli, and be swallowed.

EPIDEMIOLOGY

Trichuriasis
- There is worldwide infection, with an estimated 800 million cases. In the United States, infection is mainly in the southeastern states.
- Humans are the principal host (more prevalent in poor communities and in children ages 5–15 years).
- Swine have been noted to be infected on occasion.

Enterobiasis
- Worldwide infection of tropics and temperate zones
- Forty-two million cases in the United States
- Spans all socioeconomic levels, occurs in families and group settings, and seen mostly in children

Ascariasis
- Most common helminthic infection, with 1 billion infected
- Worldwide distribution
- Southeastern United States
- Infection seen in young children
- Eggs can survive as long as 6 years in the soil.

Hookworm
Hookworm infections exist worldwide in tropical and subtropical locations. It is estimated that as many as one-fourth of the world's population is affected. Infrequent cases are reported in the southeastern United States.

Strongyloidiasis
Worldwide distribution is noted, with those in temperate areas at risk for continual reinfection.

Incubation
- Trichuriasis
  — It takes 21 days for the eggs to embryonate in the soil and about 60 days from the time of infection to the time the first eggs appear in the stool.
- Enterobiasis
  — The entire life cycle takes 2 to 4 weeks.
- Ascariasis
  — It takes 2 months for the rhabditiform larva to develop into a mature adult worm.
  — Travel from the intestine through the lungs and back to the intestine can take 5 to 14 days.
  — The entire life cycle in humans, from ingestion to egg production, takes 60 to 70 days.
- Hookworm
  — Eggs are produced 4 to 6 weeks after initial skin contact.
- Strongyloidiasis
  — One month from the time of infection to the time eggs are passed

Clinical Manifestations

TRICHURIASIS
- Asymptomatic in most cases, with low worm burden
- Heavy infection, anemia, and diarrhea or dysentery
- On occasion, patients will have epigastric or right lower quadrant pains.
- Rectal prolapse
- Malnutrition, leading to growth retardation

ENTEROBIASIS
- Pruritus in perineal region
- Ectopic migration leads to appendicitis or salpingitis.

ASCARIASIS
- Cough and shortness of breath may occur during the pulmonary migration phase of the embryo (Loeffler's syndrome).
- Malabsorption may occur with large worm burdens.

Roundworms, Intestinal

- At times, the worms may lead to intestinal obstruction, with pain and vomiting.
- *Ascaris* has also been known to migrate into the biliary system, leading to cholangitis and, on rare occasions, obstructive jaundice.
- Twenty percent of biliary tract obstructions in the Philippines is due to *Ascaris* infections.

HOOKWORM

- Patients notice a vesicular or pustular rash at the site of skin contact (usually the hands or feet). The rash is very pruritic. Migration through the lungs causes wheezing and cough.
- The major manifestation is iron-deficiency anemia, which can be severe. Pica may be a manifestation of the iron-deficiency state.
- Patients with hookworm in the gastrointestinal tract are often asymptomatic. On occasion, diarrhea and malabsorption can occur. At times, abdominal pain is noted.

STRONGYLOIDIASIS

- A pruritic papular rash is present during skin invasion.
- Cough and wheezing occur during pulmonary migration.
- Abdominal pain and diarrhea are common with intestinal infection. Nausea, vomiting, and weight loss also occur.
- A hyperinfection syndrome seen in immunocompromised patients can produce pulmonary infiltrates with respiratory failure, or sepsis due to microperforation of the intestine secondary to larval migration.

Diagnosis

- Trichuriasis
  —In heavy infection, patients will shed some 30,000 eggs per gram of feces. Feces should be evaluated for characteristic ova (50–54 × 22 μm). Patients may have a low albumin value.

DIFFERENTIAL DIAGNOSIS
Appendicitis or Amoebic Dysentery

- Enterobiasis
  —The cellophane tape test can be performed, looking for eggs.
- Ascariasis
  —Analysis of the feces will reveal the eggs.
  —Eosinophilia is noted during the pulmonary stage of the illness.
  —X-rays with contrast may reveal the worms within the intestine.
- Hookworm
  —Diagnosis is made by stool analysis.
  —Eosinophilia is common during the migration phase.
  —Severe iron-deficiency anemia occurs with worm burdens of over 500. The average blood loss is 0.03 to 0.15 mL/d per day.
- Strongyloidiasis
  —Eosinophilia is noted in most cases.

Treatment

- Trichuriasis
  —Albendazole 400 mg orally one dose, or mebendazole 100 mg orally tid for 3 days
- Enterobiasis
  —Albendazole 400 mg orally one dose, with repeat dose in 2 weeks; or mebendazole 100 mg orally one dose, with repeat in 2 weeks
  —*Alternative*: pyrantel pamoate 11 mg/kg every day for 3 days
- Ascariasis
  —Albendazole 400 mg orally one dose, or mebendazole 100 mg orally for 3 days
  —*Alternative*: pyrantel pamoate 11 mg/kg for 1 day. With intestinal obstruction or ectopic disease in the biliary tract, use piperazine citrate 75 mg/kg once a day for 2 days.
- Hookworm
  —Albendazole 400 mg one dose, repeated in 2 weeks; or mebendazole 100 mg orally one dose, repeated in 2 weeks
  —*Alternative*: pyrantel pamoate 11 mg/kg every day for 3 days
- Strongyloidiasis
  —Ivermectin 200 μg/kg/d for 2 days, or albendazole 400 mg every day for 3 days
  —*Alternative*: thiabendazole 25 mg/kg orally bid for 2 days. Hyperinfection cases should be treated with thiabendazole for 7 to 10 days

COMPLICATIONS

- Trichuriasis
  —Patients may develop painful prolapse of the rectum in heavy worm infections.
- Enterobiasis
  —Ectopic disease can occur in the female genital tract, ear, nose, and abdominal cavity.
- Hookworm
  —Infection can lead to severe iron-deficiency anemia, malabsorption, and failure to thrive.
- Strongyloidiasis
  —Patients with immunodeficiency and AIDS may have hyperinfection syndrome. Patients may have massive infection of the lungs, with infiltrates and respiratory failure.
  —Abdominal pain is noted, and patients may have sepsis (often with multiple bacteria) due to microperforations of the intestine by the larvae.

Follow-Up

- Enterobiasis
  —Patients must wash their hands thoroughly; bed sheets and clothing must be properly cleaned.
  —Fingernails must be kept cut, and gloves are recommended.
  —At times, all family members should be treated.
- Other roundworm infections
  —Follow-up stool analysis is often needed to be sure the worm has been eradicated or the patient has not been reinfected. In addition, some patients may have more than one species of roundworm present in the gut at the same time.

PREVENTION

Good hygiene is needed to avoid contact with soil contaminated with human feces. Children should wear shoes to prevent hookworm infection. Most roundworm infections are present in humans only.

Selected Readings

Gompels MM, Todd J, Peters BS, et al. Disseminated strongyloidiasis in AIDS: Uncommon but important. *AIDS* 1991;5:329.

Khuroo MS. Ascariasis. *Gastroenterol Clin North Am* 1996;25:553–557.

Mahmoud AAF. Strongyloidiasis. *Clin Infect Dis* 1996;23:949–952.

Rubella (German Measles)

Basics

DEFINITION
Rubella, or German measles, is an enveloped RNA virus of the togavirus family.

ETIOLOGY
- Rubella is spread as an upper respiratory infection.
- It is a childhood disease, with a peak incidence between the ages of 5 and 14 years.
- The disease is mild in nature, but it can be devastating to the fetus *in utero*.
- The risk of developing congenital rubella is greatest in the first 16 weeks of gestation. The mother may be asymptomatic.
- Disease in the fetus or neonate can be transient, permanent, or delayed.
- Infants with congenital rubella shed virus for as long as 2 years after birth.

EPIDEMIOLOGY
- Rubella is found worldwide.
- Since 1969, when the vaccine for rubella became available, it has become a rare disease.
- In areas where vaccination is not adhered to, the disease is often seen in young adults.
- In the United States, disease is seen in groups of people who are unvaccinated (e.g., the Amish) or in people who immigrate from developing countries.

Risk Factors
The greatest risk factor is not having been vaccinated for this disease.

Incubation
Incubation is from 2 to 3 weeks.

Clinical Manifestations

- Patients note a mild, nonspecific upper respiratory infection syndrome with fevers and coryza.
- After this acute phase, patients may have red macules on the soft palate, followed by a morbilliform rash on the face, often starting in the posterior auricular region. This spreads down over the entire body over the next 2 days and coalesces. The rash may be pruritic. Lymphadenopathy in the postauricular and occipital regions is common early in the infection.
- Following the rash, the patient may develop arthralgias, which last 5 to 10 days or longer.

CONGENITAL RUBELLA
- Manifestations of congenital rubella syndrome, which may be progressive over the first 5 years of life, include the following:
  - Stillbirth
  - Growth retardation
  - Mental retardation
  - Deafness
  - Cataracts
  - Retinopathy
  - Patent ductus arteriosus
  - Pulmonary artery hypoplasia
  - Hepatosplenomegaly
  - Diabetes
  - Thyroid disorders

Diagnosis

Diagnosis is made on clinical grounds; a high index of suspicion is needed.

DIFFERENTIAL DIAGNOSIS
- Enterovirus
- Parvovirus B19
- HIV
- Measles
- Scarlet fever
- Drug reactions

Rubella (German Measles)

LABORATORY

- The white blood cell count may be low, with increased atypical lymphocytes.
- Cultures of the throat or nasopharynx can be performed in some laboratories.
- Serology is used most often for diagnosis.
- IgM antibodies can be detected a few days into the illness and for up to 1 month following the rash.
- False-positives may be noted for most serologic tests.
- A PCR assay for detection of viral RNA in amniotic fluid is available.

Treatment

There is no treatment for rubella or congenital rubella.

COMPLICATIONS

- Congenital rubella is a serious multisystem disease, and the option of therapeutic abortion should be considered when a pregnant woman develops disease; a firm and rapid diagnosis is needed.
- Deafness is the most common complication.

Follow-Up

- Children with the congenital rubella syndrome require close follow-up by pediatric specialists.
- In addition, when hospitalized, patients need to be isolated until the virus is no longer being shed.

PREVENTION

- Live attenuated vaccine was licensed in 1969.
- At present, vaccine is given twice in childhood as a measles–mumps–rubella vaccine: at age 1 year, and again when starting school, at age 4 to 6 years.
- Serologic screening should be done for women prior to marriage and at the first prenatal visit.
- If the prenatal serology reveals no history of previous infection or immunization, the patient should be checked again after delivery and revaccinated if it still negative.
- The vaccine is not given to seronegative pregnant women.
- The vaccine is safe for HIV-positive women, but it should not be given to women on chemotherapy or those having bone marrow transplants.
- Patients with rubella should be isolated for up to 1 week after the rash appears.

Selected Readings

Centers for Disease Control and Prevention. Increase in rubella and congenital rubella—United States. *MMWR Morbid Mortal Wkly Rep* 1991;40:93–99.

Chantler JK, Ford DK, Tingle AJ. Persistent rubella infection and rubella-associated arthritis. *Lancet* 1982;1:1323–1325.

Fleet WF, Benz EW, Karzon DT, et al. Fetal consequences of maternal rubella immunization. *JAMA* 1974;227:621.

Levin MJ, Oxman MN, Moore MG, et al. Diagnosis of congenital rubella in utero. *N Engl J Med* 1974;290:1187.

Scabies

Basics

DEFINITION
- Parasitic infection of the skin
- Transmitted by close personal contact, sexual and nonsexual

ETIOLOGY
- *Sarcoptes scabiei* (variety hominis)

EPIDEMIOLOGY
Incidence
- Worldwide, more frequent in the tropics
- In United States, most common in children
- Two percent to 5% of dermatology visits
- Mostly person-to-person transmission

Risk Factors
- Contact with infected person
- Less common in the elderly
- Frequent nosocomial infections
- HIV, more severe and in skin cleavage lines

Incubation
- Four to 6 weeks for symptoms to develop, but highly variable

Clinical Manifestations

SYMPTOMS AND SIGNS
- Itching, especially at night or when hot
- Scratch marks, erythematous papules, linear burrows
- Marks found on fingers, interdigital areas, wrists, penis, scrotum, buttocks, periumbilical skin, pelvic girdle, extensor aspects of elbows, feet, ankles, and axillae
- A secondary bacterial skin infection may be present.
- HIV or immunosuppressed patients: atypical crusted (Norwegian) scabies

Diagnosis

- Based on clinical manifestations and microscopic examination of skin for presence of mites, mite eggs, or feces in a person complaining of pruritus and rash

LABORATORY
- Microscopic examination of skin scrapings

Scabies

TESTING PROCEDURES

- Use a needle or blade to scrape skin from linear burrows on interdigital areas, wrists, ankles, or penis.
- Suspend the specimen in immersion oil.
- Cover with a glass coverslip.
- Examine under a high, dry microscope lens.

Treatment

MAIN TREATMENT

- Permethrin 5% (30-g cream).
  —Apply it once from the neck down; wash it off after 8 to 14 hours.
- Lindane 1% (30-g cream or 1-oz lotion)
  —Apply it once from neck down; wash after 8 hours.
  —Lindane is contraindicated after bathing, in pregnant/lactating women, and in children under the age of 2 years.
- Decontaminate clothing and bed linens used within 48 hours of onset of symptoms by machine washing and drying in a hot temperature or by dry cleaning.
- Treat all close personal or household contacts of patients.

SEX PARTNERS

- Avoid direct contact with an infected person.
- Treat all sexual partners of the patient who have had contact within 1 month of the patient's onset of symptoms.

COMPLICATIONS

N/A

Follow-Up

- Itching may continue several weeks after treatment and after killing all mites and ova.
- Treat with topical corticosteroids and antihistamines to relieve itching.
- Retreat with the main treatment if live mites are observed.

PREVENTION

- Observe safe-sex precautions.
- Avoid contact with an infected person.

Selected Readings

Angel TA, Nigro J, Levy ML. Infestations in the pediatric patient. *Pediatr Clin North Am* 2000;47(4):921–935, viii.

Burkhart CG, Burkhart CN, Burkhart KM. An epidemiologic and therapeutic reassessment of scabies. *Cutis* 2000;65(4):233–240.

Chosidow O. Scabies and pediculosis. *Lancet* 2000;355(9206):819–826.

Scarlet Fever

Basics

DEFINITION
- Rash produced by erythrogenic toxin of group A *Streptococcus* during a typical case of pharyngitis

ETIOLOGY
- Pyrogenic exotoxin or erythrogenic toxin A, B, C at times is produced by group A *Streptococcus*.
- The initial infection is often pharyngitis; however, skin infections may produce the syndrome.

EPIDEMIOLOGY
- Scarlet fever often occurs in children ages 2 to 10 years. It is rare in adults.
- The epidemiology is similar to that of streptococcal pharyngitis.

Incubation
- Incubation of streptococcal pharyngitis is approximately 2 to 4 days.
- Rash occurs on the second day of illness.

Clinical Manifestations

- Patients have pharyngitis or tonsillitis, with exudate and petechia over the soft palate.
- Rash begins on the neck and upper chest and spreads over the body. Hands and feet are spared.
- When the rash is present on the face, it spares the area around the lips.
- Rash is erythematous and blanches with pressure.
- Petechiae may be present.
- Pastia's lines are linear areas of deeper erythema (confluent areas of petechia) around skin folds.
- Occasionally, a sandpaper texture is noted over the rash.
- A red "strawberry" tongue is noted in some patients.
- Rash lasts 6 to 9 days.
- Desquamation occurs when the rash fades, and can last for weeks.

Scarlet Fever

- Desquamation starts on the face and progresses down the trunk.
- Desquamation occurs on the hands and feet last.

Diagnosis

- Clinical diagnosis in a patient with culture-positive *Streptococcus* pharyngitis
- Serology may help to make the diagnosis.

LABORATORY

- Leukocytosis can be present during the acute stages of illness.
- Eosinophilia of 5% to 10% is present during the desquamative phase.

DIFFERENTIAL DIAGNOSIS

- Viral rash
- Drug rash
- Toxic shock syndrome
- Kawasaki syndrome
- Sunburn

Treatment

- Antibiotics directed against *Streptococcus*
- For pharyngitis, penicillin for 10 days or erythromycin for 10 days is sufficient.

COMPLICATIONS

- There are no long-term consequences of scarlet fever; however, acute rheumatic fever can occur after any streptococcal pharyngitis.
- Severe illness leading to death is very rare if antibiotics are given early in the disease.

Follow-Up

- None needed

PREVENTION

Early treatment of streptococcal pharyngitis may abort scarlet fever.

Selected Readings

Chiesa C, Pacifico L, Nanni F, et al. Recurrent attacks of scarlet fever. *Arch Pediatr Adolesc Med* 1994;148(6):656–660.

Duncan CJ, Duncan SR, Scott S. The dynamics of scarlet fever epidemics in England and Wales in the 19th century. *Epidemiol Infect* 1996;117(3):493–499.

Schistosomiasis

Basics

DEFINITION
Schistosomiasis is one of the most widespread parasitic infections in humans. Humans are the principal hosts for a number of blood flukes of the class Trematoda. *Schistosoma mansoni, Schistosoma japonicum, Schistosoma mekongi, Schistosoma haematobium,* and *Schistosoma intercalatum* make up the group that infects humans.

ETIOLOGY
- Human schistosomiasis occurs in about 200 million people worldwide.
- The disease is present in freshwater areas of Africa, Asia, and South America.
- Method of transmittal:
  —Worms are about 1 to 2 cm in length and are of separate sex. It is estimated that the worm can survive for as long as 30 years.
  —*S. mansoni, S. japonicum,* and *S. mekongi* worms live in the terminal venules of the portal and mesenteric blood vessels.
  —*S. haematobium* lives within the vesical plexus around the bladder.
  —Half of the eggs pass through the bladder wall or the intestinal wall, out into the environment.
  —The remainder of the eggs stay locally or pass along the blood vessels.
  —Once eggs are passed into fresh water, they develop into motile miracidia that live within snails.
  —After 4 to 6 weeks, the miracidia evolve into cercariae, by which they can pass into the water and infect humans.
  —Infection in humans occurs through the skin, where the cercariae then migrate to the liver.
  —After 6 weeks of development, the adult worm descends into the portal veins or the vesical plexus.

EPIDEMIOLOGY
- The life cycle of this organism depends on the population of snails within fresh water.
- *S. mansoni* is present in Africa, South America, many islands in the Caribbean, and the Middle East, especially in the Nile Valley.
- *S. japonicum* is present in China.
- *S. mekongi* is present in Laos and Kampuchea in Southeast Asia.
  S. haematobium occurs in the Middle East and in parts of Africa.
- *S. intercalatum* occurs in Africa.

Clinical Manifestations

- A papular skin rash, lasting 24 to 48 hours, occurs in the location of the skin penetration by the cercariae.
- Four to 8 weeks after infection, patients develop fevers associated with chills, headaches, and cough. This occurs during oviposition and is known as Katayama fever. It occurs due to the antigenic stimulation produced by the laying of the eggs, and resembles serum sickness.
- Symptoms regress after 2 to 4 weeks.
- During the chronic phase, which may last many years, patients may note abdominal pain and diarrhea.
- Over years, eggs that pass through the liver lead to granulomata formation and portal hypertension, and liver enlargement.
- Over many years, patients develop decompensated liver disease, ascites, and death due to liver failure or due to variceal bleeding.
- Eggs that bypass the liver in patients with portal hypertension can lodge in the lungs and produce pulmonary hypertension.
- Patients with *S. haematobium* pass eggs into the genitourinary system. Reaction to the eggs can lead to urinary obstruction, bladder dysfunction, and hematuria. Renal failure may occur as a late event.

Schistosomiasis

- Eggs of *S. japonicum* can pass into vessels of the brain, causing seizures of vessels, or into the spinal cord, causing transverse myelitis.

Diagnosis

LABORATORY

- Eggs can be isolated from the feces or urine of infected patients.
- Serologic tests are available to diagnose light infections.
- Liver function tests are frequently normal.
- Eosinophilia is observed in most cases.
- Anemia due to chronic blood loss is mild.

IMAGING

- Ultrasound
  —May reveal periportal fibrosis and hepatosplenomegaly
  —May reveal hydroureter and hydronephrosis

DIFFERENTIAL DIAGNOSIS

- Visceral larva migrans
- Paragonimus
- Clonorchis
- Visceral leishmaniasis

Treatment

- Praziquantel 20 mg/kg twice per day in 4-hour intervals for 1 day for *S. mansoni* and *S. haematobium*
- Praziquantel 20 mg/kg three times per day in 4-hour intervals for 1 day for *S. mekongi* and *S. japonica*

ALTERNATIVE TREATMENT

- Metrifonate 10 mg/kg orally every 14 days for three doses
- Oxamniquine 15 mg/kg orally twice daily for 2 days

COMPLICATIONS

- It is postulated that chronic infection with *S. haematobium* leads to bladder cancer.
- Colonic polyposis may be caused by infection with *S. mansoni*.
- Periportal hepatic fibrosis may occur due to granulomata formation within the portal veins.
- Eggs can travel through Batson's plexus into the central nervous system and lead to myelitis.

Follow-Up

Following treatment, patients should be observed for ongoing liver disease and genitourinary dysfunction.

PREVENTION

- Improve sanitation so that eggs do not pass into areas where snails reside.
- Reduce snail populations with molluscicides.
- Prohibit swimming in contaminated waters.

Selected Readings

Doherty JF, Moody AH, Wright SG. Katayama fever: An acute manifestation of schistosomiasis. *BMJ* 1996;313:1071–1072.

Siongok TKA, Mahmoud AAF, Ouma JH, et al. Morbidity in schistosomiasis mansoni in relation to intensity of infection. Study of a community in Machakos, Kenya. *Am J Trop Med Hyg* 1976;25:273.

Septic Arthritis

Basics

DEFINITION
- Joint inflammation caused by various infectious agents: viruses, bacteria, mycobacteria, and fungi.

ETIOLOGY
Bacterial
- Hematogenous spread of bacteria, especially in cases of endocarditis
- *Staphylococcus aureus* leads to both monoarticular and polyarticular disease.
- Group A *Streptococcus* often leads to monoarticular disease.
- Group B *Streptococcus* is seen in diabetics and in elderly patients.
- Gram-negative organisms are seen in elderly patients who may have had an episode of bacteremia.
- *Neisseria gonorrhoeae* is the most common cause of septic arthritis in young adults.
  —Patients often present with a monoarticular process.
  —Arthralgias without frank arthritis are seen in the disseminated gonococcal syndrome.
- Lyme arthritis must be considered in patients who have had a history of tick bites and who live in endemic areas.
- Chronic monoarticular arthritis can be seen with tuberculosis, atypical mycobacterial infections, and chronic fungal infections such as *Coccidioides immitis* and *Sporothrix schenckii*.
- Predisposing conditions associated with septic arthritis include the following:
  —Arthritis
  —Trauma
  —Intraarticular injections
  —Joint surgery

Viral
- Hepatitis B virus
- Rubella
- Mumps
- Varicella
- Rubeola
- Adenovirus
- Parvovirus B19

EPIDEMIOLOGY
This is a diverse group of diseases seen in patients from childhood to old age.

RISK FACTORS
- Prior arthritic condition
- Trauma or animal bites
- Diabetes
- Cancer
- Immunosuppression

Clinical Manifestations

- Pain with limitation of joint motion
- Fevers
- Swelling with effusions and erythema and warmth
- Knee joint affected most, followed by hip and shoulder joints
- Infection of joints in the wrist associated with tenosynovitis suggests gonorrhea.
- Solitary joint infection in the hand may be the result of cat or other animal bites.
- Infection of the sternoclavicular of sacroiliac joints is seen in intravenous drug users.
  —*Pseudomonas* is often isolated.
- Children often present with fevers and one affected joint.
- Viral etiology often affects multiple joints.

Diagnosis

DIFFERENTIAL DIAGNOSIS
- Acute arthritis
- Trauma
- Crystal induced (pseudogout)
- Gout

Septic Arthritis

LABORATORY

- Elevated erythrocyte sedimentation rate
- Normal white blood cell count in many infections in adults
- Anemia if infection is chronic
- Turbid synovial fluid with leukocyte count in synovial fluid greater than 50,000 cells/mm^3, with greater than 75% of the cells polymorphonuclear in origin
- Synovial fluid with Gram stains revealing organisms in one-third of patients
- Synovial fluid cultures are positive in 90% of patients.
- Blood cultures are positive for the organism causing the septic arthritis in one-third of patients.
- Synovial fluid cultures are positive for the organism in 90% of patients.
- X-rays show
  —Periarticular soft-tissue swelling
  —Fat-pad edema
  —Joint-space widening or narrowing
  —Bone destruction is rarely noted, except when the infection is chronic.
- Positive triple-phase bone scan
  —*Note*: The scan can reveal a probable osteomyelitis, but it cannot resolve whether the process is infectious (neoplastic or traumatic) or whether the process has entered the joint.
- Computed tomography and magnetic resonance imaging are helpful in revealing joint effusions.

Treatment

- Joint aspiration for recurrent effusions for the first 5 to 7 days, if necessary. This is a mainstay of therapy.
- Surgical drainage must be considered if effusions persist for over 1 week.
- For *acute monoarticular arthritis* or for septic arthritis in a *patient with rheumatoid arthritis*:
  —If Gram stain suggests *S. aureus*: nafcillin or a second-generation cephalosporin empirically until cultures are available
  —If Gram stains are negative: a third-generation cephalosporin such as ceftriaxone or cefotaxime
- For *gonococcal* arthritis
  —Ceftriaxone for 7 to 10 days
- For *animal-bite* infections
  —Ampicillin/sulbactam
- For *Lyme* arthritis
  —Doxycycline for 1 month or ceftriaxone for 14 days

COMPLICATIONS

- Long-term complications
  —Worsening of arthritis
  —Joint-space narrowing
  —Articular dysfunction
- In adults, chronic disability occurs in 50% of patients.

Follow-Up

- Patients should have follow-up with physical therapy.
- Any recurrence of effusions should be tapped and recurrent arthritis ruled out,

PREVENTION

There is no way to prevent septic arthritis.

Selected Readings

Bower AC, Septic arthritis. *Radiol Clin North Am* 1996;34:293–309.

Goldenberg DL, Reed JI. Bacterial arthritis. *N Engl J Med* 1985;312:746–771.

Smith JW, Piercy EA. Infectious arthritis. *Clin Infect Dis* 1995;20:225–231.

Shigellosis

Basics

DEFINITION
Shigellosis is an enteral infection of variable severity, caused by the bacterium *Shigella*, which is characterized by diarrhea, fever, nausea, cramps, and tenesmus.

ETIOLOGY
- *Shigella* species are small, gram-negative rods that are members of the family Enterobacteriaceae. They are nonmotile and nonencapsulated.
- The approximately 40 serotypes of *Shigella* are divided into four groups, depending on serologic similarity and fermentation reaction: group A (*Shigella dysenteriae*), group B (*Shigella flexneri*), group C (*Shigella boydii*), and group D (*Shigella sonnei*).
- People can carry *Shigella* in their feces without having any symptoms.
- *S. boydii*, *S. dysenteriae*, and *S. flexneri* occur mostly in developing countries. *S. sonnei* is the most common, and *S. dysenteriae* is the least common in developed countries, but it may be imported by travelers.
- As few as 10 to 100 organisms can cause infection, enabling person-to-person transmission where hygienic conditions are compromised.

EPIDEMIOLOGY

Incidence
- It is estimated that *Shigella* spp infect over 200 million people and cause 650,000 deaths each year worldwide.
- *Shigella* is distributed worldwide and is the typical cause of inflammatory dysentery, responsible for 5% to 10% of diarrheal illness in many areas.
- Secondary attack rates in households may be as high as 40%.
- Direct spread is by the fecal–oral route; indirect spread is by contaminated food and inanimate objects. Water-borne disease is unusual. Flies serve as mechanical vectors.
- Epidemics occur most frequently in overcrowded populations with inadequate sanitation.
- Convalescents and subclinical carriers may be significant sources of infection. Infection imparts little or no immunity, because reinfection with the same strain is possible.
- *S. sonnei* is a common cause of gastroenteritis, accounting for 10,262 (73%) of the 14,071 laboratory-confirmed *Shigella* infections reported to Centers for Disease Control in 1996.

Risk Factors
- Those at greater risk include children in daycare centers, foreign travelers to certain countries, and persons living in institutions.
- Outbreaks commonly occur in prisons, institutions for children, childcare centers, psychiatric hospitals, crowded camps, and homosexual groups.
- The incubation period usually ranges from 12 hours to 4 days (usually 1 to 3 days) and may last 4 to 7 days.
- It is communicable during acute infection and while the infectious agent is present in feces (usually no longer than 4 weeks).
- Asymptomatic carriers may transmit infection.
- Two-thirds of the cases and most of the deaths are in children under 10 years. The disease is rare in infants under 6 months of age.

Clinical Manifestations

- Symptoms include the following:
  - Diarrhea (may be watery or contain blood, mucus, and pus)
  - Fever
  - Stomach cramps and/or
  - Nausea and/or
  - Vomiting
- Severe cases may cause dehydration (loss of fluids) or convulsions (in young children).
- In children, onset is sudden, with fever, irritability or drowsiness, anorexia, nausea or vomiting, diarrhea, abdominal pain and distention, and tenesmus. Within 3 days, blood, pus and mucus appear in the stools. The number of stools generally increases rapidly up to 20 per day, and weight loss and dehydration become severe.
- Though adults may present without fever, with nonbloody and nonmucoid diarrhea, and with little or no tenesmus, the onset of illness may be characterized by episodes of gripping abdominal pain, urgency to defecate, and passage of formed feces initially. These periods recur with increasing severity and frequency. Diarrhea becomes marked, with soft or liquid stools containing mucus, pus and, often, blood.
- Other more common extraintestinal manifestations of shigellosis include headache, meningismus, and even seizures, especially in children.
- Findings on physical examination are nonspecific and include a variable degree of systemic toxemia, fever, abdominal tenderness, especially over the lower abdominal quadrants, and hyperactive bowel sounds. Rectal examination or proctoscopy is generally painful. Sigmoidoscopy reveals a friable, hyperemic rectal mucosa, increased mucus secretion, and areas of ecchymosis. Ulcerations of the rectal mucosa are seen after several days of illness.

Diagnosis

DIFFERENTIAL DIAGNOSIS
- In the most common form, watery diarrhea, the illness is indistinguishable from other bacterial, viral, and protozoan infections that induce secretory activity of intestinal epithelial cells.
- In patients who develop the acute form of bacillary dysentery (i.e., small-volume stools containing blood and mucus), the differential diagnosis includes invasive *Escherichia coli*, *Salmonella*, *Yersinia*, *Campylobacter*, and amebiasis.

LABORATORY
- The total white blood cell count demonstrates no consistent findings, although either leukopenia or brisk leukocytosis is seen on occasion.

Shigellosis

- In severe forms of the disease, a leukemoid reaction is seen. Thrombocytopenia also can be observed.
- Diarrhea usually causes isomotic dehydration with metabolic acidosis and significant potassium loss. Thirst from dehydration can lead to a proportionately excessive water intake, causing hypotonicity.
- Most people pass *Shigella* in their feces for 1 to 2 weeks (without treatment).

Treatment

MAIN TREATMENT

- In shigellosis, as in any diarrheal illness, proper fluid replacement is the mainstay of treatment. In addition, the symptoms and shedding of *Shigella* can be significantly reduced by early treatment with an absorbable antimicrobial agent to which the *Shigella* strain is sensitive.
- The patient's progress should be followed until the stools are consistently free of Shigella.
- Antibiotics can be prescribed to shorten both the duration of illness and the length of time bacteria are passed in the stool. Ciprofloxacin 500 mg PO or norfloxacin 400 mg PO bid for three doses is most commonly used.
- Loperamide decreases the number of unformed stools and shortens the duration of diarrhea in dysentery caused by *Shigella* in adults with mild to moderate disease, but it must be used in conjunction with an antibiotic.

ALTERNATIVE TREATMENT

- Azithromycin (500 mg of azithromycin on day 1, followed by 250 mg once daily for 4 days) is effective in the treatment of moderate to severe shigellosis caused by multidrug-resistant *Shigella* strains.
- Trimethoprim–sulfamethoxazole, double-strength, bid PO for three doses is another alternative, although many strains are resistant.

TREATMENT FAILURE

Shigellosis imported from South and East Asia is often drug resistant. A history of international travel is the strongest risk factor for *Shigella* infection resistant to trimethoprim–sulfamethoxazole and ampicillin.

COMPLICATIONS

- The severity of the infection depends on the age and state of nutrition of the patient and the serotype of *Shigella*; for example, many infections with *S. sonnei* result in a short clinical course, and a very low case fatality rate. In contrast, *S. dysenteriae* is associated with serious disease and a high case fatality rate.
- Rectal prolapse and fecal incontinence may result from severe tenesmus.
- Intestinal obstruction, which occurs in about 3% of patients, is a poor prognostic sign, not infrequently associated with death or the development of haemolytic–uremic syndrome (HUS).
- HUS is a well-described complication of *S. dysenteriae* type I infection in childhood.

Follow-Up

- Significant dehydration and electrolyte loss with circulatory collapse and death are limited mainly to infants less than 2 year of age and to debilitated adults.
- If untreated, a child may die in the first 12 days; if the child survives, acute symptoms subside by the second week.

PREVENTION

- Symptomatic contacts of shigellosis patients should be excluded from food handling and the care of children or patients until investigated.
- Stool cultures from contacts need only be confined to food-handlers and those in situations in which the spread of infection is particularly likely (childcare centers, hospitals, institutions).
- Infected food-handlers and childcare workers, children attending childcare, and patient care providers should stay away from their regular activities until they have completed at least 5 days of an appropriate antibiotic treatment or until two stool samples have been tested and are negative for *Shigella*.
- It is important that thorough handwashing and hand-cleaning procedures be followed in child-care centers to control the spread of bacteria.
- One study reported a 23% reduction in diarrheal illness associated with successful fly control.

Selected Readings

Anonymous. From the Centers for Disease Control and Prevention. Outbreaks of *Shigella sonnei* infection associated with eating fresh parsley—United States and Canada, July–August 1998. *JAMA* 1999;281:1785–1787.

Bloom PD, MacPhail AP, Klugman K, et al. Haemolytic–uraemic syndrome in adults with resistant *Shigella dysenteriae* type I [Letter]. *Lancet* 1994;344:206.

DuPont HL. *Shigella* species (bacillary dysentery). In: Mandell GL, Bennett JE, Dolin R, eds. *Principles and practice of infectious diseases*. New York: Churchill Livingstone, 1995:2033–2039.

Hossain S, Biswas R, Kabir I, et al. Single-dose vitamin A treatment in acute shigellosis in Bangladeshi children: Randomised double blind controlled trial. *BMJ* 1998;316:422–426.

Khan WA, Seas C, Dhar U, et al. Treatment of shigellosis: V. Comparison of azithromycin and ciprofloxacin. A double-blind, randomized, controlled trial. *Ann Intern Med* 1997;126:697–703.

Levine MM, Cohen D, Green M, et al. Fly control and shigellosis [Letter]. *Lancet* 1999;353:1020.

Murphy GS, Bodhidatta L, Echeverria P, et al. Ciprofloxacin and loperamide in the treatment of bacillary dysentery. *Ann Intern Med* 1993;118:582–586.

Salam MA, Khan WA, Dhar U, et al. Vitamin A for treating shigellosis. Study did not prove benefit [Letter]. *BMJ* 1999;318:939–940.

Salam MA, Seas C, Khan WA, et al. Treatment of shigellosis: IV. Cefixime is ineffective in shigellosis in adults. *Ann Intern Med* 1995;123:505–508.

Sinusitis

Basics

DEFINITION
- Sinusitis is inflammation of the paranasal sinuses. It is classified as acute, subacute, and chronic, depending on duration of infection (anatomically, subdivided into maxillary, ethmoid, frontal, and sphenoid sinusitis).
  - Acute sinusitis: characterized by symptoms and signs of sinus inflammation lasting less than 2 weeks.
  - Subacute sinusitis: inflammation lasting 2 weeks or longer and less than 3 months
  - Chronic sinusitis: duration of the infection 3 months or longer
  - Recurrent sinusitis: the acute exacerbations of chronic sinusitis or relapses in inadequately treated patients
- Other special subgroups of sinus infection are *nosocomial* sinusitis and *fungal* sinusitis.

ETIOLOGY
- Most acute sinusitis cases are thought to be bacterial complications of viral upper respiratory infections, which frequently produce conditions in the ostiomeatal area and sinuses that favor a secondary bacterial infection. Five percent to 10% of cases of acute maxillary sinusitis are originated from a dental source.
- In chronic sinus disease, the prolonged infection leads to irreversible changes in the mucosa of the sinus, resulting in a loss of the sinus capacity for self-cleansing. Thus, sterility is no longer maintained in the sinus cavity.

Bacteriology
- Acute sinusitis (community-acquired)
  - Bacteria: *Streptococcus pneumoniae* (~30%), *Haemophilus influenzae* (~20%), (nontypable strains). In children *Moraxella catarrhalis* is also important, accounting for approximately ~20% of cases (in adults, ~2%). In adults, gram-negative bacilli play a role (~9%), and anaerobes (~6%) are important causes in cases associated with dental infections. Rare causes are *Staphylococcus aureus* (~4%) and *Streptococcus pyogenes* (~2%).
  - Viruses: Rhinovirus, influenza virus, and parainfluenza virus are recovered alone or in combination with bacteria in one-fifth of the adult cases of acute sinusitis.
  - *Chlamydia pneumoniae* (strain TWAR) should be considered among the etiologic causes of community-acquired acute sinus infection.
- Subacute and recurrent sinusitis
  - The bacteria are similar to those for acute sinusitis, including anaerobes (*Peptostreptococcus*, *Fusobacterium*, *Bacteroides* spp, *Prevotella* spp, and *Porphyromonas* spp).
- Chronic sinusitis
  - Cultures of surgical specimens have grown a wide variety of gram-positive and gram-negative bacteria, which often represent colonization rather than infection.
- Nosocomial sinusitis
  - Gram-negative bacilli (~40%) (*Pseudomonas aeruginosa*, *Klebsiella pneumoniae*, *Enterobacter* spp, and *Proteus mirabilis*), *S. aureus* (~30%), and yeasts (~15%)
  - Often polymicrobic
- Fungal sinusitis
  - Categorized as noninvasive or invasive
    - The noninvasive is chronic, occurs in immunocompetent hosts, and has two forms: the noninvasive fungus sinus disease (fungus ball) and the allergic fungal sinusitis. *Aspergillus* spp and members of the zygomycosis group are the causes.
    - The invasive fungal sinusitis has a different presentation in immunocompetent and immunocompromised hosts. Zygomycetes (*Mucor* spp, *Rhizopus* spp), *Aspergillus* spp, and other fungi are the causes. In immunocompromised hosts, fungal sinusitis has an acute onset, but in immunocompetent hosts, the disease is slowly progressive.
- In patients with cystic fibrosis, *P. aeruginosa* is the most frequent isolate, and in patients with AIDS, *Legionella pneumophila* was also identified.

EPIDEMIOLOGY

Incidence and Prevalence
- Of the acute upper respiratory infections, 0.5% are complicated by acute sinusitis. It is most prevalent during the fall, winter, and spring months.
- The most common type is maxillary sinusitis.
- Predominant age: more common in adults than in children
- Predominant sex: occurs equally in males and females

Risk Factors
- Anatomic abnormalities (congenital choanal atresia, septal deviation, foreign bodies, tumors)
- Nasal allergic reactions
- Dental infections
- Barotrauma from deep diving or airplane travel
- Mucus abnormalities (e.g., cystic fibrosis)
- Granulomatous disease (e.g., Wegener's granulomatosis)
- Nasotracheal or nasogastric intubation: a major risk factor for nosocomial sinusitis
- Chemical irritants
- Immunodeficiency

Sinusitis

Clinical Manifestations

SYMPTOMS AND SIGNS

- Acute sinusitis
  - Persistence of upper respiratory symptoms (nasal congestion) longer than 7 to 10 days
  - Purulent nasal and postnasal discharge
  - Cough
  - Feeling of pressure over sinus areas
  - Fever (in one-half of the cases)
  - Headache, nasal obstruction, disorders of smell, nasal quality of the voice
  - Erythema and tenderness often present over the involved sinus
  - Pain over cheeks and upper teeth (maxillary sinusitis) worse with bending over
  - Pain over eyebrows (frontal sinusitis)
  - Pain retro-orbital, with radiation to the occiput
  - Pain over eyes, edema of the eyelids, excessive tearing (ethmoid sinusitis)
- Chronic sinusitis
  - Constant sinus pressure, nasal congestion, and postnasal drainage
  - Fever over 38°C is rare and may signify an acute exacerbation.
  - In acute exacerbations, also note a change in nasal drainage
- Nosocomial sinusitis
  - Often during the second week of hospitalization
  - Maxillary sinusitis and pansinusitis most common
  - Often unexplained fever in patients with indwelling nasal tubes
- Fungal sinusitis
  - Noninvasive disease
    - Fungus ball: Usually only one sinus is affected; it causes symptoms of obstruction.
  - Allergic fungal sinusitis: It is seen mainly in patients with a history of nasal polyps and asthma; it is characterized by extremely thick sinus mucus, "allergic mucin," a pale material containing eosinophils, Charcot-Leyden crystals, and rare fungal hyphae.
- Invasive fungal sinusitis
  - In immunocompromised hosts, it is a life-threatening infection. It affects more frequently diabetic patients with ketoacidosis, leukemic patients with neutropenia, transplant recipients, and patients under treatment with desferrioxamine. The affected patients have facial pain, fever, and, often, orbital cellulitis, and black eschars overlying necrotic tissue ("peanut butter–like appearance") may be seen in the nasal passages.
  - In immunocompetent hosts, it has a slowly progressive course; bone erosion may be present. In ethmoid and sphenoid sinuses, it may invade the orbital apex, causing chemosis, proptosis, and limitation of eye movements.

Diagnosis

- Acute sinusitis
  - History: In any acute upper respiratory illness that lasts longer than 7 to 10 days, the diagnosis of acute sinusitis should be considered.
  - Clinical examination: the finding of purulent nasal or postnasal secretions
  - Transillumination (maxillary and frontal sinuses): Complete opacification is good evidence of sinusitis. Normal light transmission is equally good evidence that no infection is present. Dullness indicates infection in only one-fourth of cases.
  - Four-view sinus x-rays are helpful: Radiologic opacity, an air–fluid level, and sinus mucosal thickening (4 mm or more) are suggestive of active infection.
  - A CT scan of the sinus is much more sensitive than routine radiography, particularly for ethmoid and sphenoid disease. CT often shows reversible acute changes in patients with the common cold. Subsequently, CT should not be used early (within 2 weeks of disease onset). It is especially helpful for detection of extension of the disease.
  - Laboratory findings: WBC may be elevated.
  - Pathologic findings: inflammation, edema of the sinus mucosal lining. An exudate from acutely infected sinuses contains polymorphonuclear leukocytes in concentrations greater than 5,000 cells/mm^3.
  - Sinus puncture for bacterial identification should be performed in patients with unusually severe sinusitis, those who have not responded to empiric antimicrobial therapy, those with severe immunosuppression, and those with nosocomial sinusitis when identity and antimicrobial sensitivity of the causative microorganism are unpredictable. (Most bacteria causing active sinus infection are present in titers of at least 100,000 CFU/mL.)
  - The differential diagnoses include common cold, allergic rhinitis, and vasomotor rhinitis.
- Chronic sinusitis
  - A sinus CT scan should be performed in all cases of chronic sinusitis to define the extent of disease and to exclude other diagnoses.
  - Endoscopy should be used for diagnosis (exclude other conditions, biopsy) and treatment (correction of obstruction in the ostiomeatal complex that is a major contributing factor to the development of chronic sinus disease).

Sinusitis

- —Pathologic findings: The normal ciliated epithelium is replaced by stratified squamous epithelium that may eventually fill the sinus lumen.
- —The differential diagnoses include foreign bodies, polyps, tumors, granulomatous disease (Wegener's granulomatosis, rhinoscleroma, midline granuloma), and fungus sinus disease.
- Fungus sinusitis
  - —Noninvasive disease: CT scan and histopathologic examination of sinus mucus
  - —Invasive fungus sinusitis: CT scan and histopathologic examination of the tissue

Treatment

ACUTE (BACTERIAL) SINUSITIS (COMMUNITY-ACQUIRED)

- The antimicrobial chemotherapy must be selected on an empirical basis, because, in every case, sinus puncture to determine a specific microbe is not indicated.
- Treatment should ideally cover all possible causes, but primarily, it should be effective against *S. pneumoniae* and *H. influenzae*.
- The recommended duration is 10 to 14 days.
- Drugs of choice
  - —Amoxicillin 40 mg/kg/d divided q8h, or 1 g tid in adults
  - —Amoxicillin-clavulanate: 40 mg/kg/d for amoxicillin component divided q8h, or 625 mg tid in adults
  - —Cefaclor: 40 mg/kg/d divided q8h, or 500 mg tid in adults
  - —Cefuroxime axetil: 30 mg/kg/d divided q12h, or 250 mg bid in adults
  - —Cefprozil: 30 mg/kg/d divided q12h, or 500 mg bid in adults
  - —Loracarbef: 30 mg/kg/d divided q12h, or 400 mg bid in adults
  - —Clarithromycin: 15 mg/kg/d divided q12h, or 500 mg bid in adults
  - —Azithromycin: 10 mg/kg qd on day 1 and then 5 mg/kg qd on days 2 to 5; in adults, 500 mg qd on day 1 and then 250 mg qd on days 2 to 5
  - —Trimethoprim-sulfamethoxazole (TMP/SMX): 8 mg TMP/kg/d divided q12h, or 160 mg TMP/800 mg SMX bid in adults
- Intravenous administration may be necessary in patients with severe infection and for those in whom intracranial extension is a consideration.
- In acute sinusitis associated with dental infection, the therapy also should cover anaerobes.
- Ancillary treatment: (1) oral decongestant, antihistamine; (2) topical and/or steroids not recommended unless there is evidence of allergic disease
- Surgical drainage is recommended only when there is evidence of extension to the orbit or intracranial sites.

SUBACUTE AND RECURRENT SINUSITIS

- Drugs of choice
  - —Amoxicillin-clavulanate: 40 mg/kg/d for amoxicillin component divided q8h, or 625 mg tid in adults
  - —One of the other antibiotics of the acute sinusitis plus either of the following:
    - —Metronidazole 15 to 35 mg/kg/d divided q8h, or 500 mg tid in adults
    - —Clindamycin 20 to 30 mg/kg/d divided q6h, or 600 mg tid in adults
- The duration is 4 to 6 weeks.
- If symptoms persists, sinus irrigation can be performed.

CHRONIC SINUSITIS

- Antibiotics usually are not effective. Antimicrobial therapy is needed in acute exacerbations (see above, Subacute and Recurrent Sinusitis).
- Because the primary problem is impaired drainage of the sinus cavity, the correction of obstruction in the ostiomeatal complex endoscopically or surgically is necessary.

NOSOCOMIAL SINUSITIS

- Removal of the nasotracheal or nasogastric tube and sinus aspiration for culture
- Initial broad-spectrum intravenous antimicrobial chemotherapy (imipenem or ceftazidime plus vancomycin or cefepime) should be adjusted on the basis of culture results.
- The patient may need fluconazole if yeast is revealed from Gram stain of aspirate.

Sinusitis

FUNGAL SINUS DISEASE

- Noninvasive disease: Treatment is surgical only, although some recommend the use of topical or systemic glucocorticoids to prevent recurrences.
- Invasive fungal sinusitis: surgical debridement of the involved sinus and prolonged therapy with amphotericin B. Follow-up CT and MRI should be used to evaluate the progression of the disease.

COMPLICATIONS

- Orbital cellulitis: usually secondary to ethmoid sinusitis. Intravenous antibiotic therapy should be started immediately, and if there is no improvement within 24 hours, the sinus should be drained.
- Frontal subperiosteal abscess (Pott's puffy tumor) from frontal sinusitis: The treatment is surgical drainage of the abscess and the frontal sinus and intravenous antibiotic therapy lasting 6 weeks.
- Intracranial complications (epidural abscess, subdural empyema, meningitis, cerebral abscess, dural vein thrombophlebitis)

Follow-Up

Review of the patient's health status is advisable 2 weeks after the discontinuation of treatment to detect cases of early-recurrence sinusitis.

PREVENTION

Efforts to decrease the time of the use of nasotracheal and nasogastric tubes reduce the incidence of nosocomial sinusitis.

Selected Readings

Caplan ES, Hoyt NJ. Nosocomial sinusitis. *JAMA* 1982;247:639–641.

Diament MJ. The diagnosis of sinusitis in infants and children: X-ray, computed tomography, and magnetic resonance imaging. *J Allergy Clin Immunol* 1992;90:442–444.

Gwaltney JM Jr, Phillips CD, Miller RD, et al. Computed tomographic study of the common cold. *N Engl J Med* 1994;330:25–30.

Gwaltney JM Jr, Scheld WM, Sande MA, et al. The microbial etiology and antimicrobial therapy of adults with acute community-acquired sinusitis: A fifteen-year experience at the University of Virginia and review of other selected studies. *J Allergy Clin Immunol* 1992;90:457–462.

Hahn DL, Dodge RW, Goubjatnikov R. Association of *Chlamydia pneumoniae* (strain TWAR) infection with wheezing, asthmatic bronchitis, and adult-onset asthma. *JAMA* 1991;266:225–230.

Lanza DC, Kennedy DW. Current concepts in the surgical management of chronic and recurrent acute sinusitis. *J Allergy Clin Immunol* 1992;90:505–511.

McGuirt WF, Harril JA. Paranasal sinus aspergillosis. *Laryngoscope* 1979;89:1563.

Spector SL. The role of allergy in sinusitis in adults. *J Allergy Clin Immunol* 1992;90:515–517.

Sporotrichosis

Basics

DEFINITION

Sporotrichosis is an endemic fungal infection caused by *Sporothrix schenckii*, and it occurs in four forms: lymphocutaneous, fixed cutaneous, cutaneous disseminated, and systemic. The most common clinical presentations are those of the lymphocutaneous or fixed cutaneous form.

ETIOLOGY

S. schenckii is a dimorphic fungus that, at room temperature, exists as branching hyphae, and in tissue, the organism exists as a yeast that is 4 to 6 μm in diameter, sometimes with a single bud or, infrequently, with multiple buds.

EPIDEMIOLOGY

Incidence

- Most case reports come from the tropical and subtropical regions of the Americas.
- Exposure to such plants as rosebushes, barberry, sphagnum moss, contaminated mine timbers, hay, and other sharp vegetation; or contact with horses, fish, birds, reptiles, cats, dogs, and rats is a possible source of sporotrichosis.
- An outbreak was associated with stored hay or hay bales harvested in the United States Plains states. Outbreaks are possible, given adequate intensity of exposure, and may be difficult to recognize because of the delayed presentation of clinical illness.

Risk Factors

- Cutaneous disease arises at sites of minor trauma and inoculation of the fungus into the skin. Patients with fixed cutaneous sporotrichosis usually live in endemic areas and have a high degree of immunity.

Lymphocutaneous sporotrichosis is more common among the following:
—Farmers
—Florists
—Gardeners
—Horticulturists
—Veterinarians (usually because of possible spread from cats)

- The extracutaneous and disseminated forms of the disease are uncommon and occur in immunocompromised individuals; exposure to plant matter may not precede the infection. Systemic sporotrichosis is more common among persons with the following:
—Alcoholism
—Diabetes mellitus
—Immunosuppression (due to steroid use, HIV, chemotherapy, etc.)
—Lymphoma or other malignancy
—Pulmonary tuberculosis
—Sarcoidosis
- Outbreaks of sporotrichosis have been reported. The most recent outbreak was traced to contaminated sphagnum moss originating in Wisconsin. Because this product was shipped to at least 15 states, people in many different areas of the country became infected and presented with typical manifestations of cutaneous sporotrichosis.

Clinical Manifestations

- After a variable incubation period, usually 1 to 12 weeks, a papular lesion develops and may change from red to violaceous. Ulceration follows, with discharge of a serosanguineous exudate. If the initial lesion remains the only one, the term *fixed* cutaneous or *plaque* sporotrichosis has been used. The solitary lesion can persist for decades without spread. Spontaneous resolution is uncommon.
- Secondary lesions develop proximally along lymphatic channels. These secondary lesions evolve in the same fashion as the primary lesion. Lymphadenopathy may develop.
- Once the skin has been inoculated, a papule will form that progresses to form a pustule and then a nodule with ragged undetermined borders and a central ulcer. The nodule is mobile and not tender unless it is secondarily infected with bacteria. With lymphatic spread, more proximal subcutaneous nodules will appear in a linear fashion. If not treated, secondary sporotrichosis nodules may be gummatous and may persist for months to years.
- In the cutaneous disseminated form, numerous crusted, necrotic, granulomatous, ulcerated papules and nodules are irregularly distributed over the body.
- Some patients present with involvement of a single joint, with an insidious onset without previous sporotrichosis at another site. The joint is swollen and painful on motion, an effusion is present, and, after weeks or months, a sinus tract may develop.
- Pulmonary infection results from inhalation or aspiration of the fungus, causing pneumonitis with fibrocavitary disease that progressively worsens.
- Dissemination of the infection may develop from the lymphocutaneous form or the fixed cutaneous form.

Diagnosis

DIFFERENTIAL DIAGNOSIS

- Cutaneous sporotrichosis can mimic infection due to nocardia, mycobacteria, leishmaniasis, lymphocutaneous disease due to *Staphylococcus aureus* or *Streptococcus pyogenes*, and other pathogens.
- The differential diagnosis of pulmonary sporotrichosis includes mycobacterial infections due to both *Mycobacterium tuberculosis* and other mycobacteria, histoplasmosis, and coccidioidomycosis.

LABORATORY

- For the diagnosis of cutaneous and systemic sporotrichosis, culture of biopsy material is preferred and is diagnostic when positive. However, repeated attempts at culture may have to be made.

Sporotrichosis

- Serologic assays remain in the research area and are of uncertain use in clinical practice.

DIAGNOSTIC/TESTING PROCEDURES

- The diagnosis is based on clinical findings, a history of exposure, and identification of the fungus in biopsy material.
- The number of yeast forms present in the skin is usually small, accounting for the relatively large number of biopsy specimens in which no organisms are detected. They can be stained with periodic acid–Schiff and Gomori-methenamine silver but are difficult to see on hematoxylin and eosin staining.
- The histopathologic findings of sporotrichosis include the identification of round to oval spores measuring 4 to 6 μm in diameter on periodic acid–Schiff stain; the spores stain stronger in the periphery of the lesion.

Treatment

MAIN TREATMENT

- Potassium iodide has been the mainstay of therapy over the years. Increasing numbers of drops of the drug are prescribed, up to a maximum of 120 per day.
- Therapy is begun with 5 to 10 drops taken orally three times per day. The dosage is gradually advanced to 25 to 40 drops three times per day (for children) or 40 to 50 drops three times per day (for adults).
- Typical toxic effects of the iodide include nausea, anorexia, excessive lacrimation, lacrimal gland and parotid gland enlargement, acneiform rashes, and gastrointestinal problems.

ALTERNATIVE TREATMENT

- Itraconazole has proved effective in the treatment of cutaneous sporotrichosis. In one study, the usual dose was 200 to 400 mg per day, and 27 patients received 30 courses of therapy. Nine of those patients had lymphocutaneous sporotrichosis and received ten courses of therapy. All the patients had a response to the therapy, although one had a relapse and later had a response to an additional course of the drug.
- Itraconazole: The duration of therapy that would be most appropriate is poorly documented in the literature. Treatment for approximately 8 weeks after resolution of the cutaneous lesions may minimize the risk of relapse.
- Experience with ketoconazole and fluconazole has been limited, but they appear to be less efficacious than itraconazole.

TREATMENT FAILURE

- It is rarely necessary to resort to intravenous administration of amphotericin B in treating lymphocutaneous sporotrichosis.
- Disseminated and systemic forms of sporotrichosis are treated with intravenous amphotericin B, and a course of up to 2.0 to 2.5 g can be needed for osteoarticular infection.
- *S. schenckii* meningitis does not consistently respond to amphotericin B, and the addition of 5-fluorocytosine may be warranted. There are no data on the use of the azoles. The number of reported cases of involvement of other specific sites is too limited to permit generalization.
- Surgery is not necessary if the disease is limited to the cutaneous structures; however, if there is invasion into the joint that causes arthritis or tenosynovitis, debridement and repair are required.

COMPLICATIONS

Cutaneous sporotrichosis responds well to therapy.

Follow-Up

Osteoarticular sporotrichosis may require prolonged therapy.

PREVENTION

It is important to recognize the disease in animals, because they are presumably a source of the disease in human beings who have contact with them.

Selected Readings

Anonymous. Case records of the Massachusetts General Hospital. Weekly clinicopathological exercises. Case 28-1994. A 51-year-old man with a nonhealing finger wound and regional lymphadenopathy. *N Engl J Med* 1994;331:181–187.

Dooley DP, Bostic PS, Beckius ML. Spook house sporotrichosis. A point-source outbreak of sporotrichosis associated with hay bale props in a Halloween haunted-house. *Arch Intern Med* 1997;157:1885–1887.

Rex JH. Sporothrix schenckii. In: Mandell GL, Bennett JE, Dolin R, eds. *Principles and practice of infectious diseases*. New York: Churchill Livingstone, 1995:2321–2324.

Saxena M, Rest EB. An ulcerating nodule on the arm. Lymphocutaneous sporotrichosis. *Arch Dermatol* 1998;134:1281–1284.

Sharkey-Mathis PK, Kauffman CA, Graybill JR, et al. Treatment of sporotrichosis with itraconazole. NIAID Mycoses Study Group. *Am J Med* 1993;95:279–285.

Ticoras CJ, Schroeter AL, Hornbeck KL. Disseminated ulcerated papules and nodules. Cutaneous disseminated sporotrichosis. *Arch Dermatol* 1996;132:963–964, 966–967.

Stomatitis

Basics

DEFINITION
- Generalized or local inflammation of the oral mucosa of infectious or noninfectious etiology
- May be a manifestation of systemic disease

ETIOLOGY
- Several infectious causes
  - *Candida* infection (thrush) of the oral mucosa (tongue, buccal mucosa, palate, gums) is frequently seen in patients who receive corticosteroids, antibiotics, and/or chemotherapy drugs or in immunocompromised hosts.
  - The cause of recurrent aphthous stomatitis is unknown. The most accepted hypothesis is that of autoimmune origin. However, a few infectious agents, including viruses, have been associated with apthous stomatitis.
  - Viruses, such as herpes simplex virus 1 and 2 and coxsackievirus A (herpangina and hand-foot-and-mouth disease) are common causes of stomatitis.
  - Necrotizing ulcerative gingivitis/stomatitis and noma are considered to be caused by spirochetes and fusiform bacilli, such as *Borrelia vincentii* and *Fusobacterium nucleatum*. *Prevotella melaninogenica* may also be present in cultures.
- Noninfectious causes
  - Allergy (drugs, contact, food)
  - Vitamin deficiency: Riboflavin (vitamin B$_2$) deficiency causes angular stomatitis; niacin deficiency causes pellagra.
  - Smoking (nicotinic stomatitis)
  - Traumatic (e.g., dentures)
  - Systemic diseases (Behçet's disease, uremia, collagen diseases, vascular disease, anemia)

Incidence and Prevalence (United States)
- Recurrent aphthous stomatitis, herpetic stomatitis, and hand-foot-and-mouth disease are common.
- Other infections are uncommon, except oral candidiasis in immunocompromised hosts or patients who receive broad-spectrum antibiotics.

Risk Factors
- Smoking
- Antibiotics, immunosuppressive agents
- HIV infection and neoplastic causes of immunosuppression
- Alcohol

Predominant Age
- Herpangina, hand-foot-and-mouth disease, and primary herpetic stomatitis are more common in children.
- Acute necrotizing ulcerative gingivitis/stomatitis (or trench mouth or Vincent's stomatitis) usually affects teen-agers and young adults.
- Noma (or gangrenous stomatitis or cancrum oris) is more common in children.

Clinical Manifestations

SYMPTOMS AND SIGNS
- Clinical manifestations vary, depending on the cause of stomatitis.
- Oral/gingival pain or tenderness may be present. Oral lesions depend on the etiology of the stomatitis. Some patients may present with intraoral ulcers. Others may present with acute gingival/oral inflammation or necrosis (Vincent's stomatitis and noma, respectively). Grayish white palatal and tonsillar ulcerations appear in herpangina. Buccal and lip ulcers are seen in hand-foot-and-mouth disease.
- Oral candidiasis (thrush) may appear as removable, creamy-white, curdlike patches (pseudomembranous type) or red, friable plaques (erythematous type).
- Some patients may complain of general symptoms, such as fever and malaise.
- Primary herpetic stomatitis is characterized by fever, malaise, and fatigue, followed by the appearance of vesicular oral lesions after 12 days. Mucocutaneous herpes simplex virus infection (usually type 1) may appear as vesicles, which form moist ulcers a few days later.

Diagnosis

DIFFERENTIAL DIAGNOSIS
- Herpetic stomatitis
- Herpangina, hand-foot-and-mouth disease (coxsackievirus A)
- Recurrent aphthous stomatitis
- Necrotizing ulcerative gingivitis/stomatitis and noma
- Thrush (candidal stomatitis)
- Cultures and stains of abnormal exudate specimens may be of diagnostic help. However, diagnosis should be based on clinical manifestations.

PATHOLOGY
Biopsy and histologic examination should be performed on all suspicious or chronically recurrent oral lesions, or if lesions fail to heal, to rule out oral malignancies.

Treatment

MAIN TREATMENT
- Treatment is usually symptomatic.
- Antiseptic mouthwashes may be of help to reduce secondary infection of recurrent aphthous stomatitis. Local anesthetics may be used for pain relief.

Stomatitis

- Oral acyclovir (200 mg five times a day) may be necessary for treatment of herpetic stomatitis in immunosuppressed patients. (Intravenous acyclovir should be considered in severely immunosuppressed patients.)
- Coxsackievirus A oral lesions usually require no specific treatment.
- Severe facial deformity and mutilation in noma require cosmetic surgery.
- Loose teeth and sequestra may need to be removed.
- Necrotizing ulcerative gingivitis/stomatitis requires antibiotic therapy, using penicillin or metronidazole.
- Fluconazole (100 mg daily for 7–14 days), ketoconazole (200–400 mg daily for 7–14 days), or nystatin mouth rinses (500,000 U held in mouth before swallowing, tid for 7–14 days) provide effective antifungal therapy in cases of oral candidiasis. Local relief may be achieved by chlorhexidine mouth rinses.

ALTERNATIVE TREATMENT

- Acyclovir-resistant herpes simplex virus isolates in HIV-positive patients should be treated with foscarnet (40–60 mg/kg i.v. tid, adjusted for renal function).
- Acyclovir 200 mg tid, famciclovir 250 mg bid, or valacyclovir 500 mg bid is used in cases of recurrent herpetic stomatitis (when there are more than five episodes per year).
- Topical or systemic steroids are used for extensive recurrent aphthous stomatitis.

APPROPRIATE HEALTH CARE

- Usually outpatient
- If stomatitis is severe, hospitalization may be needed.
- Hospitalization may be needed if stomatitis appears as a complication of severe immunosuppression.

GENERAL MEASURES

- Cessation of smoking
- Care of problematic denture
- Topical anesthesia/analgesics

DIET

- If the oral lesions are severe and make chewing impossible, the administration of liquids (orally or intravenously) may be necessary.
- Spicy foods may need to be avoided.

COMPLICATIONS

- CNS or ocular involvement in herpetic infection
- Noma may be life-threatening if underlying conditions are severe.

Follow-Up

- Viral (herpetic or coxsackievirus A stomatitis) and episodes of recurrent apthous stomatitis usually resolve in 7 to 14 days.
- Persistent, recurrent, or suspicious lesions require biopsy.

PREVENTION

- Avoidance of smoking
- Careful oral hygiene of dentures; removal of complete dentures during sleep

Selected Readings

Eversole LR. Immunopathogenesis of oral lichen planus and recurrent aphthous stomatitis. *Semin Cutan Med Surg* 1997;16:284–294.

Higgins CR, Schoefield JK, Tatnall FM, et al. Natural history, management and complications of herpes labialis. *J Med Virol* 1993;1:22–26.

Ndiaye FC, Bourgeois D, Leclercq MH, et al. Noma: Public health problem in Senegal and epidemiological surveillance. *Oral Dis* 1999;5:163–166.

Poland JM. Current therapeutic management of recurrent herpes labialis. *Gen Dent* 1994;42:46–50.

Ramos-Vara JA, Duran O, Render JA, et al. Necrotising stomatitis associated with *Fusobacterium necrophorum* in three sows. *Vet Rec* 1998;143:282–283.

Rossie K, Guggenheimer J. Oral candidiasis: Clinical manifestations, diagnosis, and treatment. *Pract Periodon Aesthet Dent* 1997;9:635–641.

Wilson J. The etiology, diagnosis and management of denture stomatitis. *Br Dent J* 1998;185:380–384.

Strongyloidiasis

Basics

DEFINITION
The intestinal nematode *Strongyloides stercoralis* is common worldwide and causes reinfection in the human host that persists for years.

ETIOLOGY
- *S. stercoralis* is a nematode that is 2 mm in length.
- There are two forms of nematode: parasitic and free-living.
  —Both have separate sexual cycles.

Parasitic
- Adult worms live within the human intestinal wall, at the level of the duodenum and jejunum.
- Eggs hatch in the intestine, and rhabditiform larvae pass in the stool or transform into filariform larvae within the intestine.

Free-living
- Worms produce eggs that hatch into filariform larvae; these larvae may live for weeks in the soil.
- Filariform larvae may invade the skin, the intestinal mucosa, or perianal skin to produce autoinfection.

EPIDEMIOLOGY

Incidence and Prevalence
- One hundred million to 200 million people may be infected.
- Usual locations for infection are tropical, poor, and underdeveloped countries.
- There is a high prevalence in parts of Brazil, Columbia, and Southeast Asia.
- Autoinfection of people in developed countries may occur for up to 40 years.

Risk Factors
- Persons residing in or visiting endemic areas
- People who walk barefoot or in other ways are in contact with contaminated soil where larvae may reside

Incubation
It takes 25 to 30 days for the worm to invade the skin, travel to the intestine via the lungs, and start to produce eggs.

Clinical Manifestations

- Gastrointestinal symptoms are mild and may include diarrhea, cramping, and diffuse pain and weight loss.
  —Symptoms may be more severe in children, with signs of malabsorption and vitamin B12 deficiency on rare occasions.
- Cutaneous manifestations include a slightly raised, pruritic, and irregular track under the skin, resembling cutaneous larva migrans.
  —Rash due to autoinfection, which often appears around the buttocks, is known as larva currens.
  —Larvae migrate into cutaneous blood vessels to gain access to the lungs.
- Pulmonary disease is associated with a Loeffler-like syndrome. The patient has bronchospasm and cough.
- In patients who are immunocompromised or on steroids, a hyperinfection syndrome occurs and can produce overwhelming pneumonitis, leading to acute respiratory distress syndrome or multibacterial sepsis. Both lead to death.

Strongyloidiasis

Diagnosis

DIFFERENTIAL DIAGNOSIS
- Ascaris, ancylostomiasis, cutaneous larva migrans
- Disseminated disease may resemble atypical pneumonia or tropical pulmonary eosinophilia.

LABORATORY
- Moderate eosinophilia may be seen in the 10% to 25% range, but may be absent in overwhelming disease states.
- Identify adult worms or rhabditiform larvae in stool and duodenal aspirates. Shedding of the larvae may be light and require many attempts to make the diagnosis.
- Identify larvae in a duodenal biopsy.
- Gram-negative or multibacterial sepsis with enteric organisms with no obvious source
- Serology is available.

IMAGING
- Upper gastrointestinal series are usually nonspecific but may show mucosal edema of the small intestine.
- Chest x-ray findings range from lobar pneumonia, interstitial infiltrates, or, in cases of massive infection, acute respiratory distress syndrome.

DIAGNOSTIC PROCEDURES
Duodenal aspirate, biopsy, or the string test may be needed to find the larvae.

Treatment

- Albendazole 400 mg oral for 3 days
- Ivermectin 200 μg/kg/d for 2 days
- Thiabendazole 25 mg/kg bid for 2 days
- Hyperinfection syndrome may require a 7- to 10-day regimen.
- Hyperinfection syndrome requires supportive care.

COMPLICATIONS
Hyperinfection syndrome may lead to respiratory failure or sepsis.

Follow-Up

PREVENTION
Adequate sanitation can prevent many cases of this disease.

Selected Readings

Grove DI. Human strongyloidiasis. *Adv Parasitol* 1996;38:251–309.

Heyworth MF. Parasitic diseases in immunocompromised hosts. Cryptosporidiosis, isosporiasis and strongyloidiasis. *Gastroenterol Clin North Am* 1996;25:691–707.

Wehner JH, Kirsch CM. Pulmonary manifestations of strongyloidiasis. *Semin Respir Infect* 1997;12:122–129.

Superficial Skin and Soft-Tissue Infections

Basics

DEFINITION
Superficial skin and soft-tissue infections occur just below the stratum corneum, in the hair follicles or apocrine glands, and below the epidermis, penetrating the dermis to subcutaneous tissues. The superficial infections manifest as impetigo, cellulitis, pyodermas, erysipelas, and recurring erysipelas.

ETIOLOGY
- *Staphylococcus aureus*: pyodermas (folliculitis, furuncle, carbuncle)
- Group A *Streptococcus* (GAS): erysipelas, recurrent erysipelas
- Group A *Streptococcus* and *S. aureus*, either separately or together (staphylococcal form becoming most common agent of infection): impetigo
- Group A *Streptococcus pyogenes* (GAS) or *S. aureus, Staphylococcus epidermidis, Erysipelothrix rhusiopathiae, Pseudomonas aeruginosa* (gram-negative): cellulitis

EPIDEMIOLOGY
Incidence
- Diabetics
- The immunocompromised
- The elderly
- Children

Risk Factors
- Diabetic patients and immunocompromised persons are at risk for pyodermas.
- Persons using contaminated hot tubs, whirlpools, or swimming pools are at risk for pyodermas.
- Persons with diabetes, venous stasis, underlying skin ulcers, and nephrotic syndrome and those who abuse alcohol are at risk for erysipelas.
- School children and persons living in close proximity in unsanitary conditions are predisposed to impetigo.

Incubation
- Depends on the specific infection

Clinical Manifestations

SYMPTOMS AND SIGNS
- Folliculitis: vesicles and lesions involving hair follicles
- Furuncle (boil): firm, discrete nodules
- Carbuncle: extensive, multiloculated lesion occurring on back of neck, the back, or thighs, with abundant pus
- Erysipelas: raised, bright red, indurated painful lesion with advancing red border and a *peau d'orange* appearance. It most commonly occurs in the extremities, followed by the face, especially over the bridge of the nose or the cheeks. Systemic manifestations (fever, shaking chills, altered mental status) commonly accompany the skin symptoms.
- Recurrent erysipelas: chronic edema from lymphatic or venous obstruction; begins with painful red lesion advancing rapidly up the limb. Systemic manifestations (fever with shaking chills) accompany the skin lesions.
- Impetigo: bullous (superficial flaccid bullae) or nonbullous (thin-walled vesicles and pustules on an erythematous base); itching; lesions appear on face or extremities; common in hot, humid conditions
- Cellulitis: spreading inflammation that occurs acutely, then proceeds to chronic phase, associated with a break in the skin from trauma, puncture, insect bite, or surgical incision

Diagnosis

- Based on history and physical examination and direct observation of the lesions

DIFFERENTIAL DIAGNOSIS
Infectious
- Erysipelas
  —Cellulitis, necrotizing fasciitis, streptococcal gangrene, contact dermatitis, giant urticaria, erythema chronicum migrans

Superficial Skin and Soft-Tissue Infections

Noninfectious
- Pyodermas (folliculitis, furuncles, carbuncles)
  — Acne vulgaris

LABORATORY

Many lesions do not yield a positive culture, such as in cellulitis. Laboratory testing results are predictable in pyodermas.

Treatment

MAIN TREATMENT

- Warm, moist packs on milder lesions to stimulate drainage and to encourage localization for folliculitis
- Surgery for folliculitis
  — Drainage with wick after incision
- Antibiotics
  — Pyodermas
    — Cloxacillin orally
    — Oxacillin intravenously
    — Nafcillin intravenously
    — Cephalosporin
  — Erysipelas
    — Penicillin V-K orally
    — Hospitalization: penicillin intravenously in high doses
  — Recurrent erysipelas
    — Hospitalization: penicillin G intravenously in high doses
  — Cellulitis
    — Penicillin or ampicillin intravenously in high doses for streptococcal infection
    — Oxacillin or nafcillin or first-generation cephalosporin for staphylococcal infection
    — Combined ampicillin and oxacillin if infection type is unclear
    — Quinolone alone or with an aminoglycoside for *Pseudomonas* infection
    — Quinolone or tetracycline for *Aeromonas* and *Vibrio* infections
    — Quinolone intravenously with an aminoglycoside for life-threatening forms of infection

ALTERNATIVE TREATMENT

- Recurrent erysipelas
  — Cephalosporins
  — Erythromycin or clindamycin for penicillin-allergic patients

COMPLICATIONS

- Relapses of erysipelas
- Bacteremia
- Sepsis
- Spread of infection to other organs

Follow-Up

Erysipelas and cellulitis have a tendency to recur, so patients should be followed for at least 3 months.

PREVENTION

- For recurrent erysipelas
  — Physiotherapy to improve muscle tone in affected limbs
  — Use of pressure devices to reduce edema to the affected limb during the night

Selected Readings

Baddour LM, Bisno AL. Infection of the skin and subcutaneous tissue. In: Schlossberg D, ed. *Infections of the head and neck.* New York: Springer Verlag, 1987:1.

Gorbach SL. Necrotizing skin and soft tissue infections. In: Gorbach S, Bartlett J, Blacklow N, eds. *Infectious diseases.* Philadelphia: WB Saunders, 1998:922.

Schwartz MN. Cellulitis and subcutaneous tissue infections. In: Mandell GL, Bennett JE, Dolin R, eds. *Principles and practice of infectious diseases,* 4th ed. New York: Churchill Livingstone, 1995:926.

Surgical Site Infections (Surgical Wound Infections)

Basics

DEFINITION

Surgical site infection (formerly termed *surgical wound infection*) is characterized as the following:
- *Superficial incisional* when it occurs within 30 days after the operation, and it involves only skin or subcutaneous tissue and one of the following:
  - Purulent drainage from the superficial incision
  - Organisms isolated from an aseptically obtained sample from the superficial incision
  - Clinical diagnosis by a senior physician
- *Deep superficial incisional* when it occurs within 30 days after the operation (or up to 1 year if implant is in place), it appears to be related to the operation, and it involves deep soft tissues and one of the following:
  - Purulent drainage from the deep tissues of the surgical site
  - Signs of abscess or other signs (e.g., radiologic) of infection involving the deep tissues
  - Clinical diagnosis by a senior physician
- *Organ/space* when it occurs within 30 days after the operation (or up to 1 year if implant is in place), it appears to be related to the operation, and it involves any parts of the anatomy except the incision and one of the following:
  - Purulent drainage from a drain that is placed into the organ/space
  - Organisms isolated from an aseptically obtained sample from the organ/space
  - Signs of abscess or other signs (e.g., radiologic) of infection involving the organ/space
  - Clinical diagnosis by a senior physician

ETIOLOGY

- For most surgical site infections, the source of pathogens is the endogenous flora.
- The dose of contaminating microorganisms required to produce infection may be much lower when foreign material is present at the site.
- Pathogens isolated from surgical site infections mainly include the following:
  - *Staphylococcus aureus*
  - Coagulase-negative staphylococci
  - *Streptococcus* spp
  - Enterobacteriaceae (usually *Escherichia coli*)
  - *Enterococcus* spp
- *Bacteroides* spp and other anaerobes are associated with surgery involving the gastrointestinal and female genital tracts.
- An increasing proportion of surgical site infections are caused by antimicrobial-resistant pathogens, such as methicillin-resistant *S. aureus* (MRSA) or *Candida albicans*.
- Outbreaks or clusters of surgical site infections have also been caused by unusual pathogens, such as *Rhizopus oryzae, Clostridium perfringens, Rhodococcus bronchialis, Nocardia* spp, and *Legionella* spp. These rare outbreaks have been traced to contaminated adhesive dressings, elastic bandages, colonized surgical personnel, tap water, or contaminated disinfectant solutions.

EPIDEMIOLOLGY

Incidence

- Surgical site infections account for approximately 15% of all nosocomial infections.
- Among surgical patients, surgical site infections are the most common nosocomial infections, accounting for approximately 40% of all such infections. Of these surgical site infections, two-thirds are confined to the incision, and one-third involve organs or spaces accessed during the operation.
- A 1992 analysis showed that each surgical site infection resulted in 7.3 additional postoperative hospital days, adding $3,152 in extra charges.
- Many surgical site infections are detected after the patient is discharged from the hospital.
- From 1991 to 1995, the incidence of surgical site infections caused by fungi increased from 0.1 to 0.3 per 1,000 discharges.

Risk Factors

- Patient characteristics associated with an increased risk of a surgical site infection include the following:
  - Cigarette smoking
  - Coincident remote site infections or colonization
  - Diabetes
  - Extremes of age
  - Long duration of surgery
  - Long preoperative length of stay
  - Obesity
  - Poor nutritional status
  - Preoperative shaving of the field, especially if performed 24 hours or more prior to the operation
  - Presence of a drain
  - Presence of an untreated remote infection
  - Systemic steroid use

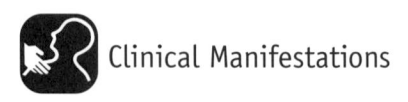

Clinical Manifestations

- Fever is often present, especially in deep incisional or organ/space surgical site infections, and it can be the only presenting symptom.
- A surgical wound should be examined for erythema extending more than 2 cm beyond the margin of the wound, localized tenderness and induration, fluctuans, drainage of purulent material, and dehiscence of sutures.
- Mechanical factors, as well as infection, can cause wound dehiscence.
- Sternal wounds following cardiac surgery are of special concern because the consequences of infection can be severe. The surface of the wound may not present an obvious cause for concern, but, in some patients, ongoing fevers and especially the development of rocking or instability of the sternum may be sufficient cause for surgical exploration of the wound.

Surgical Site Infections (Surgical Wound Infections)

Diagnosis

- Persistent leukocytosis is a common laboratory finding.
- Imaging of the surgical area (usually with the use of computed tomography) is often helpful in evaluating the presence and the extent of collection(s).
- Drainage and microbiologic evaluation of the exudate (Gram stain and aerobic and anaerobic cultures) as well as blood cultures can help identify the pathogen(s).

Treatment

- Superficial incisional surgical site infection: amoxicillin/clavulanate (500 mg tid) or dicloxacillin (100 mg PO bid), with or without fluoroquinolone (e.g., levofloxacillin 500 mg PO once daily)
- Deep superficial or organ/space surgical site infection: ampicillin–sulbactam (3 g i.v. qid), or piperacillin–tazobactam (3.375 g i.v. tid; higher doses are needed for covering *Pseudomonas* spp), or ticarcillin–clavulanate. For surgery involving the gastrointestinal or female genital tracts, consider also cefoxitin (1 g i.v. tid) or imipenem (500 mg i.v. q6h).
- Surgical drainage is often necessary.
- Duration of treatment depends on the site and extent of infection, presence of drains, response to treatment, surgical management, and the causative microorganism.

COMPLICATIONS

- Patients with a deep surgical site infection have a significantly increased mortality rate, with a risk ratio of 1.7.
- Mediastinitis or sternal osteomyelitis is a severe complication of cardiac surgery.
- Infection of wounds associated with the placement of prosthetic devices can lead to infection of the prosthesis, and generally requires surgical removal of the device.

Follow-Up

- If gastrointestinal leakage is identified at the time of the operation, then the continuation of the antibiotic agents from 1 to 3 days is usually recommended.
- Leaving the operative wound open, packed with saline-soaked gauze, decreases the incidence of postoperative wound infection in high-risk patients.

PREVENTION

- Advances in infection control practices include improved operating room ventilation, sterilization methods, barriers, surgical technique, and availability of antimicrobial prophylaxis.
- Preventive antibiotics (usually administered once, within 2 hours prior to the operation)
  - Hysterectomy: cefazolin 1 to 2 g i.v. or cefoxitin 1 to 2 g i.v.
  - Upper gastrointestinal tract: cefazolin 1 to 2 g i.v. or cefoxitin 1 to 2 g i.v.
  - Lower gastrointestinal tract
    - Elective: The vast majority of surgeons use antibiotics and mechanical cleansing for preoperative preparation for elective colon resection. The most popular regimen in the United States has been oral neomycin–erythromycin base, along with cefoxitin i.v.
    - Emergency: cefoxitin 1 to 2 g i.v. or cefoxitin 1 to 2 g i.v., and metronidazole 500 mg i.v. or cefotetan 1 to 2 g i.v.
  - Cardiovascular: cefazolin 1 g tid for up to 24 to 48 hours or vancomycin 1 g i.v. bid for up to 48 hours (the use of vancomycin is also discussed below)
- A preoperative antiseptic shower or bath decreases skin microbial colony counts.
- The routine use of vancomycin in surgical antibiotic prophylaxis is not recommended. However, vancomycin may be the agent of choice in certain clinical circumstances, such as when a cluster of MRSA mediastinitis or incisional surgical site infections due to methicillin-resistant, coagulase-negative staphylococci has been detected.
- Preventing hypothermia can prevent surgical site infections.
- The Centers for Disease Control and Prevention recommendations for the prevention of surgical site infection include the following:
  - Whenever possible, identify and treat all infections remote to the surgical site before elective operation.
  - Adequately control serum blood glucose levels in all diabetic patients and avoid hyperglycemia perioperatively.
  - Encourage tobacco cessation.
  - Keep the preoperative hospital stay as short as possible while allowing for adequate preoperative preparation of the patient.
  - Administer a prophylactic antimicrobial agent only when indicated.
  - Use delayed primary skin closure or leave an incision open to heal by second intention if the surgeon considers the surgical site to be heavily contaminated.

Selected Readings

Kurz A, Sessler DI, Lenhardt R. Perioperative normothermia to reduce the incidence of surgical-wound infection and shorten hospitalization. Study of Wound Infection and Temperature Group. *N Engl J Med* 1996;334:1209–1215.

Mangram AJ, Horan TC, Pearson ML, et al. Guideline for prevention of surgical site infection, 1999. Centers for Disease Control and Prevention (CDC) Hospital Infection Control Practices Advisory Committee. *Am J Infect Control* 1999;27:97–132; quiz 133–134; discussion 96.

Nichols RL. Surgical infections: Prevention and treatment—1965 to 1995. *Am J Surg* 1996;172:68–74.

Poulsen KB, Wachmann CH, Bremmelgaard A, et al. Survival of patients with surgical wound infection: A case-control study of common surgical interventions. *Br J Surg* 1995;82:2089, 1995.

Weinstein RA. Infection control in the hospital. In: Fauci AS, Braunwald E, Isselbacher KJ, et al., eds. *Harrison's principles of internal medicine,* 14th ed. New York: McGraw-Hill, 1998:849–852.

Syphilis

Basics

DEFINITION
Syphilis is a sexually transmitted disease manifested initially as papule at the site of inoculation. The disease is also transmitted transplacentally. It is rarely transmitted via blood product transfusion. Disease progression is divided into overlapping stages of primary, secondary, latent, and tertiary.

ETIOLOGY
- *Treponema pallidum* spirochete
- Only mucocutaneous lesions are infectious; they are seen in primary and secondary stages.

EPIDEMIOLOGY

Incidence
- United States: highest in African Americans, Hispanics, inner-city residents
- High in drug abusers (sex-for-drugs exchanges)

Risk Factors
- Unsafe sexual practices
- Multiple partners
- Drug abuse

Incubation
- Primary: 2 to 4 weeks
- Secondary: 3 to 6 weeks after disappearance of primary lesion
- Latent: after resolution of secondary signs
- Tertiary: 5 to 25 years of latent syphilis

Clinical Manifestations

SYMPTOMS AND SIGNS

Primary
- Red papule, 5- to 15-mm diameter, sharply demarcated, elevated, smooth, firm, nonpurulent
- Papule generally painless; appears at site of inoculation: external genitalia, anal area, lips, oral cavity, breasts, or fingers

Secondary
- Three to 6 weeks after disappearance of primary lesion, but, occasionally, primary lesion still present
- Malaise, headaches, sore throat, fever, weight loss, musculoskeletal pain
- Rash in approximately 90% of patients
  —Begins as faint, rose-pink, macular, rounded lesion up to 1-cm diameter
  —Gradually becomes red and papular, spreading to entire body, including palms and soles
- Lymphadenopathy (70% of patients)
- Mucosal lesions, mainly oral patches (20% of patients)
- Condylomata lata (broad, flat, exophytic lesions) in warm, moist areas; typically perianal
- Focal alopecia
- Asymptomatic acute meningitis (1%–2% of patients)
- Hepatitis
- Uveitis, iritis
- Arthritis, osteitis, periosteitis
- Glomerulonephritis

Latent
- Begins after resolution of secondary phase
- Asymptomatic
- Disease can still progress.

Tertiary
- Usually after 5 years of latent stage; sometimes 25 years or more later
- Neurosyphilis
- Pupil abnormalities
- Auditory involvement
- Cardiovascular involvement of ascending aorta, leading to aortic aneurysm and aortic valve regurgitation
- Nodules, most typically in skin and in bone

Diagnosis

History and physical examination alone often lead to an inaccurate diagnosis. Serology is needed for a definitive diagnosis.

DIFFERENTIAL DIAGNOSIS

Evaluation of the patient with genital ulcers should include the three main possibilities: genital herpes, syphilis, and chancroid.

Infectious
- Genital herpes
- Chancroid
- Acute HIV infection
- Venereal warts
- Scabies
- Molluscum contagiosum
- Folliculitis
- Lymphogranuloma venereum (rare)
- Granuloma inguinale/donovanosis (rare)
- Mycobacteria (rare)
- Fungi (rare)
- Parasites (rare)

Noninfectious
- Malignancy
- Benign lesions
- Fixed drug eruption
- Erythema multiforme
- Dermatitis herpetiformis
- Behçet's syndrome

LABORATORY
- Microscopy: dark-field examination
  —Three carefully collected specimens, collected on consecutive days, should be negative before considering syphilis unlikely in a patient with a suspicious lesion.
- Serology: Nontreponemal is recommended for screening in pregnancy, HIV infection, blood screening, intravenous drug abusers, patients with history of multiple sex partners, patients with exposure to person(s) with syphilis, and follow-up of syphilis disease activity.
- Nontreponemal
- Venereal Disease Research Laboratory (VDRL)
- Rapid plasma reagin
- Nonspecific for syphilis
- Yields false positives in the following:
  —Viral disease
  —Bacterial disease
  —Parasitic disease
  —Pregnancy
- Yields false negatives in the following:
  —The elderly
  —Intravenous drug abusers
  —Patients with chronic rheumatic or liver disease
- Inexpensive
- Titer correlates with disease activity.
- Treponemal: recommended for confirmatory testing

Syphilis

- Fluorescent treponemal antibody absorption
- Microhemagglutination assay for antibody to *T. pallidum*
  —More specific than nontreponemal tests
  —Expensive
  —Titers do not correlate with disease activity

TESTING PROCEDURES

- Gently abrade the lesion with a sterile gauze pad to provoke oozing but not gross bleeding.
- Squeeze the lesion between a gloved thumb and forefinger to increase exudate from lesion.
- Apply the exudate directly onto a microscope slide if used for dark-field and direct immunofluorescence tests.

Treatment

MAIN TREATMENT

- Primary syphilis: benzathine penicillin
  —Initial: 2.4×10^6 U i.m. one time
  —Retreatment: 2.4×10^6 U i.m. weekly for 3 weeks
- Secondary syphilis: benzathine penicillin
  —Initial: 2.4×10^6 U i.m. one time
  —Retreatment: 2.4×10^6 U i.m. weekly for 3 weeks
- Latent syphilis: benzathine penicillin
  —Latent stage less than 1 year—Initial: 2.4×10^6 U i.m. one time
  —Latent stage less than 1 year—Retreatment: 2.4×10^6 U i.m. weekly for 3 weeks
  —Latent stage greater than 1 year or unknown duration—Initial: 2.4×10^6 U i.m. weekly for 3 weeks
- Tertiary syphilis: benzathine penicillin
  —2.4×10^6 U i.m. weekly for 3 weeks
- Neurosyphilis: aqueous penicillin G and lumbar puncture
  —12 to 24×10^6 U per day for 10 to 14 days
- Lumbar puncture is appropriate at all stages if penicillin treatment is ineffective or if neurologic symptoms are present.
- Lumbar puncture is also appropriate at the latent stage if HIV infection is present.

SEX PARTNERS

- Evaluate clinically and serologically.
- Treat as appropriate to stage of disease if seropositive.

COMPLICATIONS

- HIV infection: All patients with syphilis should be tested for HIV.
- Pregnancy

Follow-Up

- Primary: at 3 and 6 months; if HIV-positive, at 1, 2, 3, 6, and 12 months
  —Fourfold decrease in titer at 3 months expected
  —Retreatment indicated if
    —Titer increases fourfold or fails to decrease fourfold at 3 months
    —Noncompliance
    —HIV infection
    —Persistent or recurrent symptoms
- Secondary at 3 and 6 months; if HIV-positive, at 1, 2, 3, 6, and 12 months
  —Fourfold decrease in titer at 6 months expected
  —Retreatment indicated if
    —Titer increases fourfold or fails to decrease fourfold at 6 months
    —Noncompliance
    —HIV infection
    —Persistent or recurrent symptoms
- Latent at 6 and 12 months
  —Fourfold decrease of titer greater than or equal to 1:32 within 6 months expected, or
  —Fourfold decrease of titer greater than or equal to 1:4 at 1 year expected
  —Retreatment indicated if
    —Titer of greater than or equal to 1:16 fails to decrease fourfold at 12 months with lower initial titer
- Tertiary at 6 and 12 months
  —Fourfold decrease of titer greater than or equal to 1:32 within 6 months expected, or
  —Fourfold decrease of titer greater than or equal to 1:4 at 1 year expected
  —Granulomatous lesions should heal.
  —Retreatment indicated if
    —Titer of greater than or equal to 1:16 fails to decrease fourfold at 12 months with lower initial titer
    —Documentation of *T. pallidum* or other histologic feature of late syphilis
- Neurosyphilis (or ocular) every 6 months until negative
  —Cerebrospinal fluid white blood cell decrease at 6 months
  —Cerebrospinal fluid normal at 1 year
  —Retreatment indicated if
    —CSF WBC decrease at 6 months
    —CSF still abnormal at 2 years
    —Persistent signs and symptoms of inflammatory response at 3 months or later
    —Fourfold increase in CSF VDRL at 6 months or later
    —Failure of CSF VDRL of greater than or equal to 1:16 to decrease by twofold at 6 months or by fourfold by 12 months

PREVENTION

- Safe-sex precautions

Selected Readings

1998 Guidelines for treatment of sexually transmitted diseases. Centers for Disease Control and Prevention. *MMWR Morb Mortal Wkly Rep* 1998;47(RR-1):28.

Hook EW III, Marra CM. Acquired syphilis in adults. *N Engl J Med* 1992;326:1060.

Musher DM. Biology of *Treponema pallidum*. In: Holmes KK, Mardh PA, Sparling PF, et al., eds. *Sexually transmitted diseases*. New York: McGraw-Hill, 1990:205.

Sparling PF. Natural history of syphilis. In: Holmes KK, Mardh PA, Sparling PF, et al., eds. *Sexually transmitted diseases*. New York: McGraw-Hill, 1990:213.

Tetanus

Basics

DEFINITION

- Tetanus is a disease of the neurologic system, characterized by persistent tonic spasm with violent brief exacerbation and caused by *Clostridium tetani*.
- Tetanus is divided into four clinical types:
  —Generalized
  —Localized
  —Cephalic
  —Neonatal

ETIOLOGY

- Under anaerobic conditions, the spores of *Clostridium tetani* germinate and produce two toxins: tetanolysin (a hemolysin with no recognized pathologic activity) and tetanospasmin, which is responsible for tetanus.
- The toxin reaches the spinal cord in a process that takes 2 to 14 days. Localized or cephalic tetanus may occur initially, followed by generalized tetanus.
- Once the toxin enters the central nervous system, it diffuses to the terminals of inhibitory cells. By preventing transmitter release from these cells, tetanospasmin leaves the motor neurons without inhibition. This produces muscular rigidity by raising the resting firing rate of motor neurons. The autonomic nervous system is affected as well.

EPIDEMIOLOGY

Incidence

- In the developed countries of the world, tetanus has become a rare disease not as a result of the elimination of *C. tetani* from soil or the interruption of disease transmission, but as a result of immunization. In the United States, only 36 cases of tetanus were reported in 1994. It has been estimated that 22% to 46% were reported, suggesting that the total number of cases was less than 170. Also, since the introduction of immunization in Israel, the annual incidence of tetanus fell from 2 in 100 000 in the 1950s to 0.1 in 100 000 in 1988.
- The development of tetanus despite full immunization is extremely rare; it is estimated at 4 per 100 million immunocompetent vaccinated subjects.
- Neonatal tetanus caused an estimated 490,000 deaths in 1994, and in developing countries, at least 730,000 deaths were prevented by protection of infants at birth through vaccination of their mothers or by clean delivery and umbilical cord care practices.
- An estimated 8 million babies and 2 million children and adults died of tetanus during the 1990s, mostly in developing countries.

Risk Factors

- Most cases of tetanus occur among adults who are unvaccinated or whose history of vaccination is unknown.
- There is an excellent correlation between vaccination rates (96%) and immunity (96%) among 6-year-olds. However, antibody levels decline over time, and one-fifth of older children (10–16 years of age) do not have protective antibody levels.
- Tetanus among injecting drug users has been reported.

Clinical Manifestations

- Generalized tetanus is the most commonly recognized form and often begins with trismus ("lockjaw"), which causes a smile or grimace ("risus sardonicus"). Abdominal rigidity is present. The patient does not lose consciousness, and experiences severe pain during each spasm. During the spasm, the upper airway can be obstructed, or the diaphragm may participate in the general muscular contraction.
- Localized tetanus involves rigidity of the muscles associated with the site of spore inoculation.
- The initial manifestation may be of "local tetanus," in which the rigidity affects only one limb or area of the body in which the *Clostridium*-containing wound is located. This mild picture may progress to generalized rigidity, with reflex spasms and dysphagia.
- The wound may seem insignificant at the time of the injury and may even appear well healed at the time of the neurologic disease.
- Early on, the patient may report a "sore throat" with dysphagia.
- With severe tetanus, there is opisthotonos, flexion of the arms, extension of the legs, periods of apnea due to spasm of the intercostal muscles and diaphragm, and rigidity of the abdominal wall.
- Late in the disease, autonomic dysfunction develops, with hypertension and tachycardia alternating with hypotension and bradycardia.

Diagnosis

DIFFERENTIAL DIAGNOSIS

- Strychnine poisoning is the only condition that truly mimics tetanus.
- Dystonic reactions to neuroleptic drugs or other central dopamine antagonists may be confused with the neck stiffness of tetanus.
- A number of conditions (including dental and other local infections, hysteria, neoplasms, encephalitis, etc.) may produce trismus, and should be sought, but do not cause the other manifestations of tetanus.

LABORATORY AND IMAGING

- Tetanus has to be diagnosed clinically. A history of a soil-contaminated puncture wound should be sought, as there are no specific diagnostic laboratory tests.
- Blood counts and blood chemical findings are unremarkable. Imaging studies of the head and spine reveal no abnormalities.

Tetanus

Treatment

- Supportive therapy includes ventilatory support and pharmacologic agents that treat reflex muscle spasms, rigidity, and tetanic seizures.
- Benzodiazepines have emerged as the mainstay of symptomatic therapy for tetanus.
- To prevent spasms that last more than 5 to 10 seconds, diazepam is administered intravenously. The usual dosage is 10 to 40 mg every 1 to 8 hours.
- Vecuronium (by continuous infusion) or pancuronium (by intermittent injection) are adequate choices.
- Passive immunization with human tetanus immunoglobulin shortens the course of tetanus and may lessen its severity. A dose of 500 U appears as effective as larger doses.
- A study comparing oral metronidazole with intramuscular penicillin showed better survival, shorter hospitalization, and less progression of disease in the metronidazole group (0.5 g every 6 hours or 1.0 g every 12 hours i.v. for 7–10 days).
- Sedative-hypnotics, narcotics, inhalational anesthetics, neuromuscular blocking agents, and centrally acting muscle relaxants, such as intrathecal baclofen, have been used.
- A dose of tetanus–diphtheria vaccine should be administered (usually one upon discharge), with another dose of toxoid 4 weeks later.

COMPLICATIONS

- The mortality rate in mild and moderate tetanus is presently about 6%, and, for severe tetanus, it may reach as high as 60%.
- During 1982 to 1990, reports from the Centers for Disease Control and Prevention showed that the overall case fatality rate in the United States was 21% to 31%.
- Sympathetic overactivity has become the major cause of death in the intensive care unit. Sympathetic hyperactivity is usually managed with labetalol 0.25 to 1.0 mg/min, as needed for blood pressure control; or morphine 0.5 to 1.0 mg/kg/h by continuous infusion.
- Neonatal tetanus follows infection of the umbilical stump, most commonly due to a failure of aseptic technique, in which mothers are inadequately immunized. The mortality rate exceeds 90%, and developmental delays are common among survivors.

Follow-Up

Tetanus survivors often have serious psychological problems related to the disease and its treatment that persist after recovery and that may require psychotherapy.

PREVENTION

- Given the risk of tetanus after bites of all kinds, tetanus immune globulin and tetanus toxoid should be administered to patients who have had two or fewer primary immunizations. Tetanus toxoid alone can be given to those who have completed a primary immunization series but who have not received a booster for more than 5 years.
- Almost 70% of a random sample of Americans 6 or more years of age have protective levels of tetanus antibodies. However, by the age of 60 to 69 years, the prevalence of protective antibodies is less than 50% and, by the age of 70, about 30%. Tetanus toxoid is a very effective immunogen that stimulates a protective response in virtually all immunocompetent subjects to whom it is administered. Studies in former military personnel have shown that up to 88% have protective antibody levels 15 years after vaccination.
- The World Health Organization is now promoting vaccination of all women of childbearing age by screening a woman's tetanus toxoid vaccine status at every contact with the health services.
- Some patients with humoral immune deficiencies may not respond adequately to toxoid injection and should receive passive immunization for tetanus-prone injuries, regardless of the period since the last booster.

Selected Readings

Anonymous. From the Centers for Disease Control and Prevention. Tetanus among injecting-drug users—California, 1997. *JAMA* 1998;279:987.

Bleck TP. *Clostridium tetani*. In: Mandell GL, Bennett JE, Dolin R, eds. *Principles and practice of infectious diseases.* New York: Churchill Livingstone, 1995:2373–2378.

Bowie C. Tetanus toxoid for adults—Too much of a good thing. *Lancet* 1996;348:1185–1186.

Brabin L, Kemp J, Maxwell SM, et al. Protecting adolescent girls against tetanus. *BMJ* 1995;311:73–74.

Gergen PJ, McQuillan GM, Kiely M, et al. A population-based serologic survey of immunity to tetanus in the United States. *N Engl J Med* 1995;332:761–766.

Glezen WP. Prevention of neonatal tetanus. *Am J Public Health* 1998;88:871–872.

Nishanian E. Can epidural anesthesia change the mortality rate of tetanus? *Crit Care Med* 1999;27:2025–2026.

Sanford JP. Tetanus—Forgotten but not gone. *N Engl J Med* 1995;332:812–813.

Shimoni Z, Dobrousin A, Cohen J, et al. Tetanus in an immunised patient. *BMJ* 1999;319:1049.

Thrombophlebitis, Suppurative

Basics

DEFINITION

- Suppurative, or septic, thrombophlebitis is inflammation of a vein due to microorganisms associated with thrombus formation and bacteremia.
- Suppurative thrombophlebitis is divided into the following categories:
  —Superficial
  —Central (including pelvic)
  —Intracranial, that is, defined by the simultaneous presence of venous thrombosis and suppuration in the intracranial compartment
  —Portal vein
- Suppuration is uncommon in bacteremia associated with central venous catheters, and such infections are discussed in more detail in a separate chapter.

ETIOLOGY

- The pathogenesis of suppurative thrombophlebitis is unclear, but probably a thrombus acts as a nidus for bacteria that gain access to the site from another focus. The route of spread of organisms to the inflamed vein may be through migration from the skin between the catheter wall and perivascular tissue, from contaminated intravenous fluid, or through hematogenous dissemination from an infected focus elsewhere. The relative contribution of these three routes, however, is unknown.
- In pelvic suppurative thrombophlebitis, the ovarian vein and the inferior vena cava are usually affected. Thrombus formation may result from stasis and/or be due to the hypercoagulable state of parturition. In a second stage, microorganisms (such as *Bacteroides* spp, *Streptococcus* spp, and Enterobacteriaceae such as *Escherichia coli*) from the vaginal or the perineal flora gain access to the thrombus.
- Septic thrombosis of the portal vein is usually associated with hepatic abscess, and the obvious extrahepatic source is often absent.
- Suppurative intracranial thrombophlebitis may begin in veins and/or venous sinuses and can occur in the following ways:
  —Following infection of the paranasal sinuses, middle ear, mastoid, facial skin, or oropharynx
  —In the presence of epidural abscess, subdural empyema, or bacterial meningitis
  —After metastatic spread of infection from a distant site
- The usual predisposing conditions for the development of cavernous sinus thrombosis are paranasal sinusitis or infections of the face or mouth.
- The organisms most often isolated from superficial suppurative thrombophlebitis are the following:
  —*Staphylococcus aureus*
  —Coagulase-negative staphylococci
  —Enterobacteriaceae
  —*Pseudomonas aeruginosa*
  —*Enterococcus* spp
  —*Candida* spp
- The recovery of anaerobic bacteria is rarely reported.
- In suppurative intracranial thrombophlebitis, the most common bacterial pathogens depend on the initial source of infection; with sinusitis, they are staphylococci, aerobic and/or microaerophilic streptococci, gram-negative bacilli, and/or anaerobes, whereas *S. aureus* predominates when a facial infection is the source.
- *S. aureus* is the most important associated pathogen in patients with cavernous sinus thrombosis and is isolated in more than two-thirds of cases. Less common isolates include streptococci, pneumococci, gram-negative bacilli, and *Bacteroides* spp. In the appropriate clinical setting, fungal pathogens, such as *Aspergillus, Mucor,* and *Rhizopus* spp, should be considered. (See the Section II chapter, "Sinusitis," for details.)

EPIDEMIOLOGY

- Superficial suppurative thrombophlebitis accounts for up to 10% of nosocomial infections, and the estimated incidence is about 88 cases per 100,000 discharges. It is usually a result of a skin and soft-tissue infection or an indwelling intravenous catheter. Most common culprits are indwelling intravenous catheters that have been in place for 3 or more days.
- The incidence is higher when indwelling intravenous catheters are inserted in the lower extremities.
- Burn patients are at highest risk for developing suppurative thrombophlebitis, followed by patients with neoplastic diseases and those on steroid therapy.
- The overall incidence of septic pelvic thrombophlebitis is 1 in 2,000 to 1 in 3,000 deliveries. The incidence is about 1 in 9,000 after vaginal delivery, 1 in 800 after cesarean section or major gynecologic surgery, and 1 in 200 after septic abortion.
- Pelvic suppurative thrombophlebitis usually presents 1 to 2 weeks postpartum or postoperatively.

Clinical Manifestations

- Fever is present in 70% of the cases of suppurative thrombophlebitis, but rigors are rare.
- Local findings are usually present in superficial suppurative thrombophlebitis and include erythema, lymphangitis, tenderness, and warmth. However, these signs can be difficult to identify, especially in burn patients.
- Patients with suppurative thrombophlebitis of the thoracic central veins usually present with systemic symptoms of bacteremia and sepsis and with minor or no local findings.
- Pelvic suppurative thrombophlebitis usually presents with high fever, chills, anorexia, nausea, and vomiting. Flank or lower abdominal tenderness can be present. Small pulmonary septic emboli may be seen on chest x-ray.
- The clinical presentation of suppurative intracranial thrombophlebitis is variable and can include focal or generalized seizures, symptoms of increased intracranial pressure, and various focal neurologic findings.
- The most common complaints in patients with cavernous sinus thrombosis include fever, periorbital swelling, and headache. Other symptoms include change in mental status, diplopia, papilledema, tearing, photophobia, drowsiness, ptosis, proptosis, chemosis, periorbital edema, and weakness of the extraocular muscles. Lateral gaze palsy may be an early neurologic finding.

Thrombophlebitis, Suppurative

Diagnosis

LABORATORY

Superficial suppurative thrombophlebitis can induce bacteremia in 80% to 90% of the cases.

Imaging

- Throughout the 1980s, the utility of computed tomography and magnetic resonance imaging in the diagnosis of septic phlebitis was shown in a number of reports. Especially, computed tomography with intravenous contrast has been found useful in the diagnosis of suppurative thrombophlebitis of the great veins (including pelvic suppurative thrombophlebitis) and the portal vein.
- Magnetic resonance imaging is the diagnostic procedure of choice for the evaluation of patients with suspected suppurative intracranial thrombophlebitis, and yield can probably improve with magnetic resonance angiography.

Diagnostic/Testing Procedures

The diagnosis of deep central vein suppurative thrombophlebitis in the thorax can be established by venography.

Treatment

MAIN TREATMENT

- Superficial suppurative thrombophlebitis can be fatal, and prompt treatment is indicated. Most patients respond to antimicrobial treatment. Excision of the infected vein is indicated only when persistent bacteremia, despite antibiotics, is present.
- Surgical exploration with drainage of all collections is needed. Radical surgeries can be required in burn patients.
- When infection of a venous catheter is suspected, it should be removed and cultured.
- Empiric antibiotic therapy
  —Superficial suppurative thrombophlebitis: vancomycin. A third-generation cephalosporin with activity against *Pseudomonas* (such as ceftazidime) or an aminoglycoside should be added in immunocompromised or burn patients.
  —Septic pelvic vein thrombophlebitis: metronidazole (500 mg i.v. qid) with a third-generation cephalosporin; or monotherapy with imipenem (500 mg i.v. qid) or cefoxitin. If fever persists, intravenous heparin is indicated.
  —Suppurative intracranial thrombophlebitis: nafcillin or oxacillin (2 g every 4 hours i.v.) and a third-generation cephalosporin with activity against *Pseudomonas* (such as ceftazidime 2 g every 8 hours i.v.). Vancomycin can replace nafcillin for the management of methicillin-resistant staphylococci.
- Concomitant use of heparin is indicated in suppurative intracranial thrombophlebitis.

COMPLICATIONS

Acute bacterial endocarditis, sepsis, pneumonia, or metastatic abscess can result from suppurative thrombophlebitis.

Follow-Up

All patients and especially those at higher risk, such as burn patients, who develop bacteremia or other systemic infection, should undergo careful examination of all previously cannulated veins.

PREVENTION

- The cannulation of the lower extremity should be avoided. Cannulae, intravenous fluid bottles, and connecting tubing should be replaced every 48 to 72 hours.
- Strategies to block microbial access to the transcutaneous tract, such as use of more potent cutaneous antiseptic agents, topical application of antimicrobial agents, use of central venous catheters coated with antibiotics (such as minocycline and rifampin), or attachment of a subcutaneous silver-impregnated cuff, have helped prevent catheter-related infection.
- The recent Centers for Disease Control and Prevention guidelines for the prevention of catheter-related infections recommend the use of antimicrobe-impregnated venous catheters for patients with a high rate of infection after full adherence to other infection-control measures, such as maximal sterile barrier precautions.

Selected Readings

Brook I, Frazier EH. Aerobic and anaerobic microbiology of superficial suppurative thrombophlebitis. *Arch Surg* 1996;131:95–97.

Brown CE, Stettler RW, Twickler D, et al. Puerperal septic pelvic thrombophlebitis: Incidence and response to heparin therapy. *Am J Obstet Gynecol* 1999;181:143–148.

Raad I, Darouiche R, Dupuis J, et al., and the Texas Medical Center Catheter Study Group. Central venous catheters coated with minocycline and rifampin for the prevention of catheter-related colonization and bloodstream infections. A randomized, double-blind trial. *Ann Intern Med* 1997;127:267–274.

Scheld WM, Sande MA. Endocarditis and intravascular infections. In: Mandell GL, Bennett JE, Dolin R, eds. *Principles and practice of infectious diseases,* 4th ed. New York: Churchill Livingstone, 1995:740–783.

Thyroiditis, Infectious

Basics

DEFINITION

- Infections can involve the thyroid and cause either of the following:
  — Acute suppurative thyroiditis, which is a painful inflammation with suppuration and abscess formation
  — Subacute granulomatous thyroiditis (also termed *granulomatous, giant-cell,* or *de Quervain's*), a condition characterized by fever and painful enlargement of the thyroid gland

ETIOLOGY

- Pyogenic thyroiditis is usually preceded by infection in other organs. It usually arises from adjacent structures, such as the oropharynx or lymph nodes, or from congenital abnormalities, such as a persistent thyroglossal duct or piriform sinus fistula. However, infection can also occur by means of hematogenous spread associated with pyelonephritis, prostatitis, esophageal perforation, otitis, postpartum infection or dental infection, or after direct trauma.
- The most common pathogens associated with pyogenic thyroiditis are the following:
  — *Streptococcus pyogenes*
  — *Staphylococcus* spp
  — *Streptococcus pneumoniae*
- Less common organisms that lead to pyogenic thyroiditis include the following:
  — *Actinomyces* spp
  — *Aspergillus* spp
  — *Bacteroides* spp
  — *Candida* spp
  — *Coccidioides immitis*
  — *Echinococcus* spp
  — *Escherichia coli*
  — *Haemophilus influenzae*
  — *Histoplasma* spp
  — *Klebsiella* spp
  — *Mycobacterium tuberculosis*
  — *Peptostreptococcus* spp
  — *Pseudallescheria boydii*
  — *Streptococcus viridans*
  — *Salmonella* spp
- Patients with AIDS may present with thyroiditis due to unusual organisms, such as *Pneumocystis carinii*.
- Subacute thyroiditis often follows a viral infection.

EPIDEMIOLOGY

Normal thyroid glands can be involved, but patients with underlying disorders are much more susceptible to pyogenic thyroiditis. Nodular goiters also predispose to bacterial thyroiditis. In childhood, it is often linked to local anatomic defects.

Clinical Manifestations

SYMPTOMS

- Pyogenic thyroiditis is characterized by anterior neck pain (present in almost 100% of cases), dysphagia (91%), swelling of the thyroid, and constitutional signs of infection.
- Subacute thyroiditis presents with the slow onset of severe thyroid pain and tenderness, along with marked nonspecific symptoms such as myalgia and fatigue. Referred pain may predominate. These symptoms may smolder for weeks before the diagnosis is suspected. Less commonly, the onset is acute, with severe pain over the thyroid, fever, and occasionally symptoms of thyrotoxicosis. Some patients have other features typical of the disease but no pain.
- Tuberculous infection is less likely than acute bacterial thyroiditis to produce fever, pain, and tenderness.
- Echinococcosis of the thyroid is a chronic process that is generally diagnosed only following excision.

SIGNS

- Clinical signs of pyogenic thyroiditis include the following:
  — Tenderness (94%)
  — Fever (92%)
  — Erythema (82%)
  — Dysphonia (82%)
  — Warmth (70%)
  — Pharyngitis (69%).
- Physical findings in subacute thyroiditis include tenderness and nodularity of the thyroid, which may be unilateral but usually involves other areas of the gland.

Diagnosis

DIFFERENTIAL DIAGNOSIS

- The other forms of thyroiditis (such as Hashimoto's thyroiditis and chronic thyroiditis with transient thyrotoxicosis) are more common and are notable for their different clinical courses and the lack of local signs associated with inflammation.
- Demonstration of a low thyroid radioactive iodine uptake (RAIU) usually serves to differentiate subacute thyroiditis from these other causes of hyperthyroidism.
- Riedel's thyroiditis is a disorder in which intense fibrosis of the thyroid and surrounding structures causes induration of the neck and may be associated with mediastinal and retroperitoneal fibrosis.

Thyroiditis, Infectious

LABORATORY

- Usual findings in subacute thyroiditis include a high erythrocyte sedimentation rate and a depressed thyroid RAIU. Early in the course, many patients are mildly thyrotoxic, the serum T_4 and T_3 are high, and TSH is undetectable. Later, as glandular hormone is depleted, the patient may pass through a hypothyroid phase.
- In pyogenic thyroiditis, leukocytosis is often present, and thyroid function tests are frequently normal.

IMAGING

Studies useful in diagnosing acute suppurative thyroiditis include lateral neck radiographs, computed tomography scan of the neck, and ultrasonography.

DIAGNOSTIC/TESTING PROCEDURES

In pyogenic thyroiditis, needle biopsy can help in the identification of the pathogen.

Treatment

MAIN TREATMENT

- Treatment in the initial phase of pyogenic thyroiditis should include intravenous antibiotics directed against staphylococci, streptococci, and anaerobes. When culture and sensitivity reports are available, antibiotics should be changed accordingly. Improvement usually occurs within 48 to 72 hours, and complete resolution is often obtained in 2 to 4 weeks.
- Thyroid abscesses should be drained; fistulas require excision to prevent recurrences.
- There is no definitive therapy for painful subacute thyroiditis, but there is effective treatment that will ameliorate the symptoms and allow the disease to run its spontaneous course in an asymptomatic fashion. Salicylates and nonsteroidal antiinflammatory drugs can be used in patients with mild or moderate forms of the disorder. In more severe forms of the condition, corticosteroids in a suitable pharmacologic dosage will generally cause a rapid relief of symptoms within 24 to 48 hours. Prednisone may be initiated in dosages of 20 to 40 mg daily, with a gradual reduction in dosage thereafter over several weeks. When the thyroid RAIU and serum T_4 return to normal, therapy can be withdrawn.

ALTERNATIVE TREATMENT

Other less common forms of treatment for subacute thyroiditis include triiodothyronine or thyroxine, generally to prevent repeated exacerbations. Irradiation is no longer used.

TREATMENT FAILURE

Thyroidectomy should be considered only in that very small minority of patients with subacute thyroiditis who have repeated relapses despite appropriate treatment.

COMPLICATIONS

- Outcome in pyogenic thyroiditis is usually favorable, with complete recovery expected in most cases. Most fatal cases have been associated with delays in diagnosis.
- Complications of pyogenic thyroiditis are unusual and include vocal cord paralysis, hypothyroidism (usually transient), tracheal involvement, and recurrent infection.

Follow-Up

- A hypothyroid phase often follows subacute thyroiditis. During the period of transient hypothyroidism, thyroxine may be provided but can usually be discontinued subsequently. Recovery is almost the universal rule, and only 1% or fewer become permanently hypothyroid.
- Recurrences do appear in a small percentage of patients with subacute thyroiditis. Repeat exacerbations are uncommon.

PREVENTION

N/A

Selected Readings

Andres JC, Nagalla R. Acute bacterial thyroiditis secondary to urosepsis. *J Am Board Fam Pract* 1995;8:128–129.

Smilack JD, Argueta R. Coccidioidal infection of the thyroid. *Arch Intern Med* 1998;158:89–92.

Volpe R. The management of subacute (DeQuervain's) thyroiditis. *Thyroid* 1993;3:253–255.

Wartofsky L. Diseases of the thyroid. In: Fauci AS, Braunwald E, Isselbacher KJ, et al., eds. *Harrison's principles of internal medicine*, 14th ed. New York: McGraw-Hill Co, 1998:2012–2035.

Toxic Shock Syndrome

Basics

DEFINITION

- Toxic shock syndrome (TSS) is a severe, life-threatening illness due to *Staphylococcus aureus,* and is characterized by sudden onset of rash, fever, vomiting, diarrhea, and myalgia, followed by hypotension, multiorgan dysfunction, and desquamation during the early convalescent period.
- Streptococcal infections can also cause a toxic shock–like syndrome (TSLS), associated with explosive, often life-threatening disease characterized by shock and multisystem organ failure.

ETIOLOGY

- Staphylococcal TSS is caused by infection or colonization with toxin-producing *S. aureus.*
- For illness to develop, an individual must be colonized or infected with a toxigenic strain of *S. aureus* and must lack a protective level of antibody to the toxin made by that strain.
- The key toxins causing this multisystem disease are TSS toxin 1 and staphylococcal enterotoxins B and C.
- TSLS is usually caused by infection with group A *Streptococcus* and the production of streptococcal pyrogenic exotoxins A, B, and C.
- Like staphylococcal toxin, streptococcal pyrogenic exotoxins A and B can induce the synthesis of cytokines such as tumor necrosis factor-alpha, interleukin-1beta, and interleukin-6. These cytokines are known to mediate fever, shock, and tissue injury.

EPIDEMIOLOGY

Incidence

TSS is a relatively uncommon illness, with a reported incidence (among menstruating women) of 1 case per 100,000; it is likely, however, that the disease is substantially underreported.

Risk Factors

- Menstruation and tampon use remain the most common settings for TSS, but the disease can also complicate the use of barrier contraceptives, the puerperium, septic abortion, and nonobstetric gynecologic surgery.
- About half of all cases occur in settings other than menstruation and are distributed among individuals of both sexes and all ages. Nonmenstrual TSS can complicate skin lesions of many types (such as chemical or thermal burns, insect bites, etc.), surgical wound infections, nasal packing, bacteremia, musculoskeletal infections, and respiratory infections.
- Menstrual and nonmenstrual cases are clinically indistinguishable.
- TSLS occurs most commonly in the setting of invasive soft-tissue infections (80% of cases), such as necrotizing fasciitis, myonecrosis, and cellulitis; however, association with streptococcal pneumonia, sinusitis, and pharyngitis has been reported.

Clinical Manifestations

SYMPTOMS

In TSS, the onset of symptoms is typically acute and rapidly progressive over a period of 48 to 72 hours.

Case Definition of Toxic Shock Syndrome

- Fever: temperature of 38.9°C (102°F) or higher
- Rash: diffuse macular erythroderma ("sunburn" rash)
- Hypotension: systolic blood pressure of less than 90 mmHg, or orthostatic hypotension
- Involvement of at least three of the following organ systems:
  —Gastrointestinal: vomiting or diarrhea at onset of illness
  —Muscular: severe myalgias or serum creatine phosphokinase level at least twice the upper limit of normal
  —Mucous membranes: vaginal, oropharyngeal, or conjunctival hyperemia
  —Renal: blood urea nitrogen or creatinine level at least twice the upper limit of normal, or pyuria
  —Hepatic: total serum bilirubin or aminotransferase level at least twice the upper limit of normal
  —Hematologic: thrombocytopenia
  —Central nervous: disorientation or alteration in consciousness but no focal neurologic signs at a time when fever and hypotension are absent
  —Desquamation: 1 to 2 weeks after the onset of illness (typically palms and soles)
  —Evidence against an alternative diagnosis: negative results of cultures of blood, throat, or CSF (if performed); no rise in titers of antibody to the agents of Rocky Mountain spotted fever, leptospirosis, and rubeola (if obtained)
- TSLS usually occurs in a young, previously healthy person who seeks medical attention because of fever, hypotension, cutaneous findings, and severe local pain. The pain is typically localized to an extremity and is often disproportionate to the findings on examination. The cutaneous signs are protean and may be subtle or absent. Desquamating erythroderma may be present but is less common than in staphylococcal TSS.
- The general features of TSLS include fever, hypotension, renal impairment, and respiratory distress syndrome. Various types of rash have been described, but rash usually does not develop.

Clinical Criteria for Diagnosis of Toxic Shock–like Syndrome

- I. Isolation of group A *Streptococcus* (*Streptococcus pyogenes*)
  —A. From a normally sterile site
  —B. From a nonsterile site (e.g., throat, vagina, superficial skin lesion)
- II. Clinical signs of severity
  —A. Hypotension *and* (B.) two or more of the following signs:
    —Renal impairment: serum creatinine level of 177 mol/L (2 mg/dL) for adults or at least twice the upper limit of normal for age; in patients with preexisting renal disease, an elevation over the baseline level by a factor of 2 or more

Toxic Shock Syndrome

- —Coagulopathy: platelet count of less than or equal to 100×10^9/L (100,000/μL) or disseminated intravascular coagulation
- —Liver involvement: alanine aminotransferase (SGOT), aspartate aminotransferase (SGPT), or total bilirubin level at least twice the upper limit of normal
- —Adult respiratory distress syndrome, or evidence of diffuse capillary leakage manifested by acute onset of generalized edema, or pleural or peritoneal effusions with hypoalbuminemia
- —Generalized erythematous macular rash that may desquamate
- —Soft-tissue necrosis, including necrotizing fasciitis or myositis, or gangrene
- —An illness fulfilling criteria IA, IIA, and IIB is defined as a *definite* case. An illness fulfilling criteria IB, IIA, and IIB is defined as a *probable* case if no other etiology is identified.

Diagnosis

DIFFERENTIAL DIAGNOSIS

- The differential diagnosis of TSS is that of a severe febrile exanthem with hypotension. Infections to consider include staphylococcal scalded-skin syndrome, Kawasaki syndrome, Rocky Mountain spotted fever, leptospirosis, meningococcemia, gram-negative sepsis, exanthematous viral syndromes, and severe drug reactions. Staphylococcal TSS and streptococcal TSS can be clinically indistinguishable.
- The clinical presentations of TSS and TSLS are frequently similar; however, TSLS is associated with extensive soft-tissue infection, bullae formation, and bacteremia, but these findings are uncommon in staphylococcal toxic shock.

LABORATORY

- Usual laboratory abnormalities of both TSS and TSLS include azotemia, hypoalbuminemia, hypocalcemia, hypophosphatemia, creatine phosphokinase elevation, leukocytosis or leukopenia with a left shift, thrombocytopenia, and pyuria.
- In contrast to TSS, more than 60% of patients with TSLS have bacteremia.

Treatment

MAIN TREATMENT

- Treatment of TSS and TSLS involves identification and removal of the source of the infection (surgical debridement or drainage, or removal of nasal packing or tampon), initiation of effective antibiotic therapy, and appropriate supportive care.
- Empiric treatment for TSS includes semisynthetic penicillins (nafcillin or oxacillin 2 g i.v. every 6 hours); some authors suggest the additional use of clindamycin (900 mg i.v. every 8 hours) to reduce toxin production. Vancomycin can be an alternative to the β-lactam antibiotic.
- Empiric treatment for TSLS consists of penicillin G (24 million units/d i.v.) and clindamycin (900 mg i.v. every 8 hours). Erythromycin or ceftriaxone (2 g i.v. qd) can be a less-well-studied alternative to penicillin G.
- Duration of therapy varies, but, in uncomplicated cases, a 14-day course of therapy is reasonable.
- In patients with severe illness consider intravenous immunoglobulin (150 mg/kg/d for 5 days or 400 mg/kg in a single dose), which contains high levels of neutralizing antibody to TSS toxins.
- Steroids should not be administered routinely.

COMPLICATIONS

- The early signs and symptoms of TSS resolve within the first few days of illness, after which, complications of organ hypoperfusion, such as renal and myocardial dysfunction, massive edema, and adult respiratory distress syndrome, dominate the picture.
- The mortality rate of TSS is less than 5% in menstrual-related cases but is twofold to threefold higher in nonmenstrual cases.
- The overall mortality rate in TSLS has been 30%, despite aggressive medical and surgical intervention.

Follow-Up

TSS recurs in as many as 40% of cases.

PREVENTION

Among patients with TSS, tampons and barrier contraceptives should be avoided in women in whom seroconversion does not occur after an acute illness.

Selected Readings

Davies HD, McGeer A, Schwartz B, et al. Invasive group A streptococcal infections in Ontario, Canada. Ontario Group A Streptococcal Study Group. *N Engl J Med* 1996;335:547–554.

Deresiewicz RL, Parsonnet J. Staphylococcal infection. In: Fauci AS, Braunwald E, Isselbacher KJ, et al., eds. *Harrison's principles of internal medicine,* 14th ed. New York: McGraw-Hill, 1998:875–885.

Drage LA. Life-threatening rashes: Dermatologic signs of four infectious diseases. *Mayo Clin Proc* 1999;74:68–72.

Wessels MR. Streptococcal and enterococcal infection. In: Fauci AS, Braunwald E, Isselbacher KJ, et al., eds. *Harrison's principles of internal medicine,* 14th ed. New York: McGraw-Hill, 1998:885–892.

Wolf JE, Rabinowitz LG. Streptococcal toxic shock–like syndrome. *Arch Dermatol* 1995;131:73–77.

Toxoplasmosis

Basics

DEFINITION

- An acute or chronic infection caused by the obligate intracellular protozoan *Toxoplasma gondii*.
- Infection in humans is usually asymptomatic.
- When symptoms occur, they range from a mild, self-limited disease to a fulminant disseminated disease that usually involves the following:
  - Central nervous system
  - Eyes
  - Skeletal or cardiac muscles
  - Lymph nodes
  - Liver
  - Lungs
- Severe infections usually occur in an immunocompromised patient or by the transplacental passage of parasites from an infected mother to the fetus (congenital toxoplasmosis).

ETIOLOGY

- Cats are the definitive hosts for *T. gondii*.
- There are two stages in the life cycle of *T. gondii*:
  - The sexual phase results in the formation of oocysts in the cat's intestine. They are excreted in the feces, sporulation occurs, and they may remain infectious for many months.
  - The sporulated oocysts are ingested by an intermediate host (e.g., a human). Bradyzoites or sporozoites are released and transformed to rapidly dividing tachyzoites, which can infect any organ. Immune responses are able to eliminate most of the tachyzoites, and a tissue cyst is formed. Active infection usually occurs due to release of encysted parasites.

EPIDEMIOLOGY

- The seroprevalence depends on geographic location and the age of the population. In the United States, it varies between 3% and 67%, while in tropical countries and in areas of western Europe, it is up to 90%.
- Cases are caused by eating undercooked meat or contaminated vegetables or by ingestion of sporulated oocysts from contaminated soil.
- Congenital toxoplasmosis
  - Incidence in the United States is 1 in 1,000 to 1 in 8,000 cases.
  - Only one of five pregnant women infected with *T. gondii* develop clinical signs.
  - Women who are seropositive before pregnancy usually are protected against acute infection and do not give birth to congenitally infected neonates.
  - If the acute infection in the mother goes untreated, congenital infection occurs in approximately 15% of the fetuses during the first trimester, 30% of the fetuses during the second trimester, and 60% of the fetuses during the third trimester.
  - However, the earlier the transmission, the more severe the outcome.
- Toxoplasmosis and HIV infection
  - The greatest incidence is seen among patients with a low CD4 count (<100 cells/mm^3)
  - In areas with high seroprevalence for toxoplasmosis, 25% to 50% of all AIDS patients, who are not receiving antiretroviral therapy, will develop CNS toxoplasmosis.

Clinical Manifestations

SYMPTOMS AND SIGNS

Immunocompetent Persons

- Asymptomatic in 80% to 90% of cases. Among symptomatic patients, lymphadenopathy is the most common presentation.
- Cervical lymph nodes are most commonly involved, but any or all lymph node groups may be enlarged. Nodes are usually discrete, nontender, less than 3 cm in diameter, and nonsuppurative.
- Less common presenting symptoms
  - Fever
  - Myalgias
  - Arthralgias
  - Malaise
  - Sore throat
  - Maculopapular rash
  - Nightsweats
  - Hepatosplenomegaly
  - Atypical lymphadenopathy (<10% of lymphocytes)
  - Abdominal pain
  - Meningoencephalitis
  - Myocarditis
  - Pericarditis
  - Polymyositis
- *Toxoplasma* causes one in three cases of chorioretinitis in the United States. Most cases are from congenital infection. Patients usually develop symptoms during the second and third decades of life. Patients may present with the following:
  - Blurred vision
  - Scotoma
  - Ocular pain
  - Photophobia
  - Epiphora
- Ophthalmologic examination reveals yellow-white, cotton-like patches with indistinct margins of hyperemia. Lesions are usually multiple and develop distinct borders and black spots within the retina.

Immunocompromised Patients

- The infection usually involves the CNS and, less often, the lung (pneumonitis), the eye (chorioretinitis), or the heart. Cases of gastrointestinal, liver, skin, or multiorgan involvement also have been reported.
- Extracerebral toxoplasmosis is less common among patients with HIV infection. The prevalence is estimated at 1.5% to 2.0%. Age, gender, and HIV risk factors are probably similar to those of the general AIDS population. Extracerebral toxoplasmosis involves the eyes and/or the lungs in more than 75% of the cases, and it may develop among patients seronegative for *T. gondii*.
- Clinical manifestations of CNS infection include the following:
  - Headache
  - Seizures
  - Weakness
  - Cranial nerve abnormalities
  - Visual field defects
  - Mental status changes
  - Cerebellar signs
  - Speech abnormalities
  - Meningism
  - Sensory or motor disorders
- Toxoplasmic pneumonitis usually presents with fever, dyspnea, and nonproductive cough.
- Ocular toxoplasmosis presents with the same symptoms as in immunocompetent patients, but it can progress more rapidly.

Congenital Toxoplasmosis

- Clinical findings are variable. There may be no sequelae, or sequelae may develop at various times after birth.
- Premature infants may present with CNS or ocular disease.
- Full-term infants usually develop milder disease, with hepatosplenomegaly and lymphadenopathy.

Diagnosis

- Diagnosis is based on compatible clinical picture, neuroimaging findings, and serology; definitive diagnosis is based on pathology.
- Microbiology
- Parasitemia may also be detected in a high proportion of patients with the infection.
- Evaluation of bronchoalveolar lavage with direct examination (by Giemsa and indirect immunofluorescence with monoclonal antibody to membrane antigen P-30) and/or tissue culture is the procedure of choice for diagnosing pulmonary toxoplasmosis.

Toxoplasmosis

OTHER LABORATORY METHODS

- Approximately 20% of patients have no detectable antibodies, and the titer does not always rise during infection. Negative serology does not rule out infection, but a rising titer may be of diagnostic significance.
- Preliminary results from the use of polymerase chain reaction (PCR) in blood samples suggest that, at present, this modality has limited diagnostic value in cases of cerebral toxoplasmosis.
- Usually cerebrospinal fluid (CSF) is also nonpathognomonic and reveals elevated protein and mild pleocytosis.
- Diagnosis of ocular toxoplasmosis is usually based on a suggestive ophthalmoscopic picture. Histopathologic identification of *T. gondii* in the eye can establish the diagnosis.
- Extracerebral toxoplasmosis involving, simultaneously, other organs among HIV-infected patients is rare, and diagnosis is usually based on biopsy.

IMAGING

- On neuroimaging, the abscesses of cerebral toxoplasmosis are typically multiple, are located in the cortex or deep nuclei (thalamus and basal ganglia), are surrounded by edema, and enhance in a ringlike pattern with contrast.
- Magnetic resonance imaging (MRI) has greater sensitivity than computed tomography (CT) for detection of smaller lesions in this population.
- Definitive diagnosis of cerebral toxoplasmosis requires brain biopsy or identification of the microorganism in CSF (by Wright-Giemsa stain).
- Currently, brain biopsy is indicated for patients with focal enhancing cerebral lesions seen on CT and MRI who do not respond to an appropriate trial of empiric antitoxoplasmosis therapy, for patients who are showing rapid clinical deterioration with neuroimaging, and for serology that is not suggestive of toxoplasmosis.
- Chest roentgenographs are abnormal in more than half of the patients with pulmonary toxoplasmosis.

Treatment

MAIN TREATMENT

- Drugs, dosages, and treatment duration for extracerebral toxoplasmosis, such as ocular, pulmonary, or disseminated, are usually the same as in cerebral involvement.
- The combination of pyrimethamine plus sulfadiazine is the regimen of choice for acute therapy.
- For acute therapy, the usual dose is 4 to 8 g/d of sulfadiazine and a loading dose of 100 to 200 mg, followed by 50 to 75 mg/d of pyrimethamine. Lower dosages are under evaluation.
- Leucovorin should always be coadministered with pyrimethamine to prevent the folinic acid deficiency and ameliorate the hematologic toxicity of pyrimethamine.
- Duration of treatment should be individualized, but it usually is for 6 to 8 weeks.

ALTERNATIVE TREATMENT

- Pyrimethamine (accompanied by folinic acid) combined with clindamycin is clearly an effective and acceptable alternative.
- For maintenance therapy, data are limited, but the current recommendation is to administer 1,200 mg/day of clindamycin in three to four doses, combined with pyrimethamine and folinic acid.
- Atovaquone has been studied in preclinical preliminary studies (750 mg orally four times a day) and was effective as a single agent during acute infection. Additional studies are needed to evaluate the efficacy of atovaquone alone or in combination with pyrimethamine.
- Clarithromycin has been found effective in preclinical studies. The combination of clarithromycin with pyrimethamine also seems effective but is probably associated with frequent adverse reactions.
- Azithromycin may have a role in combination with pyrimethamine.
- Limited clinical experience suggests that trimethoprim–sulfamethoxazole (TMP-SMX) may be an effective therapy.
- Steroids may produce transient clinical and radiographic improvement in CNS lymphoma and are not recommended for patients undergoing a therapeutic trial for cerebral toxoplasmosis, except for patients with probable impending herniation.

COMPLICATIONS

- Ocular toxoplasmosis can lead to loss of central vision, nystagmus, or strabismus.
- The incidence of adverse reactions to sulfadiazine is high, especially among HIV-infected patients, and includes urticaria, rash, gastrointestinal disturbances, myelosuppression, crystalluria that may lead to acute renal failure, and Stevens-Johnson syndrome.
- Pyrimethamine is associated with dose-related cytopenia and rash.

Follow-Up

TYPICAL PROGRESSION/PROGNOSIS

Eighty percent to 90% of patients with AIDS will have a radiographic and/or clinical response. Relapses of ocular toxoplasmosis occur in up to one-third of patients.

PATIENT FOLLOW-UP

- After induction treatment, HIV-infected patients should receive lifelong suppression therapy with pyrimethamine (25–50 mg/d) and sulfadiazine (2–4 g/d).
- Careful ophthalmologic examination is essential for newborns with suspected congenital infection.

PREVENTION

- All HIV-infected persons should be tested for IgG antibody to *T. gondii* soon after the diagnosis of HIV infection.
- Seronegative pregnant women and other individuals at risk should be advised not to eat raw or undercooked ("pink") meat and should wash fruits and vegetables well.
- They should wash their hands after contact with raw meat and after contact with soil.
- They should wash their hands after changing a cat litter box, or, preferably, it should be changed by a nonpregnant, HIV-negative person.
- *Toxoplasma*-seropositive patients with CD4 counts less than 100 cells/mm^3 should receive prophylaxis against toxoplasmosis.
- The doses of TMP/SMX recommended for *P. carinii* pneumonia appear to be effective.
- A combination of dapsone and pyrimethamine is an alternative.
- Prophylactic monotherapy with dapsone, pyrimethamine, azithromycin, clarithromycin, or atovaquone is not recommended.
- Aerosolized pentamidine does not offer protection against toxoplasmosis.

Selected Readings

Cohen BA. Neurologic manifestations of toxoplasmosis in AIDS. *Seminars in Neurology* 1999;19(2):201–211.

Foulon W, Naessens A, Ho-Yen D. Prevention of congenital toxoplasmosis. *Journal of Perinatal Medicine* 2000;28(5):337–345.

Patel R. Disseminated toxoplasmosis after liver transplantation. *Clinical Infectious Diseases* 1999;29(3):705–706.

Trachoma and Inclusion Conjunctivitis

Basics

DEFINITION

- Trachoma is a chronic follicular conjunctivitis associated with infection by *Chlamydia trachomatis*.
- In trachoma-endemic areas where the classic eye disease is seen, infection is due to *C. trachomatis*. In nonendemic areas, organisms can be transmitted from the genital tract to the eye, usually causing only the inclusion conjunctivitis syndrome, occasionally with keratitis. These cases may be referred to as *paratrachoma* to differentiate them epidemiologically from eye-to-eye–transmitted endemic trachoma.

ETIOLOGY

- *C. trachomatis* has a predilection for cells of the conjunctiva.
- Serovars A, B, Ba, or C are associated with trachoma, and serovars D through K cause the inclusion conjunctivitis syndrome.

EPIDEMIOLOGY

Incidence

- One hundred fifty million children have the active, infectious form of trachoma.
- Of the 38 million blind people in the world, 6 million (15.5%) are blind because of trachoma.
- An estimated 30 million adults, mostly women, have in-turning of the eyelid margin due to trachoma.
- Transmission of trachoma is from eye to eye via hands (particularly among young children and the women who look after them), flies, towels, and other fomites.
- In younger children, boys and girls are equally affected.
- Repeated reinfections from siblings cause the formation of follicles and inflammation of the conjunctiva, with ocular irritation and mucopurulent discharge. In children and adolescents, scar tissue begins to form on the upper tarsal conjunctiva.
- Young children are the main reservoir of infection in the community.

Risk Factors

- Blinding trachoma is found where the environment is typically hot, dry, and dusty. This includes large areas of Africa, the Middle East, parts of India and central and south Asia, Indonesia, and North Australia, and foci in Central and South America.
- Children with faces that are dirty from nasal, ocular, and aural discharges are at increased risk of severe inflammatory trachoma. Other risk factors for trachoma infection include overcrowding, proximity to cattle, the absence of latrines, high densities of flies, seasonal epidemics of bacterial or viral conjunctivitis, and dry, dusty environments in communities with an inadequate supply of water.
- Eye infection with genital *C. trachomatis* strains occur among sexually active young adults.

Clinical Manifestations

SYMPTOMS

- Both endemic trachoma and adult inclusion conjunctivitis present initially as conjunctivitis characterized by small lymphoid follicles in the conjunctiva.
- In regions with hyperendemic, classic blinding trachoma, the disease usually starts insidiously before the age of 2 years.
- Patients with trachoma can develop dryness of the eyes, due to destruction of the lacrimal ducts, and lacrimal gland.
- Neonatal chlamydial conjunctivitis has an acute onset and often produces a profuse mucopurulent discharge.

Signs

- In trachoma, the cornea becomes involved, with inflammatory leukocytic infiltrations and superficial vascularization (pannus formation). In children and adolescents, scar tissue begins to form on the upper tarsal conjunctiva. These scars may lead to in-turning of the eyelid margin (entropion) and eyelashes (trichiasis). Eventually, the corneal epithelium is abraded and may ulcerate, with subsequent corneal scarring and blindness.
- Paratrachoma is frequently associated with corneal inflammation in the form of discrete opacities ("infiltrates"), punctate epithelial erosions, and minor degrees of superficial corneal vascularization.

Diagnosis

DIFFERENTIAL DIAGNOSIS

- The clinical diagnosis of classic trachoma can be made if two of the following signs are present:
  - Lymphoid follicles on the upper tarsal conjunctiva
  - Typical conjunctival scarring
  - Vascular pannus
  - Limbal follicles
- The differential diagnosis of trachoma is discussed elsewhere and includes multiple infections due to viruses, bacteria, parasites, and fungi (see Section II chapter, "Conjunctivitis").
- In the newborn, chlamydial conjunctivitis generally has a longer incubation period than does gonococcal conjunctivitis (usually 5–14 days vs. 1–3 days).
- In addition to *C. trachomatis* and *Neisseria gonorrhoeae*, the other important infectious causes of conjunctivitis in newborns include *Haemophilus influenzae*, *Streptococcus pneumoniae*, and herpes simplex virus.

Trachoma and Inclusion Conjunctivitis

LABORATORY

- Demonstration of chlamydiae by Giemsa- or immunofluorescent-stained smears, by isolation in cell cultures, or by newer nonculture tests constitutes definitive evidence of infection.
- DNA amplification techniques to detect chlamydial infections and identify groups that should receive treatment may be used.

Treatment

MAIN TREATMENT

- Single-dose azithromycin therapy (20 mg/kg orally) is the treatment of choice for trachoma. It has an efficacy of 78% at 6-month follow-up.
- Because concomitant pharyngeal infection is often present, neonatal chlamydial conjunctivitis should be treated with oral antimicrobials in order to prevent chlamydial pneumonia.

ALTERNATIVE TREATMENT

Topical tetracycline eye ointment 1% for at least 6 weeks, or on 5 consecutive days a month for 6 months, can be administered. Oral doxycycline 100 mg once daily for 4 weeks can be added for very severe infection.

COMPLICATIONS

- Entropion and trichiasis lead to corneal ulceration, scarring, and vascularization, resulting visual loss.
- If untreated, inclusion conjunctivitis may persist for 6 weeks to 2 years.
- Inclusion conjunctivitis can lead to conjunctival scarring and eyelid distortion, particularly in patients treated for many months with topical glucocorticoids. Recurrent eye infections develop most often in patients whose sexual consorts are not treated with antimicrobials.

Follow-Up

- Acute relapse of old trachoma occasionally follows treatment with cortisone eye ointment or develops in very old persons who were exposed in their youth.
- A considerable percentage of the patients with inclusion conjunctivitis have a concomitant genital chlamydial infection, and a majority of them have no genital symptoms. Because patients with chlamydial conjunctivitis and/or their partners possibly have a concomitant genital chlamydial infection, it is recommended that both patients and their sexual partners be referred for routine examination and systemic treatment when indicated.

PREVENTION

- Community-based strategies for improving hygiene in children in trachoma-endemic villages can reduce the prevalence of trachoma.
- Health education focusing on the need for daily facewashing, the use of latrines, and the proper disposal of refuse—directed at communities with a high prevalence of inflammatory disease—is very important. School teachers, traditional healers, religious leaders, and village health workers should be encouraged to propagate this message.
- In communities where more than 5% of children have severe inflammatory trachoma, chemotherapy is indicated.
- In communities with a prevalence of trichiasis of over 1% in women, a campaign of surgical intervention to correct entropion is indicated.
- The World Health Organization has formed the Global Elimination of Trachoma by the Year 2020 campaign. This campaign is based on the SAFE strategy:
  — Surgery for in-turned eyelids with simplified procedures, often performed by nonspecialist personnel
  — Antibiotic treatment (either oral azithromycin dihydrate or topical oxytetracycline hydrochloride) for entire communities to reduce the prevalence of *C. trachomatis* and to lower transmission rates
  — Facewashing and improved hygiene in young children
  — Environmental improvements: providing safe water and better disposal of animal and human feces to reduce the population of eye-seeking flies that transmit infections

Selected Readings

Bailey RL, Arullendran P, Whittle HC, et al. Randomised controlled trial of single-dose azithromycin in treatment of trachoma. *Lancet* 1993;342:453–456.

Dawson C, Schachter J. Can blinding trachoma be eliminated worldwide? *Arch Ophthalmol* 1999;117:974.

Postema EJ, Remeijer L, van der Meijden WI. Epidemiology of genital chlamydial infections in patients with chlamydial conjunctivitis; a retrospective study. *Genitourin Med* 1996;72:203–205.

Potter AR. Combating blinding trachoma. *BMJ* 1993;307:213–214.

Stamm WE. Chlamydial infections. In: Fauci AS, Braunwald E, Isselbacher KJ, et al., eds. *Harrison's principles of internal medicine*, 14th ed. New York: McGraw-Hill, 1998:1045–1064.

West S, Munoz B, Lynch M, et al. Impact of face-washing on trachoma in Kongwa, Tanzania. *Lancet* 1995;345:155–158.

Traveler's Diarrhea

Basics

DEFINITION
Traveler's diarrhea is loose, watery bowel movements occurring three or more times in a 24-hour period, typically among travelers to less-developed countries. It is most frequently transmitted via the fecal–oral route: human to human, animal to human, water-borne, or food-borne. The average duration of illness is 3 to 5 days.

ETIOLOGY
- Bacterial
  - *E. coli*
  - *Campylobacter*
  - *Salmonella*
  - *Shigella*
  - *Plesiomonas shigelloides*
- Viral
  - Rotavirus
  - Calicivirus
- Parasitic
  - *Giardia lamblia*
  - *Entamoeba histolytica*
  - *Cryptosporidium parvum*
  - *Cyclospora cayetanesis*
  - *Isospora belli*
  - *Balantidium coli*

EPIDEMIOLOGY
Incidence
— One-fourth of a billion people travel from one country to another annually; 16 million people travel from industrialized countries to developing countries.
— High risk: greater than 50% occurrence
  — Latin America (21%–80%)
  — Asia (21%–80%)
  — Africa (36%–62%)
- Intermediate risk: 10% to 20%
  — Southern Europe
  — Israel
  — Select Caribbean islands
- Low risk: less than 8%
  — Canada
  — United States
  — Northern Europe
  — Australia
  — New Zealand
  — Japan
  — Majority of the Caribbean islands

Infection Prevalence
- Toxigenic *E. coli*: contaminated food and beverages
- Rotavirus: endemic in tropics
- Caliciviruses: camps, cruise ships
- *Giardia*: protozoa in contaminated water and food prevalent in developing countries, wilderness
- *E. histolytica*: amoeba in contaminated water or vegetables prevalent in developing countries
- *Cryptosporidium*: protozoa parasite in contaminated water prevalent in developing countries and young animals, farm animals
- *Cyclospora*: protozoa in food and water worldwide
- *I. belli*: subtropical climates and developing countries

Risk Factors
- Travel to higher risk countries
- Students, itinerant tourists
- Failure to adhere to dietary precautions
  — Undercooked or raw vegetables, meat, or seafood
  — Tap water, ice, unpasteurized milk, and other daily products

Incubation
- One to 3 days

Clinical Manifestations

Symptoms and Signs
- Watery, loose stools; usually three to five per day

Traveler's Diarrhea

- Gas
- Fatigue
- Cramps
- Nausea
- Fever
- Abdominal pain
- Anorexia
- Headache
- Chills
- Vomiting
- Malaise
- Arthralgias
- Bloody stools (2%–10%)

Diagnosis

Diagnosis is based on clinical symptoms. There is high suspicion in recent travelers to less-developed regions of the world. In severe cases, and when a laboratory is available, obtain a stool specimen for culture and parasitic examination.

Treatment

MAIN TREATMENT

- Replacement of fluids and electrolytes
- Refeeding with slight restrictions (avoid coffee, alcohol, carbonated beverages, dairy products)
- Ciprofloxacin 500 mg twice per day PO for 3 days

Parasitic Diarrhea

- Amebiasis: metronidazole 750 mg tid PO for 10 days, then iodoquinol 650 mg tid PO for 20 days, or paromomycin 500 mg tid PO for 7 days
- Giardiasis: metronidazole 250 mg tid PO for 5 days

ALTERNATIVE TREATMENT

- Trimethoprim–sulfamethoxazole, other fluoroquinolones
- Amebiasis: tetracycline 500 mg qid PO for 14 days, plus dehydroemetine 0.5 to 0.75 mg/kg every 12 hours i.m. for 5 days (maximum 90 mg/d)
- Giardiasis: furazolidone, paromomycin
- Other treatments
  —Loperamide 2 mg, up to two tablets qid; can be taken with ciprofloxacin for moderate to severe cases
  —Pepto-Bismol: 60 mL up to 4 times per day

COMPLICATIONS

N/A

Follow-Up

PREVENTION

- Avoid tap water, unpasteurized dairy products, unpeeled or uncooked fruits, and vegetables.
- Prophylactic antibiotics are successful but not generally recommended due to their side effects. The drug of choice is ciprofloxacin 500 mg/d for the duration of the trip.

Selected Readings

DuPont HL, Ericsson CD. Prevention and treatment of traveler's diarrhea. *N Engl J Med* 1993;328:1821.

Hamer DH, Gorbach SL. Infectious diarrhea and bacterial food poisoning. In: Feldman M, Scharschmildt BF, Sleisenger MH, eds. *Sleisenger & Fordtran's Gastrointestinal and liver disease pathophysiology, diagnosis, and management*, 6th ed, vol 2. Philadelphia: WB Saunders, 1997:1594–1632.

Peltola H, Gorbach SL. Travelers' diarrhea. In: DuPont HL, Steffen R, eds. *Travel medicine and health*. Toronto: BC Decker, 1997:78–86.

Trichinosis

Basics

DEFINITION
Trichinella spiralis is a nematode that infects domestic and wild pigs, polar bears, walruses, and foxes. Infection in humans is due to larvae migration into striated muscle, the brain, and the heart.

ETIOLOGY
- *T. spiralis* is a small worm (males, 1.6 mm; females, 3.0 mm) that lives in the small intestine of carnivores such as swine.
- Larvae produced by the adult worms penetrate the intestines and travel via lymphatics and the blood into striated muscles, where they encyst.
- Upon ingestion, the larvae develop into adults in 36 hours.
- Within 2 to 3 weeks, new larvae are produced that disseminate throughout the striated muscle, heart, and brain.
- Infection in humans is the result of eating undercooked meat, usually pork or bear meat, containing the larvae of the worm.

EPIDEMIOLOGY
Incidence
- Disease is found worldwide but is principally seen in North America and Europe.
- Fewer than 100 symptomatic cases occur in the United States each year.

Risk Factors
- Eating undercooked pork; outbreaks have been noted due to eating undercooked sausages

Incubation
Larval invasion generally occurs 2 to 3 weeks after intestinal infection.

Clinical Manifestations

- Most infections are asymptomatic.
- Diarrhea of varying severity occurs after the adult worm enters the intestine.
- On occasion, the patient has nausea and vomiting.
- At the time of larval invasion, the patient may have high fevers, severe myalgias, headache, and periorbital edema.
- Pain in the extraocular muscles is noted frequently.
- Peripheral muscles may appear swollen.
- A macular rash along with subconjunctival hemorrhage may be noted.
- Symptoms often last for weeks, and may last 2 to 3 months.
- Migration of the larvae through the heart may lead to congestive heart failure and sudden death.
- Larval passage through the central nervous system leads to meningitis and encephalitis.

Diagnosis

Patients that present with myositis and eosinophilia should be considered to have trichinosis.

Trichinosis

DIFFERENTIAL DIAGNOSIS

- A wide variety of infectious and noninfectious illnesses may mimic trichinosis.
- Viral infections with influenza A, measles, and bacterial infections such as group A *Streptococcus* with scarlet fever, typhoid fever, and typhus may appear clinically similar.
- Angioneurotic edema can be confused with the periorbital edema.
- Infection may resemble schistosomiasis or strongyloidiasis.

LABORATORY

- Eosinophilia is present.
- Muscle enzymes, such as creatine phosphokinase and aldolase, are elevated in severe illness.
- Serology can take 3 weeks to become positive after ingestion of the larvae.
- On occasion, a muscle biopsy reveals the organism.

Treatment

- Albendazole 400 mg orally bid for 14 days

ALTERNATIVE TREATMENT

- Mebendazole 5 mg/kg orally bid for 10 days
- Prednisone 60 mg orally every day for 14 days can be used in patients with very severe disease, especially those with heart failure or encephalitis.

TREATMENT FAILURE

- Medications given are active against the adult worm, not the larvae.
- In patients with symptoms of myositis, bed rest with supportive care is necessary.

COMPLICATIONS

- Rare
  - Pneumonia
  - Heart failure
  - Nephritis

Follow-Up

PREVENTION

- Pork should be cooked properly at all times.
- Cysts in pork will not survive freezing at −15°C for 20 days.

Selected Readings

Cabie A, Bouchaud O, Houze S, et al. Albendazole versus thiabendazole as therapy for trichinosis: A retrospective study. *Clin Infect Dis* 1996;22:1033–1035.

McAuley JB, Michelson MK, Schantz PM. Trichinosis surveillance, United States, 1987–1990. *MMWR Morb Mortal Wkly Rep* 1991;40:35–42.

Trichomoniasis

Basics

DEFINITION
- Disease caused by infection with a species of protozoan of the genus *Trichomonas* or related genera; often used to designate trichomoniasis vaginitis

ETIOLOGY
- *Trichomonas vaginalis*, a flagellated protozoan that is highly motile in vaginal secretions

EPIDEMIOLOGY
Incidence and Prevalence
- Trichomoniasis is a sexually transmitted disease that accounts for 25% of vaginitis.
- Most women are asymptomatic when the organism is discovered, but 30% will develop symptoms within 6 months.
- *T. vaginalis* is isolated from prostatic secretions of 70% of male consorts of infected women.

Risk Factors
- Multiple sex partners
- Coexistence of bacterial vaginosis (BV)

Clinical Manifestations

- Vulvar erythema, pruritus, edema
- Vaginal discharge
  - Purulent: 60%
  - Frothy: 10% to 35%
  - Gray: 45%
  - Yellow-green: 35%
- Strawberry or "flea-bitten" cervix, which can be seen by colposcopy

Diagnosis

- Examination of a wet saline mount of vaginal discharge under a microscope shows motile, flagellated protozoa in a background of many polymorphonuclear leukocytes.
- The pH of vaginal discharge is greater than 4.5.
- Culture for *Trichomonas* in special medium has a high yield of positives, but is unnecessary if direct examination shows the organism.
- Direct examination and culture of urine sediment is the test of choice for diagnosing males.

DIFFERENTIAL DIAGNOSIS
- Other forms of vaginitis (e.g., *Candida*, herpes, and BV)

Treatment

- The cure rate is approximately 95% if both sex partners are treated simultaneously.
- The preferred treatment is a single 2-g dose of metronidazole. Alternately, 500 mg bid for 7 days can be used.

Trichomoniasis

- Coitus should be avoided until treatment is complete and both partners are asymptomatic.
- A single dose of 2 g of metronidazole may be given to pregnant women only after the first trimester.
- Treatment failure occurs in up to 30% when the male partner is not treated. Causes of treatment failure include the following:
  —Metronidazole-resistant strains: Retreat with metronidazole 500 mg bid for 7 days. If repeat failure occurs, a single 2-g dose should be given once daily for 3 to 5 days. (*Caution*: A dose greater than 3 g per day can cause irreversible neurologic damage.)
  —Noncompliance or vomiting
  —Drug interactions: Metronidazole is more rapidly metabolized when given with a drug that increases hepatic microsomal enzyme activity, such as phenytoin or phenobarbital.
  —Reinfection from a sexual partner

COMPLICATIONS

- Trichomoniasis is linked to BV and may increase the risk of acquiring this infection.
- Adverse pregnancy outcomes and preterm birth are associated with trichomoniasis, but the cause-and-effect relationship has not been fully established.

Follow-Up

Because of risk of recurrences and reinfection, periodic checkups and pelvic examinations should be obtained.

PREVENTION

- Safe-sex practices
- Treatment of both infected sexual partners

Selected Readings

Carr PL, Felsenstein D, Friedman RH. Evaluation and management of vaginitis. *J Gen Intern Med* 1998;13(5):335–346.

Patel K. Sexually transmitted diseases in adolescents: Focus on gonorrhea, chlamydia, and trichomoniasis—issues and treatment guidelines. *J Pediatr Health Care* 1998;12(4):211–215; quiz 216–217.

Petrin D, Delgaty K, Bhatt R, et al. Clinical and microbiological aspects of *Trichomonas vaginalis*. *Clin Microbiol Rev* 1998;11(2):300–317.

Trypanosomiasis

Basics

DEFINITION
Trypanosomiasis is a zoonotic protozoal disease transmitted to humans via blood-sucking insect vectors. It produces various acute and chronic diseases in humans.

ETIOLOGY
- *Trypanosoma cruzi* causes Chagas' disease in 10% to 30% of those infected.
  - It is transmitted via blood-sucking insects (kissing bugs), in the insects' feces. From there, the infectious trypomastigotes enter the human body through breaks in the skin and are transformed into amastigotes.
  - *T. cruzi* also can be transmitted via blood transfusions.
  - *T. cruzi* has been transmitted *in utero*, and is associated with fetal demise and fetal abnormalities.
- *Trypanosoma brucei brucei, T. brucei rhodesiense,* and *T. brucei gambiense* cause African sleeping sickness.
  - They are transmitted by the blood-sucking tsetse fly.
  - Trypomastigotes are transmitted from the salivary glands of the fly to the human during a blood meal.
  - The organism can multiply within the bloodstream and evade the host defenses by undergoing antigenic variation.
  - Congenital and blood transfusion infections are rare.

EPIDEMIOLOGY
- *T. cruzi* is present in South America, Central America, and Mexico.
  - It is present in many species of wild and domestic mammals.
  - Most cases in humans occur during childhood, and the disease is much more common in areas of poverty and in rural areas.
  - An estimated 16 to 18 million people are currently infected with *T. cruzi* in Latin America.
- *T. brucei brucei, T. brucei rhodesiense,* and *T. brucei gambiense* occur in Africa.
  - They are present in a variety of mammals, both wild and domestic.
  - West African disease is caused by *T. brucei gambiense*. It is present in tropical rain forests and rural regions in Central and West Africa, and disease is greatest in the dry seasons.
  - East African disease is caused mostly by *T. brucei rhodesiense*. Because the reservoir of disease is mostly in wild game such as antelope, infection in humans is limited.

Incubation
- Acute symptoms of Chagas' disease occur 1 week after contact with the parasite.
- Chronic Chagas' disease takes years to decades to cause significant illness.
- Symptoms of West African trypanosomiasis occur 1 to 2 weeks following the insect bite.
- Symptoms of East African trypanosomiasis occur a few days following the insect bite.

Clinical Manifestations

ACUTE CHAGAS' DISEASE
- A small, indurated papule with erythema and local lymphadenopathy occurs at the site of invasion by the organism. It is termed a *chagoma*.
- When contact is made from the organism to the conjunctiva, periocular edema occurs (Romaña sign), or swelling and closure of the eye.
- Fevers, constitutional symptoms, lymphadenopathy, and splenomegaly can occur and usually resolve within weeks.
- Central nervous system (CNS) symptoms and myocarditis are rare complications at this stage.

CHRONIC CHAGAS' DISEASE
- Develops years after the initial infection
- Patients develop megaesophagus and dysphagia.
- Aspiration is common.
- Colonic dysfunction with megacolon occurs.
- Cardiomyopathy develops and is associated with heart failure and/or arrhythmias, which are often fatal.

WEST AFRICAN TRYPANOSOMIASIS
- A chancre develops within 1 to 2 weeks following the tsetse fly bite.
- Several weeks to several months after the initial infection, patients develop fevers associated with lymphadenopathy.
- Massive enlargement of the cervical lymph nodes is seen (Winterbottom's sign).
- Marked constitutional signs occur at this stage, along with pruritus, arthralgias, transient edema of the face and extremities, and round erythematous rashes with internal clearing.
- Several months to years after the initial infections, patients can develop CNS signs of lethargy, somnolence, and personality changes. Ataxia, fasciculations, and choreiform movements occur at this stage.
- Neurologic signs progress slowly to stupor, coma, and death.

EAST AFRICAN TRYPANOSOMIASIS
- This disease follows that of the West African disease, but it is much more acute in nature.
- Patients develop fevers and rash within weeks, as opposed to months, after the tsetse fly bite.
- Lymphadenopathy is less apparent.
- Patients often die of cardiac failure or arrhythmias due to pancarditis.
- CNS signs may occur at the time that fevers are present.

Trypanosomiasis

Diagnosis

ACUTE CHAGAS' DISEASE

- Finding circulating parasites in the blood confirms the diagnosis.
- Wet preparations and Giemsa stains of anticoagulated blood (thin and thick smears) should be obtained.
- The organisms are motile. Detection occurs 50% of the time.

CHRONIC CHAGAS' DISEASE

- Serology is used to detect antibodies to the organism.
- Many false-positive tests occur.

AFRICAN TRYPANOSOMIASIS

- Fluid from chancres or aspirated fluid from lymph nodes should be prepared with Giemsa stains to search for organisms.
- Wet preparations and Giemsa stains of blood may reveal the organism.
- Concentrated cerebrospinal fluid in patients with neurologic abnormalities often reveals the organism.

Treatment

CHAGAS' DISEASE: ACUTE OR CHRONIC

- Nifurtimox 8 to 10 mg/kg/d orally in four divided doses over a 90- to 120-day period
- Benzimidazole 5 mg/kg/d orally for 60 days
- Pacemaker insertion is warranted in patients with arrhythmias and heart block.
- Management of congestive heart failure

AFRICAN TRYPANOSOMIASIS

- *T. brucei gambiense* infection without CNS abnormalities
  —Suramin 100 mg test dose, followed by 1 g i.v. days 2, 3, 7, 14, and 21, or
  —Pentamidine 4 mg/kg/d i.m. each day for 10 days
- *T. brucei gambiense* with or without CNS involvement
  —Eflornithine 400 mg/kg/d i.v. in four divided doses for 14 days, followed by a dose of 300 mg/kg/d in four divided doses for 30 days
- Alternative for *T. brucei gambiense* with CNS abnormalities
  —Tryparsamide 30 mg/kg i.m. every 5 days for 12 doses, with suramin 10 mg/kg i.v. every 5 days for a total of 12 doses.
- *T. brucei rhodesiense*
  —Patients with infection without CNS disease, nonresponsive to suramin or pentamidine, or patients with CNS disease
  —Melarsoprol 2.0 to 3.6 mg/kg/d i.v. in three doses for 3 days. This can be repeated in 10 to 21 days.

COMPLICATIONS

- Chronic Chagas' disease causes cardiomyopathy and megaesophagus and megacolon.
- African trypanosomiasis causes carditis and neurologic conditions such as meningoencephalitis, leading to death.

Follow-Up

- Patients who have not been treated, and who are at risk for Chagas' disease, should be followed closely for signs of cardiac dysfunction, arrhythmias, and signs of achalasia and megacolon.
- Adults should have comprehensive evaluations that include electrocardiograms.

PREVENTION

Chagas' Disease

- Adequate housing and avoidance of infestations of the insect vectors, especially in bedrooms, are needed in Latin America, primarily in the poor rural areas.
- Blood for transfusion should be screened for *T. cruzi* in high-risk areas. Blood in the United States presently is not screened; however, blood for transfusions is not taken from people who are at high risk of infection, as determined by a pre-donation questionnaire.

African Trypanosomiasis

- Decrease contact with vectors by wearing occlusive clothes.
- Avoid areas of transmission.
- Use insect repellants.

Selected Readings

Ekwanzala M, Pepin J, Khonde N, et al. In the heart of darkness: Sleeping sickness in Zaire. *Lancet* 1996;348:1427–1430.

Freilij A, Altcheh J. Congenital Chagas' disease: Diagnostic and clinical aspects. *Clin Infect Dis* 1995;21:551–555.

Grant IH, Gold JWM, Wittner M, et al. Transfusion-associated acute Chagas' disease acquired in the United States. *Ann Intern Med* 1989;111:849–851.

Marr JJ, Docampo R. Chemotherapy for Chagas' disease: A perspective on current therapy and considerations for future research. *Rev Infect Dis* 1986;8:884–903.

Panosian CB, Cohen L, Bruckner D, et al. Fever, leukopenia and a cutaneous lesion in a man who recently traveled in Africa. *Rev Infect Dis* 1991;13:1131–1138.

Tuberculosis

Basics

DEFINITION

Tuberculosis is an infection caused by *Mycobacterium tuberculosis*. Tuberculosis (TB) is one of the world's greatest public health problems. The bacterium is highly contagious and leads to a number of serious medical syndromes affecting, at times, most of the organ systems.

ETIOLOGY

The organism is a small aerobic bacillus. It is slow-growing in the laboratory. Upon staining, the organism is acid-fast, appearing red on a Ziehl-Neelsen stain. Mycobacteria can produce mutations, leading to resistance to anti-TB medications.

EPIDEMIOLOGY

- Humans are the only reservoirs of TB.
- TB is the leading cause of death due to infection worldwide.
- One-third of the world's population is infected with TB. Disease occurs in over 6 million people worldwide each year.
- TB is seen frequently in urban populations where overcrowding is present.
- Disease is spread by the respiratory route; coughing, sneezing, or even talking can aerosolize organisms from patients with cavitary disease or TB pneumonia.
- HIV infection has had a big impact in increasing the numbers of patients affected with disease caused by TB.
- In the United States, TB remains one of the top public health priorities. This follows a rise in the number of cases detected between the years 1987 and 1992.
- Homelessness, drug abuse, and poverty, along with HIV infection, are major factors in the recent rise in cases.
- Institutions such as shelters, nursing homes, and prisons have contributed to the rise in numbers affected.
- Immigrants are also responsible for as many as 30% of TB cases within the United States.

Clinical Manifestations

INCUBATION

- It takes 3 to 8 weeks for the tuberculin test to become positive after exposure.
- Most cases go unrecognized.
- In the first year after infection, fewer than 5% of people exposed to *M. tuberculosis* develop active disease. During the lifetime of the individual, only 15% develop active disease.
- In patients with abnormal chest x-rays, debilitating diseases, or HIV, or those on chronic steroids, the percentage of those developing active disease is higher. As many as 10% per year of those exposed or infected develop active disease in the HIV-infected group.

PULMONARY TUBERCULOSIS

Primary Tuberculosis

- Often asymptomatic, never coming to the attention of medical providers
- May present as a typical pneumonia, with fevers and cough
- X-rays often reveal pneumonitis that, at times, resembles community-acquired pneumonia.
- More commonly, the infiltrates are associated with hilar and mediastinal adenopathy, and appear atypical at presentation.

Postprimary Tuberculosis

- Associated with cough, fevers, and nightsweats
- Weight loss may be dramatic.
- Hemoptysis is common, and can be massive in some instances.
- Patients often complain of pleuritic chest pains.
- Chest x-rays reveal upper lobe and apical cavitary disease, lymphadenopathy, and, at times, effusions.

EXTRAPULMONARY TUBERCULOSIS

- *Adenitis* is the most common form of extrapulmonary disease.
  —Cervical adenitis is most common ("scrofula"). The nodes are firm, erythematous, and often painless.
  —In HIV-infected patients, multiple nodes can be involved.
  —In AIDS patients, the differential diagnosis includes lymphoma, atypical mycobacteria, and Kaposi's sarcoma.
- TB may also affect the *tissues of the upper airway*.
  —Otitis media can present with perforation and otorrhea.
  —Laryngitis can present with dysphagia and hoarseness.
- *Miliary* TB is often associated with fevers, weight loss, and nightsweats.
- It may be associated with *TB meningitis*.
  —Patients with TB meningitis often present with headaches and fevers, followed by meningismus and cranial neuropathies.
  —In 25% of cases, evidence of TB outside of the central nervous system is lacking.
- *Skeletal TB* often presents in the thoracic spine, and is termed *Pott's disease*.
  —Patients present with fever and tenderness over the affected region.
  —Abscess formation associated with disease can spread through fascial spaces to the groin.
- Involvement of the *gastrointestinal tract* usually involves the ileocecal region.
  —Patients may have diarrhea, obstruction, and abdominal pain.
- *Renal TB* presents with few symptoms and signs.
  —Patients often have sterile pyuria.

Diagnosis

- Diagnosis is made by finding characteristic organisms on acid-fast smears of sputum or biopsy specimens.
- Cultures often take weeks to grow, because the doubling time of the organism is 12 to 18 hours.
- A number of laboratory techniques have been developed to identify, within 1 to 2 weeks of inoculation, the organisms growing in culture.
- Diagnosis of TB can be considered by finding caseating granulomata on histologic specimens.
- Typical radiographic findings of apical infiltrates with cavitation are seen in postprimary infection.

DIFFERENTIAL DIAGNOSIS

- Sarcoidosis
- Atypical mycobacteria
- Lung abscess due to necrotizing pneumonias
- Lymphoma

LABORATORY

Tuberculin Tests

- Immunocompetent patients with tuberculin tests revealing induration greater than

Tuberculosis

- 15 mm in diameter have a very high likelihood of having TB.
- Patients with induration greater than 10 mm have a 90% chance of having TB.
- False-positives can occur with cross-reaction to the bacille Calmette-Guerin strain of mycobacteria used in immunization; however, anyone at risk for infection with a tuberculin test greater than 10 mm should be considered infected.
- As many as 50% of patients with overwhelming disease have false-negative tuberculin tests (anergy).

Treatment

- Positive tuberculin test without evidence of disease
  - Isoniazid 300 mg/d orally for 6 months
  - Pyridoxine supplements 50 mg/d orally are often given.
  - Alternatives to daily INH therapy
    - INH 900 mg orally, two times per week for 12 months
    - Rifampin 600 mg orally per day, plus ethambutol 15 mg/kg orally per day for 9 to 12 months
    - Rifampin 600 mg orally per day, plus pyrazinamide 20 mg/kg/d for 6 to 12 months
    - Shorter courses of rifampin and pyrazinamide for 2 months have proved effective in HIV-infected patients.
- Positive tuberculin test with abnormal chest x-ray or in an HIV-positive patient
  - Isoniazid 300 mg/d orally for 12 months
  - Pyridoxine supplements 50 mg a day orally are often given.
- Pulmonary TB
  - The total duration of drug therapy is 6 months.
  - Generally, four drugs for the first 2 months of treatment. Start with the following:
    - INH 300 mg orally every day
    - Rifampin 600 mg orally every day
    - PZA 15 to 30 mg/kg every day
    - Ethambutol 15 to 25 mg/kg every day
  - Followed by the following:
    - INH and rifampin for 4 more months (total treatment of 6 months)
  - Alternative: Streptomycin 15 mg/kg i.v. or i.m. may be used along with three or four other drugs in the treatment of TB.
- Extrapulmonary TB
  - Same as for pulmonary TB, but the duration of therapy should be at least 12 months (INH plus rifampin for the last 10 months).
- Immunocompromised patients/HIV-infected patients with pulmonary disease or extrapulmonary disease
  - Same as for HIV-negative patients. Some suggest treating extrapulmonary disease for at least 18 months.

COMPLICATIONS

- Complications of *therapy* include the following:
  - *INH hepatitis*: Risks approach 1% for patients above the age of 35 years. It is because of this that prophylaxis is often omitted in older patients with positive tuberculin tests.
  - *Ethambutol ophthalmic toxicity*: Optic neuritis can develop during treatment with ethambutol. Green-red discrimination should be tested on a monthly basis during therapy.
  - *Streptomycin-induced ototoxicity*: Ototoxicity, along with vestibular dysfunction, may occur and be permanent following treatment with aminoglycosides. Care must be taken to ensure that these symptoms are not present on monthly visits.
  - Rifamycins interact with many drugs that require cytochrome P-450 metabolism.

Follow-Up

- Patients often require close follow-up years after what is felt to be successful treatment of TB.
- Reinfection, especially in patients that are immunocompromised, has been documented.
- There is no need for lifetime treatment with INH for patients who are HIV-positive and have recovered from TB.

PREVENTION

- Infection control programs as part of state and city public health departments have reduced the number of active cases of TB in the United States.
- Tuberculin testing should be performed on every patient. High-risk patients and hospital workers should be checked annually.
- Improvement in living conditions, with less overcrowding, is vital to limiting the spread of disease.
- Treating those at high risk for active disease and those with active disease is effective in reducing spread of infection. At times, state health authorities may need to confine high-risk, noncompliant patients.
- Directly observed therapy is crucial for many who may be noncompliant with medications.
- Respiratory prevention with ultraviolet lights, negative-pressure rooms, and masks has decreased the rates of nosocomial infections.
- Vaccination with bacille Calmette-Guerin is not performed in the United States at this time. Protection rates vary, and immunization may lead to confusion regarding results of tuberculin testing.

Selected Readings

Daley CL, Small PM, Schecter GF. An outbreak of tuberculosis with accelerated progression among persons infected with the human immunodeficiency virus. *N Engl J Med* 1992;36:231–235.

Freden TR, Sherman LF, Maw KL, et al. A multi-institutional outbreak of highly drug-resistant tuberculosis: Epidemiology and clinical outcomes. *JAMA* 1996;275:452–457.

Iseman MD. Treatment of multi-drug resistant tuberculosis. *N Engl J Med* 1993;329:784–791.

Kopanoff DE, Snider DE Jr, Caras GJ. Isoniazid-related hepatitis. A US Public Health Service cooperative surveillance study. *Am Rev Respir Dis* 1978;117:991–1001.

Tularemia

Basics

DEFINITION
Tularemia is a zoonotic infection caused by *Francisella tularensis*. The organism is responsible for a number of syndromes in humans that range from a plaguelike ulceroglandular illness to pneumonia.

ETIOLOGY
- *F. tularensis* is an aerobic gram-negative rod.
- The organism is virulent, and small numbers of organisms on the skin can invade and lead to systemic illness
- The organism
  - Requires cysteine for growth
  - Produces a β-lactamase
  - Is resistant to freezing, and may persist for weeks in dead animals
  - Is inactivated by heat

EPIDEMIOLOGY

Incidence
- This is a rare disease, with fewer than 300 cases reported in the United States annually.
- The disease occurs mainly in the Northern Hemisphere; it is not found in the United Kingdom.
- Most cases in the United States occur in Arkansas, Oklahoma, and Missouri.
- Tick-borne cases occur in the summer.
- Disease in the winter months is usually associated with skin contact with infectious organisms.
- Infection may occur in over 100 species of small and large mammals, 25 species of birds, and 50 species of insects.
- Fish and amphibians may be infected.
- In the United States, the rabbit is the most important reservoir of infection.
- Insects such as ticks, flies, and mosquitos serve as vectors for disease in humans.
- Commonly found wood ticks, dog ticks, and Lone Star ticks are responsible for a majority of transmission in the United States.

Risk Factors
- Infection in humans occurs via an arthropod vector (tick or mosquito).
- Skin contact with an infected carcass
- Inhalation of the organism
- Ingestion via eating contaminated meat infected with the bacterium
- Bite from an animal that harbors the organism in the oropharynx
- High-risk professions include hunters, farm workers, veterinarians, and laboratory workers.

Incubation
The incubation period varies, and averages 3 to 5 days.

Clinical Manifestations

- In most cases, cutaneous infection disseminates to regional lymph nodes prior to bacteremia.
- Bacteremia is associated with fever, chills, myalgias, headache, sore throat, and cough that continue for 1 to 4 days.
- Fever may be associated with a pulse–temperature deficit.
- Remission occurs for 1 to 3 days, followed by recurrent symptoms that can continue for several weeks.
- Ulceroglandular
  - Most patients have an ulceroglandular form of illness.
  - Ulcers appear at the skin site of inoculation, and start as a red, painful papule, progressing to necrotic ulcers, which leave a scar.
  - Regional lymph nodes become markedly enlarged and tender during this stage. They may stay enlarged for months.
  - Half of patients with the ulceroglandular form have evidence of pneumonia, effusions, or hilar adenopathy on chest x-ray.
- Oculoglandular
  - Inoculation in the eye may lead to an oculoglandular form of the illness.
  - Painful conjunctivitis with yellow conjunctival ulcers and preauricular or cervical lymphadenopathy occurs.

Tularemia

- Oropharyngeal
  - Ingestion of the bacteria may lead to an oropharyngeal form of disease.
  - The throat may contain a membrane that resembles diphtheria.
  - Cervical lymphadenopathy is extensive.
- Typhoidal
  - Typhoidal disease may lead to fever of unknown origin.
  - Presumably, the organism is ingested, but tick exposure may initiate the disease.
  - There is no adenopathy.
  - Diarrhea is usually prominent.
  - Most patients with the typhoidal form have abnormalities on chest x-ray and pneumonitis.
- Pneumonic
  - Associated with inhalation of the organism
  - Patients present with a dry cough, fevers, and myalgias.

Diagnosis

DIFFERENTIAL DIAGNOSIS

- Plague
- Typhoid
- Atypical pneumonia

LABORATORY

- Modest elevation of the leukocyte count may occur.
- Mild elevations of transaminases can be noted.
- Diagnosis is often made serologically.
- Cultures require a media that contains cysteine.

IMAGING

- Chest x-rays often show infiltrates with pleural effusions.
- Hilar adenopathy is often associated.
- Nodular infiltrates 2 to 8 cm in size may be observed.

Treatment

- Streptomycin 7.5 to 10.0 mg/kg every 12 hours; intravenous or intramuscular delivery for 7 to 14 days
- Gentamicin 3 to 5 mg/kg/d, divided every 8 hours i.v. for 7 to 14 days
- Chloramphenicol used with central nervous system involvement
- Third-generation cephalosporins may be effective.

ALTERNATIVE TREATMENT

The following alternatives are to be used with caution:
  - Tetracycline 1 g every day for 15 days has been associated with recurrences.
  - Erythromycin is possibly effective, but resistance has been noted.
  - Quinolones are possibly effective; however, clinical experience is lacking. The in *vitro* data appear good.

COMPLICATIONS

- Disseminated disease may lead to renal or hepatic failure, meningitis, disseminated intravascular coagulation, shock, and death.
- Suppuration of lymph nodes may occur and be prolonged.

Follow-Up

PREVENTION

- A live attenuated vaccine is available for people at high risk of infection.
- Protection from ticks is important.
- People who skin animals (hunters, trappers) should wear gloves.

Selected Readings

Evans ME, Gregory DW, Schaffner W, et al. Tularemia: A 30-year experience. *Medicine* 1985;64:251–269.

Sanford JP. Tularemia. *JAMA* 1983;250:3225–3226.

Typhoid Fever

Basics

DEFINITION
Typhoid fever is a severe systemic infection with *Salmonella typhi*. At times, other organisms, such as *Salmonella paratyphi A, Salmonella schottmuelleri,* and *Salmonella hirschfeldii,* can lead to a typhoid-like illness.

ETIOLOGY
- *S. typhi* is gram-negative rod within the family Enterobacteriaceae.
- Transmission of disease is caused by exposure to food and water contaminated by feces from either patients with acute infection or persons who carry the organism in the stool for long periods of time.

EPIDEMIOLOGY
- Infection with *S. typhi* is rare in the United States, with fewer than 500 cases occurring each year.
- Most of these cases occur in immigrants or travelers returning from less-developed countries.
- In developing countries, the disease is endemic and remains a public health problem.
- In developing countries, most cases occur in children.
- In the United States, most cases occur in older travelers.
- There are no zoonotic reservoirs for this organism.

Clinical Manifestations

- The incubation period depends on the initial inoculum; it averages 1 to 2 weeks.
- Diarrhea is noted in a minority of patients during the first week after exposure.
- Fever of 40°C is the first manifestation of disease.
- Patients note chills, myalgias, headache, sore throat, and cough.
- A faint rash on the trunk, termed *rose spots*, can be noted in some patients.
- Examination will reveal a relative bradycardia despite high fevers.
- Abdominal tenderness is also noted.
- If untreated, the patient may develop intestinal perforations at the level of the terminal ileum.
- Suppurative complications such as pericarditis, meningitis, and pneumonitis can occur.
- Hepatitis and splenomegaly are noted.

Diagnosis

- Patients may have leukopenia.
- LFTs are frequently abnormal.
- Cultures of the stool and blood should reveal the organism.
- Blood cultures are positive in 50% to 75% of patients.
- Bone marrow cultures are positive in 90% of cases.

Typhoid Fever

- Stool cultures should be positive in 90% of cases.
- Serology to the organism should be positive and is available.

DIFFERENTIAL DIAGNOSIS

- In a patient returning from a developing country, the differential diagnosis includes the following:
  - Malaria
  - Tuberculosis
  - Acute HIV infection
  - Typhus

Treatment

- Ciprofloxacin 500 mg orally twice per day for 10 days
- Ceftriaxone 2 g i.v. every day for 5 days

ALTERNATIVE TREATMENT

- Chloramphenicol 500 mg orally or intravenously every day for 14 days
- Cefixime 10 to 15 mg/kg orally every 8 hours for 8 days
- With signs of shock
  - Add dexamethasone 3 mg/kg, one dose prior to first antibiotic dose, than give dexamethasone 1 mg/kg every 6 hours for 2 days

COMPLICATIONS

N/A

Follow-Up

Patients undergoing treatment for typhoid fever should have follow-up stool cultures.

PREVENTION

- Two vaccines are available for people traveling into endemic areas:
  - Typhoid (Typhim Vi) is given in a single intramuscular dose.
  - An oral attenuated strain of typhoid (Ty21a) is given every other day for four doses. It should not be given to children under 6 years of age, and it should not be given to immunocompromised patients.
- Food and water precautions should be adhered to when traveling in developing countries.

Selected Readings

Hornick RB, Greisman SE, Woodward TE, et al. Typhoid fever: Pathogenesis and immunologic control. *N Engl J Med* 1970;283:686–691.

Mermin JH, Townes JM, Gerber M, et al. Typhoid fever in the United States, 1985–1994: Changing risks of international travel and increasing antibiotic resistance. *Arch Intern Med* 1998;158:633–638.

Typhus

Basics

DEFINITION

Typhus comprises a group of diseases caused by rickettsias, characterized by fever and rash. These include murine (endemic), epidemic (louse-borne, classic), and scrub typhus, as well as Brill-Zinsser disease.

ETIOLOGY

- Rickettsias are small, pleomorphic, fastidious, obligate intracellular bacterial organisms.
- *Rickettsia typhi, Rickettsia prowazekii*, and *Rickettsia tsutsugamushi* are the causative agents of murine, epidemic, and scrub typhus, respectively. Brill-Zinsser disease represents recurrence of epidemic typhus, years after the initial attack.
- All have a natural cycle involving an arthropod vector (fleas for *R. typhi*, lice, for *R. prowazekii*, mites for *R. tsutsugamushi*) and a vertebrate host (*R. typhi* for small rodents, *R. prowazekii* for humans and flying squirrels, *R. tsutsugamushi* for wild rodents).

EPIDEMIOLOGY

- The typhus group of rickettsioses (especially epidemic typhus) has been a major global health problem since the beginning of the twentieth century, particularly in Eastern Europe during the two world wars. Spread of epidemics, depending on the spread of the arthropod vectors and the animal reservoirs, is favored by bad sanitary conditions and crowding, as happens during wars and among refugee populations.
- Brill-Zinsser disease constitutes the recurrence of epidemic typhus, years after the primary attack. It mainly occurs among immigrant populations, particularly those originating from Eastern Europe. Brill-Zinsser disease patients may serve as a pool for recurrent epidemic typhus epidemics.
- Epidemic typhus still occurs in the highlands of South America, Africa, and Asia; murine typhus has an endemic worldwide distribution, and scrub typhus occurs in the South Pacific, Asia, and Australia.
- Effective improvement in sanitary conditions and animal and insect control programs have led to almost complete elimination of epidemic typhus in the United States during past decades. Murine typhus is still prevalent in the southeastern and Gulf Coast states.
- All these diseases are transmitted to humans via arthropod bites (via contaminated insect feces, as the latter defecate during feeding, with the exception of mites, which directly inoculate *R. tsutsugamushi* during feeding); mites and fleas pass the rickettsias to their progeny, but infected lice die of intestinal obstruction within 1 to 3 weeks.

Incubation Period and Natural History

- The abrupt clinical presentation of louse-borne typhus starts about a week after the challenge, and, if untreated, the illness lasts for 2 weeks; the patient may recover fully after approximately 2 months.
- The incubation period ranges from 1 to 2 weeks for murine typhus and from 6 to 18 days for scrub typhus. Brill-Zinsser disease may appear years after the primary epidemic typhus attack.
- Organisms multiply at the site of entry before entering the bloodstream. Despite that, the initial local lesion can be seen only in scrub typhus.
- Rickettsemia develops late in the incubation period and precedes the onset of pyrexia.
- Vascular endothelial cell destruction and consequent damage in several organ systems (notably skin, cardiovascular, respiratory, central nervous, and liver) is the primary pathology found.

Clinical Manifestations

SYMPTOMS

- The following are common in all forms of typhus:
  —Abrupt onset
  —Fever (102°F–104°F), chills and myalgias
  —Severe frontal headache
  —Altered mentation and neurologic signs
  —Severe nausea and vomiting
  —Anorexia
  —Nonproductive cough and, occasionally, moderate hemoptysis
  —Tinnitus, transient deafness
  —The patient may recall lice, fleas, or mite exposure.

SIGNS

- Epidemic typhus
  —A macular rash that fades on pressure presents on about the fifth day of illness, starting from the axillary folds and the upper trunk and spreading centrifugally, becoming petechial and confluent, sparing the face, palms, and soles. There is no visible eschar.
- Murine typhus
  —Rash develops in only about 50% of patients between the third and fifth day of illness, and may involve both the trunk and extremities. It is usually macular or maculopapular; petechiae are rare (<10%). There is no visible eschar.
  —Splenomegaly may occur in about 25% of the patients.
- Scrub typhus
  —An erythematous, indurated lesion, surrounded by vesicles that subsequently ulcerate and form a black eschar, may be present at the inoculation site (<50% of cases); regional lymphadenopathy also may occur.
  —Ocular pain and conjunctival injection
  —A maculopapular rash appears about the fifth day of illness, involving the trunk and extremities.
  —Splenomegaly and generalized lymphadenopathy
  —In critically ill patients, signs of cardiovascular collapse (edema, hypovolemia) and severe neurologic signs may be prominent.
  —Brill-Zinsser disease is generally milder than epidemic typhus, resembling murine typhus in presentation.

Diagnosis

DIFFERENTIAL DIAGNOSIS

- Other rickettsial infections (i.e., Rocky Mountain spotted fever)
- Meningococcemia/bacterial meningitis
- Typhoid
- Secondary syphilis
- Leptospirosis
- Lyme disease
- Infectious mononucleosis
- Rubella
- Measles
- Flavivirus infections

DIAGNOSIS

- Given the relevant epidemiologic factors present, diagnosis can be clinical.
- Isolation of rickettsias is expensive, time consuming, and dangerous, and should be performed only in reference laboratories. Thus, isolation is not necessary to confirm diagnosis.
- Confirmation and identification are usually done retrospectively by serology (rising of specific group- and type-specific antibody titers during convalescence).

Typhus

LABORATORY

- Normochromic anemia and mild thrombocytopenia may be present.
- The white blood cell count is usually normal or slightly decreased.
- Clotting disorders may be present.
- Hypoproteinemia, hyponatremia, hypochloremia, and azotemia are the hallmarks of fulminant disease.

SEROLOGY

- Positive after the second week of illness
- The Weil-Felix reaction and complement fixation tests can be used for routine diagnosis; but they are not very sensitive and specific.
- The Weil-Felix reaction, employing OX-19 and OX-2 *Proteus* strains, is positive in epidemic, murine, and scrub typhus. A positive test is defined by either determination of a titer of 1 in 320 or greater or a fourfold rise in titer. The OX-19 reaction is negative or low-titer-positive in Brill-Zinsser disease.
- Further confirmation and specific identification can be made by indirect fluorescent antibody (IFA) and the latex agglutination test (LA), and by direct immunofluorescent tests.
- Tissue immunofluorescence can detect rickettsias several days after the initiation of specific antibiotic therapy.
- Early and effective antibiotic therapy may delay the maximum antibody response.

MOLECULAR BIOLOGY

PCR tests to diagnose acute *R. prowazekii*, *R. typhi*, and *R. tsutsugamushi* infection have been developed and are under clinical evaluation.

Treatment

MAIN TREATMENT

- Supportive treatment may be necessary in moderate and severe cases.
- Careful nursing care to prevent aspiration pneumonia and xerostomia
- Nutritional and blood transfusion support, careful management of electrolyte abnormalities, and dialysis if renal failure occurs
- Specific antibiotic chemotherapy
  —Chloramphenicol 50 to 75 mg/kg/d in four equally divided oral or intravenous doses, or
  —Tetracycline 25 to 50 mg/kg/d in four equally divided oral or intravenous doses
- Treatment should be continued for 2 to 3 days after the resolution of fever in epidemic and murine typhus and in Brill-Zinsser disease. In scrub typhus, treatment should be continued for 3 to 7 days, and for 2 weeks in case treatment starts during the first 4 to 5 days of illness, to prevent relapse
- Steroids may be useful in critical cases (a 3-day, high-dose course is recommended).

ALTERNATIVE TREATMENT

- Epidemic typhus
  —Doxycycline 100 mg bid for 7 days
  —Single-dose doxycycline (100 mg PO)
- Murine typhus
  —Doxycycline 100 mg bid for 7 days
  —Ciprofloxacin, pefloxacin, and ofloxacin also may be used.
- Scrub typhus
  —Single-dose doxycycline (200 mg PO)
  —Ciprofloxacin also may be used.

TREATMENT FAILURE

Relapses occur if treatment is delayed. A second course of treatment is usually effective.

COMPLICATIONS

- Cardiovascular collapse
- Renal impairment (prerenal azotemia), resulting occasionally in overt renal failure
- Hepatic insufficiency
- Rickettsial pneumonitis, pulmonary edema, respiratory failure
- Rickettsial endocarditis
- Upper gastrointestinal bleeding
- Superinfections (aspiration pneumonia, parotitis, gingivitis)
- Coma

Follow-Up

- Epidemic typhus is the most severe of the typhus group rickettsioses. If untreated, fever subsides after about 2 weeks, but the convalescence period may last up to 2 to 3 months. The mortality rate in untreated disease may be high (up to 60%), with a peak incidence in elderly patients.
- Brill-Zinsser disease resembles epidemic typhus but is generally more benign.
- Murine typhus is a more benign illness, and the mortality rate, even before the introduction of specific antibiotic therapy, may be as low as 1%.
- The mortality rate in untreated scrub typhus ranges from 1% to 60% in different series.
- Antibiotic therapy dramatically alters the prognosis of this disease. After initiation of therapy, patients become afebrile within 2 to 3 days. There may be recurrence if treatment is delayed. In this case, retreatment is effective.

PREVENTION

- Control of animal reservoirs in high-prevalence areas
- Elimination of insect vectors
- Primary chemoprophylaxis has proved to be effective in preventing scrub typhus attacks and mounting an active immune response (single-dose chloramphenicol or tetracycline every 5 days, for an overall duration of 35 days)
- An effective vaccine against epidemic typhus is commercially available.

Selected Readings

Carl M, Tibbs CW, Dobson ME, et al. Diagnosis of acute typhus infection using the polymerase chain reaction. *J Infect Dis* 1990;161:791–793.

Dumler JS, Taylor JP, Walker DH. Clinical and laboratory features of marine typhus in south Texas, 1980 through 1987. *JAMA* 1991;266:1365–1370.

McClain JB, Joshi B, Rice R. Chloramphenicol, gentamicin, and ciprofloxacin against marine scrub typhus. *Antimicrob Agents Chemother* 1988;32:285–286.

Olson JG, Bourgeois AL, Fang RCY, et al. Prevention of scrub typhus: Prophylactic administration of doxycycline in a randomized double blind trial. *Am J Trop Med Hyg* 1980;29:989–997.

Perine PL, Chandler BP, Krause DK, et al. A clinicoepidemiological study of epidemic typhus in Africa. *Clin Infect Dis* 1992;14:1149–1158.

Perine PL, Krause DW, Awoke A, et al. Single-dose doxycycline treatment of louse-borne relapsing fever and epidemic typhus. *Lancet* 1974;2:742–744.

Strand O, Stromber A. Case report. Ciprofloxacin treatment of marine typhus. *Scand J Infect Dis* 1990;22:503–504.

Sugita Y, Nagatani T, Okuda K, et al. Diagnosis of typhus infection with Rickettsia tsutsugamushi by polymerase chain reaction. *J Med Microbiol* 1992;37:257–260.

Warts

Basics

DEFINITION
Warts are benign viral tumors of the skin and mucous membranes and include cutaneous warts and genital warts. The virus is transmitted by direct contact, sexual contact, and autoinoculation.

ETIOLOGY
- Human papillomavirus (HPV)
- Epitheliotropic DNA virus with more than 60 types

EPIDEMIOLOGY
Incidence

- Seven percent to 10% of the population has warts.
- Less common in Blacks than in Whites
- Cutaneous warts
  —Spread by direct contact with infected person or touch of contaminated material
  —Occur primarily in children and young adults
  —Especially common in handlers of meat, poultry, and fish (50%)
  —Fomites may be involved in transmission of HPV types that are associated with cutaneous warts.
- Anogenital warts
  —Most common viral sexually transmitted disease (STD)

Risk Factors

- Unprotected sex with partner with anogenital HPV
- Children
- Meat, poultry, fish-handlers: infection rates up to 50%

Incubation

- One to 20 months after exposure

Clinical Manifestations

SYMPTOMS AND SIGNS
Cutaneous

- Common warts: hyperkeratotic papules with rough surface commonly seen on hands, fingers, elbows, but may be seen anywhere on the body
- Plantar warts: painful; thrombosed capillaries beneath surface; bleed easily
- Juvenile/flat warts: multiple papules with smooth surface and irregular contour

Anogenital

- Condylomata acuminata: exophytic lesions varying in size and morphology
- Cervical, vaginal, vulvar: Exophytic lesions varying in size and morphology
- Cervical intraepithelial neoplasia: nonadvanced lesion, often not visible to naked eye
- Respiratory papillomatosis: usually seen in children; can recur

Diagnosis

- Based on typical appearance upon visual examination

DIFFERENTIAL DIAGNOSIS
Infectious

- Fungal infection
- Molluscum contagiosum
- Secondary syphilis (anogenital only)

Noninfectious

- Squamous cell malignancies
- Skin cancer
- Actinic keratosis
- Callus (plantar only)

LABORATORY

- Pap smear annually to detect cervical cancer associated with anogenital warts
- To identify specific HPV type, a Southern blot, *in situ* hybridization, or polymerase chain reaction is used.

Treatment

- HPV is not clearly eradicated by any treatment.
- Warts often regress spontaneously.
  —Anogenital warts, within 4 months (20%)
  —Cutaneous warts in children, between 1 and 5 years (50% and 90%, respectively)
- The rate of recurrence of the anogenital type after treatment is high (<25% at 3 months).
- Most currently available therapies are not specific antiviral regimens, but rather are physically destructive or chemically cytotoxic to the superficial wart; some cause scarring.

MAIN TREATMENT
Anogenital

- External genital
  —Cryotherapy with liquid nitrogen or cryoprobe is effective: 63% to 88%, with recurrence in 21% to 39%.

Warts

- Podofilox 0.5% applied twice per day for 3 days, repeated for 4 weeks if required, is effective: 45% to 88%.
  - The health care provider should give the initial application or instruct the patient on how to do the initial application.
- Podophyllin 10% to 25% in a compound tincture of benzoin is effective: 32% to 79%, with recurrences of 27% to 65%.
  - Must wash off thoroughly 1 to 4 hours after application
- Trichloracetic acid: 80% to 90%
  - Powder with talc or baking soda after application to remove untreated acid; pain common in treatment
- Electrodesiccation or electrocautery
  - Contraindicated in patients with pacemakers
  - Local anesthesia required; pain common in treatment
- Carbon dioxide laser or surgery used for extensive warts
- Intralesional interferon-alpha used for refractory warts; effective 44% to 61%, with recurrence up to 67%
- 5-Fluorouracil (topical) causes local irritation and is not studied extensively.
- Perianal
  - Treat as for anogenital (discussed previously), except that podofilox is contraindicated.
- Anal
  - Patients with warts on rectal mucosa should be referred to an expert.
  - Cryotherapy with liquid nitrogen or trichloroacetic acid: 80% to 90%
    - Cryoprobe is contraindicated.
  - Surgery
- Urethral meatus
  - Cryotherapy with liquid nitrogen
  - Podophyllin: 10% to 25%
    - Wash off thoroughly 1 to 2 hours after application.
    - Contraindicated in pregnancy
- Cervical
  - Consult with an expert.
- Vaginal
  - Cryotherapy with liquid nitrogen, not cryoprobe
  - Trichloracetic acid: 80% to 90%
  - Podophyllin: 10% to 25%

Oral

- Treatment is not necessary unless warts are painful or cause a cosmetic problem.
- Cryotherapy with liquid nitrogen, not cryoprobe
- Electrodesiccation or electrocautery
- Surgery

Cutaneous

- Common
  - Cryotherapy with liquid nitrogen
    - Pain during and after procedure
    - Apply with a cotton swab, and retreat in 2 to 3 weeks, if necessary.
    - Contraindicated in patients with Raynaud's phenomenon
- Plantar
  - Salicylic acid plaster: 40%
    - Self-treatment after demonstration by health care provider
    - Pare lesions before applying plaster; remove after 1 to 3 days; scrape off macerated skin for 2 to 3 weeks.
- Flat
  - Topical 5-fluorouracil or retinoin acid

SEX PARTNERS

- May benefit from evaluation for other STDs and education about HPV and STDs in general

COMPLICATIONS

- Pregnancy: Anogenital warts tend to enlarge and become friable; cesarean section may be required if the size of genital warts obstructs the birth canal.
- Cervical cancer is associated with anogenital warts.
- Recurrences result from reactivation of subclinical HPV rather than from reinfection.

Follow-Up

The initial Pap smear for women with genital warts should be followed at 6 months, then annually if the smear is negative.

PREVENTION

- Safe-sex precautions to prevent anogenital warts
- Avoidance of direct contact with persons with cutaneous warts

Selected Readings

Bonnez W, Reichman RC. Papillomaviruses. In: Mandell GL, Bennett JE, Dolin R, eds. *Principles and practice of infectious diseases*, 5th ed. Philadelphia: Churchill Livingstone, 2000:1630.

Grussendorf-Conen E-I. Papillomavirus-induced tumors of the skin: Cutaneous warts and epidermodysplasia verruciformis. In: Syrjanen K, Gissmann L, Koss LG, eds. *Papillomaviruses and human disease*. Berlin: Springer Verlag, 1987:158.

Jablonska S, Orth G, Obalek S, et al. Cutaneous warts: Clinical, histologic, and virologic correlations. *Clin Dermatol* 1985;3:71.

Yellow Fever

Basics

DEFINITION
Yellow fever virus is responsible for a severe systemic illness associated with hemorrhage, liver dysfunction, and fevers. The case fatality rate is greater than 10%. Yellow fever has great historic significance, causing disease in both northern and southern urban areas throughout the United States in the 1700s to 1800s.

ETIOLOGY
- Yellow fever virus is an RNA virus in the family Flaviviridae.
- The virus is enveloped and spherical.

EPIDEMIOLOGY
- Yellow fever virus is present in the tropical forests of Africa and South America, between 15 degrees North and South latitudes.
- Transmission to humans is via *Aedes aegypti* mosquitos.
- Humans, along with nonhuman primates, comprise a reservoir of infection.
- Disease may be sporadic or part of an outbreak.
- Underreporting of disease occurs.

Risk Factors
- Travel in endemic areas, especially during the rainy season
- Mosquito bites occurring while in endemic regions
- No prior immunization

Incubation
- Three to 6 days

Clinical Manifestations

- The spectrum of disease ranges from asymptomatic to severe illness with death.
- The disease has three stages:
  —Infection
  —Remission
  —Intoxication
- The infection stage is noted by the onset of fever, chills, myalgias, and headache. The patient is noted to have relative bradycardia despite high fevers.
- Remission of symptoms occurs after 3 to 4 days of fever and lasts for hours to days.
- The intoxication stage has a mortality rate of close to 50%. It is associated with recurrent fevers, mucosal hemorrhage, liver failure, renal failure, and myocarditis. Disseminated intravascular coagulation (DIC) may occur. Signs of meningitis and encephalitis occur.

Diagnosis

DIFFERENTIAL DIAGNOSIS
- Hemorrhagic fevers caused by a wide array of viruses, such as Ebola, Lassa fever, Rift Valley fever, and Congo-Crimean hemorrhagic fever.
- Acute hepatitis
- Dengue

Yellow Fever

- Malaria
- Typhoid
- Leptospirosis

LABORATORY

- Nonspecific leukopenia and thrombocytopenia are often seen.
- Evidence of DIC and severe elevations of transaminases and bilirubin are seen in severe cases.
- Diagnosis is made by serology, but this may be misleading due to cross-reactive antibodies.
- Virus can be grown in cell culture.
- A polymerase chain reaction may be performed on blood samples of patients felt to be viremic.

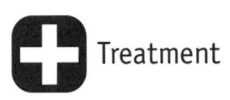

Treatment

- Supportive measures in the intensive care unit are needed for the sickest patients.
- There is no specific treatment.

COMPLICATIONS

Bacterial infections in acutely ill patients account for much of the mortality associated with the infection.

Follow-Up

- Patients surviving the illness have high antibody levels and are thus immune to recurrence of disease.
- Myocarditis may lead to arrhythmias.

PREVENTION

- Eradication of the A. *aegypti* mosquito in tropical areas
- Avoidance of mosquito bites in endemic areas, especially during the rainy seasons
- Vaccination with a live attenuated virus is effective.
- Postvaccination encephalitis occurs in infants younger than 4 months.
- Patients should not be immunized if less than 4 months of age.
- HIV-positive patients may be immunized if the CD4 count is greater than 200/mm^3.
- Immunization takes 7 to 10 days to be effective and is effective for 10 years.

Selected Readings

Monath TP. Yellow fever: A medically neglected disease. *Rev Infect Dis* 1987;9:165.

Yersinia enterocolitica Infections

Basics

DEFINITION

The genus *Yersinia* includes the pathogens *Yersinia pestis* (the cause of plague), *Yersinia enterocolitica*, and *Yersinia pseudotuberculosis*. (The topic of plague is discussed in a separate chapter.)

ETIOLOGY

- *Y. enterocolitica* and *Y. pseudotuberculosis* are gram-negative, non–lactose-fermenting, urease-positive bacilli.
- The natural reservoirs of *Y. enterocolitica* are animals, including rodents, rabbits, pigs, sheep, cattle, horses, dogs, and cats.
- Infection due to *Y. pseudotuberculosis* is also a zoonotic infection.
- Plague is usually contracted by bites from fleas found on rodents, occasionally by direct contact with infectious tissues or exudates, and rarely by respiratory droplets from a person or animal with pneumonic plague.

EPIDEMIOLOGY

Incidence

- From 1947 through 1996, a total of 390 cases of plague were reported in the United States, resulting in 60 (15.4%) deaths. Of these, bubonic plague accounted for 327 (83.9%) cases and 44 (13.5%) deaths; primary septicemic plague, for 49 (12.6%) cases and 11 (22.4%) deaths; and primary pneumonic plague, for seven (1.8%) cases and four (57.1%) deaths. Seven (1.8%) cases were unclassified.
- In the United States, most cases of human plague are reported from New Mexico, Arizona, Colorado, and California.
- From 1980 through 1994, 18,739 cases of plague and 1,853 deaths (10%) were reported to the World Health Organization (WHO) by 24 countries in Africa, the Americas, and Asia.
- *Y. enterocolitica* is more common in Northern Europe. Infections have been documented in other parts of the world, including South America, Africa, and Asia.
- Between 1967 and 1996, more than 18,700 strains of *Yersinia* species, excluding *Y. pestis*, were recovered in Belgium from a variety of gastrointestinal and extraintestinal sites in patients. Acute enterocolitis was the most common clinical form of *Y. enterocolitica* infection, affecting primarily children younger than 5 years of age. Starting in 1967, there was a steady increase in isolations every year, with 305 cases in 1975 and up to 1,469 in 1986. From 1987 on, there was a clear decrease in the number of reported cases, although the number of participating laboratories and culture techniques remained constant. This significant decrease in the occurrence of *Y. enterocolitica* infections may be explained by changes in the slaughtering procedures and eating habits of the population.
- *Y. enterocolitica* is transmitted through food, animal contact, and contaminated blood products.

Risk Factors

- A prospective case control study in Auckland, New Zealand, concluded that the risk of illness due to *Y. enterocolitica* is increased by contact with untreated water, nonreticulated sewerage, and consumption of pork.
- Patients with iron excess (such as those with beta-thalassemia) and those receiving desferrioxamine are at a higher risk for serious infection due to *Y. enterocolitica*.
- *Y. enterocolitica* septicemia is more common among patients with diabetes mellitus, severe anemia, hemochromatosis, cirrhosis, and malignancy, and in elderly patients.
- The increased number of reported transfusion complications during recent years, caused by *Y. enterocolitica*–infected blood components, is probably related to the use of additive solutions for red-cell storage, which brings about a decrease in complement activity.

Clinical Manifestations

- The incubation period for plague is 1 to 7 days. Manifestations of the illness include acute onset of fever, chills, malaise, myalgias, and prostration, often with nausea. In particular, bubonic plague is characterized by painfully swollen regional lymph nodes (buboes) draining from the cutaneous inoculation site. Pneumonic plague is characterized by a productive cough, often with hemoptysis, and pulmonary infiltrates. Septicemic plague may result in endotoxic shock and disseminated intravascular coagulation without localized signs of infection. Plague meningitis is a less common presentation.
- *Y. enterocolitica* produces a spectrum of disease, including acute enterocolitis, terminal ileitis, and mesenteric adenitis. *Y. pseudotuberculosis*, which commonly infects animals, is a less frequent cause of human disease. When it infects humans, it usually produces mesenteric adenitis, especially in older children and adults.
- By far, the most common manifestation of *Y. pseudotuberculosis* infection in humans is mesenteric adenitis, which causes an acute appendicitis-like syndrome, with fever and right lower quadrant abdominal pain.
- Patients with mesenteric adenitis and/or terminal ileitis have fever, right lower quadrant pain, and leukocytosis. This syndrome is most common in older children and adolescents and may be indistinguishable from acute appendicitis.
- *Y. pseudotuberculosis* or *Y. enterocolitica* infection in mesenteric lymph nodes can also cause necrotizing lymphadenitis.
- *Y. enterocolitica* and *Y. pseudotuberculosis* can each produce an enteric fever–like illness, characterized by fever, headache, and abdominal pain.
- A reactive polyarthritis is seen in 10% to 30% of adults with *Y. enterocolitica* infection.

Diagnosis

- Stool, mesenteric lymph node, pharyngeal exudate, peritoneal fluid, or blood cultures may yield *Yersinia*, depending on the clinical syndrome.
- Plague bacteriologic diagnosis is readily made by smear and culture of a bubo aspirate. The aspirate is obtained by

Yersinia enterocolitica Infections

inserting a 20-gauge needle on a 10-mL syringe containing 1 mL of sterile saline into the bubo and withdrawing it several times until the saline becomes blood-tinged. Drops of the aspirate should be placed onto microscopic slides and air-dried for both Gram and Wayson stains.
- Fecal excretion of *Yersinia* may continue for weeks after symptoms have subsided. Leukocytes and, less commonly, blood or mucus may be present in the stool. Most patients with this syndrome are less than 5 years of age.
- Serologic tests are useful in diagnosing *Yersinia* infections. *Y. enterocolitica* and *Y. pseudotuberculosis* cross-react with each other and with other organisms. Agglutinating antibodies appear soon after onset of illness but generally disappear within 2 to 6 months.

Treatment

- For patients with plague, streptomycin should be administered intramuscularly in two divided doses daily, totaling 30 mg/kg of body weight per day for 10 days.
- The 10-day course of streptomycin is recommended to prevent relapses. Tetracycline is a satisfactory alternative. It is administered orally in a dose of 2 to 4 g/d in four divided doses for 10 days.
- The value of antimicrobial therapy in cases of enterocolitis and mesenteric adenitis due to *Y. enterocolitica* is unclear, because these infections are usually self-limited.
- Patients with *Y. enterocolitica*–induced septicemia should receive antibiotic therapy. The drug of choice has not yet been identified, but gentamicin (5 mg/kg/d i.v.) or chloramphenicol is suggested.
- *Y. pseudotuberculosis* is usually sensitive *in vitro* to ampicillin, tetracycline, chloramphenicol, cephalosporins, and aminoglycosides. Although antibiotic therapy is probably not warranted in most patients with mesenteric adenitis, patients with septicemia should receive ampicillin 100 to 200 mg/kg/d i.v., or streptomycin 20 to 30 mg/kg/d i.m., or tetracycline.

COMPLICATIONS

- Prompt and specific treatment of plague reduces the case fatality rates from 60% or more to less than 15%.
- The case fatality rate for untreated septicemic and pneumonic plague approaches 100%.
- Erythema nodosum and polyarthritis have also been described in patients with *Y. pseudotuberculosis* infection.
- Patients with *Y. enterocolitica*–induced septicemia, which has a mortality of 50% despite treatment, should receive antibiotic therapy. Arthritis or ankylosing spondylitis rarely occurs. This complication is much more likely to develop in individuals with the HLA-B27 antigen.
- The mortality rate in *Y. pseudotuberculosis* septicemia is up to 75%.

Follow-Up

- Untreated, bubonic plague progresses to septicemic plague within 2 to 6 days. Patients exhibit shock, ecchymoses, and small artery thromboses, resulting in digital gangrene.
- In serious cases of *Y. pseudotuberculosis* enterocolitis, rectal bleeding and perforation of the ileum may occur.
- Patients with suspected *Y. pestis* infections should be reported immediately to local or state health departments to enable prompt initiation of appropriate public health control and prevention activities. In the United States, testing of clinical specimens and isolates from suspected plague patients should be coordinated through state health departments and sent to CDC's Diagnostic and Reference Laboratory Section, Division of Vector-Borne Infectious Diseases, National Center for Infectious Diseases (telephone: [970] 221-6400), for confirmation of *Y. pestis*.

PREVENTION

- Plague would likely be released as an aerosol during a modern biologic-warfare attack and could generate many cases of highly lethal and contagious pneumonia.
- The currently licensed, inactivated, whole-cell vaccine prevents bubonic plague. However, animal challenge studies suggest that it does not reliably protect against primary pneumonic plague.
- Public health measures to control *Yersinia* infection should focus on the animal reservoirs in any particular location.
- The prevention of plague in humans depends primarily on the maintenance of public sanitation and hygiene, national programs for surveillance and control, and adherence to international health regulations.

Selected Readings

Adamkiewicz TV, Berkovitch M, Krishnan C, et al. Infection due to *Yersinia enterocolitica* in a series of patients with beta-thalassemia: Incidence and predisposing factors. *Clin Infect Dis* 1998;27:1362–1366.

Anonymous. From the Centers for Disease Control and Prevention. Fatal human plague–Arizona and Colorado, 1996. *JAMA* 1997;278:380–382.

Butler T. *Yersinia* species (including plague). In: Mandell GL, Bennett JE, Dolin R, eds. *Principles and practice of infectious diseases*. New York: Churchill Livingstone, 1995:2070–2078.

Dennis DT, Hughes JM. Multidrug resistance in plague. *N Engl J Med* 1997;337:702–704.

Hogman CF. Killing *Yersinia enterocolitica*. *J Clin Pathol* 1996;49:955.

McGovern TW, Christopher GW, Eitzen EM. Cutaneous manifestations of biological warfare and related threat agents. *Arch Dermatol* 1999;135:311–322.

Satterthwaite P, Pritchard K, Floyd D, et al. A case-control study of *Yersinia enterocolitica* infections in Auckland. *Aust N Z J Public Health* 1999;23:482–485.

Swanink CM, Stolk-Engelaar VM, van der Meer JW, et al. Surveillance of human *Yersinia enterocolitica* infections in Belgium: 1967–1996. *Clin Infect Dis* 1998;27:59–64.

SECTION III
Microorganisms

Microorganisms

Absidia corymbifera

GENUS Absidia

SPECIES
- *A. corymbifera* is the only human pathogenic species of Absidia.
- *A. corymbifera* was previously named *A. ramosa*.

MICROBIOLOGIC CHARACTERISTICS
- Filamentous fungus (mold)
- Similar to *Rhizopus* species
- Hyaline nonseptate hyphae
- Hyphae are wide (6–15 mm in diameter).
- Rapid growth in cultures (within 4 days); light gray to grayish-brown
- Grows at 25°C to 45°C
- Belongs to the order Mucorales

EPIDEMIOLOGY
- Inhalation of sporangiospores is the most probable cause of infection.
- Ubiquitous
- May be a contaminant in cultures
- May cause severe infections, especially in immunocompromised patients
- Immunocompromised patients are at higher risk to develop infections.

INFECTIONS
- An infrequent cause of zygomycosis
- Zygomycosis may affect a wide range of anatomic sites.
- The most common forms of the infection are rhinocerebral, pulmonary, cutaneous, and disseminated.
- Infrequent agent of mucormycosis in humans
- Meningitis (after head injury); rare
- Cutaneous infections
- Infections in patients with AIDS or other causes of immunosuppression

DIAGNOSIS
- Culture

TREATMENT
- Amphotericin B 0.7 to 1.2 mg/kg/d
- Appropriate total dose not known (2–4 g recommended or until correction of neutropenia in neutropenic patients)

ALTERNATIVE TREATMENT
- A lipid formulation of amphotericin B 3 to 5 mg/kg/d
- There are no available clinical data to support the use of other than amphotericin B antifungal agents.

PREVENTION
- Avoidance of severe immunosuppression, if possible (e.g., appropriate management of HIV infection)

Acanthamoeba Species

GENUS Acanthamoeba

SPECIES
- *A. astronyxis*
- *A. castellanii*
- *A. culbertsoni*
- *A. glebae*
- *A. hatchetti*
- *A. palestinensis*
- *A. polyphaga*
- *A. rhysodes*

MICROBIOLOGIC CHARACTERISTICS
- Protozoon
- Free-living life cycle
- Ubiquity in the environment

EPIDEMIOLOGY
- Worldwide distribution
- Found in soil, fresh and brackish water, dust, hot tubs, and sewage
- Acquisition probably occurs by inhalation or direct contact with contaminated soil or water.
- Contaminated saline solutions or tap water rinses for care of contact lenses may transmit the pathogen.

INFECTIONS
- Granulomatous encephalitis in immunosuppressed patients
- Infections occur primarily in debilitated and immunocompromised persons; however, some patients have no demonstrable underlying disease or defect.
- Encephalitis (granulomatous) has an insidious onset and is usually chronic, lasting for more than a week and sometimes even months.
- Dendritic keratitis (mimicking herpes keratitis); trauma-related or keratitis related to infection transmitted with contact lenses contaminated by cleaning solutions
- Chronic ulcerative skin lesions, abscesses, or erythematous nodules

DIAGNOSIS
- Culture in special media
- Cysts can be visualized in sections of brain or corneal tissue or fresh cerebrospinal fluid (rarely).
- Silver-methenamine, PAS stains

TREATMENT
- Pentamidine, azoles, and 5-fluorocytosine are active against *Acanthamoeba* species *in vitro*.
- However, there is no effective treatment for encephalitis.
- Keratitis may be treated with a combination of local and systemic antifungal agents.

PREVENTION
- Standard precautions for hospitalized patients are recommended.
- Avoid swimming in hot springs and other bodies of warm, polluted, fresh water.
- *Acanthamoeba* species are resistant at the usual concentrations of chlorine found in drinking water and swimming pools.
- Only sterile solutions should be used to clean contact lenses.

Acinetobacter Species

GENUS Acinetobacter

SPECIES
- *A. baumannii*
- *A. calcoaceticus*
- *A. haemolyticus*
- *A. johnsonii*
- *A. junii*
- *A. lwoffi*

MICROBIOLOGIC CHARACTERISTICS
- Aerobic, gram-negative bacilli
- It is a constituent of the normal skin and mucosa flora.

EPIDEMIOLOGY
- Worldwide distribution
- Common cause of nosocomial infection, especially in intensive care units

INFECTIONS
- Urinary tract infection (after urinary catheterization or related to other causes of complicated UTI)
- Pneumonia (alcoholics, nosocomial)
- Tracheobronchitis (children, tracheal intubation)
- Cellulitis (line-related)
- Burn and wound infections
- Meningitis (especially after neurosurgical operations)
- Bacteremia

DIAGNOSIS
- Culture

TREATMENT
- Carbapenem (imipenem, meropenem)
- Imipenem or meropenem is almost always active against *Acinetobacter*.
- Ampicillin–sulbactam, piperacillin–tazobactam, ceftazidime, aminoglycosides, doxycycline, or a fluoroquinolone is frequently active against *Acinetobacter*.
- Local infection associated with a catheter (vascular, urinary, others) may be controlled by removing the catheter. However, antibiotics should also be given.
- *A. baumannii* is more resistant than other *Acinetobacter* species.
- In systemic or severe infections, amikacin or another active aminoglycoside may be added to the initially chosen drug.

PREVENTION
- Adherence to infection control guidelines in hospitals, especially in intensive care units

Microorganisms

Acremonium Species

GENUS Acremonium

SPECIES
- Formerly called *Cephalosporium*
- About 100 species:
  - *A. alabamense*
  - *A. falciforme*
  - *A. kiliense* (the most common, medically important species)
  - *A. recifei*
  - *A. roseogriseum*
  - *A. strictum*

MICROBIOLOGIC CHARACTERISTICS
- Filamentous fungi (mold)
- Septate hyphae
- Similar to *Fusarium,* but growth is slower
- Some species can tolerate cycloheximide.
- Colonies are often white, velvety, cottony, or fasciculate and flat or slightly raised in the center.

EPIDEMIOLOGY
- *Acremonium* is associated with soil, insects, sewage, rhizospores of plants, and other environmental substrates.

INFECTIONS
- Mycetoma (chronic skin and subcutaneous tissue infection)
- Onychomycosis
- Mycotic keratitis
- Colonization of soft contact lenses
- Rarely invasive infection
  - Invasive pulmonary disease
  - Meningitis
  - Cerebritis
  - Brain abscess
  - Prosthetic valve endocarditis
  - Midline granuloma
  - Osteomyelitis and posttraumatic arthritis
  - Postsurgery endophthalmitis
  - Peritonitis associated with peritoneal dialysis
  - Disseminated infection in neutropenic patients

DIAGNOSIS
- Culture

TREATMENT
- Amphotericin B and azoles may be effective, but experience is limited.
- Surgical drainage or resection is helpful (when possible).

Actinobacillus Species

GENUS Actinobacillus

SPECIES
- *A. actinomycetemcomitans*
- *A. equuli*
- *A. hominis*
- *A. suis*
- *A. ureae*

MICROBIOLOGIC CHARACTERISTICS
- Aerobic, gram-negative bacilli, nonmotile

EPIDEMIOLOGY
- Actinobacilli were first associated with cattle, but they have been recovered from other animals and humans.
- Several human infections occur after animal bites (e.g., horse bite).

INFECTIONS
- *A. actinomycetemcomitans*
  - Endocarditis (part of the HACEK group, which includes *Haemophilus* species, *A. actinomycetemcomitans*, *Cardiobacterium* species, *Eikenella* species, and *Kingella* species)
  - Wound infection
  - Periodontitis
  - Animal bites
  - Endophthalmitis
- *A. hominis*: bacteremia (especially in patients with chronic lung disease and hepatic failure)
- *A. ureae*: bacteremia, meningitis
- *A. suis* and *A. equuli*: animal bite–related wound infections

DIAGNOSIS
- Culture
- On 1-day-old plates, colonies are translucent and 1 to 2 mm in diameter.
- *A. actinomycetemcomitans*: relatively fastidious, obligate capnophile. Colonies on 1-day-old plates may be less than 0.5 mm in diameter but enlarge to 2 to 3 mm, sometimes with rough surfaces and pitting after several days of incubation.

TREATMENT
- Ampicillin or penicillin G plus aminoglycoside

ALTERNATIVE TREATMENT
- Third-generation cephalosporins
- Trimethoprim–sulfamethoxazole (TMP-SMX)
- Ciprofloxacin
- Azithromycin shows good activity *in vitro*.

Actinomadura Species

GENUS Actinomadura

SPECIES
- *A. madurae*
- *A. pelletieri*
- Others

MICROBIOLOGIC CHARACTERISTICS
- Filamentous bacterium
- Branched
- Gram-positive
- Aerobic

EPIDEMIOLOGY
- Mainly affecting humans in tropical and subtropical regions of the world
- Rare cause of infections in the United States

INFECTIONS
- Actinomycetomas
- Chronic infection of skin, soft tissue, muscles, and bone
- Occasionally a cause of pulmonary or disseminated disease

DIAGNOSIS
- Culture

TREATMENT
- Infections due to *Actinomadura* are frequently refractory to antimicrobial therapy.
- Pulmonary or disseminated infection is managed with aggressive antimicrobial treatment. Streptomycin, with trimethoprim–sulfamethoxazole or dapsone, has been associated with moderate success.
- Surgical resection is used in several cases to manage actinomycetomas.

ALTERNATIVE TREATMENT
- Carbapenems

Actinomyces Species

See Section II, "Actinomycosis"

Aeromonas Species

GENUS Aeromonas

SPECIES
- *A. caviae*
- *A. hydrophila*
- *A. schubertii*
- *A. veronii*
- Others

MICROBIOLOGIC CHARACTERISTICS
- Aerobic, gram-negative bacilli

EPIDEMIOLOGY
- Ubiquitous in fresh and brackish water and soil
- May be isolated from stools of asymptomatic carriers

INFECTIONS
- Gastroenteritis (usually mild but sometimes severe)
- Intraabdominal abscess
- Acute enteritis is common in patients with AIDS.
- Wound infection after exposure to contaminated water or bleeding with leeches (cellulitis, osteomyelitis, myonecrosis)
- Sepsis and necrotizing myositis or ecthyma gangrenosum in patients who are immunosuppressed
- Aspiration pneumonia (after drowning)
- Bacteremia and spontaneous peritonitis in patients with cirrhosis

DIAGNOSIS
- Culture

TREATMENT
- Third-generation cephalosporin, with or without an aminoglycoside
- In patients with enteritis, appropriate volume and salt repletion is important.

ALTERNATIVE TREATMENT
- Imipenem
- Meropenem
- Aztreonam
- Trimethoprim–sulfamethoxazole
- Fluoroquinolone
- Aminoglycoside

Microorganisms

Afipia Species

GENUS Afipia
SPECIES
- A. broomeae
- A. clevelandensis
- A. felis

MICROBIOLOGIC CHARACTERISTICS
- Pleomorphic, aerobic, gram-negative bacilli
- Better seen with silver strains

INFECTIONS
- Its role in human disease is unclear.
- It was thought to be the cause of cat-scratch disease for some time, but more recent data have proved that other agents (mainly Rochalimaea species) cause most cases of this infection.
- It may cause a minority of cases of cat-scratch disease.

DIAGNOSIS
- Histology of affected lymph nodes

TREATMENT
- A macrolide antibiotic may be beneficial (no clear data).

Agrobacterium radiobacter

GENUS Agrobacterium
SPECIES
- A. radiobacter

MICROBIOLOGIC CHARACTERISTICS
- Aerobic, gram-negative bacilli

INFECTIONS
- Rare cause of infections
- Prosthetic valve endocarditis
- Line-related sepsis or bacteremia
- Peritonitis
- Urinary tract infection

DIAGNOSIS
- Culture

TREATMENT
- Trimethoprim–sulfamethoxazole
- Chloramphenicol

ALTERNATIVE TREATMENT
- Aminoglycosides
- Ciprofloxacin

Alcaligenes Species

GENUS Alcaligenes
SPECIES
- A. denitrificans
- A. faecalis
- A. piechaudii
- A. xylosoxidans (previously classified as Achromobacter)

MICROBIOLOGIC CHARACTERISTICS
- Aerobic, gram-negative bacilli

EPIDEMIOLOGY
- Worldwide, rare infection

INFECTIONS
- Sepsis
- Localized infections
- It has been reported to be a rare cause of bacteremia secondary to contaminated intravenous fluids.

DIAGNOSIS
- Culture

TREATMENT
- Carbapenem (imipenem, meropenem)
- Ureidopenicillins

ALTERNATIVE TREATMENT
- Antimicrobial treatment may need to be modified based on results of in vitro susceptibility testing.
- Ceftazidime
- Trimethoprim–sulfamethoxazole
- Fluoroquinolone

Alphavirus

GROUP Alphavirus
SUBGROUPS
- Eastern equine encephalitis
- Western equine encephalitis
- Venezuelan equine encephalitis
- Ross River
- Chikungunya
- Mayaro
- O'nyong-nyong
- Others

MICROBIOLOGIC CHARACTERISTICS
- These viruses belong to the arboviruses group A.
- Single-stranded, positive RNA virus
- Icosahedral symmetry
- Enveloped

EPIDEMIOLOGY
- Alphaviruses cause vector-borne infections.
- Infections are usually transmitted to humans via mosquito bites.
- Rare infections
- Specific subgroups of alphaviruses are associated with infection in different parts of the world.
- Ross River virus is found in Australia and Tasmania, Papua-New Guinea, Indonesia, and the South Pacific Islands.
- Sindbis virus is found throughout Africa, Europe, and Australia.
- Barmah Forest virus is found in Australia.
- Chikungunya and O'nyong viruses are found in the sub-Saharan region in Africa.
- Mayaro virus is found in the forests of South America.

Microorganisms

INFECTIONS
- Eastern equine, Western equine, and Venezuelan alphaviruses cause encephalitis.
- Other subgroups of alphaviruses, such as Chikungunya, usually cause epidemic outbreaks, with fever, vesicular rash, and polyarthralgia/polyarthritis.

DIAGNOSIS
- Cell culture
- Serology

TREATMENT
- Symptomatic
- There is no specific treatment.
- Ribavirin has some activity *in vitro* against alphaviruses, but there is no controlled, published experience from clinical use.

PREVENTION
- Control of mosquitoes and other arthropods

Alternaria Species

GENUS Alternaria

SPECIES
- A. alternata
- A. longipes
- A. tenuissima

MICROBIOLOGIC CHARACTERISTIC
- Dematiaceous, filamentous fungi (mold)
- In histologic specimens, *Alternaria* may be found in several forms: yeasts, pseudohyphae, or pigmented septate hyphae *in vivo*.
- Hyphae at 30°C in culture

EPIDEMIOLOGY
- Worldwide infection

INFECTIONS
- Phaeohyphomycosis involving skin and subcutaneous tissue
- Sinusitis and osteomyelitis in immunosuppressed patients
- Peritonitis in patients undergoing peritoneal dialysis
- Corneal infections (keratitis)

DIAGNOSIS
- Identification of *Alternaria* from clinical specimens
- Isolation from culture

TREATMENT
- Amphotericin B intravenously
- Itraconazole

ALTERNATIVE TREATMENT
- Surgical management may be beneficial in cases of skin, subcutaneus tissue, or bone involvement.

Anaerobiospirillum

GENUS Anaerobiospirillum

SPECIES
- A. succiniciproducens
- A. thomasii

MICROBIOLOGIC CHARACTERISTICS
- Anaerobic, gram-negative bacilli

EPIDEMIOLOGY
- Rare cause of infections

INFECTIONS
- Bacteremia
- Intestinal infection, especially in immunosuppressed persons

DIAGNOSIS
- Anaerobic culture

TREATMENT
- There are no good data for the optimal treatment.
- Chloramphenicol
- Metronidazole

ALTERNATIVE TREATMENT
- Doxycycline

Ancylostoma

GENUS Ancylostoma

SPECIES
- A. braziliense (hookworm of dogs and cats)
- A. ceylanicum
- A. duodenale

MICROBIOLOGIC CHARACTERISTICS
- Round worms (nematode helminths)

EPIDEMIOLOGY
- A. duodenale: Mediterranean coast of Europe and Africa, South America, India (especially in the northern part of the country), China, Southeast Asia, South Pacific
- A. braziliense: tropical and subtropical regions
- A. ceylanicum: more rare than the other two species (occurs in Southeast Asia)

INFECTIONS
- A. duodenale: hookworm (anemia, dyspepsia, diarrhea)
- Larva migrans cutanea: A syndrome manifested by dermatitis, causing significant pruritus, may be the result of A. braziliense infection.

DIAGNOSIS
- Stool examination after concentration

TREATMENT
- A. braziliense: albendazole 400 mg q12h for 3 days
- A. duodenale: mebendazole 100 mg PO q12h for 3 days

ALTERNATIVE TREATMENT
- Thiabendazole 25 mg/kg PO q12h for 5 days also may be given for A. braziliense.
- Pyrantel pamoate 11 mg/d PO for 3 days also may be given for A. duodenale.
- In severe parasitosis with anemia, repeat the same dose 8 to 14 days later.

Microorganisms

Angiostrongylus Species

GENUS Angiostrongylus
SPECIES
- A. cantonensis
- A. costaricensis

MICROBIOLOGIC CHARACTERISTICS
- Nematode helminth (round worm)

EPIDEMIOLOGY
- Southeast Asia and South Pacific for A. cantonensis
- Central and South America for A. costaricensis

INFECTIONS
- Angiostrongylosis, which is manifested by eosinophilic meningoencephalitis, keratitis, iritis, and blepharospasm, may be the result of A. cantonensis infection.
- A. costaricensis may lead to intestinal infection of varying severity, which ranges from an asymptomatic infection to persistent abdominal discomfort due to abdominal masses.

DIAGNOSIS
- CSF examination
- Serology

TREATMENT
- Mebendazole 100 mg PO q12h for 5 days for A. cantonensis
- Surgical management may be necessary to remove abdominal masses for some patients with A. costaricensis infections.

ALTERNATIVE TREATMENT
- Thiabendazole 25 mg/kg PO q12h for 7 days is an alternative regimen for A. cantonensis.

Anisakis Species

GENUS Anisakis
SPECIES
- Several species

MICROBIOLOGIC CHARACTERISTICS
- Nematode helminth (round worm)

INCUBATION PERIOD
- The patient may develop gastric symptoms a few hours after ingestion of infective larvae.
- It takes a few days to weeks after infection for small- and large-bowel symptoms to develop.

EPIDEMIOLOGY
- The infection occurs in people who eat raw, inadequately cooked, or inadequately treated (smoked, marinated, salted) saltwater fish, squid, or octopus.
- Common in Japan, Scandinavian countries, the Netherlands, and the Pacific coast of Latin America
- Increasing incidence in the United States and Europe

INFECTIONS
- Anisakiasis
- The motile parasite invades the gastric wall and causes symptoms sometimes due to ulceration.

DIAGNOSIS
- Recognition of the parasite (a 2-cm-long larvae invading the oropharynx or the stomach)

TREATMENT
- Endoscopic removal of the parasite

ALTERNATIVE TREATMENT
- Surgical excision of the lesions

Apophysomyces elegans

GENUS Apophysomyces
SPECIES
- A. elegans

MICROBIOLOGIC CHARACTERISTICS
- Filamentous fungi (mold) with hyaline, nonseptate hyphae

EPIDEMIOLOGY
- Worldwide, rare infection

INFECTIONS
- Zygomycosis (mucormycosis, phycomycosis): wound infection with secondary spread

DIAGNOSIS
- Culture
- Identification of the fungus in tissue biopsies

TREATMENT
- Amphotericin B

ALTERNATIVE TREATMENT
- There are no clear data for the effectiveness of itraconazole or other azoles.

Arcanobacterium Species

GENUS Arcanobacterium
SPECIES
- A. haemolyticum
- A. pyogenes

MICROBIOLOGIC CHARACTERISTICS
- Aerobic, gram-positive bacilli

INCUBATION PERIOD
- Unknown

EPIDEMIOLOGY
- Worldwide, rare infection

INFECTIONS
- Pharyngitis (with exanthematic rash in about 50% of cases)
- Arcanobacterium haemolyticum may also cause endocarditis.

DIAGNOSIS
- Culture

TREATMENT
- Macrolides

ALTERNATIVE TREATMENT
- Clindamycin
- Tetracycline

Microorganisms

Arenaviral Hemorrhagic Fevers in South America

GROUP Arena virus

STRAINS
- Junin virus (Argentinian hemorrhagic fever)
- Machupo virus (Bolivian hemorrhagic fever)
- Guanarito virus (Venezuelan hemorrhagic fever)
- Sabia virus (Brazilian hemorrhagic fever)

MICROBIOLOGIC CHARACTERISTICS
- These viruses belong to the Tacaribe complex of arena viruses.
- They are Arena viruses.
- They are related to the viruses of Lassa fever and lymphocytic choriomeningitis.

INCUBATION PERIOD
- Seven to 16 days

EPIDEMIOLOGY
- Occasional outbreaks have been reported from South American countries.
- They may be directly transmitted from person to person (rarely).
- Transmission to humans usually occurs via the inhalation of small-particle aerosols derived from contaminated excreta and saliva of rodents.

INFECTIONS
- These viruses cause acute illness, manifested by fever, headache, retro-orbital pain, sweating, conjunctival infection, myalgias, malaise, and prostration. In severe cases, hemorrhagic manifestations, central nervous system dysfunction, bradycardia, and hypotension may appear.
- Case fatality rates range from 10% to 30%.

DIAGNOSIS
- Isolation of the virus (virologic culture)
- Detection of viral antigens in blood or affected organs
- Serology tests, which identify serum antibody against the causative virus

TREATMENT
- There are only few reported data on the treatment of these syndromes.
- Ribavirin is useful in all four hemorrhagic fevers caused by Arena viruses.

ALTERNATIVE TREATMENT
- Specific immune plasma was shown to be effective in the treatment of Junin virus (Argentinian hemorrhagic fever) if given within 8 days of onset of disease.

PREVENTION
- Strict isolation of affected persons during the acute febrile period
- Rodent control

Ascaris lumbricoides

GENUS Ascaris

SPECIES
- A. lumbricoides

MICROBIOLOGIC CHARACTERISTICS
- Nematode helminth (round worm, about 15–35 cm in length)

INCUBATION PERIOD
- The incubation period is prolonged. The life cycle of A. lumbricoides is 4 to 8 weeks.
- Feces contain eggs about 2 months after ingestion of embryonated eggs.

EPIDEMIOLOGY
- Very common infection worldwide, mainly in developing countries (and especially in tropical areas)
- Estimated prevalence of infected people about 1 billion worldwide

INFECTIONS
- Ascariasis (abdominal pain, pulmonary infiltrates, biliary tract obstruction, and eosinophilia)
- Heavy infection may lead to severe nutritional problems.
- Transmission is usually by hand to mouth.

DIAGNOSIS
- Stool examination after concentration

TREATMENT
- Mebendazole 100 mg PO q12h for 3 days

ALTERNATIVE TREATMENT:
- Pyrantel pamoate 11 mg/kg (maximum dose 1 g) in a single dose
- Albendazole 400 mg (single dose)
- Ivermectin 12 mg (single dose)

Aspergillus Species

See Section II, "Aspergillosis"

Aureobasidium pullulans

GENUS Aureobasidium

SPECIES
- A. pullulans

MICROBIOLOGIC CHARACTERISTICS
- Dematiaceous, filamentous fungus (mold)
- Yeasts, pseudohyphae, or pigmented septate hyphae *in vivo*
- Hyphae in cultures at 30°C

EPIDEMIOLOGY
- Worldwide, rare infection

INFECTIONS
- Phaeohyphomycosis in immunosuppressed individuals
- Peritonitis in patients under peritoneal dialysis

DIAGNOSIS
- Culture
- Identification of the fungus in tissue biopsies

TREATMENT
- There are no good data for treatment.
- Amphotericin B is probably effective.
- Removal of the peritoneal dialysis catheter helps in the management of this fungal infection (in patients with peritonitis related to peritoneal dialysis).

ALTERNATIVE TREATMENT
- No data for clinical efficacy of azoles

Babesia Species

See Section II, "Babesiosis"

Microorganisms

Bacillus Species

GENUS Bacillus

SPECIES
- B. alvei
- B. anthracis (the cause of anthrax, discussed in Section II)
- B. cereus
- B. circulans
- B. laterosporus
- B. pseudoanthracis
- B. pumilus
- B. sphaericus
- B. subtilis
- Others

MICROBIOLOGIC CHARACTERISTICS
- Aerobic, gram-positive bacillus

INCUBATION PERIOD
- For the food poisoning syndrome, causing mainly vomiting, the incubation period is 1 to 6 hours; for the diarrhea syndrome, it is 6 to 24 hours.

EPIDEMIOLOGY
- Rice is the usual food related to Bacillus species food poisoning (emetic form).
- Meat or a vegetable is usually associated with the diarrhea syndrome caused by Bacillus species.

INFECTIONS
- Food poisoning and enterotoxic gastroenteritis (B. cereus)
- Meningitis, brain abscess
- Bacteremia (in intravenous drug users or associated with intravenous lines)
- Endocarditis
- Pneumonia
- Soft-tissue infections
- Conjunctivitis, keratitis ulcers, panophthalmitis

DIAGNOSIS
- Culture

TREATMENT
- There is no need for a specific antimicrobial treatment in patients with gastroenteritis due to Bacillus species.
- Vancomycin, with or without an aminoglycoside

ALTERNATIVE TREATMENT
- Imipenem
- Ciprofloxacin
- Tetracycline
- Chloramphenicol
- Clindamycin
- Macrolide
- B. cereus is resistant to most β-lactam antibiotics.

PREVENTION
- Proper food handling reduces the risk of food poisoning due to Bacillus species.

Bacteroides Species

GENUS Bacteroides

SPECIES
- B. caccae
- B. capillosus
- B. distasonis
- B. eggerthii
- B. forsythus
- B. fragilis
- B. gracilis
- B. merdae
- B. ovatus
- B. putredinis
- B. stercoris
- B. tectum
- B. thetaiotaomicron
- B. uniformis
- B. ureolyticus
- B. vulgatus
- Others

MICROBIOLOGIC CHARACTERISTICS
- Anaerobic, gram-negative bacilli
- Bacteroides species are classified in the B. fragilis group and others.

EPIDEMIOLOGY
- Usual cause of infection where there is mixed etiology with aerobic and anaerobic organisms
- Many of the Bacteroides species are part of the normal gastrointestinal flora (i.e., B. fragilis).

INFECTIONS
- Intraabdominal and pelvic infections
- Pleuropulmonary
- Cervicofacial infection
- Brain abscess
- Sepsis
- Skin and soft-tissue infections (including surgical wounds)

DIAGNOSIS
- Anaerobic culture

TREATMENT
- Metronidazole or clindamycin
- In case of infection caused by B. gracilis, imipenem or chloramphenicol is the first choice.

ALTERNATIVE TREATMENT
- Imipenem
- Meropenem
- Cephamycin (cefoxitin, cefotetan, cefmetazole)
- Piperacillin–tazobactam
- Ticarcillin–clavulanate
- Ampicillin–sulbactam
- Chloramphenicol
- There is an increasing incidence of resistance in Bacteroides species.
- Twenty percent of the B. fragilis group (particularly B. distasonis and B. thetaiotaomicron) and nearly 30% of B. gracilis are resistant to the cephamycins.
- Ten percent of B. gracilis are resistant to metronidazole.

Microorganisms

Balantidium coli

GENUS Balantidium
SPECIES
- B. coli

MICROBIOLOGIC CHARACTERISTICS
- Protozoon

INCUBATION PERIOD
- Unknown, but may be only several days

EPIDEMIOLOGY
- Worldwide

INFECTIONS
- Balantidiasis (colitis, dysentery)

DIAGNOSIS
- Stool examination (fresh and after concentration)

TREATMENT
- Metronidazole 750 mg q8h for 5 to 10 days

ALTERNATIVE TREATMENT
- Oxytetracycline 500 mg q6h for 10 days

Bartonella bacilliformis

See Section II, "Bartonellosis"

Bartonella (Rochalimaea) henselae

GENUS Bartonella
SPECIES
- Bartonella (Rochalimaea) henselae

MICROBIOLOGIC CHARACTERISTICS
- Gram-negative coccobacillus, probably of intracellular location

INCUBATION PERIOD
- Usually 2 to 14 days from inoculation of the pathogen to primary skin lesion and 5 to 60 days from inoculation to lymphadenopathy

EPIDEMIOLOGY
- Worldwide infection

INFECTIONS
- Bacillary angiomatosis (skin lesions due to vascular proliferation), peliosis hepatica or splenic involvement, CNS lesions, lymph node involvement (especially in AIDS patients)
- Cat-scratch disease (local process with regional adenopathy, oculoglandular syndrome)
- Endocarditis
- Bacteremia

DIAGNOSIS
- Blood cultures using lysis-centrifugation methods
- Optimal growth in blood-enriched media
- Prolonged incubation (minimum, 2 weeks)
- Histopathology of cutaneous lesions is characteristic.
- Serology

TREATMENT
- Erythromycin (1-4 months) (unclear efficacy)
- Cat-scratch disease usually has a benign course, with spontaneous improvement in a few weeks.

ALTERNATIVE TREATMENT
- Doxycycline, azithromycin, clarithromycin

PREVENTION
- Avoid cat scratches.

Bartonella (Rochalimaea) quintana

GENUS Bartonella
SPECIES
- B. (Rochalimaea) quintana

MICROBIOLOGIC CHARACTERISTICS
- Small coccobacillus of intracellular growth

INCUBATION PERIOD
- Usually 7 to 30 days

EPIDEMIOLOGY
- There are several endemic foci of the infection in many countries, including Poland, the former Soviet Union, and several African and South American countries.

INFECTIONS
- Trench fever
- Bacillary angiomatosis in immunosuppressed patients
- Bacteremia
- Endocarditis

DIAGNOSIS
- Blood cultures using lysis-centrifugation systems
- Cell cultures

TREATMENT
- Doxycycline 100 mg PO q12h for 7 days

ALTERNATIVE TREATMENT
- Chloramphenicol
- Erythromycin (500 mg q6h)

PREVENTION
- Destroy the vector (louse) to prevent transmission to humans.

Basidiobolus ranarum

GENUS Basidiobolus
SPECIES
- B. ranarum

MICROBIOLOGIC CHARACTERISTICS
- Filamentous fungus (mold)

EPIDEMIOLOGY
- Worldwide, rare infection
- More common in India, Indonesia, and Africa

INFECTIONS
- Nodular skin lesions in the subcutaneous tissue of trunk or extremities

DIAGNOSIS
- Culture
- Identification of the fungus in tissue (biopsy)

TREATMENT
- Potassium iodide-saturated solution, 30 mg/kg/d for 6 to 12 months
- Spontaneous resolution has been observed occasionally.
- Surgical management may be helpful in difficult-to-treat cases with the use of antifungal agents

ALTERNATIVE TREATMENT
- Ketoconazole
- Amphotericin B i.v.
- Trimethoprim-sulfamethoxazole

Microorganisms

Baylisascaris procyonis

GENUS Baylisascaris
SPECIES
- B. procyonis

MICROBIOLOGIC CHARACTERISTICS
- Anematode parasite (round worm)

EPIDEMIOLOGY
- Rare infection in the United States
- Humans are infected accidentally when they ingest infective eggs found in soil.
- Intestinal round worm of raccoon

INFECTIONS
- Larva migrans visceral
- Meningoencephalitic complications

DIAGNOSIS
- Histologic examination of surgically removed tissues

TREATMENT
- Directed laser therapy (ocular infection)
- Corticosteroids

ALTERNATIVE TREATMENT
- Diethylcarbamazine or ivermectin may be tried.

Bilophila wadsworthia

GENUS Bilophila
SPECIES
- B. wadsworthia

MICROBIOLOGIC CHARACTERISTICS
- Anaerobic, gram-negative bacillus

EPIDEMIOLOGY
- Isolated, usually, from mixed infections

INFECTIONS
- Peritonitis secondary to appendicitis
- Bacteremia
- Liver abscess

DIAGNOSIS
- Anaerobic culture

TREATMENT
- Metronidazole, clindamycin, or cefoxitin

ALTERNATIVE TREATMENT
- Carbapenem (imipenem, meropenem), piperacillin–tazobactam, or ticarcillin–clavulanate

Bipolaris Species

GENUS Bipolaris
SPECIES
- B. australiensis
- B. hawaiiensis
- B. spicifera

MICROBIOLOGIC CHARACTERISTICS
- Dematiaceous, filamentous fungus (mold)
- Colonies rapidly growing, cottony, gray to black
- Yeast, pseudohypha, or septate and pigmented hyphae *in vivo*
- Hyphae grow at 30°C in culture.

EPIDEMIOLOGY
- Usually is found in soil and plants
- Inoculation through a penetrating injury or by inhalation of conidia from the environment

INFECTIONS
- Occasionally, it causes infections in humans and animals.
- Mycotic infection in healthy and compromised hosts
- Infections of the eye (corneal)
- Subcutaneous infections
- Paranasal sinusitis in patients with allergic rhinitis and nasal polyposis
- Pulmonary infections
- Meningoencephalitis
- Disseminated manifestations in immunosuppressed patients

DIAGNOSIS
- Identification of the fungus in clinical specimens
- Culture

TREATMENT
- Infection of the cornea: topical natamycin
- Subcutaneous infection: amphotericin B i.v., flucytosine, ketoconazole, or itraconazole as complement for surgery
- Systemic infection: amphotericin B i.v.

ALTERNATIVE TREATMENT
- Subcutaneous or systemic infection: itraconazole (limited experience)
- Surgical excision of local lesions is important.

Blastocystis hominis

GENUS Blastocystis
SPECIES
- B. hominis

MICROBIOLOGIC CHARACTERISTICS
- Protozoon

EPIDEMIOLOGY
- Worldwide
- It is commonly found in stool specimens; however, its pathogenicity is unclear. It seems not to cause any disease in most cases of isolation.

INFECTIONS
- Self-limited, acute diarrhea

DIAGNOSIS
- Identification in stool specimen

TREATMENT
- Antibiotic treatment is indicated only if another enteropathogen is not isolated and a high number of *Blastocystis* is found in stools.
- Metronidazole 750 mg q8h for 10 days

ALTERNATIVE TREATMENT
- None studied

Blastomyces dermatitidis

See Section II, "Blastomycosis"

Microorganisms

Blastoschizomyces capitatus

GENUS Blastoschizomyces

SPECIES
- B. capitatus

MICROBIOLOGIC CHARACTERISTICS
- Yeast that can develop arthroconidia, hyphae, blastoconidia, and pseudohypha

EPIDEMIOLOGY
- Rare infection
- Probably worldwide

INFECTIONS
- Disseminated forms with fungemia, skin lesions, and visceral abscesses in neutropenic patients
- Fungemia in intravenous drug users
- Surgical wound infections
- Prosthetic valve endocarditis

DIAGNOSIS
- Culture
- Identification of fungus in tissue biopsies

TREATMENT
- Amphotericin B i.v.
- Flucytosine has been used in combination with amphotericin B.

ALTERNATIVE TREATMENT
- Fluconazole 800 mg/d

Bordetella bronchiseptica

GENUS Bordetella

SPECIES
- B. bronchiseptica

MICROBIOLOGIC CHARACTERISTICS
- Aerobic, gram-negative bacillus

EPIDEMIOLOGY
- Worldwide

INFECTIONS
- Pneumonia
- Tracheobronchitis
- Bacteremia

DIAGNOSIS
- Culture

TREATMENT
- In contrast to *Bordetella pertussis*, *B. bronchiseptica* is usually resistant to macrolide antibiotics.
- Antipseudomonal β-lactam agents are usually effective.

ALTERNATIVE TREATMENT
- Aminoglycoside, doxycycline, or chloramphenicol

Bordetella Species

GENUS Bordetella

SPECIES
- B. parapertussis
- B. pertussis

MICROBIOLOGIC CHARACTERISTICS
- Aerobic, gram-negative bacilli

EPIDEMIOLOGY
- Worldwide
- It may affect previously immunized patients, particularly adults.

INFECTIONS
- Whooping cough

DIAGNOSIS
- Culture in special medium (Bordet-Gengou)
- Serology may be helpful.
- Antigen detection in nasopharyngeal exudate

TREATMENT
- Cough medicines, including codeine, are usually ineffective.
- Erythromycin 40 to 50 mg/kg/d (maximum, 2 g/d) for 14 days

ALTERNATIVE TREATMENT
- Macrolides
- Trimethoprim
- Sulfamethoxazole
- Amoxicillin

PREVENTION
- Respiratory isolation is required.

Borrelia burgdorferi

See Section II, "Lyme Disease"

Borrelia Species

GENUS Borrelia

SPECIES
- B. hispanica
- B. mazzottii
- B. recurrentis
- B. venezuelensis
- Others

MICROBIOLOGIC CHARACTERISTICS
- Aerobic, gram-negative bacilli

INCUBATION PERIOD
- The incubation period is 4 to 18 days, with a mean of 7 days.

EPIDEMIOLOGY
- Worldwide infection

INFECTIONS
- Relapsing fever (discussed in Section II)

DIAGNOSIS
- Identification with Giemsa or Wright stains or dark-field examination of peripheral blood smears (not available in most laboratories)
- Intraperitoneal inoculation in rats
- Serology

TREATMENT
- Doxycycline
- The louse-borne infection may be treated with a single dose of antibiotics, whereas the tick-borne infection requires 5 to 10 days of treatment.

ALTERNATIVE TREATMENT
- Penicillin G
- Erythromycin
- Chloramphenicol

Brucella Species

See Section II, "Brucellosis"

Microorganisms

Brugia Species

GENUS Brugia
SPECIES
- B. malayi
- B. timory

MICROBIOLOGIC CHARACTERISTICS
- Nematode helminth

EPIDEMIOLOGY
- B. malayi: India, Papua New Guinea, Vietnam, Cambodia, Thailand (and other countries of Indochina), China, Korea
- B. timory: Indonesia

INFECTIONS
- Lymphatic filariasis
- Elephantiasis (lymphangitis, lymphedema, abscesses)

DIAGNOSIS
- Blood smear examination (fresh, concentrated, or filtrated specimen)
- Giemsa or H&E stain for species identification

TREATMENT
- Diethylcarbamazine 2 mg/kg q8h for 3 weeks (50 mg the first day, 50 mg q12h the second, 50 mg q8h the third, 100 mg q12h the fourth, and 100 mg q8h the fifth day, for completion for a 3-week treatment period)
- Allergic reactions may occur during treatment, especially during the first few days of treatment.

ALTERNATIVE TREATMENT
- Ivermectin 150 μg/kg (single dose)

Burkholderia (Pseudomonas) mallei

GENUS Burkholderia
SPECIES
- B. mallei

MICROBIOLOGIC CHARACTERISTICS
- Aerobic, gram-negative bacilli

INCUBATION PERIOD
- One to 5 days

EPIDEMIOLOGY
- B. mallei causes infection in equine animals. However, it is sometimes transmitted to humans.
- Rare human infection, mainly in Asia, Africa, and Central and South America
- Affected persons usually have a history of contact with horses, donkeys, or mules.

INFECTIONS
- Glanders (cutaneous infection with adenitis, pneumonia, or sepsis)

DIAGNOSIS
- Microscopic examination of exudates rarely reveals the pathogen.
- B. mallei cannot be distinguished by microscopic examination from B. pseudomallei.
- Culture or inoculation into animals
- Serology

TREATMENT
- There are limited data on the efficacy of antibiotics for glanders.
- Doxycycline or chloramphenicol may be beneficial.
- Surgical management is helpful in cases with suppurative lymphadenitis.

ALTERNATIVE TREATMENT
- Sulfadiazine 100 mg/kg/d orally for 3 weeks

PREVENTION
- Isolation of the affected person is indicated.

Burkholderia (Pseudomonas) pseudomallei

GENUS Burkholderia
SPECIES
- B. pseudomallei

MICROBIOLOGIC CHARACTERISTICS
- Aerobic, gram-negative bacilli

INCUBATION PERIOD
- The first symptoms may appear quickly after infection (2–3 days).
- Most patients develop symptoms months to years after infection.

EPIDEMIOLOGY
- B. pseudomallei is a natural saprophyte isolated from soil, ponds, and market produce.
- It is unclear how humans contract the pathogen. Some experts believe that the most common mechanism is by soil contamination of skin abrasions.
- It is a rare cause of human infection, except in Thailand. A study from northeast Thailand reported that 40% of deaths from community-acquired septicemia were attributable to melioidosis (B. pseudomallei).

INFECTIONS
- Melioidosis (skin infection, with adenitis, pneumonia, or sepsis)
- Some patients may develop a secondary abscess in several organs.

DIAGNOSIS
- The diagnosis of melioidosis should be considered in patients from endemic areas presenting with febrile illness.
- Culture or inoculation into animals
- Serology

TREATMENT
- Ceftazidime
- Chloramphenicol

ALTERNATIVE TREATMENT
- Trimethoprim–sulfamethoxazole (TMP–SMX)
- Minocycline
- A significant proportion (10%–80%) of B. pseudomallei species isolated from patients in Thailand are resistant to TMP–SMX.
- Patients with low-titer antibodies against the pathogen, but without any evidence of infection, do not require treatment.

Burkholderia (Pseudomonas) Species

GENUS Burkholderia
SPECIES
- B. cepacia
- B. gladioli
- B. pickettii
- B. stutzeri

MICROBIOLOGIC CHARACTERISTICS
- Aerobic, gram-negative bacilli

EPIDEMIOLOGY
- Recent studies in patients with cystic fibrosis have shown that B. cepacia is transmissible between humans.

INFECTIONS
- Bronchitis in patients with cystic fibrosis (B. cepacia, B. gladioli)
- Wound infection
- Sepsis in immunosuppressed patients or in association with central venous lines
- Pneumonia (B. stutzeri)

DIAGNOSIS
- Culture

TREATMENT
- Several antibiotics active against Pseudomonas species are also active against B. cepacia.
- However, strains of B. cepacia isolated from patients with cystic fibrosis have frequently high minimal inhibitory concentration (MIC) with these agents. For this reason, some experts recommend monitoring of serum levels of antibiotics in this setting.
- Ceftazidime
- Meropenem
- Piperacillin–tazobactam

ALTERNATIVE TREATMENT
- Trimethoprim–sulfamethoxazole

PREVENTION
- Patients with cystic fibrosis who are not colonized with B. cepacia should avoid contact with patients who are infected or colonized with the pathogen.

Microorganisms

Caliciviruses and Calici-like Viruses

GROUP Calicivirus

GENOGROUPS
- There are four recognized genogroups of caliciviruses causing disease in humans: Norwalk-like, Snow Mountain-like, and Sapporo-like caliciviruses, and hepatitis E virus.

MICROBIOLOGIC CHARACTERISTICS
- Single-stranded, positive RNA virus
- Icosahedral symmetry
- Naked

INCUBATION PERIOD
- Twelve hours to 4 days

EPIDEMIOLOGY
- Common cause of human disease (Norwalk-like virus)

INFECTIONS
- Calicivirus causes gastroenteritis in children and adults.
- The Norwalk-like serogroup of caliciviruses is usually detected in children younger than 4 years old.

DIAGNOSIS
- Direct visualization in stools, using electron microscopy
- Enzyme immunoassay for detection of viral antigen in stool or antibody in serum
- Reverse transcriptase polymerase chain reaction (RT-PCR) for detection of viral RNA in stool

TREATMENT
- Symptomatic

ALTERNATIVE TREATMENT
- There is no effective specific treatment with antiviral agents.

PREVENTION
- Contact precautions for diapered and/or incontinent children for the duration of illness.

Calymmatobacterium granulomatis

GENUS *Calymmatobacterium*

SPECIES
- *C. (Donovania) granulomatis*

MICROBIOLOGIC CHARACTERISTICS
- Aerobic, pleomorphic, gram-negative coccobacilli

INCUBATION PERIOD
- Unknown (probably between 1 and 16 weeks)

EPIDEMIOLOGY
- A sexually transmitted infection
- Rare in industrialized countries
- Cluster outbreaks occasionally occur in the United States.
- Endemic in tropical and subtropical areas

INFECTIONS
- Granuloma inguinale (donovanosis)
- Chronic and progressively destructive disease of the genitalia, inguinal area, and anal area

DIAGNOSIS
- Histologic examination
- A Wright or Giemsa stain of a smear of affected areas reveals the presence of intracytoplasmic, rod-shaped inclusions known as Donovan bodies.
- Culture is difficult and unreliable.

TREATMENT
- Doxycycline 100 mg q12h orally for 3 weeks

ALTERNATIVE TREATMENT
- Trimethoprim–sulfamethoxazole
- Ampicillin
- Gentamicin
- Chloramphenicol
- A macrolide antibiotic

PREVENTION
- Safe-sex practice

Campylobacter Species

See Section II, "Campylobacter Infections"

Candida Species

See Section II chapters on *Candida* infections

Capillaria Species

GENUS *Capillaria*

SPECIES
- *C. aerophila*
- *C. hepatica*
- *C. philippinensis*

MICROBIOLOGIC CHARACTERISTICS
- Nematode helminths

EPIDEMIOLOGY
- *C. philippinensis*: the Philippines, Thailand; rare elsewhere
- *C. hepatica*: sporadic cases reported in several countries worldwide
- *C. aerophila*: rare cases reported from the former Soviet Union

INFECTIONS
- *C. philippinensis*: intestinal capillariasis
- *C. hepatica*: hepatic capillariasis
- *C. aerophila*: pulmonary capillariasis

DIAGNOSIS
- Identification of ova or larvae in the stool in cases of intestinal capillariasis
- Histopathology of liver biopsy in cases of hepatic capillariasis

TREATMENT
- Intestinal capillariasis: mebendazole
- Hepatic capillariasis: thiabendazole

ALTERNATIVE TREATMENT
- Intestinal capillariasis: albendazole
- Hepatic capillariasis: albendazole

PREVENTION
- Avoid eating uncooked fish in endemic areas (for *C. philippinensis*).

Capnocytophaga Species

GENUS *Capnocytophaga*

SPECIES
- *C. canimorsus* (CDC Group Dysgonic Fermenter 2 [DF-2])
- *C. cynodegmi*
- Other *Capnocytophaga* species, such as *C. gingivalis*, *C. sputigena*, and *C. ochracea*

MICROBIOLOGIC CHARACTERISTICS
- Microaerophilic, gram-negative bacilli

INCUBATION PERIOD
- One to 5 days after inoculation

EPIDEMIOLOGY
- *Capnocytophaga* species can cause clinical infection in persons who have been bitten, scratched, or licked by dogs or cats.
- Splenectomy, alcoholism, and chronic pulmonary disease are known risk factors.
- Some *Capnocytophaga* species are part of the normal human flora.
- Neutropenic patients may develop septicemia due to these organisms.

INFECTIONS
- Wound infection after dog bite
- Sepsis (severe, with shock and diffuse intravascular coagulation in splenectomized patients)
- Purulent meningitis
- Endocarditis
- Septic arthritis
- *Capnocytophaga* species of the normal human oral flora may cause periodontitis and oral mucositis.

DIAGNOSIS
- Culture
- Finding gram-negative bacilli within neutrophils

TREATMENT
- Penicillin G or ampicillin
- A third-generation cephalosporin may be the initial drug of choice for patients with septicemia due to *Capnocytophaga* species other than *C. canimorsus*.

ALTERNATIVE TREATMENT
- Cephalosporins, carbapenem (imipenem, meropenem)

PREVENTION
- Preventive therapy with penicillin may be warranted for splenectomized patients bitten by dogs.

Microorganisms

Chlamydia Species

GENUS Chlamydia

SPECIES

- There are three clinically important *Chlamydia* species:
  — *C. pneumoniae* (TWAR), the etiologic agent in a significant proportion of cases of pneumonia
  — *C. psittaci*, the cause of psittacosis (see Section II, "Psittacosis")
  — *C. trachomatis*, including serotypes that cause trachoma, genital infections, conjunctivitis, infant pneumonia, and lymphogranuloma venereum

MICROBIOLOGIC CHARACTERISTICS

- Gram-negative bacteria
- Obligate intracellular bacteria

EPIDEMIOLOGY

- Common cause of infection worldwide

INFECTIONS

- Besides the infections presented above, there is some evidence for a role for *C. pneumoniae* in the pathogenesis of atherosclerosis.

DIAGNOSIS

- *Chlamydia* organisms may be seen with Giemsa stain or direct immunofluorescence.
- Serology
- Culture
- Molecular biology techniques (PCR)

TREATMENT

- Doxycycline for 14 days

ALTERNATIVE TREATMENT

- A macrolide or a fluoroquinolone

Chromobacterium violaceum

GENUS Chromobacterium

SPECIES

- *C. violaceum*

MICROBIOLOGIC CHARACTERISTICS

- Aerobic, gram-negative bacillus

EPIDEMIOLOGY

- Worldwide, rare infection

INFECTIONS

- Traumatic wound infections
- Sepsis (mostly in neutropenic patients and in patients with chronic granulomatous disease)
- Pneumonia (after drowning)

DIAGNOSIS

- Culture

TREATMENT

- Doxycycline or a fluoroquinolone

ALTERNATIVE TREATMENT

- Trimethoprim–sulfamethoxazole
- Aminoglycoside

Chromomycosis Agents

GENUS/SPECIES

- Chromomycosis (chromoblastomycosis or dermatitis verrucosa) may be caused by several fungal species, including the following:
  — *Cladosporium carrionii*
  — *Fonsecaea compacta*
  — *Fonsecaea (Phialophora) pedrosoi*
  — *Phialophora verrucosa*
  — *Rhinocladiella aquaspera*

MICROBIOLOGIC CHARACTERISTICS

- Dematiaceous, filamentous fungus (mold)
- Pigmented septate hyphae *in vivo*

INCUBATION PERIOD

- The incubation period is unknown; however, it is probably months.

EPIDEMIOLOGY

- Rare cause of infection
- There is a worldwide distribution of cases, although most of the cases occur in developing countries.
- It usually affects rural, barefooted agricultural workers in tropical and subtropical regions.

INFECTIONS

- Chromomycosis (chromoblastomycosis) is manifested by chronic warty nodules or tumor-like masses of the subcutaneous tissue of the lower extremities (and sometimes in other areas of the body).
- Rarely, the infection spreads to muscle, central nervous system, or the lungs.

DIAGNOSIS

- The etiologic agents of chromoblastomycosis are seen in affected tissue as sclerotic bodies.
- Identification of responsible fungus is based on morphology and culture characteristics.

TREATMENT

- Optimal management has not been defined.
- Itraconazole may benefit some patients. Long-term treatment is usually necessary (for at least 6 months).
- Oral 5-fluorocytosine also has been tried and showed moderate results.

ALTERNATIVE TREATMENT

- Intravenous 5-fluorocytosine combined with amphotericin B may be necessary in patients with large lesions due to chromomycosis.
- Small skin and subcutaneous tissue lesions may also be cured by excision.

PREVENTION

- Wearing shoes and clothes decreases the probability of small puncture wounds.

Chryseomonas luteola

GENUS Chryseomonas

SPECIES

- *C. luteola*

MICROBIOLOGIC CHARACTERISTICS

- Gram-negative bacillus

EPIDEMIOLOGY

- Worldwide, rare infection

INFECTIONS

- Septicemia, sometimes polymicrobial and in association with central venous catheters
- Wound infection
- Peritonitis in patients with peritoneal dialysis
- Prosthetic valve endocarditis
- Meningitis

DIAGNOSIS

- Culture

TREATMENT

- Ceftazidime

ALTERNATIVE TREATMENT

- Ureidopenicillins
- An aminoglycoside
- Imipenem, meropenem
- Ciprofloxacin

Microorganisms

Chrysosporium parvum

GENUS Chrysosporium
SPECIES
- C. parvum

MICROBIOLOGIC CHARACTERISTICS
- Filamentous fungus (mold)
- Septate hyaline hyphae *in vivo*

EPIDEMIOLOGY
- Worldwide, rare infection

INFECTIONS
- Osteomyelitis
- Pulmonary infection
- Prosthetic valve endocarditis
- Rhinitis–sinusitis with occasional extension to the central nervous system
- Dissemination of infection in immunocompromised patients

DIAGNOSIS
- Culture of the fungus
- Identification of the fungus in tissue biopsies

TREATMENT
- Amphotericin B i.v.

Citrobacter Species

GENUS Citrobacter
SPECIES
- C. amalonaticus
- C. freundii
- C. koseri

MICROBIOLOGIC CHARACTERISTICS
- Aerobic, gram-negative bacillus

EPIDEMIOLOGY
- Increasing importance as a cause of nosocomial infections

INFECTIONS
- Urinary tract infections
- Pulmonary infections
- Line-associated sepsis
- Surgical wound infections
- Neonatal meningitis

DIAGNOSIS
- Culture of the pathogen

TREATMENT
- Carbapenem (imipenem, meropenem)
- Fluoroquinolone
- The addition of an aminoglycoside to carbapenem or fluoroquinolone may be warranted in severe cases of *Citrobacter* infection.

ALTERNATIVE TREATMENT
- Third-generation cephalosporin, aztreonam, antipseudomonal penicillins, or an aminoglycoside

Clonorchis sinensis (Opisthorchis sinensis)

GENUS Clonorchis
SPECIES
- C. sinensis: (the chinese liver fluke)

MICROBIOLOGIC CHARACTERISTICS
- A trematode helminth

EPIDEMIOLOGY
- People are infected by eating raw or undercooked freshwater fish.
- China, Japan, Korea, Vietnam, Taiwan
- Endemic in China, especially in the southeast part of the country. The infection is also a problem in Indochina, Taiwan, and Japan.
- Imported cases occur in other countries.

INFECTIONS
- Clonorchiasis (obstructive jaundice and cholangitis)
- The symptoms sometimes appear late after infection (many years later).
- Clonorchiasis is considered to be a risk factor for cholangiocarcinoma.

DIAGNOSIS
- Examination of concentrated stools or bile obtained with a duodenal aspirate
- Serologic tests are also helpful in finding the characteristic eggs.

TREATMENT
- Praziquantel 25 mg/kg q8h PO for 2 days

PREVENTION
- Cook or irradiate freshwater fish.

Clostridium botulinum

See Section II, "Botulism"

Clostridium difficile

See Section II, "Antibiotic- and *Clostridium difficile*–associated Diarrhea and Colitis"

Clostridium Species

GENUS Clostridium
SPECIES
- C. bifermentans
- C. butyricum
- C. clostridiiforme
- C. histolyticum
- C. novyi
- C. perfringens
- C. ramosum
- C. septicum
- C. sordelli
- Other species are discussed elsewhere (*C. difficile*, *C. botulism*, and *C. tetani*)

MICROBIOLOGIC CHARACTERISTICS
- Anaerobic, gram-positive bacilli

INCUBATION PERIOD
- For cases of food poisoning due to *Clostridium* species, the incubation period is 6 to 24 hours, usually 8 to 12 hours.

EPIDEMIOLOGY
- Worldwide infections

INFECTIONS
- Food poisoning
- Bacteremia
- Localized infections (polymicrobial) involving the biliary tract, intraabdominal abscesses, and soft tissues
- Gas gangrene (see Section II, "Gas Gangrene")
- Necrotizing enteritis
- Typhlitis in neutropenic patients and patients with AIDS
- Postpartum endometritis, with hypotension and shock (*C. sordellii*)
- The isolation of *C. septicum* from blood cultures or the onset of spontaneous gas gangrene should prompt the search for a colonic neoplasia or other structural lesions.

Microorganisms

DIAGNOSIS
- Anaerobic culture
- Prolonged incubation of culture may be needed.

TREATMENT
- No antibiotic treatment is needed for cases of food poisoning.
- Penicillin G alone or with clindamycin for severe clostridial infections such as gas gangrene

ALTERNATIVE TREATMENT
- Chloramphenicol, metronidazole, carbapenem (imipenem, meropenem) clindamycin, or a tetracycline (agents with action against anaerobic bacteria)

Clostridium tetani

See Section II, "Tetanus"

Coccidioides immitis

See Section II, "Coccidioidomycosis"

Colorado Tick Fever Virus

GROUP Coltivirus

STRAINS
- Colorado tick fever virus
- Other tick-borne arboviral fevers include infections caused by Kemerova virus, Nairobi sheep disease (Canjam), Lipovnik, Quaranfil, Bhanja, Thogoto, and Dugde viruses.

MICROBIOLOGIC CHARACTERISTICS
- Double-stranded RNA
- Naked

INCUBATION PERIOD
- About 5 days

EPIDEMIOLOGY
- Colorado tick fever is endemic in the mountainous regions (altitude above 5,000 feet) of Canada and the western United States.
- Mode of transmission is by the bite of an infected tick.
- Persons engaged in recreational activities or occupations that increase the probability of tick bite in the endemic areas are at risk of developing Colorado tick fever.

INFECTIONS
- Colorado tick fever is an acute febrile illness.

DIAGNOSIS
- Cell culture
- Serology tests

TREATMENT
- Symptomatic
- There is no specific antiviral treatment.

PREVENTION
- Protective measures to avoid tick bites

Comamonas Species

GENUS Comamonas

SPECIES
- C. acidovorans
- C. terrigena
- C. testosteroni

MICROBIOLOGIC CHARACTERISTICS
- Aerobic, gram-negative bacillus
- Low pathogenicity

EPIDEMIOLOGY
- An infrequent contaminant of cultures

INFECTIONS
- Endocarditis, especially in intravenous drug abusers
- Bacteremia in immunosuppressed patients
- Rarely a cause of keratitis, leading to corneal ulcers (usually *C. acidovorans*)

DIAGNOSIS
- Culture
- The physician should consider the possibility of contamination in cases of patients with positive cultures for *Comamonas*.

TREATMENT
- Little is known about the efficacy of antibiotics of different classes against *Comamonas* species.
- Few available data support the use of antipseudomonal agents.

Conidiobolus Species

GENUS Conidiobolus

SPECIES
- C. coronatus

MICROBIOLOGIC CHARACTERISTICS
- Filamentous fungus (mold)
- Hyphae have few septa.

EPIDEMIOLOGY
- Worldwide infections
- Most reported cases are from Africa and Asia.

INFECTIONS
- Entomophthoromycosis conidiobolae is manifested with nodular lesions of the nose, mouth, and perinasal tissues, which are frequently large and disfiguring.
- Mediastinitis
- Pericarditis

DIAGNOSIS
- Identification of the fungus in biopsy
- Culture of the fungus

TREATMENT
- There are scarce published data for the management of this fungal infection.
- Saturated potassium iodide solution, with or without trimethoprim–sulfamethoxazole, may be used in cases of skin and subcutaneous tissue disease.
- Surgical management may be done in patients with large disfiguring lesions.
- Azoles (fluconazole or ketoconazole) have been reported to help and may be used in patients with severe manifestation of entomophthoromycosis conidiobolae.

Microorganisms

Coronavirus

GROUP Coronavirus

MICROBIOLOGIC CHARACTERISTICS
- Single-stranded, positive RNA virus
- Enveloped virus

INCUBATION PERIOD
- It is usually 2 to 4 days.

EPIDEMIOLOGY
- Worldwide infection

INFECTIONS
- Common cold and other upper respiratory tract infections, such as sinusitis
- Rare cause of pneumonia in children or adults

DIAGNOSIS
- Efforts for specific diagnosis of coronavirus are not warranted for patients with common cold in clinical practice.
- In research settings, a specific diagnosis may be made by detection of antigen and nucleic acid and direct visualization with electron microscopy.

TREATMENT
- Symptomatic

PREVENTION
- Avoid crowded places during winter months.

Corynebacterium diphtheriae

See Section II, "Diphtheria"

Corynebacterium jeikeium

GENUS Corynebacterium
SPECIES
- C. jeikeium

MICROBIOLOGIC CHARACTERISTICS
- Aerobic, gram-positive bacillus

EPIDEMIOLOGY
- Worldwide rare infection

INFECTIONS
- Infections due to *C. jeikeium* are mainly seen in immunosuppressed patients, especially those with neutropenia and advanced infection with HIV.
- Sepsis
- Endocarditis
- Central venous catheter–associated infections
- Pneumonia
- Meningitis

DIAGNOSIS
- Culture

TREATMENT
- Vancomycin

ALTERNATIVE TREATMENT
- Penicillin G in combination with an antipseudomonal aminoglycoside

Corynebacterium minutissimum

GENUS Corynebacterium
SPECIES
- C. minutissimum

MICROBIOLOGIC CHARACTERISTICS
- Aerobic, gram-positive bacillus

EPIDEMIOLOGY
- Common cause of skin infection

INFECTIONS
- Erythrasma
- A rare cause of endocarditis and sepsis, especially in neutropenic patients
- Subcutaneous tissue infections

DIAGNOSIS
- Culture
- Coral-red fluorescence with Wood's lamp in cases of erythrasma

TREATMENT
- Erythromycin 250 mg every 6 hours PO for 14 days
- Vancomycin for systemic infections due to *C. minutissimum*

ALTERNATIVE TREATMENT
- Local treatment with 2% aqueous clindamycin is also effective in patients with erythrasma.

Corynebacterium pseudotuberculosis

GENUS Corynebacterium
SPECIES
- C. pseudotuberculosis

MICROBIOLOGIC CHARACTERISTICS
- Aerobic, gram-positive bacillus

EPIDEMIOLOGY
- Rare cause of human infection, usually in persons exposed to animals

INFECTIONS
- Suppurative granulomatous lymphadenitis

DIAGNOSIS
- Culture in blood agar with 10% CO_2

TREATMENT
- Macrolide antibiotics

ALTERNATIVE TREATMENT
- Tetracycline or penicillin G

Microorganisms

Corynebacterium Species

GENUS Corynebacterium
SPECIES
- C. bovis
- C. pilosum
- C. pseudodiphtheriticum
- C. striatum
- C. xerosis
- Others

MICROBIOLOGIC CHARACTERISTICS
- Aerobic, gram-positive bacilli

EPIDEMIOLOGY
- Rare cause of infections

INFECTIONS
- Native or prosthetic valve endocarditis
- Rare cause of septicemia (seen more commonly in neutropenics)
- Pneumonia, tracheitis, other respiratory tract infections
- Infection of prosthetic materials

DIAGNOSIS
- Culture

TREATMENT
- Vancomycin (plus an aminoglycoside in cases of endocarditis)
- Removal of the prosthetic material is frequently necessary.

ALTERNATIVE TREATMENT
- Modification of the initially chosen empiric regimen may be needed, based on the progress of the infection and *in vitro* antimicrobial susceptibility testing.
- Penicillin G, tetracycline, a macrolide, rifampicin, first-generation cephalosporin, or teicoplanin

Corynebacterium urealyticum

GENUS Corynebacterium
SPECIES
- C. urealyticum

MICROBIOLOGIC CHARACTERISTICS
- Aerobic, gram-positive bacillus

INFECTIONS
- Rare cause of urinary tract infection
- It may cause chronic cystitis with deposits of phosphate ammonium magnesium crystals.
- Bacteremia has been reported rarely.

DIAGNOSIS
- Culture

TREATMENT
- Vancomycin

ALTERNATIVE TREATMENT
- Doxycycline

Coxiella burnetii

See Section II, "Q Fever"

Coxsackievirus

GROUP Enterovirus
TYPES
- There are several serotypes of coxsackievirus A and serotypes of coxsackievirus B.

MICROBIOLOGIC CHARACTERISTICS
- Single-stranded, positive RNA virus
- Icosahedral symmetry
- Naked

EPIDEMIOLOGY
- Worldwide, common cause of infections

INFECTIONS
- Common cause of several types of syndromes, which are manifested by enanthems and exanthems, including a herpetiform rash (mouth–hand–foot syndrome)
- Upper respiratory infection
- Herpangina
- Pleurodynia
- Myopericarditis
- Acute hemorrhagic conjunctivitis
- Disseminated infection in newborns
- Meningitis, encephalitis, and, rarely, paralytic syndromes
- Chronic meningoencephalitis in immunosuppressed persons, especially in patients with agammaglobulinemia

DIAGNOSIS
- Virologic culture
- Serology tests

TREATMENT
- Symptomatic

ALTERNATIVE TREATMENT
- There is no specific antiviral treatment.

PREVENTION
- Enteric isolation for 1 week
- Respiratory precautions in case of herpangina

Crimean–Congo Hemorrhagic Fever Virus

GROUP Nairovirus
MICROBIOLOGIC CHARACTERISTICS
- Crimean–Congo virus belongs to the *Nairovirus* genus, which belongs to the family Bunyaviridae
- Three segments of single-stranded, circular RNA
- Enveloped
- Helicoidal symmetry

EPIDEMIOLOGY
- The virus is transmitted to humans by ticks.
- Eastern Europe, Central Asia, the Balkans, the Middle East, and Africa

INFECTIONS
- Hemorrhagic fever (acute hepatitis with jaundice, disseminated intravascular coagulation, thrombocytopenia, bleeding)
- Other infections caused by other viruses of the Bunyaviridae family include California encephalitis, Rift Valley fever, hemorrhagic fever with renal syndrome, and hantavirus pulmonary syndrome.

DIAGNOSIS
- Cell culture
- Serology
- Antigen nucleic acid detection

TREATMENT
- Symptomatic
- High mortality (30%–40%) in cases of severe Crimean-Congo hemorrhagic fever

ALTERNATIVE TREATMENT
- There is no specific antiviral treatment.

PREVENTION
- Strict isolation of affected patients

Cryptococcus neoformans

See Section II, "Cryptococcal Infections"

Cryptosporidium parvum

See Section II, "Cryptosporidiosis"

Microorganisms

Cunninghamella bertholetiae

GENUS Cunninghamella
SPECIES
- C. bertholetiae

MICROBIOLOGIC CHARACTERISTICS
- Filamentous fungus (mold) with nonseptate hyaline hyphae

EPIDEMIOLOGY
- Worldwide, rare infection
- It affects more frequently immunosuppressed people and patients on hemodialysis.

INFECTIONS
- Zygomycosis (mucormycosis)

DIAGNOSIS
- Identification of the fungus in tissue biopsies
- Culture

TREATMENT
- Amphotericin B intravenously

ALTERNATIVE TREATMENT
- There are limited data for the efficacy of azoles (itraconazole).

Curvularia Species

GENUS Curvularia
SPECIES
- C. boedijn
- C. geniculata
- C. lunata
- C. pallescens
- C. senegalensis

MICROBIOLOGIC CHARACTERISTICS
- Dematiaceous, filamentous fungus (mold)
- Yeasts, pseudohypha, or septate pigmented hyphae *in vivo*

EPIDEMIOLOGY
- Rare cause of infection

INFECTIONS
- Keratitis
- Skin and subcutaneous tissue infection
- Rarely a cause of deep-tissue infection (e.g., pneumonia, endocarditis, osteomyelitis)

DIAGNOSIS
- Tissue biopsy
- Culture

TREATMENT
- Amphotericin B

ALTERNATIVE TREATMENT
- There are limited data for the efficacy of azoles.

Cyclospora cayatanensis

GENUS Cyclospora
SPECIES
- C. cayatanensis

MICROBIOLOGIC CHARACTERISTICS
- A protozoon
- Acid-fast organism
- Designated previously as coccidian-like body (CLB)

EPIDEMIOLOGY
- Found in Nepal, Caribbean, Peru, and in travelers coming from various regions (Turkey, Pakistan, Sri Lanka, India, Morocco, Mexico, Australia, Malaysia)
- Worldwide distribution
- Rare in the United States
- There are few reports from other countries but it is probably a pathogen affecting people worldwide.

INFECTIONS
- Prolonged, watery diarrhea; self-limited; with fluorescent microscopy

DIAGNOSIS
- Examination of concentrated stools, Kinyoun strain
- Fresh examination with fluorescent microscopy

TREATMENT
- Trimethoprim–sulfamethoxazole (160–800 mg q12h for 3–5 days)

Cytomegalovirus

See Section II, "Cytomegalovirus Infections"

Microorganisms

Dengue Virus

See Section II, "Dengue"

Dermatobia hominis

See "Myiasis Agents"

Dicrocoelium dendriticum

GENUS Dicrocoelium
SPECIES
- D. dendriticum

MICROBIOLOGIC CHARACTERISTICS
- A trematode helminth

EPIDEMIOLOGY
- Worldwide, rare infection

INFECTIONS
- Ova of *D. dendriticum* sometimes are seen in examination of human stool specimens. However, the parasite rarely causes a symptomatic infection.
- It occasionally causes biliary colic.

DIAGNOSIS
- Parasitology examination of stools

TREATMENT
- Praziquantel 25 mg/kg PO q8h (for three doses) for the exceptional patient with symptomatic *D. dendriticum* infection and absent other possible causes of symptoms

Dientamoeba fragilis

GENUS Dientamoeba
SPECIES
- D. fragilis

MICROBIOLOGIC CHARACTERISTICS
- Protozoon
- It should not be confused with *Entamoeba histolytica,* the cause of amebiasis.

EPIDEMIOLOGY
- Worldwide

INFECTIONS
- It leads usually to an asymptomatic infection.
- The organism sometimes causes abdominal pain and/or diarrhea.

DIAGNOSIS
- Direct stool examination and ferrous hematoxylin stain

TREATMENT
- Paromomycin 500 mg q8h for 7 days
- Iodoquinol 650 mg q8h for 20 days

ALTERNATIVE TREATMENT
- Tetracycline for 7 to 10 days
- Metronidazole for 7 days

Diphyllobothrium Species

GENUS Diphyllobothrium
SPECIES
- D. dalliae
- D. dendriticum
- D. latum
- D. pasificum
- D. ursi

MICROBIOLOGIC CHARACTERISTICS
- Cestode helminths

INCUBATION PERIOD
- Three to 6 weeks from ingestion to passage of eggs in the stool
- However, symptoms may appear months or years later (with continued infection).

EPIDEMIOLOGY
- The infection is acquired by humans by eating inadequately cooked or raw fish.
- The infection is not transmitted directly from person to person. A cycle of transmission including a first and a second intermediate host is necessary for the development of the worm.
- The first intermediate host is copepods of the genera *Cyclops* and *Diaptomus*.
- Freshwater fish (salmon, perch, pike, turbots) ingest infected copepods and become the second intermediate host.
- Humans and fish-eating mammals can then become infected by eating infected fish.
- Infection by *Diphyllobothrium* species occurs mainly in lake regions, where eating undercooked or raw fish is common. Eskimos in Alaska and Canada are more likely to be infected than are other populations, due to food preparation practices which increase the probability of infection with *Diphyllobothrium* species.

INFECTIONS
- Infection by *Diphyllobothrium* species is usually asymptomatic.
- The parasite occasionally causes diarrhea and/or abdominal discomfort (in massive infection).
- Obstruction of the bile duct or the bowel may be rarely seen.
- A small minority of infected patients develop vitamin B12 deficiency.

DIAGNOSIS
- Macroscopic stool examination (for proglottids) and examination of concentrated stools (for eggs)

TREATMENT
- Praziquantel 10 to 20 mg/kg in a single dose

ALTERNATIVE TREATMENT
- Niclosamide 2 g in a single dose
- Niclosamide tablets should be chewed completely before swallowing.

PREVENTION
- Avoid eating undercooked or raw fish.

Microorganisms

Dipylidium caninum

GENUS Dipylidium

SPECIES
- D. caninum

MICROBIOLOGIC CHARACTERISTICS
- Cestode (tapeworm) helminth

EPIDEMIOLOGY
- Adult *D. caninum* worms are found in dogs and cats worldwide.
- Children (usually toddler-aged) occasionally become infected with the parasite.

INFECTIONS
- Infected humans are usually asymptomatic.
- Humans may have seedlike proglottids in the stool or the anal area.
- The parasite may occasionally cause gastrointestinal symptoms such as abdominal discomfort in cases of massive infection.

DIAGNOSIS
- Stool examination for proglottids or eggs

TREATMENT
- Praziquantel 10 to 20 mg/kg in a single dose

ALTERNATIVE TREATMENT
- Niclosamide 2 g in a single dose

Dirofilaria Species

GENUS Dirofilaria

SPECIES
- D. immitis
- D. repens
- D. tenuis
- D. ursi

MICROBIOLOGIC CHARACTERISTICS
- A nematode helminth

EPIDEMIOLOGY
- *D. immitis* is the dog heartworm (few reported cases of human disease worldwide).
- *D. tenuis*, a raccoon parasite in the United States
- *D. repens*, a parasite of dogs and cats (Europe)
- *D. ursi*, a parasite of bears in Canada

INFECTIONS
- *D. immitis* may cause pulmonary or cutaneous disease in humans.
- Other Dirofilaria species occasionally may cause cutaneous manifestation in humans.
- Microfilaremia is rare in humans.

DIAGNOSIS
- By the finding of worms in tissue biopsies of excised lesions

TREATMENT
- Surgical removal of the affected areas

Dracunculus medinensis

GENUS Dracunculus

SPECIES
- D. medinensis

MICROBIOLOGIC CHARACTERISTICS
- A nematode helminth

INCUBATION PERIOD
- About a year

EPIDEMIOLOGY
- Infection due to *D. medinensis* is seen in sub-Saharan African countries, the Middle East, and Asia.
- Humans become infected by drinking water from infected step wells and ponds.

INFECTIONS
- Guinea worm (skin vesicle and a subsequent ulcer where the worm emerges)
- Secondary infections due to bacteria are common in skin lesions due to the Guinea worm.

DIAGNOSIS
- Identification of worms in skin lesions (adult worms may protrude from skin lesions)
- Microscopic identification of skin lesions may reveal the presence of larvae of the parasite.

TREATMENT
- Extraction of the worm

ALTERNATIVE TREATMENT
- Thiabendazole 50 mg/kg/d orally (in two doses) for 2 days, or metronidazole 10 mg/kg (divided in three doses) for 1 week to reduce the inflammation of the skin lesions (although the drugs have no effect on the worm)

PREVENTION
- Patients with skin lesions should not enter any source of drinking water.
- Drink potable, safe water.
- Immunization against tetanus reduces the risk of tetanus associated with secondary infection of Guinea worm skin lesions.

Ebola–Marburg Viral Diseases

GROUP Filovirus

SPECIES
- Ebola virus
- Marburg virus

MICROBIOLOGIC CHARACTERISTICS
- Single-stranded, RNA virus
- Helicoidal symmetry
- Enveloped

INCUBATION PERIOD
- Two days to 3 weeks for Ebola virus
- Three to 9 days for Marburg virus

EPIDEMIOLOGY
- Fortunately, a rare cause of infections
- Ebola virus outbreaks occurred in Africa.
- Marburg virus cases were reported, rarely, from Africa and Europe.

INFECTIONS
- These viruses cause severe illnesses with high case fatality rates (specifically, 50%–90% for Ebola virus and 30% for Marburg virus).
- Sudden onset of illness manifested by high fever, myalgia, headache, vomiting, diarrhea, pharyngitis, and maculopapular rash

DIAGNOSIS
- Cell culture
- Serology tests

TREATMENT
- Symptomatic

ALTERNATIVE TREATMENT
- There is no specific antiviral treatment.

PREVENTION
- Strict isolation of patients
- No sexual intercourse for 3 months (or until semen is shown to be free of virus)

Echinococcus Species

See Section II, "Echinococcosis"

Microorganisms

Echinostoma ilocanum

GENUS Echinostoma
SPECIES
- E. ilocanum

MICROBIOLOGIC CHARACTERISTICS
- A trematode helminth

EPIDEMIOLOGY
- Philippines, Indonesia, Malaysia, and China

INFECTIONS
- A rare cause of small-bowel infection

DIAGNOSIS
- Examination of concentrated stools (parasitologic examination)

TREATMENT
- Praziquantel 25 mg/kg PO q8h for 2 days

Echovirus

GROUP Enterovirus
MICROBIOLOGIC CHARACTERISTICS
- Single-stranded, RNA viruses
- Icosahedral symmetry
- Naked

INCUBATION PERIOD
- Usually a few days (depends on the syndrome caused by the virus)

EPIDEMIOLOGY
- The virus is isolated from stool specimens for a week in cases of gastroenteritis.

INFECTIONS
- Common cause of human infection manifested by different syndromes
- Exanthems and enanthems
- Upper respiratory infection
- Herpangina
- Pleurodynia
- Myopericarditis
- Disseminated infection in the newborn
- Chronic meningoencephalitis in immunosuppressed individuals, particularly those with agammaglobulinemia
- Meningitis and encephalitis, rarely paralysis

DIAGNOSIS
- Cell culture
- Serology tests

TREATMENT
- Symptomatic

ALTERNATIVE TREATMENT
- There is no specific antiviral treatment.

PREVENTION
- Enteric isolation for 7 days decreases the possibility of transmission of the virus to other people.

Edwardsiella tarda

GENUS Edwardsiella
SPECIES
- E. tarda

MICROBIOLOGIC CHARACTERISTICS
- Aerobic, gram-negative bacillus

EPIDEMIOLOGY
- Worldwide, rare infection
- Part of the normal bowel flora of animals and snakes

INFECTIONS
- Gastroenteritis
- Bacteremia

DIAGNOSIS
- Culture

TREATMENT
- Fluoroquinolone (intravenous treatment with a quinolone is needed for patients with bacteremia due to this pathogen)

ALTERNATIVE TREATMENT
- Ampicillin, aminoglycosides, or a cephalosporin

Ehrlichia Species

See Section II, "Ehrlichiosis"

Eikenella corrodens

GENUS Eikenella
SPECIES
- E. corrodens

MICROBIOLOGIC CHARACTERISTICS
- Microaerophilic, gram-negative bacillus
- Belongs to the HACEK group

EPIDEMIOLOGY
- Worldwide, rare infection

INFECTIONS
- Part of the normal oral flora
- Human bite-wound infection
- Skin infection in intravenous drug users
- Internal jugular vein thrombophlebitis
- Endocarditis
- Lung infection (pneumonia, abscess, empyema), usually polymicrobial in origin

DIAGNOSIS
- Culture

TREATMENT
- Penicillin G or amoxicillin–clavulanate

ALTERNATIVE TREATMENT
- Doxycycline, aminoglycoside, or a second- or third-generation cephalosporin
- Resistant to metronidazole, oxacillin, first-generation cephalosporins, and clindamycin
- These antibiotics should not be used empirically to treat human-bite wound infections.
- Some strains produce β-lactamases.

Microorganisms

Emmonsia parva

GENUS Emmonsia
SPECIES
- E. parva

MICROBIOLOGIC CHARACTERISTICS
- Filamentous fungus (mold)

EPIDEMIOLOGY
- Worldwide, rare infection

INFECTIONS
- Rare cases of osteomyelitis, prosthetic valve endocarditis, rhinitis, sinusitis with extension to the CNS, pneumonia, or dissemination in immunocompromised patients have been reported.

DIAGNOSIS
- Culture
- Identification of the fungus in tissue biopsies

TREATMENT
- Amphotericin B i.v.

ALTERNATIVE TREATMENT
- Surgical intervention is also helpful in most cases (removal of lesions).

Encephalitis Viruses of the Flaviviridae Family

GROUP Flavivirus
STRAINS
- Arthropod-borne viral encephalitides are classified in two categories: arboviral encephalitides and tick-borne arboviral encephalitides.
- Mosquito-borne arboviral encephalitides are caused by a specific virus in one of the following three groups: Togaviridae/Alphaviridae (Eastern equine encephalitis virus and Western equine encephalitis virus), Bunyaviridae (LaCrosse virus, California encephalitis virus, Jamestown Canyon virus, and Snowshoe hare virus), and Flaviviridae (Japanese encephalitis virus, Kunjin virus, Murray Valley encephalitis virus, St. Louis encephalitis virus, and Rocio encephalitis virus).

MICROBIOLOGIC CHARACTERISTICS
- Single-stranded, positive RNA virus
- Spheric
- Enveloped

INCUBATION PERIOD
- Five to 15 days

EPIDEMIOLOGY
- Rare cause of infection

INFECTIONS
- Epidemic outbreaks of encephalitis

DIAGNOSIS
- Cell culture
- Serology tests are helpful.

TREATMENT
- Symptomatic

ALTERNATIVE TREATMENT
- There is no specific antiviral treatment.

PREVENTION
- Avoid mosquito bites.
- Japanese encephalitis virus vaccine (inactivated) is recommended for travelers who will stay for a long time (more than 2 months) in rural areas with endemicity of the virus.

Endolimax nana

GENUS Endolimax
SPECIES
- E. nana

MICROBIOLOGIC CHARACTERISTICS
- Protozoon

EPIDEMIOLOGY
- Worldwide

INFECTIONS
- E. nana is thought to be nonpathogenic.

DIAGNOSIS
- Examination of concentrated stools

TREATMENT
- Not required because of the commensal-type nature of the parasite

Entamoeba histolytica

See Section II, "Amebiasis"

Entamoeba Species

GENUS Entamoeba
SPECIES
- E. coli
- E. hartmanni
- E. polecki

MICROBIOLOGIC CHARACTERISTICS
- Protozoon, which should not be confused with *Entamoeba histolytica*, the cause of amebiasis

EPIDEMIOLOGY
- Worldwide

INFECTIONS
- These protozoa do not appear to cause symptoms.
- Some experts support that these protozoa may rarely cause diarrhea.

DIAGNOSIS
- Parasitologic examination of stool specimens

TREATMENT
- No treatment is usually required.

ALTERNATIVE TREATMENT
- Metronidazole 500 mg q8h for 6 days or tinidazole 1 g q12h for 3 days may be given to the occasional patient with *Entamoeba* parasites and a syndrome of diarrhea with no other clear cause.

Microorganisms

Enterobacter Species

GENUS Enterobacter

SPECIES
- E. aerogenes
- E. cloacae
- E. sakazakii
- E. tayorae
- Others

MICROBIOLOGIC CHARACTERISTICS
- Aerobic, gram-negative bacillus

INCUBATION PERIOD
- Unknown

EPIDEMIOLOGY
- Part of the normal enteric flora
- Infections due to *Enterobacter* species are caused by strains that have already colonized the patient's bowel flora.
- However, there are also documented reports of nosocomial outbreaks of *Enterobacter* infections, showing that human-to-human transmission or common source (e.g., contaminated intravenous solutions) infections also occur.

INFECTIONS
- Generally, nosocomial infections
- Urinary and pulmonary infections
- Bacteremia associated with catheters
- Contamination of intravenous infusion
- Surgical wound infection
- Neonatal meningitis

DIAGNOSIS
- Culture of the pathogen

TREATMENT
- Carbapenem (imipenem, meropenem)
- Piperacillin-tazobactam
- Fluoroquinolone

ALTERNATIVE TREATMENT
- A third-generation cephalosporin
- Aztreonam
- Aminoglycoside

Enterobius vermicularis

GENUS Enterobius

SPECIES
- E. vermicularis

MICROBIOLOGIC CHARACTERISTICS
- An intestinal nematode (pinworm infection)

INCUBATION PERIOD
- The life cycle of *E. vermicularis* is 2 to 6 weeks. However, successive reinfections with the parasite are usually needed to cause symptoms.

EPIDEMIOLOGY
- Worldwide

INFECTIONS
- Enterobiasis (pinworm infection, oxyuriasis)

DIAGNOSIS
- Macroscopic examination of the stools
- Finding characteristic eggs on adhesive tape preparations taken from the perianal skin

TREATMENT
- Pyrantel pamoate 11 mg/kg in a single dose (maximum, 1 g)
- Treatment should be repeated after 2 weeks.
- Treatment of the whole family should be considered, especially if more than one family member is infected with the parasite.

ALTERNATIVE TREATMENT
- Mebendazole 100 mg PO q12h for 3 days
- Albendazole 400 mg in a single dose

PREVENTION
- Good personal hygiene practices

Enterococcus Species

GENUS Enterococcus

SPECIES
- E. avium
- E. casseliflavus
- E. durans
- E. faecalis
- E. faecium
- E. gallinarum
- E. hirae
- Others

MICROBIOLOGIC CHARACTERISTICS
- Aerobic, gram-positive coccus

INCUBATION PERIOD
- Usually, infection follows a prolonged period of colonization with *Enterococcus*.

EPIDEMIOLOGY
- Infections due to *Enterococcus* species have become more frequent the last 2 decades.
- *Enterococcus* isolates are the second most common cause of bacteremia after *Staphylococcus* species in many hospitals.

INFECTIONS
- Bacteremia (polymicrobial in some cases)
- Urinary tract infection
- Acute or subacute endocarditis
- Neonatal, intraabdominal, or pelvic infection
- Meningitis
- Pneumonia
- Skin and soft-tissue infections

DIAGNOSIS
- Culture of the pathogen

TREATMENT
- *E. faecalis:* amoxicillin, ampicillin or penicillin G
- In endocarditis or other serious infections, ampicillin 12 g or penicillin 20 to 30 million units/d with gentamicin (if the MIC is <2,000 μg/mL for gentamicin)
- Endocarditis requires 6 weeks of therapy.
- *E. faecium:* teicoplanin or vancomycin combined with gentamicin (if the MIC is <2,000 μg/mL)

ALTERNATIVE TREATMENT
- Imipenem, vancomycin, teicoplanin, or the combination of amoxicillin–clavulanate, ampicillin–sulbactam, or piperacillin–tazobactam
- For cystitis: Ciprofloxacin, trimethoprim-sulfamethoxazole, and nitrofurantoin are frequently active.

Enterocytozoon bieneusi

See "Microsporidia"

Microorganisms

Enterovirus

GROUP Enterovirus

SUBGROUPS
- Enteroviruses and rhinoviruses are the two groups of viruses in the family Picornaviridae that cause disease in humans.
- The group of enteroviruses includes polioviruses (serotypes 1–3), coxsackievirus A and B (several serotypes), enterovirus serotypes 68 to 71, and hepatitis A virus (enterovirus 72).

MICROBIOLOGIC CHARACTERISTICS
- Single-stranded, RNA viruses

INCUBATION PERIOD
- For acute hemorrhagic conjunctivitis, 12 to 72 hours

EPIDEMIOLOGY
- Worldwide, common infections

INFECTIONS
- Acute hemorrhagic conjunctivitis (serotype 70)
- Meningoencephalitis, skin rash, and a syndrome similar to poliomyelitis (serotype 71)

DIAGNOSIS
- Cell culture
- Serology may be helpful.

TREATMENT
- Symptomatic treatment

ALTERNATIVE TREATMENT
- There is no effective, specific antiviral treatment.

PREVENTION
- No sharing of towels (to avoid transmission of enterovirus); it may cause acute hemorrhagic conjunctivitis

Epidermophyton floccosum

GENUS Epidermophyton

SPECIES
- E. floccosum

MICROBIOLOGIC CHARACTERISTICS
- Filamentous fungus (mold) with septated hyaline hyphae

EPIDEMIOLOGY
- Common cause of infection worldwide

INFECTIONS
- Infection of skin (dermatomycosis, tinea)
- All types of tinea (cruris, corporis, pedis, inguinal), except capitis

DIAGNOSIS
- Finding the fungus in clinical samples
- Growth in culture

TREATMENT
- Extensive or inflammatory manifestations: itraconazole 200 mg/d for 2 to 4 weeks
- Localized, noninflammatory manifestations: cyclopyroxolomine (one application q12h)

ALTERNATIVE TREATMENT
- Onychomycosis: itraconazole 200 mg/d for 3 to 6 months

Epstein-Barr Virus

See Section II, "Infectious Mononucleosis"

Erysipelothrix rhusiopathiae

GENUS Erysipelothrix

SPECIES
- E. rhusiopathiae

MICROBIOLOGIC CHARACTERISTICS
- Aerobic, gram-positive bacillus

INCUBATION PERIOD
- Unknown

EPIDEMIOLOGY
- Rare cause of infection (worldwide)

INFECTIONS
- Skin infection (erysipeloid)
- It may also cause a diffuse cutaneous eruption accompanied by systemic symptoms (fever, myalgias, arthralgias).
- Occasionally, systemic infection with endocarditis or bacteremia
- Associated with handling fish, crustaceans, animals, or soil

DIAGNOSIS
- Culture

TREATMENT
- Penicillin G for 10 days

ALTERNATIVE TREATMENT
- Cephalosporin, clindamycin, ciprofloxacin, or carbapenem (imipenem, meropenem)

Escherichia coli

See Section II, "Escherichia coli Infections"

Eubacterium Species

GENUS Eubacterium

SPECIES
- E. lentum
- E. nodatum
- E. timidum
- others

MICROBIOLOGIC CHARACTERISTICS
- Anaerobic, pleomorphic, gram-positive bacillus

EPIDEMIOLOGY
- Eubacterium species are part of the normal human flora.
- Subsequently, culture of the organism does not necessarily mean infection due to this organism.

INFECTIONS
- Abscesses and other infections at various sites (almost always mixed infections)
- Periodontal disease
- Septic arthritis in patients with colonic lesions (E. lentum)
- Endometritis in women who wear an IUD (E. nodatum)

DIAGNOSIS
- Culture in anaerobic media

TREATMENT
- Penicillin G or a cephamycin
- Metronidazole

ALTERNATIVE TREATMENT
- Imipenem, meropenem, clindamycin, or a ureidopenicillin

Microorganisms

Ewingella americana

GENUS Ewingella
SPECIES
- E. americana

MICROBIOLOGIC CHARACTERISTICS
- Aerobic, gram-negative bacillus
- Belongs to the Enterobacteriaceae group

EPIDEMIOLOGY
- Rarely grown in cultures
- Its clinical significance is unclear.

INFECTIONS
- Bacteremia, wound infection in immunocompromised patients

DIAGNOSIS
- Culture

TREATMENT
- There are no data for the efficacy of antimicrobial agents against E. americana.
- Agents that are usually active against other Enterobacteriaceae (such as quinolones, aminoglycosides, cephalosporins) are likely to be active against this organism.

Exophiala Species

GENUS Exophiala
SPECIES
- E. dermatitidis
- E. jeanselmei
- E. moniliae
- E. pisciphila
- E. spinifera

MICROBIOLOGIC CHARACTERISTICS
- Dematiaceous, filamentous fungus (mold)
- Yeasts, pseudohypha, and septate pigmented hyphae *in vivo*

EPIDEMIOLOGY
- Worldwide

INFECTIONS
- Rare cause of infection
- Occasional cases of corneal, subcutaneous, and systemic infection (prosthetic valve endocarditis, arthritis, brain abscess, pneumonia) due to *Exophiala* species have been reported.

DIAGNOSIS
- Culture of the fungus
- Histopathology

TREATMENT
- Amphotericin B, with or without flucytosine

ALTERNATIVE TREATMENT
- Itraconazole

Fasciola Species

GENUS Fasciola
SPECIES
- F. gigantica
- F. hepatica

MICROBIOLOGIC CHARACTERISTICS
- A trematode helminth (about 3 cm long)

EPIDEMIOLOGY
- Worldwide, rare infection
- Humans are an accidental host.
- Natural parasite of sheep, cattle, and other animal worldwide
- Human disease has been reported in sheep- and/or cattle-raising areas.

INFECTIONS
- The parasites cause fascioliasis, a liver and biliary tree disease.
- Infection outside the liver and the biliary tree may be seen rarely, especially with *F. gigantica*.

DIAGNOSIS
- Similar to *Clonorchis sinensis*
- Serology

TREATMENT
- There is no satisfactory antiparasitic drug for this infection.
- Bithionol 30 to 50 mg/kg on alternate days for 10 to 14 doses has moderate results.

ALTERNATIVE TREATMENT
- Praziquantel

Fasciolopsis buski

GENUS Fasciolopsis
SPECIES
- F. buski

MICROBIOLOGIC CHARACTERISTICS
- A large (7 cm long) trematode helminth

EPIDEMIOLOGY
- Rural Southeast Asia and India

INFECTIONS
- *F. buski* causes fasciolopsiasis, a disease manifested by gastrointestinal symptoms such as diarrhea, constipation, vomiting, and anorexia. In rare cases, acute intestinal obstruction is caused by the parasites.

DIAGNOSIS
- Parasitologic stool examination

TREATMENT
- Praziquantel 25 mg/kg PO q8h for 1 day

ALTERNATIVE TREATMENT
- Niclosamide 2 g in a single dose

Microorganisms

Flavimonas oryzihabitans

GENUS Flavimonas
SPECIES
- F. oryzihabitans

MICROBIOLOGIC CHARACTERISTICS
- Aerobic, gram-negative bacillus

EPIDEMIOLOGY
- Rare cause of infection

INFECTIONS
- Bacteremia, frequently polymicrobial and associated with intravascular lines
- Peritonitis in patients undergoing peritoneal dialysis
- Central nervous system shunt infection
- Prosthetic joint infection
- Prosthetic valve endocarditis
- Meningitis
- Wound infection

DIAGNOSIS
- Culture

TREATMENT
- An antipseudomonal β-lactam
- A carbapenem (imipenem, meropenem)

ALTERNATIVE TREATMENT
- Ciprofloxacin, aminoglycoside

Flavobacterium Species

GENUS Flavobacterium
SPECIES
- F. indologenes
- F. meningosepticum
- F. odoratum
- Others

MICROBIOLOGIC CHARACTERISTICS
- Aerobic, gram-negative bacillus
- The taxonomy of these bacteria has not been settled.

INFECTIONS
- Meningitis and bacteremia (F. meningosepticum, especially in newborns)
- Endocarditis, particularly on prosthetic valve
- Few reports of nosocomial outbreaks of bacteremia due to *Flavobacterium* associated with contaminated solutions
- Wound infection

DIAGNOSIS
- Culture

TREATMENT
- Ciprofloxacin

ALTERNATIVE TREATMENT
- There are reports of successful use of vancomycin to treat meningitis due to *Flavobacterium* in neonates. This is interesting, because *Flavobacterium* is the only gram-negative organism for which vancomycin seems to be effective.

Fonsecaea Species

See "Chromomycosis Agents"

Francisella tularensis

See Section II, "Tularemia"

Fusarium Species

GENUS Fusarium
SPECIES
- F. moniliforme
- F. oxysporum
- F. solani
- Others

MICROBIOLOGIC CHARACTERISTICS
- Filamentous fungus (mold), with septate hyphae

EPIDEMIOLOGY
- Worldwide infection

INFECTIONS
- Localized infection of skin and subcutaneous tissue
- Keratitis
- Endophthalmitis
- Osteomyelitis and arthritis following trauma or surgery
- Peritonitis in peritoneal dialysis
- Disseminated infections (similar to disseminated aspergillosis, but with higher incidence of cutaneous lesions and fungemia)
- Catheter-associated infections in neutropenic patients and in patients with major burns

DIAGNOSIS
- Identification of the fungus in tissue biopsies
- Culture of the fungus

TREATMENT
- There are limited data for the efficacy of antifungal agents in patients with *Fusarium* infections.
- Amphotericin B i.v. (1.0-1.5 mg/kg/d), with or without flucytosine

ALTERNATIVE TREATMENT
- Surgical removal of operable lesions may be necessary in difficult-to-manage patients with *Fusarium* infections when using only antifungal agents.

Fusobacterium Species

GENUS Fusobacterium
SPECIES
- F. alocis
- F. mortiferum
- F. necrophorum
- F. nucleatum
- F. periodonticum
- F. sulci
- F. ulcerans
- F. varium
- Others

MICROBIOLOGIC CHARACTERISTICS
- Anaerobic, gram-negative bacilli

INCUBATION PERIOD
- Infections are usually endogenous (i.e., from the patient's microbial flora)

EPIDEMIOLOGY
- *Fusobacterium* species are found frequently as part of the normal human oral and bowel flora.

INFECTIONS
- Cervicofacial, pleuropulmonary, abdominal, or pelvis infection (abscesses, usually polymicrobial)
- Soft-tissue infections
- Wound infections (surgical or bite wound)
- Postangina sepsis
- Jugular vein thrombophlebitis and abscesses in the lungs, bones, and CNS
- Endocarditis

DIAGNOSIS
- Anaerobic culture

TREATMENT
- Metronidazole
- Penicillin G

ALTERNATIVE TREATMENT
- Clindamycin
- Cefotetan or cefoxitin
- Carbapenem (imipenem, meropenem)
- Chloramphenicol

Microorganisms

Gardnerella vaginalis

GENUS Gardnerella
SPECIES
- G. vaginalis

MICROBIOLOGIC CHARACTERISTICS
- Aerobic, gram-negative bacillus

EPIDEMIOLOGY
- Worldwide

INFECTIONS
- G. vaginalis has been implicated in the pathogenesis of bacterial vaginosis.
- Postpartum endometritis
- Urinary infection in pregnant women
- Bacteremia

DIAGNOSIS
- Culture in specific media
- Clue cells on vaginal smears are diagnostic of bacterial vaginosis.

TREATMENT
- Metronidazole is highly effective for the treatment of vaginosis, although G. vaginalis is relatively resistant in vitro.
- Metronidazole or clindamycin as a topical application

ALTERNATIVE TREATMENT
- Amoxicillin-clavulanate
- Clindamycin
- In systemic or urinary infection, ampicillin or amoxicillin should be used.

Gemella Species

GENUS Gemella
SPECIES
- G. haemolysans
- G. morbillorum

MICROBIOLOGIC CHARACTERISTICS
- Gram-positive coccus
- Gemella strains are sometimes confused with viridans streptococci.

EPIDEMIOLOGY
- Worldwide, rare cause of infection

INFECTIONS
- Endocarditis
- Bacteremia
- Gemella strains have been also isolated, rarely, from patients with pneumonia, urinary tract infection, wound infection, abscesses, total knee arthroplasty–related infection, and arteriovenous shunt infection.

DIAGNOSIS
- Culture

TREATMENT
- Penicillin G

ALTERNATIVE TREATMENT
- Vancomycin
- Macrolide

Geotrichum candidum

GENUS Geotrichum
SPECIES
- G. candidum

MICROBIOLOGIC CHARACTERISTICS
- Filamentous fungus (mold), with septate hyphae
- *In vivo*, septate hyaline hyphae with arthroconidia

EPIDEMIOLOGY
- Rare, worldwide infection

INFECTIONS
- Disseminated disease in neutropenics

DIAGNOSIS
- Finding the fungus in tissue biopsies
- Culture of the fungus

TREATMENT
- There are few data about the efficacy of antifungal agents against this fungus.
- Amphotericin B (intravenously) has been used with moderate results.

Giardia lamblia

See Section II, "Giardiasis"

Gnathostoma spinigerum

GENUS Gnathostoma
SPECIES
- G. spinigerum

MICROBIOLOGIC CHARACTERISTICS
- Most reported cases are from Thailand.
- A nematode helminth of dogs and cats

EPIDEMIOLOGY
- Japan, China, and other Southeast Asian countries
- People and animals are infected with ingestion of undercooked fish or poultry.

INFECTIONS
- The parasites migrate through several tissues of humans or animals, causing gnathostomiasis (transient pruritic, erythematous edema with eosinophilia).
- The brain may be affected, too (focal cerebral lesions and eosinophilic pleocytosis of the cerebrospinal fluid are common in patients with gnathostomiasis).

DIAGNOSIS
- Extraction and identification of the parasite

TREATMENT
- The effectiveness of antihelminthic agents is unclear. However, they are commonly used.
- Albendazole 400 mg q12h for 14 days may be given.

ALTERNATIVE TREATMENT
- Successful treatment of ocular lesions has been reported with mebendazole 200 mg q3h for 6 days.

Microorganisms

Haemophilus ducreyi

GENUS Haemophilus
SPECIES
- H. ducreyi

MICROBIOLOGIC CHARACTERISTICS
- Aerobic, gram-negative coccobacillus

INCUBATION PERIOD
- Usually 3 to 5 days (sometimes up to 2 weeks)

EPIDEMIOLOGY
- More common in tropical and subtropical climates
- Outbreaks of infections due to H. ducreyi have occurred in the United States, mainly in inner-city residents and migrant farm workers.
- Men are more likely to develop this infection.

INFECTIONS
- Chancroid (genital ulcer with inguinal adenopathy)

DIAGNOSIS
- Culture in special medium

TREATMENT
- Ceftriaxone 250 mg i.m. (single dose)
- Azithromycin 1 g (single dose)
- Ciprofloxacin 500 mg PO q12h for 3 days

ALTERNATIVE TREATMENT
- Erythromycin 0.5 g PO q6h for 7 days
- Trimethoprim–sulfamethoxazole (320 and 1,600 mg/d, respectively), for 7 days
- Ofloxacin
- Inguinal adenopathy that is fluctuant and larger than 5 cm in diameter should be drained by needle aspiration.

PREVENTION
- Safe-sex practices

Haemophilus influenzae

GENUS Haemophilus
SPECIES
- H. influenzae

MICROBIOLOGIC CHARACTERISTICS
- Aerobic, gram-negative coccobacillus

INCUBATION PERIOD
- The incubation period for meningitis due to H. influenzae is unknown; however, most data support an incubation period of 2 to 4 days.

EPIDEMIOLOGY
- Worldwide
- Vaccination programs against H. influenzae have led to a dramatic decrease of infections due to this pathogen.

INFECTIONS
- In children, epiglottitis, meningitis, cellulitis, and arthritis are caused by encapsulated strains (serotype b) and are often associated with bacteremia.
- Nonencapsulated strains cause otitis, sinusitis, exacerbations of chronic bronchitis, pneumonia, and, less often, bacteremia; it is seen more frequently in adults.
- In splenectomized patients, it may cause a severe sepsis with a fulminant course.
- Epididymitis
- Orchitis

DIAGNOSIS
- Antigen detection techniques (coagglutination, CIE, latex) in secretions or body fluids

TREATMENT
- Amoxicillin–clavulanate or a second- or third-generation cephalosporin

ALTERNATIVE TREATMENT
- Trimethoprim–sulfamethoxazole, fluoroquinolones, azithromycin, aztreonam, or carbapenem (imipenem or meropenem)

PREVENTION
- There are several protein–polysaccharide vaccines against H. influenzae type B that have been proved effective in children older than 2 months.
- Rifampin and ciprofloxacin have been used as protective measures for close household contacts of patients with H. influenza meningitis.

Haemophilus Species

GENUS Haemophilus
SPECIES
- H. aegyptius
- H. aphrophilus
- H. haemolyticus
- H. parahaemolyticus
- H. parainfluenzae
- H. paraphrophilus
- H. segnis

MICROBIOLOGIC CHARACTERISTICS
- Aerobic, gram-negative coccobacilli

EPIDEMIOLOGY
- Worldwide infections

INFECTIONS
- Bacteremia
- Upper respiratory infection
- Epiglottitis
- Pneumonia exacerbation of chronic bronchitis
- Soft-tissue infection
- Endocarditis
- Meningitis
- Brain abscess
- Urinary tract infection
- Conjunctivitis, sepsis with purpuric manifestations (H. aegyptius)

DIAGNOSIS
- Culture

TREATMENT
- Ampicillin (combined with an aminoglycoside in case of endocarditis or sepsis)

ALTERNATIVE TREATMENT
- Third-generation cephalosporin or carbapenem (imipenem or meropenem)

Hafnia alvei

GENUS Hafnia
SPECIES
- H. alvei

MICROBIOLOGIC CHARACTERISTICS
- Aerobic, gram-negative bacillus

INCUBATION PERIOD
- Usually an endogenous infection (H. alvei may be a part of the normal human bowel flora)
- In cases of infection associated with contaminated intravenous fluids, symptoms usually start within 1 to 2 days.

EPIDEMIOLOGY
- The incidence of infections due to H. alvei has increased during the past two decades (usually nosocomial infections).

INFECTIONS
- Generally nosocomial infections
- Urinary tract infections
- Pneumonia
- Bacteremia associated with intravenous catheters

DIAGNOSIS
- Culture

TREATMENT
- Third-generation cephalosporin
- Aztreonam
- The combination of β-lactam agent (with antipseudomonal action) with an aminoglycoside is frequently done in severe infections due to gram-negative bacilli, including H. alvei.

ALTERNATIVE TREATMENT
- Carbapenem (imipenem or meropenem)
- Ureidopenicillins
- Ciprofloxacin
- Aminoglycoside

Microorganisms

Hansenula Species

GENUS Hansenula
SPECIES
- H. anomala
- H. polymorpha

MICROBIOLOGIC CHARACTERISTICS
- Yeast

EPIDEMIOLOGY
- Culture
- Identification of the fungus in clinical biopsy specimens

INFECTIONS
- Fungemia
- Endocarditis
- Meningitis
- Mediastinal lymphadenitis (usually in immunocompromised patients)

DIAGNOSIS
- Rare infection

TREATMENT
- Amphotericin B i.v., with or without flucytosine

Hantaan Virus

GROUP Hantavirus
SPECIES
- Several (see below)

MICROBIOLOGIC CHARACTERISTICS
- Three circular segments of single-stranded, negative RNA virus
- Helicoidal symmetry
- Enveloped

EPIDEMIOLOGY
- Rare viral infections

INFECTIONS
- Sin nombre virus, Muerto Canyon virus (in southwestern United States)
- Fever and pulmonary disease with respiratory failure
- May be associated with hemorrhagic manifestations and renal failure
- In Far East, epidemic hemorrhagic fever, hemorrhagic fever with renal syndrome
- The genus *Hantavirus* includes several species (Seoul, Belgrade, Puumala, Prospect Hill) that are the agents of less severe hemorrhagic fever with renal syndrome.

DIAGNOSIS
- Cell culture serology

TREATMENT
- Ribavirin, 33 mg/kg i.v. initially, followed by 16 mg/kg for 4 days, followed by 8 mg/kg q8h for 6 more days, has been used in China.
- This regimen has been disappointing in early trials in the United States.

PREVENTION
- Strict isolation during the entire illness

Helicobacter Species

See Section II, "*Helicobacter pylori* Infection"

Hendersonula toruloidea

GENUS Hendersonula
SPECIES
- H. toruloidea

MICROBIOLOGIC CHARACTERISTICS
- Filamentous fungus (mold) with septate hyphae

INCUBATION PERIOD
- Unknown

EPIDEMIOLOGY
- Worldwide

INFECTIONS
- Similar to tinea (dermatomycosis), affecting the hands, feet, and nails
- Traumatic wound infections
- Sinusitis in diabetics

DIAGNOSIS
- Finding of the fungus in specimens of affected tissue
- Culture of the fungus

TREATMENT
- There are limited reported data for the optimal treatment of this fungal infection.
- Surgical removal of the affected nail may be necessary to eradicate the infection in cases of onychomycosis.
- Amphotericin B should be given in cases of severe, invasive disease.

Hepatitis Viruses

See Section II, "Hepatitis"

Herpes Simplex Virus Type 1 and 2

See Section II, "Herpes Simplex Virus Infections"

Human Herpesvirus Type 6

GROUP Herpesvirus
SPECIES
- N/A

MICROBIOLOGIC CHARACTERISTICS
- Double-stranded DNA virus
- Icosahedral symmetry
- Enveloped

INCUBATION PERIOD
- The mean incubation period, based on experimental infection, is estimated to be approximately 9 to 10 days.

EPIDEMIOLOGY
- Worldwide

INFECTIONS
- Roseola infantum or exanthem subitum (a febrile infection with or without a rash after defervescence)
- Interstitial pneumonitis
- Mononucleosis-like syndrome in adults with primary infection
- Bone marrow suppression, encephalitis, pneumonia, hepatitis, and exanthem, in bone marrow transplant recipients and immunocompromised patients
- Spontaneous abortion in primary infection during the first trimester of pregnancy

DIAGNOSIS
- Cell culture and serology

TREATMENT
- Symptomatic

Microorganisms

Human Herpesvirus Type 8

GROUP Herpesvirus
SPECIES
- N/A

MICROBIOLOGIC CHARACTERISTICS
- Double-stranded DNA virus

INCUBATION PERIOD
- Unknown

INFECTIONS
- The virus is associated with Kaposi's sarcoma.

DIAGNOSIS
- Cell culture and serology

TREATMENT
- Foscarnet

ALTERNATIVE TREATMENT
- Symptomatic treatment only

Herpes Zoster Virus

See Section II, "Herpes Zoster"

Heterophyes heterophyes

GENUS Heterophyes
SPECIES
- H. heterophyes

MICROBIOLOGIC CHARACTERISTICS
- A nematode helminth
- Small size (2 mm in length)

INCUBATION PERIOD
- Unknown

EPIDEMIOLOGY
- Egypt (Nile delta), Israel, Russia, Japan, Southeast Asia
- Infection is acquired by consumption of undercooked or salted fish.

INFECTIONS
- Heterophyiasis (frequently asymptomatic, but patients sometimes complain of dyspepsia, mucous diarrhea, and abdominal pain)

DIAGNOSIS
- Parasitologic examination of stools (identification 30 × 15-μm eggs)

TREATMENT
- Praziquantel 25 mg/kg PO q8h for 1 day
- No treatment is necessary for asymptomatic patients.

PREVENTION
- Avoid consumption of undercooked fish.

Hymenolepsis Species

GENUS Hymenolepsis
SPECIES
- H. diminuta
- H. nana

MICROBIOLOGIC CHARACTERISTICS
- Very small tapeworms
- H. nana is the only human tapeworm without an obligatory intermediate host.
- H. diminuta is a rat tapeworm (with accidental infection in humans).

INCUBATION PERIOD
- The development of mature worms of H. nana takes about 2 weeks. However, the time to symptoms is variable and depends on the number of worms in the person's bowel.

EPIDEMIOLOGY
- A worldwide infection
- More common in warm than in cold climates
- The most common tapeworm infection the United States
- Infection is usually acquired by ingestion of eggs via contaminated foods or water or directly from fecally contaminated fingers (person-to-person transmission or autoinfection).

INFECTIONS
- Light infection (small number of worms) usually causes no symptoms.
- Heavy infection may cause dyspepsia, abdominal discomfort, and/or diarrhea.

DIAGNOSIS
- Examination of concentrated stools (eggs)

TREATMENT
- Praziquantel 25 mg/kg in a single dose

ALTERNATIVE TREATMENT
- Niclosamide 2 g in a single dose is also effective.

PREVENTION
- Protect food and water from contamination with human and rodent feces.

Hypoderma Species

See "Myiasis Agents"

Influenza A, B, and C Virus

See Section II, "Influenza"

Isospora belli

GENUS Isospora
SPECIES
- I. belli

MICROBIOLOGIC CHARACTERISTICS
- A protozoon

INCUBATION PERIOD
- Unknown

EPIDEMIOLOGY
- Worldwide

INFECTIONS
- Isosporiasis (diarrhea, malabsorption, eosinophilia), particularly in patients with AIDS

DIAGNOSIS
- Examination of concentrated stools (parasitologic examination)
- Kinyoun stain

TREATMENT
- Two tablets of trimethoprim-sulfamethoxazole (160 mg and 800 mg, respectively) q6h for 10 days, followed by same dose q12h for 3 weeks

ALTERNATIVE TREATMENT
- Pyrimethamine 75 mg/d PO and folinic acid 10 mg/d for 2 weeks.
- Doxycycline combined with nitrofurantoin

Junin Virus (Argentine Hemorrhagic Fever)

See "Arenaviral Hemorrhagic Fevers in South America"

Microorganisms

Kingella Species

GENUS Kingella
SPECIES
- K. denitrificans
- K. kingae

MICROBIOLOGIC CHARACTERISTICS
- Aerobic, gram-negative coccobacillus
- Facultative, anaerobic bacterium
- The organism belongs to the HACEK group of bacteria.

INCUBATION PERIOD
- Unknown

EPIDEMIOLOGY
- Usually an endogenous infection (Kingella species may be a part of the normal human flora)

INFECTIONS
- Endocarditis
- Arthritis and osteomyelitis
- Bacteremia (more frequently in children)
- Suttonella indologenes, a bacterium previously called Kingella indologenes, has been associated with eye infections.

DIAGNOSIS
- Culture

TREATMENT
- Penicillin G combined with an aminoglycoside

Klebsiella Species

GENUS Klebsiella
SPECIES
- K. oxytoca
- K. pneumoniae

MICROBIOLOGIC CHARACTERISTICS
- Aerobic, gram-negative bacillus

INCUBATION PERIOD
- Usually an endogenous infection (from strains that are part of the normal human flora)

EPIDEMIOLOGY
- Worldwide

INFECTIONS
- Pneumonia, urinary infection, bacteremia
- Atrophic rhinitis
- Rhinoscleroma

DIAGNOSIS
- Culture

TREATMENT
- Third-generation cephalosporin
- Aztreonam

ALTERNATIVE TREATMENT
- Ciprofloxacin
- Carbapenem (imipenem or meropenem)
- Amoxicillin–clavulanate
- Piperacillin–tazobactam
- Aminoglycoside

Kluyvera Species

GENUS Kluyvera
SPECIES
- K. ascorbata
- K. cryorencens

MICROBIOLOGIC CHARACTERISTICS
- Aerobic, gram-negative bacilli

INCUBATION PERIOD
- Usually an endogenous infection

EPIDEMIOLOGY
- Rare cause of infection
- Worldwide distribution

INFECTIONS
- Bacteremia
- Soft-tissue infection
- Urinary infection
- Pneumonia in immunosuppressed persons

DIAGNOSIS
- Culture

TREATMENT
- There are limited data for *in vitro* susceptibility of Kluyvera species to antimicrobial agents.
- Antipseudomonal antibiotics are probably active against Kluyvera species.

ALTERNATIVE TREATMENT
- Chloramphenicol

Kurthia Species

GENUS Kurthia
SPECIES
- K. gibsonii
- K. sibirica
- K. zopfii

MICROBIOLOGIC CHARACTERISTICS
- Aerobic, gram-positive bacilli

INCUBATION PERIOD
- Unknown

EPIDEMIOLOGY
- Rare cause of infections
- Worldwide distribution
- Intravenous drug users are at higher risk for developing infections due to aerobic, gram-positive bacilli, including Kurthia species.

INFECTIONS
- Endocarditis
- Bacteremia

DIAGNOSIS
- Culture

TREATMENT
- Penicillin G associated with an aminoglycoside (in case of endocarditis)

ALTERNATIVE TREATMENT
- Trimethoprim–sulfamethoxazole
- Chloramphenicol
- Erythromycin

PREVENTION
- Social programs to decrease the number of intravenous drug users

Microorganisms

Kyasanur Forest Disease Virus

GENUS Flavivirus
SPECIES
- N/A

MICROBIOLOGIC CHARACTERISTICS
- Single stranded, positive RNA virus
- Spheric
- Enveloped

EPIDEMIOLOGY
- Found in several parts of India

INFECTIONS
- Hemorrhagic fever with renal syndrome

DIAGNOSIS
- Cell culture and serology

TREATMENT
- Symptomatic

Lactobacillus Species

GENUS Lactobacillus
SPECIES
- L. acidophilus
- L. casei
- L. plantarum
- L. rhamnosus
- L. salivarius
- Others

MICROBIOLOGIC CHARACTERISTICS
- Gram-positive bacilli
- Microaerophilic

INCUBATION PERIOD
- Usually an endogenous infection

EPIDEMIOLOGY
- *Lactobacillus* strains are part of the normal human vaginal, oral, and bowel flora.
- *Lactobacillus* strains also are found in a variety of food products.
- Changes of the hormonic environment of the vagina leads to changes of the number of lactobacilli locally, which is implicated in the pathogenesis of urinary tract infections (because it permits the overgrowth of other bacteria such as Enterobacteriaceae).

INFECTIONS
- Endocarditis
- Neonatal meningitis
- Amnionitis
- Bacteremia (especially in neutropenic patients)
- Mediastinitis

DIAGNOSIS
- Culture

TREATMENT
- Penicillin G

ALTERNATIVE TREATMENT
- Amoxicillin

Lassa Virus

GROUP Arenavirus
SPECIES
- N/A

MICROBIOLOGIC CHARACTERISTICS
- Two single-stranded, circular RNA segments
- Helicoidal symmetry
- Enveloped

EPIDEMIOLOGY
- Found in West Africa

INFECTIONS
- Lassa fever (hemorrhagic fever)

DIAGNOSIS
- Cell culture and serology

TREATMENT
- Ribavirin 1 g i.v. q6h for 4 days and then 0.5 g i.v. q8h for 6 days

PREVENTION
- Strict isolation for the duration of illness

Leclercia adecarboxylata

GENUS Leclercia
SPECIES
- L. adecarboxylata

MICROBIOLOGIC CHARACTERISTICS
- Aerobic, gram-negative bacillus

INCUBATION PERIOD
- Unknown

EPIDEMIOLOGY
- Worldwide, rare cause of infection

INFECTIONS
- Bacteremia
- Respiratory tract infections

DIAGNOSIS
- Culture

TREATMENT
- Fluoroquinolone

ALTERNATIVE TREATMENT
- Trimethoprim–sulfamethoxazole
- A combination of a β-lactam agent with an inhibitor of β-lactamase

Legionella Species

See "Legionellosis"

Leishmania Species Complex

See Section II, "Leishmaniasis"

Microorganisms

Leptomyxid Species

GENUS Leptomyxid
SPECIES
- N/A

MICROBIOLOGIC CHARACTERISTICS
- A free-living amoeba (water, dust, air conditioning)
- Other free-living amoebae of clinical significance include *Naegleria* and *Acanthamoeba*.

INCUBATION PERIOD
- Unknown

EPIDEMIOLOGY
- Worldwide
- Rare cause of infection

INFECTIONS
- Meningoencephalitis
- Most patients have been diagnosed postmortem.
- Patients with AIDS have a higher risk of infection.

DIAGNOSIS
- Fresh CSF examination
- Direct immunofluorescence and immunoblot to distinguish various strains

TREATMENT
- There is no known effective treatment.

Leptospira Species

See Section II, "Leptospirosis"

Leuconostoc Species

GENUS Leuconostoc
SPECIES
- *L. citreum*
- *L. lactis*
- *L. mesenteroides*
- *L. paramesenteroides*
- Others

MICROBIOLOGIC CHARACTERISTICS
- Anaerobic, gram-positive coccus
- *Leuconostoc* species are sometimes confused with *Enterococcus* species or *viridans* streptococci.
- The growth of *Leuconostoc* species from a clinical specimen may be due to contamination of the specimen.

INCUBATION PERIOD
- Unknown

EPIDEMIOLOGY
- Worldwide distribution

INFECTIONS
- The clinical significance of *Leuconostoc* species has not been clarified.
- There are a few reports of bacteremia in newborns and immunocompromised patients.

DIAGNOSIS
- Culture

TREATMENT
- Penicillin G or ampicillin (high intravenous doses are recommended for severe cases)

ALTERNATIVE TREATMENT
- First-generation cephalosporin
- Imipenem
- *Leuconostoc* species are resistant to vancomycin.

Linguatula serrata

GENUS Linguatula
SPECIES
- *L. serrata*

MICROBIOLOGIC CHARACTERISTICS
- A pentastome helminth (tongue worm)

INCUBATION PERIOD
- Unknown

EPIDEMIOLOGY
- More frequent in the Middle East and Africa
- Parasite of reptiles, birds, and mammals

INFECTIONS
- Immature (nymphal) stages of this parasite sometimes lodge in the human nasopharynx, causing obstruction and irritation. This condition is known as halzoun ormorrara.

DIAGNOSIS
- Finding and examination of the parasite

TREATMENT
- Surgical removal

Listeria monocytogenes

See Section II, "Listeriosis"

Loa loa

GENUS Loa
SPECIES
- *L. loa*

MICROBIOLOGIC CHARACTERISTICS
- A filarial nematode helminth

INCUBATION PERIOD
- Microfilariae may appear in the peripheral blood 4 months or later after infection with Loa loa.
- Symptoms may appear as early as 4 months after infection. However, it usually takes several years for symptoms to appear.

EPIDEMIOLOGY
- A common infection in Central Africa
- Up to 90% of people in the Congo River basin are infected.
- The infectious agents are transmitted to humans by the bite of infective deer fly.

INFECTIONS
- Chronic disease (loiasis) manifested by transient swelling of potentially any part of the body (skin, subcutaneous, and deeper tissues). Pruritus and localized pain are common symptoms. These manifestations are caused by migration of the adult worm in different parts of the body.

Microorganisms

DIAGNOSIS
- Finding of microfilariae in peripheral blood smear examination

TREATMENT
- Diethylcarbamazine is the most effective agent. It leads to disappearance of microfilariae. The drug also may kill the adult worm, leading to complete cure.
- However, hypersensitivity reactions during treatment with diethylcarbamazine may become a serious problem.
- Treatment with diethylcarbamazine should be done under careful supervision, especially in cases with severe microfilaremia (>2,000/mL of blood), due to the risk of severe meningoencephalitis.

ALTERNATIVE TREATMENT
- Ivermectin
- Albendazole

Lymphocytic Choriomeningitis Virus

GROUP Arenavirus

SPECIES
- N/A

MICROBIOLOGIC CHARACTERISTICS
- Two single-stranded, circular RNA segments
- Helicoidal symmetry
- Enveloped

EPIDEMIOLOGY
- Rare cause of infection

INFECTIONS
- Fever, adenitis, skin rash, meningoencephalitis with significant lymphocytic pleocytosis

DIAGNOSIS
- Cell culture
- Serology

TREATMENT
- Symptomatic

Lymphotropic T-Cell Human Virus

GROUP Human T-lymphocyte viruses (HTLV-1 and HTLV-2)

SPECIES
- N/A

MICROBIOLOGIC CHARACTERISTICS
- Single stranded, positive RNA; retroviruses
- Enveloped

INCUBATION PERIOD
- Unknown

EPIDEMIOLOGY
- The geographic distribution of these viruses (HTLV-1 and HTLV-2) is not well known, but it is likely that they are found worldwide.
- High seropositivity rates of HTLV-1 have been found in the islands of southeastern Japan and the Caribbean basin.
- Antibodies against HTLV-2 are found in a considerable proportion of intravenous drug users in several countries.

INFECTIONS
- Adult T-cell leukemia and tropical spastic paraparesis, Jamaican infectious dermatitis
- No disease has been causally associated with HTLV-2 (the virus was initially isolated from two patients with hairy-cell leukemia).

DIAGNOSIS
- Cell culture
- Serology
- Antigen detection

TREATMENT
- Symptomatic
- There are limited data about the efficacy of antiviral agents against HTLV-1 or HTLV-2.

PREVENTION
- Methods of prevention are similar to those for HIV.

Microorganisms

Machupo Virus (Bolivian Hemorrhagic Fever)

See "Arenaviral Hemorrhagic Fevers in South America"

Madurella Species

GENUS *Madurella*

SPECIES
- *M. grisea*
- *M. mycetomatis*

MICROBIOLOGIC CHARACTERISTICS
- Filamentous fungus (mold), with septate hyaline hyphae

INCUBATION PERIOD
- Months

EPIDEMIOLOGY
- *Madurella* fungi are widespread in nature.
- However, symptomatic infection due to these organisms is rare.
- Most cases occur in tropical and subtropical areas (including Northern Africa, Southern Asia, and Central America).

INFECTIONS
- Infection with *Madurella* may lead to local chronic inflammation with formation of sinus tracts.
- Lesions usually appear on the foot or tibia.
- Lesions similar to these caused by *Madurella* fungi may be the result of infection with other fungi (such as *Scedosporium, Exophiala, Acremonium, Pyrenochaeta, Neotestudina, Leptosphaeria,* and *Pseudallescheria*) or bacteria (such as *Nocardia* and *Actinomyces*).

DIAGNOSIS
- Isolation of etiologic fungus in culture of pus from affected tissues
- Granules visible with the naked eye are frequently seen in the pus.
- The main differential diagnosis for this chronic infection (mycetoma) is chronic osteomyelitis and botryomycosis.

TREATMENT
- Ketoconazole 400 mg/d for 9 to 12 months

ALTERNATIVE TREATMENT
- Itraconazole
- Surgical removal of lesions

PREVENTION
- Avoid puncture wounds by wearing shoes and clothes.

Malassezia Species

GENUS *Malassezia*

SPECIES
- *M. furfur*
- *M. pachydermatis*
- *M. sympodialis*

MICROBIOLOGIC CHARACTERISTICS
- Lipophilic yeasts
- Supplementation of culture media with lipids help *Malassezia* grow.
- *M. furfur* was previously known as *Pityrosporum orbiculare* or *P. ovale*.

INCUBATION PERIOD
- Unknown

EPIDEMIOLOGY
- Worldwide distribution
- Patients with Cushing syndrome are at risk to develop infection.

INFECTIONS
- Pityriasis versicolor (previously called tinea versicolor)
- *M. furfur* may also cause systemic infection in patients (especially immunocompromised patients and neonates) receiving intravenous fluids with lipids.
- Patients with continuous ambulatory peritoneal dialysis catheters may develop peritonitis due to *M. furfur*.
- A few cases of pneumonia have also been reported.
- *M. pachydermatis* has been reported to cause systemic infection in low-birth-weight children receiving lipid emulsions via a central venous catheter.
- The role of *M. sympodialis* as a cause of a human disease is unclear.

DIAGNOSIS
- Finding the fungus in clinical samples
- Blood culture (preferentially obtained from catheters in cases of fungemia)
- *M. furfur* has been implicated in the pathogenesis of several diseases, including seborrheic dermatitis, dandruff, atopic dermatitis, and confluent and reticulate papillomatosis. However, data supporting a causative association between *M. furfur* and these diseases are controversial.

TREATMENT
- Pityriasis versicolor is effectively managed with local or systemic azole treatment.
- Itraconazole 200 mg/d by mouth for 7 days usually suffices. A shorter regimen (400 mg itraconazole given once) may be enough for a considerable proportion of patients.
- Some cases of pityriasis versicolor are self-limited.
- Systemic infections due to *Malassezia* need high doses of intravenous treatment with azoles (and removal of the central catheter in cases of infection related to this risk factor).

ALTERNATIVE TREATMENT
- Selenium sulfur used topically (one daily application of selenium sulfur 2.5% for half an hour for 2 weeks) is also effective for pityriasis versicolor.

Mansonella Species

GENUS *Mansonella*

SPECIES
- *M. ozzardi*
- *M. perstans*
- *M. streptocerca*

MICROBIOLOGIC CHARACTERISTICS
- Nematode helminth

INCUBATION PERIOD
- Unknown

EPIDEMIOLOGY
- *M. ozzardi* infections occur in Central and South America and in the West Indies.
- *M. perstans* infections occur in West Africa and northeastern South America. It is likely that the organism has a wider geographic distribution than is estimated.
- *M. streptocerca* infections occur in West and Central Africa.

INFECTIONS
- Hypopigmented pruritic dermatitis

DIAGNOSIS
- Histopathology of skin biopsy
- Finding of microfilariae in affected tissues

TREATMENT
- Diethylcarbamazine 50 mg on the first day, 100 mg on the second and third days, followed by 50 mg q8h for 3 weeks

Marburg Virus

See "Filoviruses"

Measles Virus

See Section II, "Measles"

Microorganisms

Metagonimus yokogawai

GENUS Metagonimus
SPECIES
- M. yokogawai

MICROBIOLOGIC CHARACTERISTICS
- A trematode helminth

INCUBATION PERIOD
- Unknown

EPIDEMIOLOGY
- Rare cause of symptomatic human infection
- Cases of *M. yokogawai* infection have been reported from several areas of the world, including Russia, the Middle East (Israel, Egypt), India, Indonesia, China, Japan, and Taiwan.

INFECTIONS
- *M. yokogawai* usually causes an asymptomatic infection.
- The parasite sometimes leads to gastrointestinal symptoms, including diarrhea, abdominal discomfort, and dyspepsia.

DIAGNOSIS
- Parasitologic examination of stool specimens

TREATMENT
- Praziquantel 25 mg/kg PO q8h for 1 day (three doses)

Methylobacterium Species

GENUS Methylobacterium
SPECIES
- M. extorquens
- M. mesophilicum
- Others

MICROBIOLOGIC CHARACTERISTICS
- Aerobic, gram-negative bacillus
- Previously named *Protomonas* species

INCUBATION PERIOD
- Unknown

EPIDEMIOLOGY
- Reports of infections due to these gram-negative bacilli, which produce pink-pigmented colonies, have increased in the recent literature.

INFECTIONS
- Bacteremia
- *Methylobacterium* species may cause infections in immunosuppressed individuals (as opportunistic pathogens).
- Peritonitis (in patients undergoing peritoneal dialysis)

DIAGNOSIS
- Culture

TREATMENT
- Trimethoprim–sulfamethoxazole

ALTERNATIVE TREATMENT
- Ciprofloxacin
- Aminoglycoside

Microsporidia

GENERA/SPECIES
- The phylum Microspora includes over 100 genera and about 1,000 species. Among them, species of certain or possible clinical significance are the following:
  - *Enterocytozoon bieneusi*
  - *Enterocytozoon cuniculi*
  - *Enterocytozoon hellem*
  - *Nosema connori*
  - *Nosema corneum*
  - *Nosema ocularum*
  - *Pleistophora* species
  - *Septata intestinalis*

MICROBIOLOGIC CHARACTERISTICS
- Microsporidia comprises a group of obligately intracellular, spore-forming protozoa.
- They should not be confused with other protozoa, such as *Cryptosporidium* and *Isospora*.

EPIDEMIOLOGY
- The significance of Microsporidia as a cause of human disease has become clear only during the past decade.
- Possible routes of transmission are the fecal–oral route and the urine–oral route.
- There is limited understanding about the epidemiology, pathogenesis, and optimal management of infections due to Microsporidia.

INFECTIONS
- Microsporidiosis may also lead to biliary tree disease and pulmonary, CNS, and cornea infections.
- Clearly, much more should be understood about the protean manifestations of the infection.

DIAGNOSIS
- Histologic examination of affected tissue, using light (and electron, if needed) microscopy

TREATMENT
- Albendazole may be effective.

ALTERNATIVE TREATMENT
- Fumagillin preparations (topical treatment) appear to be effective in patients with conjunctival and/or corneal microsporidiosis.

Microsporum Species

GENUS Microsporum
SPECIES
- M. audouinii
- M. canis
- Others

MICROBIOLOGIC CHARACTERISTICS
- Filamentous fungus (mold)

INCUBATION PERIOD
- Unknown

EPIDEMIOLOGY
- Worldwide infection

INFECTIONS
- All forms of tinea infection (fungal infection of the head, face, trunk, extremities, inguinal areas, interdigital areas, and nails)

DIAGNOSIS
- Identification of the fungus in scrapings of lesions

TREATMENT
- Topical terbinafine twice a day for 2 to 4 weeks
- Prolonged treatment is needed (3–12 months) for onychomycosis.

ALTERNATIVE TREATMENT
- Itraconazole

Microorganisms

Mobiluncus Species

GENUS Mobiluncus
SPECIES
- M. curticei
- M. mulieris

MICROBIOLOGIC CHARACTERISTICS
- Anaerobic, curved, motile, bacillus
- It may be gram-negative (it is sometimes a gram-variable organism).

INCUBATION PERIOD
- Unknown

EPIDEMIOLOGY
- Mobiluncus strains have been detected from the vaginas of about 5% of women with no evidence for bacterial vaginosis.
- However, the organism has been isolated from the great majority (about 97%) of women with bacterial vaginosis.

INFECTIONS
- An etiologic association between Mobiluncus and bacterial vaginosis has not been established.
- Other bacteria (mainly Gardnerella vaginalis) are also frequently isolated from the vaginal fluid of women with bacterial vaginosis.

DIAGNOSIS
- Culture (anaerobic)
- Direct immunofluorescence of vaginal fluid

TREATMENT
- Penicillin

ALTERNATIVE TREATMENT
- Amoxicillin–clavulanate
- Metronidazole is the drug of choice for bacterial vaginosis, regardless of the presence or absence of Mobiluncus in vaginal fluid.

Molluscum contagiosum Virus

FAMILY Poxviridae
GENUS Molluscipoxvirus

MICROBIOLOGIC CHARACTERISTICS
- Double-stranded DNA virus
- Complex symmetry

INCUBATION PERIOD
- The incubation period varies between 2 and 7 weeks but may be as long as 6 months.

EPIDEMIOLOGY
- Worldwide
- It is spread by direct contact (including sexual contact and by fomites).
- Humans are the only source of the virus.

INFECTIONS
- Molluscum contagiosum, a common disease manifested by few (usually 2–20) papular, waxy, discrete skin lesions with central umbilication
- In patients with AIDS or other causes of immunodeficiency, lesions tend to be larger and numerous and affect an extensive area of the skin.

DIAGNOSIS
- Direct visualization under electron microscopy of the poxvirus particles
- The diagnosis is usually made with no tests performed (from the characteristic appearance of lesions).
- Giemsa or Wright staining of expressed material from the center of the lesions may show intracytoplasmic inclusions.

TREATMENT
- Lesions are usually self-limited.
- However, removal of lesions is recommended because of the possibility of autoinoculation in other areas of the body of the patient and/or spread of the infection to other people.

ALTERNATIVE TREATMENT
- Topical application of several agents, including cantharidin (0.7% in collodion) or peeling agents (e.g., salicylic acid preparations) is also helpful.
- Liquid nitrogen for destruction of lesions is also successful in the management of molluscum contagiosum.

PREVENTION
- In cases of outbreaks of molluscum contagiosum (which occur commonly in tropical areas), restriction of direct body contact and avoidance of sharing of fomites are recommended.

Moraxella (Branhamella) Species

GENUS Moraxella (Branhamella)
SPECIES
- M. altantae
- M. catarrhalis
- M. lacunata
- M. nonliquefaciens
- M. osloensis
- M. phenylpyruvica

MICROBIOLOGIC CHARACTERISTICS
- Aerobic, gram-negative coccobacilli

INCUBATION PERIOD
- Unknown

EPIDEMIOLOGY
- M. catarrhalis is a common human pathogen.
- Moraxella species are part of the normal oral flora of humans and animals.

INFECTIONS
- Moraxella species may cause ear and upper and lower respiratory tract infections, including otitis media, sinusitis, laryngitis, acute bronchitis, pneumonia, and bronchopneumonia.
- Neonatal conjunctivitis (usually due to M. catarrhalis), blepharoconjunctivitis (due to several Moraxella species, usually M. lacunata)
- Bacteremia
- Endocarditis
- Arthritis

DIAGNOSIS
- Culture

TREATMENT
- Amoxicillin–clavulanate

ALTERNATIVE TREATMENT
- A macrolide antibiotic
- A second-generation cephalosporin
- Trimethoprim–sulfamethoxazole
- M. catarrhalis strains frequently produce β-lactamases.

Morganella morganii

GENUS Morganella
SPECIES
- M. morganii

MICROBIOLOGIC CHARACTERISTICS
- Aerobic, gram-negative bacillus

INCUBATION PERIOD
- Unknown

EPIDEMIOLOGY
- Worldwide

INFECTIONS
- Usually nosocomial infections: urinary, pulmonary, sepsis

DIAGNOSIS
- Culture

TREATMENT
- Carbapenem (imipenem, meropenem)
- Ciprofloxacin

ALTERNATIVE TREATMENT
- A third-generation cephalosporin
- Aztreonam
- Ofloxacin
- Piperacillin–tazobactam
- Aminoglycoside

Mucor Species

See Section II, "Mucormycosis"

Muerto Canyon Virus

See "Hantaan Virus"

Microorganisms

Multiceps multiceps

GENUS Multiceps
SPECIES
- M. multiceps

MICROBIOLOGIC CHARACTERISTICS
- A cestode helminth

INCUBATION PERIOD
- Unknown

EPIDEMIOLOGY
- *M. multiceps* is a parasite of dogs.
- Worldwide distribution

INFECTIONS
- A rare cause of human infection
- Scattered cases of cenurosis (a disease that causes cysts in the central nervous system) have been reported.

DIAGNOSIS
- Histopathology of removed affected tissues may reveal the parasite.

TREATMENT
- Surgical removal of the cysts, if possible

ALTERNATIVE TREATMENT
- Praziquantel at high doses (>50 mg/kg) may also help.

Mumps Virus

See Section II, "Mumps"

Mycobacterium, Atypical

See "Atypical Mycobacteria"

Mycobacterium bovis

GENUS Mycobacterium
SPECIES
- M. bovis

MICROBIOLOGIC CHARACTERISTICS
- Aerobic, acid-fast bacillus

EPIDEMIOLOGY
- Generally acquired by ingestion of contaminated milk

INFECTIONS
- *M. bovis* may cause lymphadenitis, pulmonary infection, and gastrointestinal tract infection.

DIAGNOSIS
- Culture

TREATMENT
- INH plus rifampin and either ethambutol or streptomycin
- Some strains have primary resistance to pyrazinamide.

Mycobacterium leprae

See Section II, "Leprosy"

Mycobacterium tuberculosis

See Section II, "Tuberculosis"

Mycoplasma Species

GENUS Mycoplasma
SPECIES
- M. buccale
- M. faucium
- M. felis
- M. genitalium
- M. hominis
- M. laidlawii
- M. lipophilum
- M. oculi
- M. orale
- M. penetrans
- M. pirum
- M. pneumoniae
- M. primatum
- M. salivarium
- M. spermatophilum
- M. urealyticum

MICROBIOLOGIC CHARACTERISTICS
- Aerobic coccoid bacteria of small size
- *Mycoplasma* strains do not have a wall.

INCUBATION PERIOD
- *M. pneumoniae* causes clinical syndromes with an incubation period of 6 to 32 days.

EPIDEMIOLOGY
- Worldwide distribution for all *Mycoplasma* species
- *Mycoplasma* species are frequently commensal organisms, which may be isolated from several human sites. *M. pneumoniae* has a predilection for the oral cavity and the respiratory tract, while *M. hominis* is usually isolated from the genitourinary tract.
- Respiratory tract infection (including pneumonia due to *M. pneumoniae*) is common, especially between the ages of 10 and 40 years.
- Infections due to *M. pneumoniae* may occur in a sporadic, endemic, or even epidemic form. Epidemics occur more frequently in military populations.
- Transmission of *M. pneumoniae* occurs, most likely, mainly by droplet inhalation.

INFECTIONS
- *M. pneumoniae* is a common cause of upper and lower respiratory tract infections, including pneumonia, bronchitis, tracheobronchitis, pharyngitis, sinusitis, and myringitis.
- *M. pneumoniae* also may cause (rarely) hemolytic anemia, pericarditis, myocarditis, meningoencephalitis, erythema multiforme, and hepatitis.
- *M. fermentans* has been associated with pneumonia, encephalitis, hepatitis, myopericarditis, sepsis, and diarrhea.
- *M. hominis* has been isolated from the endometrium and/or fallopian tubes of about 10% of women with salpingitis. However, an etiologic role cannot be certainly established for *M. hominis* in these women, especially when several microorganisms are present.
- *M. genitalium* has obtained increasing attention during the past decade as a possible cause of genitourinary tract infections, including urethritis and pelvic inflammatory disease.
- There are some data that support the role of *Mycoplasma* species in infertility.

DIAGNOSIS
- Culture
- Serology tests
- Detection of cryoagglutinins (for *M. pneumoniae*)

TREATMENT
- Doxycycline 100 mg orally q12h for 7 to 14 days

ALTERNATIVE TREATMENT
- A macrolide or a fluoroquinolone for *M. pneumoniae* infections
- A fluoroquinolone for other *Mycoplasma* species

PREVENTION
- Avoidance of crowded living and sleeping quarters may decrease the possibility of *M. pneumoniae* infections.
- Safe sexual activity (use of condoms) may decrease the possibility of transmission of *Mycoplasma* species that are part of the urethral and vaginal flora.

Microorganisms

Myiasis Agents

GENERA
- Several genera of dipterous flies may cause myiasis. Among them are the following:
  - *Calliphora*
  - *Chrysomyia*
  - *Cochliomyia*
  - *Cordylobia*
  - *Dermatobia*
  - *Gasterophilus*
  - *Lucilia*
  - *Phormia*
  - *Sarcophaga*
  - *Wohlfahrtia*

SPECIES
- There are several species in each genus of flies capable of causing myiasis.

MICROBIOLOGIC CHARACTERISTICS
- Flying larvae (arthropods)

EPIDEMIOLOGY
- Tropical and subtropical climates
- Latin America

INFECTIONS
- Myiasis
- Flying larvae parasitize skin and subcutaneous tissue and cause local inflammation.

DIAGNOSIS
- Identification of larvae in the affected area

TREATMENT
- One usually successful technique is occlusion of the orifice of the area of myiasis with Vaseline (or other petroleum jelly) or pork fat and removal of the parasite 1 to 2 hours later by using pressure. Use of these materials causes suffocation of the larva and make it emerge from the skin.

ALTERNATIVE TREATMENT
- Surgical removal of the larvae may be necessary if the previously mentioned, simpler technique is not successful.

Naegleria fowleri

GENUS *Naegleria*

SPECIES
- *N. fowleri*

MICROBIOLOGIC CHARACTERISTICS
- A protozoon

INCUBATION PERIOD
- Unknown

EPIDEMIOLOGY
- Worldwide (temperate regions)

INFECTIONS
- Meningoencephalitis (purulent meningitis and cortical hemorrhages)

DIAGNOSIS
- Fresh examination of CSF and Giemsa or Wright stain
- Culture in special medium

TREATMENT
- An effective treatment is not known.
- Intrathecal and intravenous amphotericin B (1 mg/kg), and miconazole in combination with intravenous or PO rifampin, may be tried.
- Topical propamidine isethionate has been reported to be helpful in several cases of eye infections.

Nanophyetus salmincola

GENUS *Nanophyetus*

SPECIES
- *N. salmincola*

MICROBIOLOGIC CHARACTERISTICS
- A trematode helminth

INCUBATION PERIOD
- Unknown

EPIDEMIOLOGY
- *N. salmincola* infections in humans have been reported from the northwestern United States.

INFECTIONS
- Infection of the gastrointestinal tract, presenting with various gastrointestinal symptoms

DIAGNOSIS
- Parasitologic examination of stool specimens (for identification of eggs of the parasite, 64 to 97 μm long × 43 to 55 μm wide)

TREATMENT
- Praziquantel 60 mg/kg/d in three doses for 1 day

PREVENTION
- Avoid eating raw, incompletely cooked, or smoked salmon.

Necator americanus

GENUS *Necator*

SPECIES
- *N. americanus*

MICROBIOLOGIC CHARACTERISTICS
- A nematode helminth

EPIDEMIOLOGY
- Common infection in the Americas

INFECTIONS
- Hookworm (anemia, dyspepsia, diarrhea)

DIAGNOSIS
- Parasitologic examination of stools

TREATMENT
- Mebendazole 100 mg PO q12h for 3 days
- Patients with anemia due to a large number of parasites should receive a second cycle of treatment 1 to 2 weeks after the first cycle.

ALTERNATIVE TREATMENT
- Albendazole 400 mg PO in a single dose
- In children, pyrantel pamoate for 3 days may be used.

Neisseria gonorrhoeae

See Section I, "Urethritis and Urethral Discharge"

Neisseria meningitidis

See Section II, "Meningitis, Acute"

Microorganisms

Neisseria Species

GENUS Neisseria

SPECIES
- *N. canis*
- *N. cinerea*
- *N. elongata*
- *N. flavescens*
- *N. gonorrhoeae*
- *N. lactamica*
- *N. meningitidis*
- *N. mucosa*
- *N. polysaccharea*
- *N. sicca*
- *N. subflava*
- *N. weaveri*

MICROBIOLOGIC CHARACTERISTICS
- Aerobic, gram-negative cocci

INCUBATION PERIOD
- The incubation period for gonorrhea (caused by *N. gonorrhoeae*) is usually 2 to 7 days; occasionally, a longer incubation period may be observed.
- The incubation period of meningitis due to *N. meningitidis* is usually 3 to 4 days; occasionally, a shorter (2 days) or longer (5–10 days) incubation period may be observed.
- The incubation period of infections due to other *Neisseria* species is unknown.

EPIDEMIOLOGY
- Common cause of human infections
- *N. gonorrhoeae* is usually sexually transmitted.
- *N. gonorrhoeae* also may be transmitted from mother to neonate and cause neonatal conjunctivitis.
- Other *Neisseria* species are transmitted, usually, by air droplets.

INFECTIONS
- Meningitis
- Endocarditis in intravenous drug users, immunocompromised patients, or patients with heart valve disease who undergo dental procedures
- Bacteremia
- Dog bite wound infection (*N. weaveri*)
- *N. gonorrhoeae* may cause several syndromes, including urethritis, epididymitis, prostatitis, cervicitis, pelvic inflammatory disease, proctitis, pharyngitis, perihepatitis (Fitz-Hugh–Curtis syndrome), and a systemic infection manifested by arthritis and rash.
- *N. meningitidis* may cause meningitis, bacteremia, lower and upper respiratory tract infections, conjunctivitis, and a systemic syndrome manifested by rash, fever, and arthritis.

DIAGNOSIS
- Culture

TREATMENT
- Penicillin G or ampicillin
- For urethritis, pelvic inflammatory disease, cervicitis, and meningitis, specific treatment is reviewed elsewhere in this book.

ALTERNATIVE TREATMENT
- Third-generation cephalosporin

Nocardia Species

See Section II, "Nocardiosis"

Norwalk Virus

See "Caliciviruses and Calici-like Viruses"

Nosema Species

See "Microsporidia"

Ochrobactrum anthropi

GENUS Ochrobactrum

SPECIES
- *O. anthropi*

MICROBIOLOGIC CHARACTERISTICS
- Aerobic, gram-negative bacillus

INCUBATION PERIOD
- Unknown

EPIDEMIOLOGY
- Rare cause of human infection
- This microorganism has been isolated from various environmental sources and human specimens.

INFECTIONS
- Central venous catheter–related bacteremia is the main infection caused by *O. anthropi*.

DIAGNOSIS
- Culture

TREATMENT
- Trimethoprim–sulfamethoxazole

ALTERNATIVE TREATMENT
- Imipenem
- Aminoglycosides
- Fluoroquinolone

Oerskovia Species

GENUS Oerskovia

SPECIES
- *O. turbata*
- *O. xanthineolytica*

MICROBIOLOGIC CHARACTERISTICS
- Aerobic (facultatively anaerobic), gram-positive bacillus
- Branching filamentous bacteria, which fragment into pleomorphic rods
- Catalase-positive microorganism
- Some experts believe that this genus should be combined with the genus *Cellulomonas*.

INCUBATION PERIOD
- Unknown

EPIDEMIOLOGY
- Infections due to *Oerskovia* species were underestimated until recently because of problems related to microbiologic recognition of the pathogen.
- Sources of isolation of *Oerskovia* species include cerebrospinal fluid, blood, heart tissue, ascitic fluid, and urine.
- Infection is frequently associated with a foreign body.
- Bacteremia (especially in patients with central venous catheters)
- Endocarditis
- Endophthalmitis
- Meningitis
- Peritonitis
- Urinary tract infection

INFECTIONS
- Line-associated sepsis
- Prosthetic valve endocarditis

DIAGNOSIS
- Culture

TREATMENT
- There are very limited data for the efficacy of various antimicrobial agents.
- Removal of a foreign body (e.g., central venous catheter) is frequently necessary to eradicate infection.
- Ampicillin or penicillin may be effective.

ALTERNATIVE TREATMENT
- Third-generation cephalosporin, vancomycin, aminoglycoside, imipenem, or trimethoprim–sulfamethoxazole

Microorganisms

Oligella Species

GENUS Oligella
SPECIES
- O. ureolytica
- O. urethralis

MICROBIOLOGIC CHARACTERISTICS
- Anaerobic, gram-negative coccobacilli

INCUBATION PERIOD
- Unknown

EPIDEMIOLOGY
- Most isolates of Oligella have been found in urine specimens.

INFECTIONS
- Rare cause of urinary tract infection

DIAGNOSIS
- Culture

TREATMENT
- There are very limited available data for the in vitro susceptibility of Oligella species to various antimicrobial agents.
- Penicillin may be effective.

ALTERNATIVE TREATMENT
- Cephalosporin

Omsk Virus (Hemorrhagic Fever)

See "Hantaan Virus"

Onchocerca volvulus

GENUS Onchocerca
SPECIES
- O. volvulus

MICROBIOLOGIC CHARACTERISTICS
- A filarial (nematode) worm

INCUBATION PERIOD
- The incubation period from larval inoculation to microfilariae in the skin is approximately 6 to 12 months.

EPIDEMIOLOGY
- Sub-Saharan Africa, southwestern Saudi Arabia, Yemen, Central and South America
- Infection is transmitted to humans only by the bite of infected blackflies of the genus Simulium.

INFECTIONS
- O. volvulus causes onchocerciasis, a chronic, nonfatal disease manifested by subcutaneous nodules.
- Microfilariae may reach the eye and cause visual abnormalities and even blindness.

DIAGNOSIS
- Microscopic examination of fresh skin biopsy incubated in water or saline may show the presence of microfilariae.
- Detection of microfilariae in urine specimens
- Detection of adult worms in excised nodules

TREATMENT
- Ivermectin (6-mg tablets): less than 30 kg, one-half tablet; 30 to 44 kg, 1 tablet; 45 to 64 kg, 1.5 tablets; greater than 64 kg, 2 tablets
- In a single dose, in children: 0.15 mg/kg, repeated every 6 months
- Retreatment every 6 months to 1 year is recommended.

ALTERNATIVE TREATMENT
- Suramin: Treatment with suramin should be done under close medical supervision, due to possible nephrotoxicity and other adverse effects.
- Diethylcarbamazine should not be used, due to the possible, severe adverse effects, which are observed especially in patients with heavy load of worms.

PREVENTION
- Avoid bites by species of flies.

Opisthorchis Species

GENUS Opisthorchis
SPECIES
- O. felineus
- O. viverrini

MICROBIOLOGIC CHARACTERISTICS
- Trematode helminths

INCUBATION PERIOD
- Unknown (probably months)

EPIDEMIOLOGY
- About 2 million people in the countries of the former Soviet Union are infected with O. felineus.
- High rates of infections due to O. viverrini are found in Thailand, especially in the northern part of the country.

INFECTIONS
- Opisthorchiasis is manifested by obstructive jaundice and cholangiitis.
- Opisthorchiasis is considered to be a risk factor for cholangiocarcinoma (as is thought for clonorchiasis, which is caused by Clonorchis sinensis).

DIAGNOSIS
- Parasitologic examination of stools

TREATMENT
- Praziquantel 25 mg/kg every 8 hours for 2 days

PREVENTION
- Cook or irradiate freshwater fish.

ORF Virus

GROUP Parapoxvirus (family Poxviridae)
SPECIES
- N/A

MICROBIOLOGIC CHARACTERISTICS
- Double-stranded DNA virus

INCUBATION PERIOD
- Usually 3 to 6 days

EPIDEMIOLOGY
- Worldwide infections
- Infection is usually transmitted to humans by direct contact with infected animals (usually sheep or goats; rarely deer or reindeer).
- A common infection in persons who are at risk because of their professions (shepherds, abattoir workers, and veterinarians in areas producing sheep and goats, such as New Zealand).

INFECTIONS
- Small, painless nodule(s), usually localized in the hands
- A lesion is usually solitary.
- Lesions may become pustular when secondary bacterial infection occurs.

DIAGNOSIS
- Direct identification of the virus under electron microscopy (ovoid parapoxvirus are seen in affected tissues)
- Serology tests
- Growth of virus in cell cultures of ovine, bovine, or primate origin

TREATMENT
- Usually a self-limited infection

ALTERNATIVE TREATMENT
- There is no specific antiviral treatment.

PREVENTION
- Good personal hygiene of persons exposed potentially frequently to the virus due to their professions
- General cleanliness of animal-housing areas

Microorganisms

Paecilomyces Species

GENUS Paecilomyces

SPECIES
- P. javanicus
- P. lilacinus
- P. marquandii
- P. variotii

MICROBIOLOGIC CHARACTERISTICS
- Filamentous fungus (mold)
- It resembles *Penicillium* species in morphology.

INCUBATION PERIOD
- Unknown

EPIDEMIOLOGY
- Worldwide distribution
- Rare cause of human infection

INFECTIONS
- *Paecilomyces* isolates were usually considered contaminants. However, recent data support the idea that the fungus has a pathogenetic potential and may lead to infection of several sites.
- Keratitis
- Endophthalmitis
- Sinusitis
- Fungemia
- Respiratory tract infection
- Skin and subcutaneus tissue infection
- Endocarditis

DIAGNOSIS
- Culture
- Tissue biopsy (histopathology)

TREATMENT
- Amphotericin B intravenously

ALTERNATIVE TREATMENT
- Flucytosine may be added to treatment with amphotericin B.
- Surgical management may be necessary in cases of endophthalmitis, sinusitis, or endocarditis.

Pantoea agglomerans

GENUS Pantoea

SPECIES
- P. agglomerans

MICROBIOLOGIC CHARACTERISTICS
- Aerobic, gram-negative bacillus
- Formerly called *Enterobacter agglomerans*

INCUBATION PERIOD
- Unknown

EPIDEMIOLOGY
- Rare, worldwide infection

INFECTIONS
- *P. agglomerans* is usually a cause of nosocomial infections.
- Urinary tract infection
- Bacteremia (related to central venous catheter or not)
- Pneumonia
- A rare cause of meningitis in neonates

DIAGNOSIS
- Culture

TREATMENT
- Third-generation cephalosporin or aztreonam

ALTERNATIVE TREATMENT
- Ciprofloxacin
- Carbapenem (imipenem or meropenem)
- Aminoglycoside
- Aztreonam

Papillomavirus

See Section II, "Warts" and "Cervicitis/Mucopurulent Cervicitis"

Paracoccidioides brasiliensis

GENUS Paracoccidioides

SPECIES
- P. brasiliensis

MICROBIOLOGIC CHARACTERISTICS
- Dimorphic fungus

INCUBATION PERIOD
- The incubation period is highly variable, ranging from 1 month to many years.

EPIDEMIOLOGY
- *P. brasiliensis* is endemic in tropical and subtropical areas of South America.
- The fungus is also found in Central America.
- Farmers and workers in construction are at risk to contact the fungus because of frequent contact with soil.
- The infection is more common in men than in women.

INFECTIONS
- *P. brasiliensis* causes paracoccidioidomycosis (also called South American blastomycosis).
- Paracoccidioidomycosis is a potentially fatal infection that usually affects the lungs (pneumonia) and the oral, nasal, and gastrointestinal tract mucosa (ulcerative lesions); lymphadenopathy is common.
- The infection may affect any organ.
- Adrenal glands are commonly affected.
- Bone marrow involvement is common in the acute form of the infection.

DIAGNOSIS
- Serology tests
- Identification of the fungus in tissue biopsies
- Finding the fungus in respiratory secretion specimens

TREATMENT
- Itraconazole or ketoconazole are the drugs of choice. They should be given for a prolonged period (at least 6 months).
- In cases of severe infection, amphotericin B i.v. should be given (1.5–2.0 g total dose).

ALTERNATIVE TREATMENT
- Sulfadiazine 4 to 6 g/d for several months, and then 2 to 3 g/d for 3 to 5 years

PREVENTION
- Standard precautions are recommended for hospitalized patients.

Microorganisms

Paragonimus Species

GENUS Paragonimus

SPECIES
- *P. africanus*
- *P. kellicotti*
- *P. mexicanus* (*P. peruvianus*)
- *P. skrjabini*
- *P. uterobilateralis*
- *P. westermani*

MICROBIOLOGIC CHARACTERISTICS
- A trematode helminth

INCUBATION PERIOD
- The interval between infection and symptoms is usually long (at least several months).

EPIDEMIOLOGY
- Infection is transmitted to humans by eating infected crabs or crayfish.
- *P. africanus* and *P. uterobilateralis* are endemic in Africa (especially in Central Africa).
- *P. mexicanus* is endemic in the Americas.
- *P. westermani* and *P. skrjabini* are endemic in Asia.
- *P. kellicotti* has been found in the United States and Canada.

INFECTIONS
- Lungs are usually involved in paragonimiasis (the infection caused by *Paragonimus* species).
- Paragonimiasis is usually manifested by cough, pleuritic chest pain, and hemoptysis.
- Diffuse or segmental infiltrates, cavities, ring cysts, nodules, and/or pleural effusions may be seen in lung imaging (chest x-rays or CT scan).
- Extrapulmonary manifestations of paragonimiasis are also seen frequently. The infection may affect any organ.

DIAGNOSIS
- Eggs of *Paragonimus* species may be found in sputum specimens, usually in masses.
- Eggs of the parasite also may be found in stool specimens, especially in children.
- Attention should be paid to the fact that acid-fast staining for mycobacteria may destroy the eggs of *Paragonimus* species, and thus lead to difficulties in diagnosing the infection.
- Serology tests are also available.
- Chest x-ray abnormalities due to paragonimiasis may be mistakenly attributed to tuberculosis.

TREATMENT
- Praziquantel 25 mg/kg PO q8h for 3 days

ALTERNATIVE TREATMENT
- Bithionol 15 to 25 mg/kg q12h (alternate days) for 10 to 14 doses
- Steroids may be beneficial in cases of central nervous system involvement.

PREVENTION
- Thorough cooking of crustacea

Parainfluenza Virus

GROUP/TYPES: Paramyxovirus (types 1–4)

SPECIES
- N/A

MICROBIOLOGIC CHARACTERISTICS
- Single-stranded, RNA virus (large)
- Helicoidal symmetry
- Enveloped virus

INCUBATION PERIOD
- From 2 to 6 days

EPIDEMIOLOGY
- Worldwide infection
- Parainfluenza virus infections may present in an epidemic or sporadic fashion.

INFECTIONS
- Major cause of laryngotracheobronchitis (croup)
- Frequent cause of other upper respiratory tract infections
- Rare cause of pneumonia and bronchiolitis
- Immunosuppressed individuals may develop severe parainfluenza viral infections.

DIAGNOSIS
- Serology tests
- Viral cultures

TREATMENT
- In mild infections, only symptomatic treatment suffices.
- Racemic epinephrine aerosol reduces airway obstruction in patients with severe laryngotracheobronchitis (croup).
- Intubation may be necessary in patients with severe croup.

PREVENTION
- Handwashing is emphasized in an effort to reduce nosocomial transmission rates of parainfluenza infections.

Parvovirus B-19

See Section II, "Parvovirus Infections"

Microorganisms

Pasteurella Species

GENUS *Pasteurella*

SPECIES
- *P. aerogenes*
- *P. canis*
- *P. gallinarum*
- *P. haemolytica*
- *P. multocida*
- *P. pneumotropica*
- Others

MICROBIOLOGIC CHARACTERISTICS
- Aerobic, gram-negative bacilli

INCUBATION PERIOD
- Usually less than 24 hours

EPIDEMIOLOGY
- Part of the normal oropharyngeal flora of many animals, including 70% to 90% of cats and 20% to 50% of dogs
- Transmission usually occurs to humans from animal bites.
- Respiratory spread from animals to humans also occurs.
- Human-to-human transmission has not been documented.

INFECTIONS
- Cellulitis at the site of a scratch or bite of a cat, dog, or other animal
- Regional lymphadenopathy is common.
- Septic arthritis, tenosynovitis, or osteomyelitis may occur locally at the site of the animal scratch or bite.
- *Pasteurella* species also may cause infection of other sites, including respiratory tract infections, meningitis, peritonitis, urinary tract infection, appendicitis, hepatic abscess, and ocular infections (conjunctivitis, keratitis, and endophthalmitis).

DIAGNOSIS
- Culture

TREATMENT
- Penicillin G or amoxicillin–clavulanic acid for 7 to 10 days in cases of cellulitis
- The duration of treatment should be 14 days in invasive infection.

ALTERNATIVE TREATMENT
- Doxycycline
- Third-generation cephalosporin
- Ofloxacin
- Chloramphenicol
- Trimethoprim-sulfamethoxazole

PREVENTION
- Avoid animal bites and scratches.
- Promptly clean, irrigate, and debride (if needed) areas of animal bites and scratches.
- Antibiotic prophylaxis may be given after an animal bite, but data to support its use are lacking.

Pediculus and *Phthirus* Species (Lice)

GENERA *Pediculus/Phthirus*

SPECIES
- *Pediculus humanus capitis*
- *Pediculus humanus corporis*
- *Phthirus pubis*

MICROBIOLOGIC CHARACTERISTICS
- Lice

INCUBATION PERIOD
- The life cycles of *Pediculus* and *Phthirus* species are composed of three stages: eggs, nymphs, and adults. Under optimal temperature conditions, the eggs hatch in 7 to 10 days, and the nymphal stage lasts about 7 to 13 days.
- The egg-to-egg cycle lasts about 3 weeks.

EPIDEMIOLOGY
- Worldwide distribution
- More common in populations with poor personal hygiene

INFECTIONS
- *Pediculus humanus capitis* causes head lice and is found on the hair, eyelashes, and eyebrows.
- *Pediculus humanus corporis* causes body lice.
- *Phthirus pubis* (crab lice) causes infestation on the pubic hair. In cases of heavy infestation, *P. pubis* may be found on the facial hair, axillae, and body surfaces.
- Both *Pediculus* and *Phthirus* species may cause severe itching.
- Local lymphadenitis may be caused from secondary bacterial infection.

DIAGNOSIS
- Finding and examination of the parasite

TREATMENT
- Head and pubic lice: 1% pyrethrin cream rinse or 1% gamma benzene hexachloride lotion. Retreatment may be necessary 7 to 10 days after the first treatment (if eggs of the parasite survive).
- Body lice: Clothing and bedding should be washed with the hot-water cycle of an automatic washing machine or dusted with pediculicides.

PREVENTION
- Regular inspection of children (by direct examination)
- Effective, prompt treatment of patients with lice
- Avoidance of physical contact with infected individuals

Microorganisms

Pediococcus Species

GENUS Pediococcus

SPECIES
- P. acidilactici
- P. pentosaceus

MICROBIOLOGIC CHARACTERISTICS
- Aerobic, gram-positive coccus
- May be confused with *Leuconostoc* species

INCUBATION PERIOD
- Unknown

EPIDEMIOLOGY
- Worldwide

INFECTIONS
- Isolates of *Pediococcus* have been traditionally considered contaminants.
- However, recent data support the pathogenic role of *Pediococcus* species, especially in immunosuppressed patients.
- Bacteremia
- Respiratory tract infections

DIAGNOSIS
- Culture

TREATMENT
- Penicillin G
- Ampicillin

ALTERNATIVE TREATMENT
- Aminoglycoside
- Imipenem

Penicillium Species

GENUS Penicillium

SPECIES
- P. chrysogenum
- P. commune
- P. marneffei
- Others

MICROBIOLOGIC CHARACTERISTICS
- Filamentous fungus (mold), with septate hyaline hyphae

INCUBATION PERIOD
- Unknown

EPIDEMIOLOGY
- *P. marneffei* is a common cause of infection in the Far East.

INFECTIONS
- It has been traditionally considered a contaminant.
- However, recent data support a pathogenic role for *Penicillium* species.
- *P. marneffei* usually causes disseminated infection in immunosuppressed patients.
- *Penicillium* species also may cause infection in several organs, including the heart valves (endocarditis), the cornea (keratitis), external ear (otitis externa), and the respiratory and urinary tract systems.
- *P. marneffei* has caused a significant number of infections in patients with AIDS in southern Asia.

DIAGNOSIS
- Culture
- Finding the fungus in tissue biopsies

TREATMENT
- Amphotericin B i.v. is the recommended agent for severe *Penicillium* infections.

ALTERNATIVE TREATMENT
- Itraconazole in a high dose (at least 400 mg/d) is also effective.
- Patients with AIDS and continued severe immunosuppression should receive preventive treatment with itraconazole after an episode of *Penicillium* infection.

Peptococcus niger

GENUS Peptococcus

SPECIES
- P. niger

MICROBIOLOGIC CHARACTERISTICS
- Anaerobic, gram-positive coccus
- Usually an endogenous infection: *P. niger* is part of the normal human bowel flora.

EPIDEMIOLOGY
- A frequent isolate in mixed infections (due to anaerobic and aerobic bacteria)
- Worldwide

INFECTIONS
- *P. niger* is isolated from patients with mixed infections, such as intraabdominal, pelvic, brain, and lung abscesses.
- It also may cause bacteremia of unclear etiology.
- The pathogen also may cause skin and subcutaneous tissue infections.

DIAGNOSIS
- Culture under anaerobic conditions, which may require prolonged intubation for growth of the pathogen.

TREATMENT
- Penicillin G

ALTERNATIVE TREATMENT
- Clindamycin
- Cephamycin
- Carbapenem (imipenem or meropenem)
- Vancomycin
- Piperacillin–tazobactam

Microorganisms

Peptostreptococcus Species

GENUS Peptostreptococcus

SPECIES
- *P. anaerobius*
- *P. asaccharolyticus*
- *P. magnus*
- *P. prevotii*
- Others

MICROBIOLOGIC CHARACTERISTICS
- Anaerobic, gram-positive coccus

INCUBATION PERIOD
- Usually a cause of endogenous infection

EPIDEMIOLOGY
- Part of the normal human bowel flora
- Worldwide distribution

INFECTIONS
- The pathogen is sometimes isolated from specimens of patients with mixed infections, such as intraabdominal, pelvic, lung, and brain abscess.
- Rare cause of endocarditis
- Bacteremia
- Skin and subcutaneous tissue infection
- Surgical wound infections
- Septic arthritis

DIAGNOSIS
- Culture under anaerobic conditions.

TREATMENT
- Penicillin G

ALTERNATIVE TREATMENT
- Clindamycin
- Cephamycin
- Carbapenem (imipenem or meropenem)
- Vancomycin

Phialophora Species

See "Chromomycosis Agents"

Phthirus pubis

See "*Pediculus* and *Phthirus* species"

Piedraia hortae

GENUS Piedraia

SPECIES
- *P. hortae*

MICROBIOLOGIC CHARACTERISTICS
- A fungus
- Hyphae are closely septate, dark, and thick walled.

INCUBATION PERIOD
- Unknown

EPIDEMIOLOGY
- Mainly seen in tropical countries

INFECTIONS
- *P. hortae* causes black piedra, an infection seen most commonly in the tropics.
- Black piedra is manifested by small, gritty, dark nodules along the hair shafts.
- Black piedra should be differentiated from white piedra, which is manifested by soft, pasty nodules on the hair shafts and is caused by *Trichosporon beigelii*.

DIAGNOSIS
- Finding the fungus (microscopic examination of the lesions)
- Culture of the fungus

TREATMENT
- Shaving of the affected area

ALTERNATIVE TREATMENT
- Terbinafine 250 mg/d PO for 6 weeks

Plasmodium Species

See Section II, "Malaria"

Pleistophora Species

See "Microsporidia"

Microorganisms

Plesiomonas shigelloides

GENUS Plesiomonas
SPECIES
- P. shigelloides

MICROBIOLOGIC CHARACTERISTICS
- Aerobic, gram-negative bacillus

INCUBATION PERIOD
- The exact incubation period is unclear. Evidence from patients with traveler's diarrhea supports a short incubation period (a few days).

EPIDEMIOLOGY
- Ubiquitous freshwater and soil inhabitant

INFECTIONS
- P. shigelloides may cause diarrhea of different degrees of severity, from mild self-limited disease to severe, bloody diarrhea with fever, malaise, and white blood cells in stool specimens.
- The pathogen also may rarely cause bacteremia, skin and subcutaneous tissue infection, septic arthritis, osteomyelitis, cholecystitis, endophthalmitis, and meningitis, especially in neonates.
- It is one of the causes of traveler's diarrhea.

DIAGNOSIS
- Culture

TREATMENT
- Fluoroquinolone

ALTERNATIVE TREATMENT
- Chloramphenicol
- Trimethoprim–sulfamethoxazole
- Carbapenems
- Aminoglycosides

Pneumocystis carinii

See Section II, "*Pneumocystis carinii* Infection"

Poliomyelitis Virus

See Section II, "Poliomyelitis"

Polyomaviruses

See Section II, "Progressive Multifocal Leukoencephalopathy"

Porphyromonas Species

GENUS Porphyromonas
SPECIES
- P. asaccharolytica
- P. endodontalis
- P. gingivalis
- P. salivosa

MICROBIOLOGIC CHARACTERISTICS
- Anaerobic, gram-negative bacillus
- *Porphyromonas* species were classified previously in the genus *Bacteroides*.

INCUBATION PERIOD
- Usually an endogenous infection

EPIDEMIOLOGY
- *Porphyromonas* species are part of the normal human flora of the mouth, bowel, and vagina.

INFECTIONS
- *Porphyromonas* species are isolated from mixed aerobic and anaerobic bacterial infections, such as intraabdominal, pelvic, brain, and lung abscesses, as well as empyema.
- *Porphyromonas* species also may cause root canal, periodontal, and oropharyngeal infections.
- Rare cause of bacteremia
- It may be associated with infections due to human bites.
- Skin and subcutaneous tissue infections, including diabetic foot infections

DIAGNOSIS
- Culture under anaerobic conditions.

TREATMENT
- Clindamycin or metronidazole

ALTERNATIVE TREATMENT
- Penicillin
- Amoxicillin
- Ticarcillin–clavulanate
- Piperacillin–tazobactam
- Chloramphenicol
- Carbapenem (imipenem or meropenem)

Prevotella Species

GENUS Prevotella
SPECIES
- P. bivia
- P. buccae
- P. buccalis
- P. corporis
- P. denticola
- P. disiens
- P. heparinolytica
- P. intermedia
- P. loescheii
- P. melaninogenica
- P. nigrescens
- P. oralis
- P. oulorum
- P. pallens
- Others

MICROBIOLOGIC CHARACTERISTICS
- Anaerobic, gram-negative bacillus
- *Prevotella* species were classified previously in the *Bacteroides* genus.

INCUBATION PERIOD
- Usually an endogenous infection

EPIDEMIOLOGY
- *Prevotella* species are part of the normal human flora (oral, bowel, and vagina).

INFECTIONS
- Lung, intraabdominal, brain abscess
- Dental infections
- Pelvic infections (mainly P. disiens and P. bivia)
- Human bite infections
- Skin and subcutaneous tissue infection including diabetic foot infections
- Surgical wound infections

DIAGNOSIS
- Culture under anaerobic conditions.

TREATMENT
- Clindamycin or metronidazole

ALTERNATIVE TREATMENT
- Amoxicillin
- Ampicillin–sulbactam
- Piperacillin–tazobactam
- Ticarcillin–clavulanate
- Chloramphenicol
- Cefoxitin
- Cefotetan
- Carbapenem (imipenem or meropenem)

Microorganisms

Prions

GENUS N/A
SPECIES
- N/A

MICROBIOLOGIC CHARACTERISTICS
- Prions are thought to be proteinaceous material.
- Although they lack nucleic acid, it seems that they really have an infectious capability.

INCUBATION PERIOD
- The incubation period is unknown, but it seems that it is long (at least a few years).
- Cases of a variant of Creutzfeldt-Jakob disease have recently caused considerable concern in Europe.

INFECTIONS
- Kuru
- Creutzfeldt-Jakob disease (sporadic and familial, including the variant possibly related to the agent of bovine spongiform encephalopathy [BSE]) and Gerstmann-Straussler syndrome
- Insomnia secondary to thalamic destruction
- Slow encephalopathy with a very prolonged incubation, scant inflammatory reaction and spongiform changes, and progressive, relentless deterioration and death

DIAGNOSIS
- Direct visualization of the infectious proteinaceous particles using electron microscopy

TREATMENT
- There is no effective treatment.

Propionibacterium propionicus

See Section II, "Actinomycosis"

Propionibacterium Species

GENUS *Propionibacterium*
SPECIES
- *P. ances*
- Others

MICROBIOLOGIC CHARACTERISTICS
- Anaerobic, gram-positive bacillus

INCUBATION PERIOD
- Unknown (usually an endogenous infection from the patient's flora)

EPIDEMIOLOGY
- *Propionibacterium* species are part of the normal human flora (mainly skin).

INFECTIONS
- Acne
- Infection related to prosthetic material, including arthroplasty materials, prosthetic heart valves, and shunt for the cerebrospinal fluid
- Meningitis, especially after neurosurgical procedures
- Bacteremia

DIAGNOSIS
- Culture (anaerobic)

TREATMENT
- Tetracycline or a macrolide

ALTERNATIVE TREATMENT
- Trimethoprim–sulfamethoxazole
- Vancomycin
- The pathogen is resistant to metronidazole.

PREVENTION
- Good antiseptic techniques during surgery

Proteus Species

GENUS *Proteus*
SPECIES
- *P. mirabilis*
- *P. myxofaciens*
- *P. penneri*
- *P. vulgaris*

MICROBIOLOGIC CHARACTERISTICS
- Aerobic, gram-negative bacillus

INCUBATION PERIOD
- Usually an endogenous infection

EPIDEMIOLOGY
- Worldwide distribution
- Part of the normal human bowel flora
- Common cause of infection

INFECTIONS
- *Proteus* species are a common cause of urinary tract infection, especially in patients with nephrolithiasis.
- The pathogen also has been isolated frequently from specimens of abscesses from various anatomic sites.
- Bacteremia

DIAGNOSIS
- Culture

TREATMENT
- Amoxicillin–clavulanate
- Fluoroquinolone

ALTERNATIVE TREATMENT
- Second- or third-generation cephalosporins
- Aztreonam
- Carbapenem (meropenem or imipenem)
- Ureidopenicillins
- Trimethoprim–sulfamethoxazole
- Aminoglycoside

Protomonas Species

See "Methylobacterium species"

Prototheca Species

GENUS *Prototheca*
SPECIES
- *P. stagnora*
- *P. wickerhamii*
- *P. zopfii*

MICROBIOLOGIC CHARACTERISTICS
- *Prototheca* species are unicellular, achloric algae that grow in a fungus medium as a yeast.
- It reproduces by endosporulation.

EPIDEMIOLOGY
- *Prototheca* organisms are found in several environmental sites, including foodstuffs, sewage, soil, fresh and marine water, tree slime, and so on.

INFECTIONS
- Several cases of *Prototheca* infections have been reported from around the world.
- The best-described clinical syndrome caused by *Prototheca* species is a skin and subcutaneous infection manifested by a single, painless, plaque or papulonodular lesion that sometimes ulcerates.
- A few cases of olecranon bursitis have also been reported.
- Rare cause of other infections, such as peritonitis in patients on continuous ambulatory peritoneal dialysis and meningitis in patients with AIDS

DIAGNOSIS
- Culture
- Finding the pathogen in pathology specimens of lesions

TREATMENT
- Amphotericin B i.v.

ALTERNATIVE TREATMENT
- Ketoconazole or itraconazole

Microorganisms

Providencia Species

GENUS Providencia

SPECIES
- P. alcalifaciens
- P. rettgeri
- P. rustigianii
- P. stuartii
- Others

MICROBIOLOGIC CHARACTERISTICS
- Aerobic, gram-negative bacillus

INCUBATION PERIOD
- Usually an endogenous infection

INFECTIONS
- *Providencia* species may cause infection in several sites, including the urinary tract, intraabdominal infection, central venous catheter-related infections, and bacteremia of an unclear primary source.
- The pathogen has been recognized as an important cause of nosocomial infections.

DIAGNOSIS
- Culture of the pathogen

TREATMENT
- Carbapenem (meropenem, imipenem)
- Ciprofloxacin

ALTERNATIVE TREATMENT
- Third-generation cephalosporin
- Aztreonam
- Ofloxacin
- Piperacillin-tazobactam
- Aminoglycoside

Pseudallescheria boydii

GENUS Pseudallescheria

SPECIES
- P. boydii

MICROBIOLOGIC CHARACTERISTICS
- Filamentous fungus (mold), with septate hyaline hyphae
- Fungal aggregates (granules) *in vivo* (mycetoma)
- Septate hyaline hyphae in hyalohyphomycosis

INCUBATION PERIOD
- Unknown

EPIDEMIOLOGY
- Worldwide distribution
- Mycetomas are seen more commonly in the tropics.

INFECTIONS
- *P. boydii* has been recognized recently as an important opportunistic pathogen, causing a variety of infections.
- The fungus is one of the causes of mycetoma, which is manifested by slowly growing, tumor-like skin and subcutaneous tissue lesions. Mycetoma lesions may drain granular pus through sinuses.
- Mycetomas may be caused by a variety of fungal species, as well as *Nocardia* and *Actinomyces* species.
- Mycetoma lesions usually appear on the feet and hands. However, they may occur on any exposed part of the body.
- Manifestations of *P. boydii* infections in sites other than the skin are similar to those of *Aspergillus* (clinical manifestations, histopathology findings, and appearance of hyphae).
- *P. boydii* also may cause the following:
  —Osteomyelitis
  —Brain abscess
  —Meningitis
  —Eye infections
  —Pneumonia
  —Sinusitis
  —Endocarditis
  —Fungal balls in various sites
  —Disseminated infection

DIAGNOSIS
- The granules of pus drained through mycetoma lesions contain fungal elements of various shapes.
- Culture of the fungus
- Identification of the fungus in tissue biopsy specimens

TREATMENT
- There are limited published data for the treatment of *P. boydii* infections
- Amphotericin B does not seem to be effective for this fungus.
- Azoles: High doses of itraconazole, miconazole, or ketoconazole are recommended.

Pseudomonas aeruginosa

See Section II, "*Pseudomonas* Infections/Melioidosis/Glanders"

Psychrobacter Immobilis

GENUS Psychrobacter

SPECIES
- P. immobilis

MICROBIOLOGIC CHARACTERISTICS
- Gram-negative coccobacillus
- The classification of pathogens, which may belong to the genus *Psychrobacter* or similar genera, is incomplete.

INCUBATION PERIOD
- Unknown

EPIDEMIOLOGY
- *P. immobilis* has been isolated from food.

INFECTIONS
- Isolated from blood, urine, and wound specimens
- There are only a few reports of disease due to *P. immobilis*.

DIAGNOSIS
- Culture

TREATMENT
- There are not enough published data to make solid recommendations.
- Selection of antimicrobial agents should be based on *in vitro* susceptibility results.

Microorganisms

Rabies Virus

See Section II, "Rabies"

Respiratory Syncytial Virus

See Section II, "Respiratory Syncytial Virus Infection"

Rhinocladiella aquaspera

See "Chromomycosis Agents"

Rhinosporidium seeberi

GENUS Rhinosporidium
SPECIES
- R. seeberi

MICROBIOLOGIC CHARACTERISTICS
- Sporangia containing sporangiospores (biopsy material)
- Large, round sporangia
- Mature sporangia may contain both immature and mature spores.

EPIDEMIOLOGY
- Worldwide distribution (rare infection)

INFECTIONS
- Rhinosporidiosis, which is manifested by chronic, usually painless nasal or conjunctival lesions that resemble polyps

DIAGNOSIS
- Finding the characteristic sporangia in tissue biopsies

TREATMENT
- Surgical resection of the nasal or conjunctival polyps
- Lesions may recur after surgical management.

ALTERNATIVE TREATMENT
- The efficacy of antifungal treatment is unknown.

Rhinovirus

GROUP Rhinovirus
SPECIES
- N/A

MICROBIOLOGIC CHARACTERISTICS
- Single-stranded, positive RNA virus
- There are more than 100 recognized serotypes of rhinovirus.

INCUBATION PERIOD
- Usually 2 to 3 days (range, 12 hours to 5 days)

EPIDEMIOLOGY
- Worldwide distribution

INFECTIONS
- Common cold

DIAGNOSIS
- Cell culture
- Efforts for a specific diagnosis of the virologic cause of the common cold are not warranted in clinical practice.

TREATMENT
- Symptomatic

PREVENTION
- When possible, avoid crowded areas.
- Frequent handwashing
- Covering the mouth when coughing and sneezing
- Sanitary disposal of nasal and oral secretions

Rhizomucor Species

See Section II, "Mucormycosis"

Rhizopus Species

See Section II, "Mucormycosis"

Microorganisms

Rhodococcus Species

GENUS Rhodococcus

SPECIES
- R. aurantiacus
- R. bronchialis
- R. equi (the most important species for infection in humans)
- R. erythropolis
- R. luteus
- R. rhodochrous
- R. rubropertinctus

MICROBIOLOGIC CHARACTERISTICS
- Aerobic, gram-positive bacilli
- It may be acid-fast stain–positive.
- Intracellular pathogen

EPIDEMIOLOGY
- Worldwide, rare infection

INFECTIONS
- R. equi has been isolated more frequently during the past two decades than previously. This is because the microorganism may be the cause of opportunistic infections manifested in patients with immunosuppression.
- R. equi causes mainly pulmonary infection.
- However, the pathogen has been isolated from clinical specimens of patients with a variety of infections, including the following:
  —Brain abscess
  —Osteomyelitis
  —Prostatic abscess
  —Bacteremia
  —Lymphadenitis
  —Endophthalmitis
  —Intraabdominal infections
- Pneumonia due to R. equi may take an acute, subacute, or chronic course. It may resemble tuberculosis, nocardiosis, and actinomycosis, because it may cause cavitations in the upper lung lobes.
- Isolation of R. equi from a clinical specimen should lead to an investigation for possible cellular immunity dysfunction of the patient, especially due to HIV infection.
- Rhodococcus species other than R. equi are usually associated with surgical infections.

DIAGNOSIS
- Culture of the pathogen

TREATMENT
- Vancomycin 2 g i.v. qd
- Erythromycin 500 mg PO qid with rifampicin 600 mg qd
- Ciprofloxacin 750 mg PO bid
- Imipenem 0.5 g i.v. q6h
- Treatment should be given for 4 weeks.

ALTERNATIVE TREATMENT
- Azithromycin

PREVENTION
- Avoid severe immunosuppression related to advanced HIV infection with the use of highly active antiretroviral treatment in patients with HIV infection.

Rhodotorula Species

GENUS Rhodotorula

SPECIES
- R. glutinis
- R. rubra

MICROBIOLOGIC CHARACTERISTICS
- Yeast
- Rapid growth (mature in 4 days)
- In culture, budding cells (round or oval) and few rudimentary pseudohyphae are seen.

INCUBATION PERIOD
- Unknown

EPIDEMIOLOGY
- Worldwide

INFECTIONS
- Rhodotorula species are usually contaminants of cultures.
- However, there is increasing evidence supporting a pathogenic role of Rhodotorula species, especially in immunocompromised hosts.
- Rhodotorula species may cause several infections, including fungemia, especially in patients with central venous catheters, peritonitis in patients on chronic ambulatory peritoneal dialysis, and endocarditis.

DIAGNOSIS
- Culture
- Histopathology

TREATMENT
- Amphotericin B 0.7 mg/kg/d i.v., with or without flucytosine

Rickettsia Species

GENUS Rickettsia

SPECIES
- R. akari
- R. australis
- R. conorii
- R. mooseri
- R. orientalis
- R. prowazekii
- R. rickettsii
- R. sibirica
- R. tsutsugamushi
- R. typhi

MICROBIOLOGIC CHARACTERISTICS
- Small, intracellular coccobacilli

INCUBATION PERIOD
- Depends on the specific Rickettsia species
- It is 3 to 14 days for R. rickettsii, the cause of Rocky Mountain spotted fever.
- Incubation period for other Rickettsia species:
  —R. conori: usually 5 to 7 days
  —R. sibirica: 2 to 7 days
  —R. australis: usually 7 to 10 days

EPIDEMIOLOGY
- Common cause of human infections

INFECTIONS
- Rickettsia species cause several infections, with various manifestations.
- R. rickettsii: Rocky mountain spotted fever (discussed in detail elsewhere in this book)

Microorganisms

- *R. conorii:* Boutonneuse fever (Mediterranean spotted fever, India tick typhus, African tick typhus), which is manifested frequently by fever, a primary lesion at the site of a tick bite, which ulcerates and has a black center, regional lymphadenopathy (not always present), and, later, a generalized maculopapular erythematous rash.
- *R. australis:* Queensland tick typhus (similar manifestations with *R. conorii*)
- *R. sibirica:* North Asian tick fever (similar manifestations with *R. conorii*)
- *R. akari:* rickettsialpox (transmitted to humans by mite bites and manifested with disseminated vesicular skin rash generally not involving the soles and palms, fever, and lymphadenopathy)
- *R. prowazekii:* louse-borne typhus, classic typhus fever
- *R. typhi* (*R. mooseri*): flea-borne typhus, endemic typhus fever
- *R. tsutsugamushi* (*R. orientalis*): scrub typhus

DIAGNOSIS
- Serology

TREATMENT
- Doxycycline 100 mg PO q12h for 7 days

ALTERNATIVE TREATMENT
- Chloramphenicol

PREVENTION
- Avoid tick bites (for tick-borne rickettsial infections)

Rotavirus, Human

GROUP Rotavirus

SPECIES
- N/A

MICROBIOLOGIC CHARACTERISTICS
- RNA virus that belongs to the Reoviridae family

INCUBATION PERIOD
- The incubation period is usually from 1 to 3 days.

EPIDEMIOLOGY
- Worldwide distribution
- Clinically apparent infections appear in infants and young children.

INFECTIONS
- Rotavirus causes gastroenteritis, which may be sporadic or seasonal and is manifested by fever, vomiting, and watery diarrhea.
- The infection may lead to severe dehydration, especially in infants and young children.

DIAGNOSIS
- Rotavirus antigen detection in stool specimens
- Direct visualization of the virus with electron microscopy
- Molecular biology tests

TREATMENT
- Symptomatic

ALTERNATIVE TREATMENT
- There is no specific antiviral treatment.

PREVENTION
- Effective preventive measures have not been determined.
- The efficacy of hygienic measures applicable to other infectious diseases that are transmitted via the fecal–oral route has not been established. However, these measures should be taken in all diarrheal diseases.

Rothia dentocariosa

GENUS Rothia

SPECIES
- *R. dentocariosa*

MICROBIOLOGIC CHARACTERISTICS
- Aerobic, pleomorphic, gram-positive bacillus

INCUBATION PERIOD
- Unknown

EPIDEMIOLOGY
- Worldwide

INFECTIONS
- Endocarditis
- It is implicated in the pathogenesis of dental caries.
- Periodontal disease and abscesses

DIAGNOSIS
- Culture

TREATMENT
- Penicillin with aminoglycosides in endocarditis

ALTERNATIVE TREATMENT
- Cephalosporin
- Erythromycin
- Aminoglycosides

Rubella Virus

See Section II, "Rubella (German Measles)"

Microorganisms

Saccharomyces cerevisiae

GENUS Saccharomyces

SPECIES
- S. cerevisiae

MICROBIOLOGIC CHARACTERISTICS
- Yeast
- Rapid growth

INCUBATION PERIOD
- Unknown

EPIDEMIOLOGY
- Worldwide distribution

INFECTIONS
- *S. cerevisiae* traditionally has been considered a nonpathogenic fungal organism.
- However, recent data support its pathogenicity, especially in immunocompromised patients, including those with advanced HIV infection.
- *S. cerevisiae* may cause fungemia in patients with central venous catheters, peritonitis in patients on chronic ambulatory peritoneal dialysis, septic arthritis, respiratory tract infection, and vaginitis.

DIAGNOSIS
- Culture

TREATMENT
- Amphotericin B intravenously for systemic infections
- Topical azole treatment for patients with vaginitis

Saksenaea vasiformis

GENUS Saksenaea

SPECIES
- S. vasiformis

MICROBIOLOGIC CHARACTERISTICS
- Filamentous fungus (mold), with nonseptate hyaline hyphae

INCUBATION PERIOD
- Unknown

EPIDEMIOLOGY
- The usual way of transmission of the fungus to humans is via traumatic inoculation.

INFECTIONS
- An occasional cause of zygomycosis manifested by rhinocerebral, cutaneous, subcutaneous, bone, and lung lesions
- Surgical wound infections

DIAGNOSIS
- Culture
- Histopathology

TREATMENT
- Amphotericin B intravenously is the recommended treatment.

ALTERNATIVE TREATMENT
- Itraconazole

Salmonella Species

See Section II, "Typhoid Fever"

Sarcocystis Species

GENUS Sarcocystis

SPECIES
- S. bovihominis
- S. suihominis

MICROBIOLOGIC CHARACTERISTICS
- A protozoon with characteristics similar to those of *Isospora* belli

INCUBATION PERIOD
- Unclear

EPIDEMIOLOGY
- Worldwide distribution
- However, most cases are reported from Southeast Asia.

INFECTIONS
- Muscular sarcocystosis, which is usually an asymptomatic infection but may occasionally be manifested with myalgias and muscle swelling.
- Mild intestinal disease

DIAGNOSIS
- Parasitologic examination of stool specimens

TREATMENT
- Not available

ALTERNATIVE TREATMENT
- Furazolidone may be tried.

Sarcoptes scabiei

See Section II, "Scabies"

Scedosporium prolificans

GENUS Scedosporium

SPECIES
- S. prolificans

MICROBIOLOGIC CHARACTERISTICS
- Filamentous fungus (mold) with septate hyaline hyphae
- Formerly called *Scedosporium inflatum*
- Growth is inhibited by cycloheximide.

INCUBATION PERIOD
- Unknown

EPIDEMIOLOGY
- Worldwide distribution

INFECTIONS
- It may cause invasive infection (usually arthritis and/or osteomyelitis, but it may affect various organs).
- Asymptomatic colonization with the fungus may occur.

DIAGNOSIS
- Culture
- Histopathology

TREATMENT
- Amphotericin B intravenously

ALTERNATIVE TREATMENT
- Azoles

Schistosoma Species

See Section II, "Schistosomiasis"

Microorganisms

Scopulariopsis Species

GENUS *Scopulariopsis*

SPECIES
- *S. brevicaulis*
- *S. brumptii*
- Others

MICROBIOLOGIC CHARACTERISTICS
- Filamentous fungus (mold)

INCUBATION PERIOD
- Unknown

EPIDEMIOLOGY
- Worldwide distribution

INFECTIONS
- Onychomycosis
- Locally invasive disease (otitis externa) and disseminated disease in neutropenic patients
- Cutaneous lesions in patients with advanced HIV infection

TREATMENT
- Chemical nail removal with 40% urea for patients with onychomycosis

ALTERNATIVE TREATMENT
- Surgical removal of the affected nail(s)
- There are limited data about the efficacy antifungal agents.
- Amphotericin B intravenously for invasive infections

Septata intestinalis

See "Microsporidia"

Serratia Species

GENUS *Serratia*

SPECIES
- *S. ficaria*
- *S. fonticola*
- *S. grimesii*
- *S. liquefaciens*
- *S. marcescens*
- *S. odorifera*
- *S. plymuthica*
- *S. rubidaea*
- Others

MICROBIOLOGIC CHARACTERISTICS
- Aerobic, gram-negative bacilli

INCUBATION PERIOD
- Usually an endogenous infection

EPIDEMIOLOGY
- Worldwide distribution
- Intravenous drug users are at risk for infection due to *Serratia* species.

INFECTIONS
- *Serratia* species have been isolated more frequently during the past two decades than previously.
- A common cause of nosocomial infection of various sites (bacteremia, urinary tract infections, respiratory tract infections, intraabdominal infections)

DIAGNOSIS
- Culture

TREATMENT
- Carbapenem (imipenem, meropenem)
- Ciprofloxacin

ALTERNATIVE TREATMENT
- Third-generation cephalosporin
- Aztreonam
- Ureidopenicillins
- Aminoglycosides
- Ofloxacin
- Trimethoprim–sulfamethoxazole

Shigella Species

See Section II, "Shigellosis"

Smallpox Virus

GROUP Orthopoxvirus

SPECIES
- N/A

MICROBIOLOGIC CHARACTERISTICS
- A DNA virus

INCUBATION PERIOD
- About 12 days

EPIDEMIOLOGY
- Smallpox (variola) has been eradicated. The last reported case of smallpox was in October 1977 in Somalia.
- Smallpox virus is held under tight security in two research laboratories (one in Atlanta, Georgia, and another in Koltsovo, Russia).

INFECTIONS
- Smallpox

DIAGNOSIS
- Cell culture
- Serology

TREATMENT
- Metisazone

PREVENTION
- Smallpox vaccine: Currently no vaccination is required because the infection has been eradicated.

Microorganisms

Sphingobacterium Species

GENUS Sphingobacterium
SPECIES
- S. multivorum
- S. spiritivorum
- Others

MICROBIOLOGIC CHARACTERISTICS
- Aerobic, gram-negative bacillus

INCUBATION PERIOD
- Unknown

EPIDEMIOLOGY
- Rare cause of infections (worldwide)
- Sphingobacterium species usually cause nosocomial infections.

INFECTIONS
- Peritonitis
- Bacteremia
- Respiratory tract infections
- Urinary tract infections

DIAGNOSIS
- Culture

TREATMENT
- Ampicillin

ALTERNATIVE TREATMENT
- Trimethoprim–sulfamethoxazole

Spirillum minus (minor)

GENUS Spirillum
SPECIES
- S. minus (minor)

MICROBIOLOGIC CHARACTERISTICS
- Aerobic, gram-negative bacillus

INCUBATION PERIOD
- One to 3 weeks

EPIDEMIOLOGY
- Worldwide distribution (rare in the United States)
- More common in Asia, especially in Japan

INFECTIONS
- Rat-bite fever (sodoku)
- The case fatality rate for untreated cases is about 10%.

DIAGNOSIS
- Does not grow in cultures
- Isolation after inoculation to animals
- A Giemsa or Wright stain or dark-field microscopy of peripheral blood samples may reveal the pathogen.

TREATMENT
- Procaine penicillin G 600,000 IU i.m. q12h for 10 to 14 days

ALTERNATIVE TREATMENT
- Doxycycline
- Streptomycin

Spirometra Species

GENUS Spirometra
SPECIES
- S. spargana
- S. mansonoides

MICROBIOLOGIC CHARACTERISTICS
- A cestode helminth
- The developmental stage found in humans is the larval cyst.
- The source of transmission to human is cysts from infected copepods, frogs, and snakes.

EPIDEMIOLOGY
- Most cases have been reported from Southeast Asia and Africa.

INFECTIONS
- Sparganosis (localized inflammatory edema)

DIAGNOSIS
- Parasitologic examination

TREATMENT
- Surgery

Sporobolomyces Species

GENUS Sporobolomyces
SPECIES
- S. holsaticus
- S. roseus
- S. salmonicolor

MICROBIOLOGIC CHARACTERISTICS
- Yeast

INCUBATION PERIOD
- Unknown

EPIDEMIOLOGY
- Most commonly isolated from environmental sources

INFECTIONS
- Rare cause of infections in humans (usually mycetoma)
- It may cause systemic infection in immunocompromised patients, including those with advanced HIV infection.

DIAGNOSIS
- Culture

TREATMENT
- Amphotericin B intravenously for systemic infection

Sporothrix schenckii

See Section II, "Sporotrichosis"

Microorganisms

Staphylococcus Species

GENUS Staphylococcus

SPECIES
- S. aureus
- S. capitis
- S. cohnii
- S. epidermidis
- S. galinarum
- S. haemolyticus
- S. hominis
- S. intermedius
- S. lugdunensis
- S. warneri
- S. xylosus
- Others

MICROBIOLOGIC CHARACTERISTICS
- Aerobic, gram-positive coccus
- *Staphylococcus* species are classified into two main categories:
  —Coagulase-positive (mainly *S. aureus*)
  —Coagulase-negative (most *Staphylococcus* species, including S. epidermidis)

INCUBATION PERIOD
- The incubation period for staphylococcal infections is highly variable.

EPIDEMIOLOGY
- Worldwide distribution

INFECTIONS
- *Staphylococcus* species are a common cause of human infections of practically all body sites.
- Among all *Staphylococcus* species, *S. aureus* and *S. epidermidis* are the most common isolates from clinical specimens.
- The incidence of staphylococcal infections has increased considerably recently, partly because of the frequent use of central venous catheters.
- *S. aureus* tends to cause abscesses in several sites.
- *Staphylococcus* species are a common cause of endocarditis.

DIAGNOSIS
- Culture

TREATMENT
- Antistaphylococcal penicillins (e.g., oxacillin, nafcillin, or cloxacillin) are the best drugs for *Staphylococcus* species sensitive to methicillin.
- However, a big proportion of coagulase-negative *Staphylococcus* species and a considerable proportion of *S. aureus* strains are resistant to methicillin.
- A glycopeptide (vancomycin or teicoplanin) may be needed to treat infections due to these strains.

Stenotrophomonas Species

GENUS Stenotrophomonas

SPECIES
- S. africana
- S. maltophilia

MICROBIOLOGIC CHARACTERISTICS
- Aerobic, gram-negative bacillus

INCUBATION PERIOD
- Unclear

EPIDEMIOLOGY
- Worldwide distribution
- An important cause of nosocomial infections, especially in patients who received antibiotics for prolonged periods

INFECTIONS
- Bacteremia
- Pneumonia
- Skin and soft-tissue infections

DIAGNOSIS
- Culture

TREATMENT
- Trimethoprim–sulfamethoxazole
- Infections due to *Stenotrophomonas* species have been found to have considerable mortality.

ALTERNATIVE TREATMENT
- Ceftazidime
- Ciprofloxacin
- Minocycline
- Piperacillin–tazobactam
- Ticarcillin and aztreonam–clavulanate
- *S. maltophilia* strains are resistant to carbapenems and aztreonam.

Stomatococcus mucilaginosus

GENUS Stomatococcus

SPECIES
- S. mucilaginosus

MICROBIOLOGIC CHARACTERISTICS
- Aerobic, gram-positive coccus

EPIDEMIOLOGY
- Worldwide, rare infection

INFECTIONS
- Bacteremia associated with central venous catheters
- Oral mucositis in patients with neutropenia, especially those receiving antibiotics for intestinal decontamination
- Endocarditis

DIAGNOSIS
- Culture

TREATMENT
- Vancomycin

ALTERNATIVE TREATMENT
- Penicillin G or a macrolide

Microorganisms

Streptobacillus moniliformis

GENUS Streptobacillus
SPECIES
- S. moniliformis

MICROBIOLOGIC CHARACTERISTICS
- Aerobic, pleomorphic, gram-negative bacillus

INCUBATION PERIOD
- Three to 10 days, sometimes longer

EPIDEMIOLOGY
- Worldwide distribution
- Rare cause of infection in North America and Europe
- Most patients with infection report a rat bite.

INFECTIONS
- Rat-bite fever (Haverhill fever or streptobacillosis). It is manifested by fever, headache, and malaise, followed by a maculopapular rash.
- Untreated patients with streptobacillosis may develop endocarditis, pericarditis, tenosynovitis, and abscesses in several organs, including the brain.

DIAGNOSIS
- Culture in specific medium.
- Serology

TREATMENT
- Procaine penicillin G 600,000 IU i.m. q12h for 10 to 14 days
- Higher doses of penicillin must be used in patients with endocarditis or other focal infection.

ALTERNATIVE TREATMENT
- Doxycycline

Streptococcus agalactiae (Group B)

GENUS Streptococcus
SPECIES
- S. agalactiae (group B)

MICROBIOLOGIC CHARACTERISTICS
- Aerobic, gram-positive coccus

INCUBATION PERIOD
- The incubation period of early-onset neonatal disease is less than 6 days.
- In late-onset disease, the incubation period from group B Streptococcus acquisition to disease is unclear.

EPIDEMIOLOGY
- Worldwide distribution

INFECTIONS
- Sepsis and meningitis in the newborn
- Urinary and genital tract infection (endometritis) in pregnant women
- Recent data support the increasing significance of S. agalactiae infections in men and nonpregnant women.

DIAGNOSIS
- Culture
- Antigen detection techniques in body fluids (including cerebrospinal fluid)

TREATMENT
- Penicillin G or ampicillin

ALTERNATIVE TREATMENT
- Macrolide antibiotic

Streptococcus pneumoniae

See Section II, "Pneumonia"

Streptococcus pyogenes (Group A β-Hemolytic Streptococcus)

GENUS Streptococcus
SPECIES
- S. pyogenes

MICROBIOLOGIC CHARACTERISTICS
- Aerobic, gram-positive coccus

INCUBATION PERIOD
- The incubation period of streptococcal pharyngitis is 2 to 5 days.
- For impetigo, a 7- to 10-day period between the acquisition of the pathogen on healthy skin and development of lesions has been demonstrated.

EPIDEMIOLOGY
- Worldwide distribution

INFECTIONS
- Tonsillitis, scarlet fever, otitis, sinusitis, pneumonia
- Skin and soft-tissue infections (impetigo, erysipelas, cellulitis, others)
- Bacteremia
- Necrotizing fasciitis and toxic shock syndrome (TSS)
- Late nonsuppurative (immune-mediated) complications are rheumatic fever, erythema nodosum, and acute glomerulonephritis.

DIAGNOSIS
- Culture
- Serology

TREATMENT
- Penicillin G. i.v. 16 million units (divided in 4 or 6 doses) should be used in severe cases
- Amoxicillin 500 mg every 6 hours PO or penicillin V 1.5 million units every 6 hours PO in nonsevere cases
- Clindamycin 900 mg i.v. q8h or 600 mg i.v. q6h

ALTERNATIVE TREATMENT
- Macrolide antibiotics

Strongyloides Species

See Section II, "Strongyloidiasis"

Taenia saginata

GENUS Taenia
SPECIES
- T. saginata

MICROBIOLOGIC CHARACTERISTICS
- A tapeworm

INCUBATION PERIOD
- Eggs appear in the stool 10 to 14 weeks after infection with T. saginata.
- Symptoms (if any) may delay even more.

EPIDEMIOLOGY
- Worldwide
- More frequent in populations where beef is consumed insufficiently cooked

INFECTIONS
- Beef tapeworm infection, which is usually asymptomatic. It may cause mild gastrointestinal symptoms.

DIAGNOSIS
- Parasitologic examination of the stool

TREATMENT
- Niclosamide 2 g PO in a single dose

ALTERNATIVE TREATMENT
- Praziquantel 25 mg/kg PO (children, 10–15 mg/kg) in a single dose

PREVENTION
- Thorough cooking of beef

Taenia solium

See Section II, "Cysticercosis"

Microorganisms

Toxocara Species

GENUS Toxocara
SPECIES
- T. canis
- T. cati

MICROBIOLOGIC CHARACTERISTICS
- Nematode helminth

INCUBATION PERIOD
- Weeks to months
- Manifestation from eye infection may appear several years (2–10) after infection.

EPIDEMIOLOGY
- Worldwide distribution
- Children are at risk for infection.

INFECTIONS
- *Toxocara* species may cause toxocariasis, a chronic disease that is manifested by fever, pulmonary symptoms, hepatomegaly, hyperglobulinemia, and eosinophilia.
- The eosinophil count may increase significantly (up to 80,000/mm^3 of blood) in patients with heavy infection (e.g., a large number of larvae).
- *Ocular larva migrans* refers to eye infection by *Toxocara* species.

DIAGNOSIS
- Serology

TREATMENT
- Albendazole 400 mg q12h for 3 to 5 days; mebendazole 100 to 200 mg bid for 5 days

ALTERNATIVE TREATMENT
- Diethylcarbamazine 6 mg/kg/d in three doses for 7 to 10 days

PREVENTION
- Wash hands after handling soil and before eating.
- Deworm dogs and cats.
- Educate the public about ways to decrease the possibility of infection.

Toxoplasma Gondii

See Section II, "Toxoplasmosis"

Treponema carateum

GENUS Treponema
SPECIES
- T. carateum

MICROBIOLOGIC CHARACTERISTICS
- A spirochete

INCUBATION PERIOD
- Usually 2 to 3 weeks

EPIDEMIOLOGY
- Tropical areas of South America

INFECTIONS
- Pinta, which is a nonvenereal infection with manifestations from the skin

DIAGNOSIS
- Dark-field examination of samples taken from the lesions

TREATMENT
- Benzyl penicillin G 1.2 mIU i.m. (single dose)

ALTERNATIVE TREATMENT
- A tetracycline or chloramphenicol for 14 days

Treponema pallidum

See Section II, "Syphilis"

Trichinella spiralis

GENUS Trichinella
SPECIES
- T. spiralis

MICROBIOLOGIC CHARACTERISTICS
- A nematode helminth (round worm)

INCUBATION PERIOD
- Gastrointestinal symptoms may appear within a few days after infection.
- Systemic symptoms appear 5 to 45 days after infection.

EPIDEMIOLOGY
- Worldwide
- Variable incidence, depending partially on practices of preparing and eating pork or wild animal meat

INFECTIONS
- *T. spiralis* causes an infection with variable severity, depending on the number of ingested larvae and the susceptibility of the host.
- Asymptomatic infection is common.
- Diffuse myalgias accompanied by edema of the upper eyelids are common manifestations of the infection.
- Gastrointestinal symptoms, including mild diarrhea, may precede the ocular manifestations.
- Other sites, including the heart and the central nervous system, may be affected in trichinellosis.

DIAGNOSIS
- Serology
- Muscular biopsy (deltoid)
- Marked eosinophilia may be found in *Trichinella* infections.

TREATMENT
- Mebendazole 200 to 400 mg PO q8h for 2 weeks, with corticosteroids for severe symptoms, especially from the heart and the central nervous system
- In children: 200 to 400 mg q8h for 6 days, followed by 400 to 500 mg q8h for 10 days

ALTERNATIVE TREATMENT
- Thiabendazole 25 mg/kg PO q12h for 7 days

PREVENTION
- Properly cook all fresh pork and pork products and meat from wild animals.

Trichomonas vaginalis

See Section II, "Trichomoniasis Vaginitis"

Trichophyton Species

See Section II, "Superficial Skin and Soft-Tissue Infections"

Microorganisms

Trichosporon beigelii

GENUS Trichosporon

SPECIES
- T. beigelii

MICROBIOLOGIC CHARACTERISTICS
- Yeast capable of developing arthroconidia, hyphae, blastoconidia, and pseudohyphae

INCUBATION PERIOD
- Unknown

EPIDEMIOLOGY
- It is found more commonly in the tropics but also in the temperate zones.

INFECTIONS
- White piedra (superficial infection manifested by small yellow concretions on the hair shafts)
- The fungus may also cause a systemic infection in immunocompromised patients, including transplant recipients and patients with advanced HIV infection.

DIAGNOSIS
- Culture
- A false-positive latex agglutination test for cryptococcus antigen may occur in systemic T. beigelii infections.
- Histopathology specimens

TREATMENT
- Shaving of the hair will effectively manage white piedra.
- Systemic infections should be managed with systemic antifungal agents (amphotericin B intravenously).

ALTERNATIVE TREATMENT
- Oral ketoconazole may cure white piedra.

Trichostrongylus Species

GENUS Trichostrongylus

SPECIES
- T. orientalis
- T. colubriformis

MICROBIOLOGIC CHARACTERISTICS
- Nematode helminth

INCUBATION PERIOD
- Unclear

EPIDEMIOLOGY
- Worldwide distribution
- More commonly found in rural areas where herbivorous animals are raised

INFECTIONS
- Usually an asymptomatic infection
- It may occasionally cause mild gastrointestinal symptoms (e.g., dyspepsia) and anemia.

DIAGNOSIS
- Parasitologic examination of stool
- Trichostrongylus eggs resemble hookworm eggs, but Trichostrongylus eggs are usually larger.

TREATMENT
- Mebendazole 100 mg PO q12h for 5 days

ALTERNATIVE TREATMENT
- Albendazole 400 mg PO in a single dose
- In children: pyrantel pamoate in a single dose

Trichuris trichiura

GENUS Trichuris

SPECIES
- T. trichiura

MICROBIOLOGIC CHARACTERISTICS
- Nematode helminth

INCUBATION PERIOD
- Symptoms may appear a few weeks after infection.

EPIDEMIOLOGY
- Worldwide distribution
- More common in moist and warm regions

INFECTIONS
- Trichuriasis is usually an asymptomatic infection of the large bowel.
- Heavy infections (large number of T. trichiura in the large bowel) may cause diarrhea, with mucoid and bloody stools.
- Heavy infection with T. trichiura in children may be complicated by rectal prolapse, anemia, hypoproteinemia, growth retardation, and clubbing of the fingers.

DIAGNOSIS
- Parasitologic examination of stools (detection of eggs of the parasite)
- Colonoscopy may reveal worms attached to the large bowel wall.

TREATMENT
- Mebendazole 600 mg PO (single dose) or 100 mg PO q12h for 3 days

ALTERNATIVE TREATMENT
- Albendazole 400 mg once (in heavy infection, treatment should be given for 3–5 days)

PREVENTION
- Good hygienic practices in the use of toilet facilities

Tropheryma whippelii

GENUS Tropheryma

SPECIES
- T. whippelii

MICROBIOLOGIC CHARACTERISTICS
- Intracellular, gram-positive bacillus

INCUBATION PERIOD
- Unknown

EPIDEMIOLOGY
- Probably worldwide distribution

INFECTIONS
- Whipple disease (a syndrome manifested by migratory arthralgias, diarrhea, malabsorption, fever, neurologic disorder, and lymphadenopathy)

DIAGNOSIS
- Histologic examination of intestinal biopsy or lymph node

TREATMENT
- Trimethoprim–sulfamethoxazole (160 mg and 800 mg, respectively) q12h PO for 1 year

ALTERNATIVE TREATMENT
- Penicillin V
- Chloramphenicol
- Tetracycline

Trypanosoma Species

See Section II, "Trypanosomiasis"

Microorganisms

Tunga penetrans

GENUS Tunga
SPECIES
- T. penetrans

MICROBIOLOGIC CHARACTERISTICS
- Hematophagous flea

INCUBATION PERIOD
- Unknown

EPIDEMIOLOGY
- Mainly found in developing countries of Africa, South and Central America, and the Far East

INFECTIONS
- Tungiasis, which is manifested by painful nodules, usually on the feet. The lesions may be confused with those caused by myiasis. Tungiasis is caused by invasion of the skin by the mature flea, *T. penetrans*.

DIAGNOSIS
- Finding and examination of the parasite in the lesions

TREATMENT
- Surgical excision of the lesions

Ureaplasma urealyticum

GENUS Ureaplasma
SPECIES
- U. urealyticum

MICROBIOLOGIC CHARACTERISTICS
- Small bacterium
- No cell wall

INCUBATION PERIOD
- The incubation period of nongonococcal urethritis (a common infection that is caused, in some patients, by *U. urealyticum*) after sexual transmission is 10 to 20 days.

EPIDEMIOLOGY
- Common cause of infections worldwide

INFECTIONS
- Urethritis
- Chorioamnionitis
- Disseminated infection in the newborn

DIAGNOSIS
- Culture
- Serology tests

TREATMENT
- A macrolide antibiotic for 7 to 14 days

ALTERNATIVE TREATMENT
- Doxycycline
- Ofloxacin
- Ciprofloxacin should not be used, because a large proportion (up to 50%) of *U. urealyticum* strains are resistant to this antibiotic.

Varicella Zoster Virus

See Section II, "Chickenpox" and "Herpes Zoster"

Veillonella parvula

GENUS Veillonella
SPECIES
- V. parvula

MICROBIOLOGIC CHARACTERISTICS
- Anaerobic, gram-negative coccus

INCUBATION PERIOD
- Unknown

EPIDEMIOLOGY
- Worldwide
- Part of the normal oropharyngeal flora

INFECTIONS
- It may contribute to mixed infection of the female genital tract.
- A probable cause of oral infections

DIAGNOSIS
- Culture (anaerobic conditions)
- Culture requires prolonged incubation for growth of *V. parvula*.

TREATMENT
- Clindamycin

ALTERNATIVE TREATMENT
- Penicillin G
- Metronidazole

Vibrio cholerae

See Section II, "Cholera"

Microorganisms

Vibrio Species

GENUS Vibrio

SPECIES
- V. alginolyticus
- V. cholerae non-O:1
- V. cincinnatiensis
- V. damselae
- V. fluvialis
- V. furnissii
- V. hollisae
- V. metschnikovii
- V. mimicus
- V. parahaemolyticus
- V. vulnificus

MICROBIOLOGIC CHARACTERISTICS
- Aerobic, gram-negative bacilli

INCUBATION PERIOD
- The incubation period of enteritis due to most Vibrio species is 24 hours, with a range of 5 to 92 hours.

EPIDEMIOLOGY
- Ubiquitous in sea water
- Highest risk associated with consumption of raw clams, mussels, and oysters

INFECTIONS
- Gastroenteritis
- Wound infection and secondary sepsis
- Necrotizing skin infection and severe sepsis (mainly V. vulnificus)

DIAGNOSIS
- Culture

TREATMENT
- Doxycycline
- Supportive measures (fluid and electrolytes) are necessary for patients with gastroenteritis.

ALTERNATIVE TREATMENT
- Fluoroquinolone, aminoglycoside, chloramphenicol, third-generation cephalosporin, carbapenem

Weeksella Species

GENUS Weeksella

SPECIES
- W. virosa
- W. zoohelcum

MICROBIOLOGIC CHARACTERISTICS
- Aerobic, gram-negative bacilli

EPIDEMIOLOGY
- Unclear

INFECTIONS
- Rare cause of infections
- Animal bite wound infection (W. zoohelcum)
- Urinary infection (W. virosa)
- Peritonitis in patients with peritoneal dialysis (W. virosa)

DIAGNOSIS
- Culture

TREATMENT
- There are limited data about the antimicrobial susceptibility of Weeksella species.
- Penicillin

ALTERNATIVE TREATMENT
- Ciprofloxacin
- Trimethoprim–sulfamethoxazole
- Tetracyclines
- Aminoglycoside

PREVENTION
- N/A

Wohlfahrtia magnifica

See "Myiasis Agents"

Wuchereria bancrofti

See Section II, "Filariasis"

Yellow Fever Virus

See Section II, "Yellow Fever"

Yersinia pestis

See Section II, "Plague"

Yersinia Species

See Section II, "Yersinia Infections"

SECTION IV
Drugs and Vaccines

Drugs and Vaccines

Table 1a. Adverse Reactions to Antimicrobial Agents

Reaction	Common for	Infrequent for
Hypersensitivity-allergic		
Anaphylaxis	Penicillin G	Cephalosporins, imipenem
Fever	—	All agents
SLE-like reactions	Isoniazid	Griseofulvin, nitrofurantoin
Cutaneous reactions	Sulfonamides, penicillins	All agents
Histamine reactions	Vancomycin	—
Phototoxicity	Tetracyclines	Quinolones, chloroquine, primaquine, griseofulvin
Hematopoietic		
Pancytopenia	—	Choramphenicol
Neutropenia	Sulfonamides, trimethoprim, pyrimethamine, zidovudine	Penicillins, cephalosporins, dapsone
Hemolytic anemia (G6PD-associated)	Sulfonamides, nitrofurans, chloramphenicol, sulfones, nalidixic acid, primaquine	—
Immune hemolysis	Penicillins, cephalosporins, isoniazid, rifampin	—
Sideroblastic anemia	Isoniazid	—
Thrombocytopenia	Sulfonamides, penicillins, cephalosporins, rifampin, trimethoprim, pyrimethamine	Vancomycin, teicoplanin
Platelet dysfunction	Carbenicillin, ticarcillin, moxalactam	Extended-spectrum penicillins
Hypoprothrombinemia	Moxalactam, cefoperazone, cefamandole	Cefotetan, ceftriaxone, cefmetazole
Gastrointestinal		
Nausea, emesis, abdominal pain	Erythromycin	Almost any agent, including oral penicillins, quionolones, metronidazole, clindamycin, nystatin, tetracyclines, TMP-SMX, ketoconazole
Diarrhea	Ampicillin-sulbactam, amoxicillin-clavulanate, cefixime, cefoperazone, ceftriaxone	Any agent
Pseudomembranous enterocolitis (*Clostridium difficile*)	Almost any agent, more commonly ampicillin, TMP-SMX, cefoxitin, clindamycin	Quinolones (ciprofloxacin)
Malabsorption	Neomycin	Other aminoglycosides
Hepatic		
Transaminase level increase	Penicillins, particularly oxacillin, aztreonam	Azoles
Cholestatic jaundice	Oleandomycin, erythromycin estolate, nitrofurans, sulfonamides	—
Hepatitis	Isoniazid, nitrofurantoin, trovafloxacin	Rifampin, sulfonamides, ketoconazole

Drugs and Vaccines

Table 1a. Adverse Reactions to Antimicrobial Agents (*Continued*)

Reaction	Common for	Infrequent for
Pulmonary		
Histamine release	Polymyxin by aerosol	—
Interstitial infiltrates	Nitrofurantoin	—
Cardiovascular		
Arrhythmias	Amphotericin B, miconazole	Penicillin G
Hypotension	Pentamidine, emetine	—
Metabolic		
Hypokalemia	Carbenicillin, amphotericin B	—
Hypogonadal effects	Ketoconazole	—
Hyperglycemia	Nalidixic acid	—
Pancreatitis	Pentamidine, nitrofurantoin, TMP-SMX	—
Diabetes	Pentamidine	—
Hypomagnesemia	Amphotericin B, aminoglycosides	—
Renal		
Hypersensitivity nephritis	Sulfonamides	—
Interstitial nephritis	All beta-lactams	—
Tubular toxicity	Aminoglycosides, polymyxins	Vancomycin, teicoplanin
Distal tubular acidosis	Amphotericin B, tetracyclines	—
Crystal deposition	Fluoroquinolones, acyclovir	—
Neurologic		
Peripheral neuropathy	Nitrofurans, metronidazole, polymyxins, griseofulvin, cycloserine, isoniazid	Tetracyclines
Muscular blockade	Polymyxins, aminoglycosides, capreomycin	Clindamycin, lincomycin
Central nervous excitation	—	Fluoroquinolones
Seizures	Penicillin, imipenem, cycloserine	Amantadine, isoniazid, metronidazole, fluoroquinolones, thiabendazole
Ophthalmic		
Opthalmic disturbances	Ethambutol	Isoniazid, chloramphenicol, quinolones, chloroquine
Ototoxiclty		
Deafness	Aminoglycosides, vancomycin	Erythromycin
Vestibulotoxicity	Aminoglycosides, minocycline	—

Abbreviations: SLE, systemic lupus erythematosus; G6PD, glucose-6-phosphate dehydrogenase; TMP-SMX, trimethoprim-sulfamethoxazole.

Drugs and Vaccines

Table 1b. Reported Percentage Frequency of Selected Adverse Effects after Oral Administration of Antibacterial Drugs in Different Studies

Drug	No. of patients	Nausea	Vomiting	Diarrhea	Rash	Therapy stopped	Other Adverse Effects
Cephalosporins							
Cephalexin	116	4.0	10	6.0	1.0	NP	"Serum sickness"
	305	2.3	0.7	1.3	1.0	1.3	0.02%–0.5%
Cefaclor	245	4.5	0.4	5.7	0.4	—	
	129	NP	NP	3.0	2.0	—	
	435	1.0	1.0	2.0	1.0	—	
	374	2.4	0.5	3.7	1.3	—	
	NP	NP	NP	1.0	1.5	2.4	
Cefuroxime axetil	84	5.0	1.0	8.0	0	—	
	NP	2.4	2.0	3.5	0.6	—	
Cefixime	134	NP	NP	16	3.0	—	
	NP	7.0	NP	16	<2.0	3.8	
Cefprozil	2,383	2.3	0.7	1.2	0.7	2.0	
	NP	3.5	1.0	2.9	0.9	2.0	
Cefpodoxime	762	1.0	NP	4.0	NP	2.0	
Proxetil	3,650	—	2.0	—	NP	NP	
	1,468	1.0	0.2	4.6	0.5	2.3	
Loracarbef	4,506	1.9	1.4	4.1	1.2	1.5	
Ceftibuten	1,870	1.0	2.0	4.0	<1.0	—	
Penicillins							
Penicillin V	630	3.3	1.3	3.7	0.6	2.5	
	199	0	0	5.0	0	—	
	918	NP	NP	NP	1.2–3.0	—	
	NP	NP	NP	NP	2.5–4.2	—	
Ampicillin	1,775	NP	NP	NP	5.2	—	
	2,998	NP	NP	—	5.2	—	
Amoxicillin	574	1.7	0.5	4.5	1.6	1.9	
	1,225	NP	NP	NP	3.9–6.4	—	
Amoxicillin-clavulanate	129	NP	1.6	8.5	0.8	—	
	267	NP	2.0	22.0	1.0	1.0	
	110	5.0	2.0	18.0	4.0	—	
	306	NP	9.2	24.0	NP	—	
	NP	3.0	1.0	9.0	3.0	2.0–3.0	

Drugs and Vaccines

Table 1b. Reported Percentage Frequency of Selected Adverse Effects after Oral Administration of Antibacterial Drugs in Different Studies (*Continued*)

Drug	No. of patients	Nausea	Vomiting	Diarrhea	Rash	Therapy stopped	Other Adverse Effects
Lincosamide							
Clindamycin	52	NP	NP	31.0	21.0	31.0	CDT antibiotic associated diarrhea in 0.01%–18% of treated patients
Macrolides							
Erythromycin base	128	2.0	3.0	2.0	0	NP	Rare idiosyncratic hepatitis
	147	NP	NP	NP	NP	0.4–0.6	
Enteric coated	441	5.5	2.9	5.3	0.6	4.9	
	112	—	27.0	—	0	19.0	
	21	-	52.0	—	0	14.0	
Azithromycin	3,995	2.6	0.8	3.6	0.2	0.7	
	229	2.6	NP	5.2	NP	NP	
	NP	3.0	<1.0	5.0	<1.0	0.7	
Clarithromycin	3,768	3.8	NP	3.0	NP	NP	
	NP	3.0	NP	3.0	0	4.0	
Fluoroquinolines							Symptoms referable to CNS
Ciprofloxacin	4,287	—	2.3	1.5	0.8	1.2	(i.e., headache, agitation, dizziness, sleep disturbances in 1%–4%)
	2,799	5.2	2.0	2.3	1.1	3.5	In high dose, headache, tremor
Ofloxacin	3,184	—	5.4	—	NP	—	disorientation
	15,641	—	0.9	0.4	0.3	1.5	
	NP	3.0	1.3	1.0	NP	4.0	
Lomefloxacin	2,869	3.7	<1.0	1.4	1.0	2.6	
Temafloxacin	2,602	5.6	1.1	2.8	1.5	4.1	
TMP-SMX	1,066	—	—	—	—	2.4–4.7	
	47	—	18.0	—	2.0	2.0	
	47	11.0	NP	0	6.0	11.0	
	196	8.2	—	0	5.0	4.0	
	180	—	4.0	—	2.0	3.9	
	129	—	7.0	—	7.0	NP	
	216	9.3	NP	NP	NP	5.1	

Abbreviations: NP, not provided; CNS, central nervous system; CDT, *Clostridium difficile*, toxin; TMP-SMX, trimethoprim-sulfamethoxazole.
Source: Modified from Gilbert DN. Aspects of the safety profile of oral antibacterial agents. *Infect Dis Clin Pract* 1995; 4[Suppl 2]:S103–S112.

Drugs and Vaccines

Table 1c. Selected Drug-Drug Interactions Involving an Oral Antibacterial Agent

Antibacterial Agent (A)	Other Drug (B)	Effect	Significance/Certainty
Erythromycin (includes azithromycin and clarithromycin)	Carbamazepine	↑ Levels[a] of B	Avoid combination
	Corticosteroids	↑ Levels[a] of B	Awareness
	Digoxin	↑ Levels[a] of B	Awareness
	Theophylline	↑ Levels[a] of B	Dosage adjustment
	Terfenadine or astemizole	↑ Levels[a] of B	Avoid risk of serious cardiovascular adverse drug reactions
Fluoroquinolones			
All agents	Cimetidine	↑ Levels[a] of A	Awareness
	Multivalent cations (i.e., aluminum, chromium, iron, magnesium, zinc)	↓ Absorption of A	Awareness
Ciprofloxacin	Theophylline	↑ Levels[a] of B	Dosage adjustment
	Caffeine	↑ Levels[a] of B	Awareness
	Oral anticoagulants	↑ Prothrombin time	Monitor prothrombin time
Ofloxacin	Oral anticoagulants	↑ Prothrombin time	Monitor prothrombin time
Tetracyclines (includes doxycycline)	Multivalent cations (i.e., aluminum, bismuth, iron, magnesium, and others)	↓ Absorption of A	Awareness
	Digoxin	↑ Levels[a] of B	Awareness
	Phenytoin	↓ Serum half-life of A	Awareness
Trimethoprim-sulfamethoxazole	Phenytoin	↑ Levels[a] of B	Dosage adjustment
	Oral anticoagulants	↑ Prothrombin time	Monitor prothrombin time
	Sulfonylureas	↑ Effects of B	Monitor blood glucose

[a] Serum levels.
Source: From Gilbert DN. Aspects of the safety profile of oral antibacterial agents. *Infect Dis Clin Pract* 1995;4[Suppl 2]:S103-S112.

Drugs and Vaccines

Table 2a. Antimicrobial Dosing Regimens in Renal Failure

GENERAL PRINCIPLES

The initial dose is not modified in renal failure. Adjustments in subsequent doses for renally excreted drugs may be accomplished by the following:
- Usual maintenance dose at extended intervals, usually three half-lives (extended interval method)
- Reduced doses at the usual intervals (dose reduction method)
- A combination of each

Adjustments in dose are usually based on creatinine clearance that may be estimated by the Cockroft-Gault equation that corrects for three critical variables: age, weight, and gender (Nephron 1976; 16:31)

$$\text{Male: } \frac{\text{weight (kg)} \times (140 \text{ minus age in years})}{72 \times \text{serum creatinine (mg/dL)}}$$

Female: above value $\times$ 0.85

Pitfalls and notations with calculations follow.
- Elderly patient: Serum creatinine may be deceptively low (with danger of overdosing) due to reduced muscle mass.
- Pregnancy, ascites, and other causes of volume expansion: GFR may be increased (with danger of underdosing) in the third trimester of pregnancy and in patients with normal renal function who receive massive parenteral fluids.
- Obese patients: Use lean body weight.
- Renal failure: Formulas assume stable renal function; for patients with anuria or oliguria assume creatinine clearance of 5–8 mL/min.

AMINOGLYCOSIDE DOSING

Guidelines of the Johns Hopkins Hospital Clinical Pharmacology Department

Agent	Loading Dose Regardless of Renal Function (mg/kg)	Subsequent Doses (before level measurements) CCr > 70 mL/min	Subsequent Doses (before level measurements) CCr < 70 mL/min	Therapeutic Levels 1 Hour after Start of Infusion over 20–30 Minutes (μg/mL)
Gentamicin[a]	2.0	1.7–2.0 mg/kg/8 h	0.03 CCr = mg/kg/8 h	5–10
Tobramycin[a]	2.0	1.7–2.0 mg/kg/8 h	0.03 CCr = mg/kg/8 h	5–10
Netilmicin[a]	2.2	2.0–2.2 mg/kg/8 h	0.03 CCr = mg/kg/8 h	5–10
Amikacin	7.5	7.5–8.0 mg/kg/8 h	0.12 CCr = mg/kg/8 h	20–40
Kanamycin	7.5	7.5–8.0 mg/kg/8 h	0.12 CCr = mg/kg/8 h	20–40

Initial dose: gentamicin, tobramycin, netilmicin 1.5–2.0 mg/kg; amikacin, kanamycin 5.0–7.5 mg/kg.
Maintenance dose: usual daily dose creatinine clearance/100. CCr, creatinine clearance.

[a] Doses should be written in multiples of 5 mg; doses of amikacin and kanamycin should be written in multiples of 25 mg. For obese patients use calculated lean body weight plus 40% of excess adipose tissue. For patients who are oliguric or anuric, use CCr of 5–8 mL/min. Seriously ill patients with sepsis often need higher loading doses to achieve rapid therapeutic levels despite third spacing, for example, 3 mg/kg for gentamicin and tobramycin.

Mayo clinic guidelines follow Van Scoy RE, Wilson WR. *Mayo Clin Proc* 1987;62:1142.

ONCE-DAILY AMINOGLYCOSIDES

Rationale

Efficacy.

High serum levels achieve concentration-dependent killing properties; the postantibiotic effect (PAE) refers to continued bacterial growth suppression when the serum concentration is below the MIC. The PAE usually lasts 2 to 4 hours. The implication is that therapeutic levels are readily achieved and the antibiotic continues to suppress bacteria at concentrations below the MIC. Meta-analysis of 17 studies showed that clinical outcome is comparable with once-daily aminoglycosides and standard treatment with multiple daily doses.

(Continued)

Drugs and Vaccines

Table 2a. Antimicrobial Dosing Regimens in Renal Failure (*Continued*)

Toxicity.
- Renal: Longer dosing intervals are associated with reduced renal cortical accumulation and a trend toward reduced nephrotoxicity.
- Ototoxicity: This side effect is related to perilymph accumulation of aminoglycoside rather than to concentration. Meta-analysis of 17 reports showed a 33% reduction in ototoxicity.

Clinical Trials

A review of 24 published trials involving once-daily aminoglycoside compared with standard multiple dosing treatment showed the following.

	Once-Daily Dosing	Multiple Dosing
Favorable outcome		
Clinical	1,041/1,163 (90%)	929/1,097 (84%)
Bacteriologic	636/718 (89%)	557/668 (83%)
Toxicity		
Nephrotoxicity	73/1,617 (5%)	86/1,564 (6%)
Ototoxicity	28/674 (4%)	34/636 (5%)

Contraindications

Patients receiving aminoglycosides for synergy with β-lactam agents versus enterococcus (enterococcal endocarditis) should receive standard multiple daily-dosing regimens. There is limited experience with once-daily aminoglycosides in selected clinical settings, such that some authorities consider them relative contraindications in the following settings: neutropenic patients, critically ill or septic patients, pregnant patients, renal failure, elderly and pediatric patients, infections involving gram-positive bacteria, endocarditis or burn patients.

Monitoring

Some authorities suggest monitoring predose levels (18 hours) that should show gentamicin or tobramycin levels <0.5 μg/mL and amikacin levels <4–5 μg/mL; higher levels should lead to dose reduction.

Regimen

- Standard dose: gentamicin and tobramycin 5–6 mg/kg/d (some use a range of 4–7 mg/kg); amikacin and streptomycin 15–20 mg/kg/d
- Dose adjustment based on trough levels; gentamicin and tobramycin $\leq$0.5 μg/mL; amikacin <5 μg/mL.
- Dose adjustment is based on renal function.

	Creatinine clearance (mL/min)			
Agent	>80	60–80	40–60	30–40
Gentamicin or tobramycin (mg/kg/d)	5	4	3.5	2.5
Amikacin (mg/kg/d)	15	12	7.5	4.0

Dose may be based on anatomic site of infection: high dose for pneumonia; low dose for urinary tract infection.

Hartford Hospital Regimen

Creatinine Clearance (mL/min)	Aminoglycoside Dosage	
	Gentamicin or Tobramycin	Amikacin
>60	7 mg/kg[a] q24 h	15 mg/kg q24 h
40–59	7 mg/kg q36 h	15 mg/kg q36 h
20–39	7 mg/kg q48 h	15 mg/kg q48 h

Experience with 2,184 patients: mean dose, 450 mg; mean peak serum level, 26 μg/mL (gentamicin, tobramycin); frequency of nephrotoxocity (creatinine increase of 0.5 mg/dL above baseline), 1.2%; nephrotoxicity with >6 days of therapy, 2.0%; nephrotoxicity with >13 days of therapy, 3.3%; ototoxicity, 0.2%.

[a] Obese patients >20% above ideal body weight: ideal weight +0.4 (actual weight-ideal weight); aminoglycoside was delivered over 60 min in 50-mL increments.

Source: See article in *Antimicrob Agents Chemother* 1995;39:650.

Table 2b. Drug Therapy Dosing Guidelines

Drug	Major Excretory Route	Half-life (hr) Normal	Half-life (hr) Anuria	Usual regimen Oral	Usual regimen Parenteral	Maintenance regimen renal failure glomerular filtration rate (mL/min) 50–80	10–50	<10
Acyclovir	Renal	2.0–2.5	20	200 mg 3–5 times/d	—	Usual	Usual	200 mg q12h
				400 mg bid	—	Usual	Usual	200 mg q12h
				800 mg 5 times/d	—	Usual	800 mg q8h	800 mg q12h
				—	5–10 mg/kg q8h	Usual	5–12 mg/kg q12–24h	2.5–6.0 mg/kg q24h
Albendazole	Hepatic	8	8	400–800 mg bid	—	Usual	Usual	Usual
Amantadine	Renal	15–20	170	100 mg bid	—	100–150 mg qd	100–200 mg 2–3 times/wk	100–200 mg qwk
Amikacin	Renal	2	30	—	7.5 mg/kg q12h	12 mg/kg q24h (60–80CCr) 7.5 mg/kg q24h (40–60CCr)	7.5 mg/kg q48–72h	7.5 mg/kg q24h (40–60CCr) 4 mg/kg q24h (30–40CCr)
Amoxicillin	Renal	1	15–20	250–500 mg q8h	—	0.25–0.5 g q12–24h	0.25–0.5 g q12–24h	0.25–0.5 g q12–24h
Amoxicillin-clavulanic acid	Renal	1	8–16	250–500 mg q8h	—	Usual	0.25–0.5 g q12h	0.25–0.5 g q24–36h
Amphotericin B	Hepatic	15 d	15 d	—	0.3–1.4 mg/kg/d	Usual	Usual	Usual
Amphotericin B lipid complex	Hepatic	8 d	8 d	—	5 mg/kg	Usual	Usual	Usual
Ampicillin	Renal	1	8–12	0.25–0.5 g q6h	1–3 g q4–6h	Usual	0.5 g q8h	0.5 g q12h
				—	1–2 g q6h	Usual	1–2 g i.v. q8h	1–2 g i.v. q12h
Ampicillin-sulbactam	Renal	1	8–12	—	—	1–2 g i.v. q8h	1–2 g i.v. q8h	1–2 g i.v. q12h
Atovaquone	Gut	70	70	750 mg bid suspension	—	Usual	Usual	Unknown
Azithromycin	Hepatic	68	68	250 mg/d	—	Usual	No data; use caution	—
Aztreonam	Renal	1.7–2.0	6–9	—	1–2 g q6h	1–2 g q8–12h	1–2 g q12–18h	1–2 g q24h
Bacampicillin	Renal	1	8–12	0.4–0.8 g q12h	—	Usual	Usual	0.4–0.8 g 24h
Capreomycin	Renal	4–6	50–100	—	1 g qd (i.m.)	—	Usual	Usual
Carbenicillin	Renal	1	13–16	0.5–1.0 g q6h	—	Usual	0.5–1.0 g q8h	Avoid
Cefaclor	Renal	0.75	2.8	0.25–0.5 g q8h	—	Usual	Usual	Usual
Cefadroxil	Renal	1.4	20–25	0.5–1.0 g q12–24h	—	Usual	0.5 g q12–24h	0.5 g q36h
Cefamandole	Renal	0.5–2.1	10	—	0.5–2.0 g q6h	0.5–2.0 g q6h	1–2 g q8h	0.5–0.75 g q12h
Cefazolin	Renal	1.8	18–36	—	0.5–2.0 g q8h	0.5–1.5 q8h	0.5–1.0 g q8–12h	0.25–0.75 g q18–24h
Cefepime	Renal	2	13	—	0.5–2.0 g q12h	0.5–2.0 g q24h	0.5–1.0 g q24h	250–500 mg q24h
Cefixime	Renal	3–4	12	200 mg q12h	—	Usual	300 mg/d	200 mg/d
Cefmetazole	Renal	1.2	—	—	2 g q6–12h	1–2 g q12h	1–2 g q18–24h	1–2 g q48h
Cefonicid	Renal	4–5	50–60	—	0.5–2.0 g q24h	8–25 mg/kg q24h	4–8 mg/kg q24h	4 mg/kg q3–5d
Cefoperazone	Gut	1.9–2.5	2.0–2.5	—	1–2 g q6–12h	Usual	Usual	Usual
Ceforanide	Renal	3	20–40	—	0.5–1.0 g q12h	Usual	0.5–1.0 g q24h	0.5–1.0 g q48–72h
Cefotaxime	Renal	1.1	3	—	1–2 g q4–8h	Usual	1–2 g q6–12h	1–2 g q12h
Cefotetan	Renal	3–4	12–30	—	1–2 g q12h	Usual	1–2 g q24h	1–2 g q48h
Cefoxitin	Renal	0.7	13–22	—	1–2 g q6–8h	Usual	1–2 g q12–24h	0.5–1.0 g q12–48h
Cefpodoxime	Renal	2.4	10	200–400 mg q12h	—	200–400 mg q24h	200–400 mg 3 times/wk	200–400 mg/wk
Cefprozil	Renal	1.3	5–6	0.25–0.5 g q12h	—	Usual	0.25–0.5 g q24h	0.25 g q12–24h

(Continued)

Table 2b. Drug Therapy Dosing Guidelines (*Continued*)

Drug	Major Excretory Route	Half-life (hr) Normal	Half-life (hr) Anuria	Usual regimen Oral	Usual regimen Parenteral	Maintenance regimen renal failure glomerular filtration rate (mL/min) 50–80	10–50	<10
Ceftazidime	Renal	0.9–1.7	15–25	—	1–2 g q8–12h	Usual	1 g q12–24h	0.5 g q24–48h
Ceftibuten	Renal	2.4	22	400 mg/d	—	Usual	200 mg/d	100 mg/d
Ceftizoxime	Renal	1.4–1.8	25–35	—	1–3 g q6–8h	0.5–1.5 g q8h	0.25–1.0 g q12h	0.25–0.5 g q24h
Ceftriaxone	Renal and gut	6–9	12–15	—	0.5–1.0 g q12–24h	Usual	Usual	Usual
Cefuroxime	Renal	1.3–1.7	20	—	0.75–1.5 g q8h	Usual	0.75–1.5 g q8–12h	0.75 g q24h
Cefuroxime axetil	Renal	1.2	20	250 mg q12h	—	Usual	Usual	250 mg q24h
Cephalexin	Renal	0.9	5–30	0.25–1.0 g q6h	—	Usual	0.25–1.0 g q8–12h	0.25–1.0 g q24–48h
Cephalothin	Renal	0.5–0.9	3–8	—	0.5–2.0 g q4–8h	Usual	1.0–1.5 g q6h	0.5 g q8h
Cephapirin	Renal	0.6–0.9	2.4	—	0.5–2.0 g q4–6h	0.5–2.0 g q6h	0.5–2.0 g q8h	0.5–2.0 g q12h
Cephradine	Renal	0.7–2.0	8–15	0.25–1.0 g q6h	—	Usual	0.5 g q6h	0.25 g q12h
Chloramphenicol	Hepatic	2.5	3–7	0.25–0.75 g q6h	0.25–1.0 g q6h	Usual	Usual	Usual
Chloroquine	Renal and metabolized	48–120	?	300–600 mg PO qd	—	Usual	Usual	150–300 mg PO qd
Cidofovir	Renal	17–65	↑	—	5 mg/kg qwk for 2 wk (induction); 5 mg/kg qwk for 22 wk (maintenance)	Usual	Dosage titrated to creatinine clearance	Contraindicated
Cinoxacin	Renal	1.5	8.5	0.25–0.5 g q12h	—	0.25 g q8h	0.25 g q12h	0.25 g q24h
Ciprofloxacin	Renal and hepatic metabolism	4	5–10	0.25–0.75 g q12h	—	Usual	0.25–0.5 g q12h	0.25–0.5 g q18h
Clarithromycin	Hepatic and renal metabolism	4	↑	250–500 mg q12h	400 mg q12h	Usual	0.4 g q18h	0.4 g q24h
					—	Usual	Usual	250–500 mg q24h
Clindamycin	Hepatic	2.0–2.5	2.0–3.5	150–300 mg q6h	300–900 mg q6–8h	Usual	Usual	Usual
Clofazimine	Hepatic	8 d	8 d	50 mg qd 100 mg tid	—	Usual	Usual	Usual
Cloxacillin	Renal	0.5	0.8	0.5–1.0 g q6h	—	Usual	Usual	Usual
Colistin	Renal	3–8	10–20	—	1.5 mg/kg q6–12h	2.5–3.8 mg/kg q24h	1.5–2.5 mg/kg q24–36h	0.6 mg/kg q24h
Cycloserine	Renal	8–12	?	250–500 mg bid	—	Usual	250–500 mg q24h	250 mg q24h
Dapsone	Hepatic metabolism	30	↑	50–100 mg/d	—	Usual	Usual	No data
Dicloxacillin	Renal	0.5–0.9	1.0–1.6	0.25–0.5 g q6h	—	Usual	Usual	Usual
D₄T (see Stavudine)								
Dideoxyinosine (ddI, didanosine)	Renal, nonrenal	1.3–1.6	?	200 mg bid	—	Usual	Consider dose reduction; note Mg load—60 mEq/tablet	
Dideoxychytidine (ddC, zalcitabine)	Renal	1.2–1.6	4–6	0.75 mg tid	—	Usual	0.75 mg bid	0.75 mg
Dirithromycin	Bile	2	8	500 mg q24h	—	Usual	Usual	Usual
Doxycycline	Renal and gut	30–44	30–44	100 mg bid	100 mg bid	Usual	Usual	Usual
Enoxacin	Renal and hepatic metabolism	14–25	15–36	200–400 mg bid	—	Usual	Half usual dose	Half usual dose
Erythromycin	Hepatic	3–6	—	—	1 g q6h	Usual	Usual	Usual
Ethambutol	Renal	3–4	8	15–25 mg/kg q24h	—	15 mg/kg q24h	15 mg/kg q24–36h	15 mg/kg q48h

490

Drug	Route of Elimination	Half-life (normal)	Half-life (ESRD)	Dose (normal)	Dose (CCr >50)	Dose (CCr 10-50)	Dose (CCr <10)
Ethionamide	Metabolized	4	9	0.5–1.0g q24h (in 1-3 doses)	—	Usual	Usual	5 mg/kg q48h
Famciclovir	Renal	2.3	13	125 mg q12h	—	Usual	125 mg q24h	125 mg q48h
				500 mg q8h	—	Usual	500 mg q12–24h	250 mg q48h
Fluconazole	Renal	20–50	100	100–200 mg q24h	100–400 mg q24h	Usual	One-half usual dose	25–50 mg q24h
Flucytosine	Renal	3–6	70	37 mg/kg q6h	—	Usual	37 mg/kg q12–24h	Adjust to keep 2-hr concentration at 50–100 μg/mL
Foscarnet								
Induction	Renal	3	8	—	60 mg/kg q8h	40–50 mg/kg q8h	20–30 mg/kg q8h	Contraindicated (CCr <20 mL/min)
Maintenance				—	90 mg/kg/qd	60–70 mg/kg qd	50–70 mg/kg qd	Contraindicated (CCr <20 mL/min)
Maintenance				—	120 mg/kg/qd	80–90 mg/kg qd	60–80 mg/kg qd	Contraindicated (CCr <20 mL/min)
Ganciclovir								
Induction	Renal	2.5–3.6	10	—	5 mg/kg bid	2.5 mg/kg bid	2.5 mg/kg qd	1.25 mg/kg qd
Maintenance (half of induction dose)				—	5 mg/kg qd	2.5 mg/kg/qd	1.2 mg/kg/qd	0.6 mg/kg/qd
Ganciclovir (oral)	GI	3–7	10	1,000 mg tid	—	500 mg tid	500 mg qd	500 mg 3 times/wk
Gentamicin	Renal	2	48	—	1.7 mg/kg q8h	4 mg/kg q24h (60–80 CCr)	3.5 mg/kg q24h (40–60 CCr)	
						3.5 mg/kg q24h (40–60 CCr)	2.5 mg/kg q24h (30–40 CCr)	
Griseofulvin	Hepatic metabolism							
Microsize		24	24	0.5–1.0 g q24h	—	Usual	Usual	Usual
Ultramicrosize	Same	24	24	0.33–0.66 g q24h	—	Usual	Usual	Usual
Imipenem-cilastatin	Renal	0.8–1.0	3.5	—	0.5–1.0 g q6h	0.5 g q6–8h	0.5 g q8–12h	0.25–0.5 mg q12h
Indinavir	Hepatic metabolism	1.5–2.0	?	800 mg tid	—	Usual	Usual	Usual
Isoniazid	Hepatic	0.5–4.0	2–10	300 mg q24h	300 mg q24h	Usual	Usual	Slow acetylators, half-dose
Itraconazole	Hepatic	20–60	20–60	100–200 mg/d	—	Usual	Usual	Usual
Ketoconazole	Hepatic metabolism	1–4	1–4	200–400 mg q12–24h	—	Usual	Usual	Usual
Lamivudine (3TC)	Renal	3–6h	?	150 mg bid	—	Usual	100–150 mg/d	25–50 mg/d
Levofloxacin	Renal	6.3	35	500 mg q24h	500 mg q24h	Usual	250 mg q24h	250 mg q48h
Lomefloxacin	Renal	8	45	400 mg q24h	—	Usual	400 mg q24h; then 200 mg q24h	
Loracarbef	Renal	1	32	200–400 mg q12h	—	Usual	200–400 mg q24h	200–400 mg q3–5d
Mefloquine	Hepatic	2–4 wk	2–4 wk	250 mg/wk	—	Usual	Usual	Usual
Meropenem	Renal	1	↑	—	1 g q8h	Usual	500 mg q12h	500 mg q24h

(Continued)

Table 2b. Drug Therapy Dosing Guidelines (*Continued*)

Drug	Major Excretory Route	Half-life (hr) Normal	Half-life (hr) Anuria	Usual regimen Oral	Usual regimen Parenteral	Maintenance regimen renal failure glomerular filtration rate (mL/min) 50–80	10–50	<10
Methenamine Hippurate	Renal	3–6	?	1 g q12h	—	Usual	Avoid	Avoid
Mandelate	Renal	3–6	?	1 g q6h	—	Usual	Avoid	Avoid
Metronidazole	Hepatic	6–14	8–15	0.25–0.75 g tid	0.5 g q6h	Usual	Usual	Usual
Mezlocillin	Renal	1	1.5	—	3–4 g q4–6h	Usual	3 mg q8h	2 g q8h
Miconazole	Hepatic	0.5–1	0.5–1.0	—	0.4–1.2 g q8h	Usual	Usual	Usual
Minocycline	Hepatic and metabolized	11–26	17–30	100 mg q12h	100 mg q12h	Usual	Usual	Usual or slight decrease
Nafcillin	Hepatic metabolism	0.5	1.2	0.5–1.0 g q6h	0.5–2.0 g q4–6h	Usual	Usual	Usual
Nalidixic acid	Renal and hepatic metabolism	1.5	21	1 g q6h	—	Usual	Usual	Avoid
Nelfinavir	Hepatic metabolism	3.5–5.0	3.5–5.0	750 mg tid	—	Usual	Usual	Usual
Netilmicin	Renal	2.5	35	—	2 mg/kg q8h	0.03 × CCr mg/Kg/8h	0.03 × CCr mg/Kg/8h	0.03 × CCr mg/Kg/8h
Nevirapine	Hepatic	25	?	200 mg bid	—	Usual	Usual	Usual, "with caution"
Nitrofurantoin	Renal	0.3	1	50–100 mg q6–8h	—	Usual	Avoid	Avoid
Norfloxacin	Renal and hepatic metabolism	3.5	8	400 mg bid	—	Usual	400 mg qd	400 mg qd
Nystatin	Not absorbed	—	—	0.4–1.0 million units 3–5 times/d	—	Usual	Usual	Usual
Ofloxacin	Renal	6	40	200–400 mg bid	—	Usual	200–400 mg qd	100–200 mg qd
					200–400 mg q12h	Usual	200–400 mg q24h	100–200 mg q24h
Oxacillin	Renal	0.5	1	0.5–1.0 g q6h	1–3 g q6h	Usual	Usual	Usual
Penicillin Crystalline (G)	Renal	0.5	7–10	—	1–4 million units q4–6h	Usual	Usual	Half usual dose
Procaine	Renal	24	—	—	0.6–1.2 million units i.m. q12h	Usual	Usual	Usual
Benzathine	Renal	Days	—	—	0.6–1.2 million units i.m.	Usual	Usual	Usual
V	Renal	0.5–1.0	7–10	0.4–0.8 million units q6h	—	Usual	Usual	Usual
Pentamidine	Nonrenal	6	6–8	—	4 mg/kg q24h	Usual	4 mg/kg q24–36h	4 mg/kg q 48h
Piperacillin	Renal	1	3	—	3–4 g q4–6h	Usual	3 g q8h	3 g q12h
Piperacillin + Tazobactam	Renal	1	3	—	3/0.375 g q6h	Usual	2/0.25 g q6g	2/0.25 g q 8h
Praziquantel	Hepatic metabolism	0.8–1.5	?	10–25 mg/kg tid	—	Usual	Usual	Usual
Pyrazinamide	Metabolized	10–16	?	15–35 mg/kg/d	—	Usual	Usual	12–20 mg/kg/d
Pyrimethamine	Hepatic metabolism	1.5–5.0 d	?	25–75 mg/d	—	Usual	Usual	Usual
Quinacrine	Renal	5 d	—	100–200 mg q6–8h	—	Usual	?	?
Quinine	Hepatic metabolism	4–5	4–5	650 mg tid	7.5–10.0 mg/kg q8h	Usual	Usual	Usual

Drug	Metabolism	Half-life (h) normal	Half-life (h) ESRD	Usual dose	CCr >50	CCr 10-50	CCr <10
Rifampin	Hepatic	Early 2-5, Late 2	2-5	600 mg/d	Usual	Usual	Usual
Rimantadine	Hepatic	24-30	48-60	100 mg bid	Usual	Usual	100 mg/d
Ritonavir	Hepatic metabolism	3-4	?	600 mg bid	Usual	Usual	Usual
Saquinavir	Hepatic metabolism	1-2	1-2	600 mg tid	Usual	Usual	Usual
Sparfloxacin	Renal	20	↑	200 mg q24h	Usual	200 mg q48h	200 mg q48h
Spectinomycin	Renal	1-3	?	—	Usual	Usual	Usual
Stavudine	Renal and hepatic metabolism	1	?	40 mg bid	Usual	20 mg 1-2 times/d	No data
Streptomycin	Renal	2-5	100-110	—	15 mg/kg q24-72h	15 mg/kg q72-96h	7.5 mg/kg q72-96h
Sulfadiazine	Renal	8-17	22-34	0.5-1.5 g q4-6h	Usual	0.5-1.5 g q8-12h	0.5-1.5 g q12-24h
Sulfisoxazole	Renal			30-50 mg/kg q6-8h	Usual	30-50 mg/kg q12-18h	30-50 mg/kg q18-24h
Sulfisoxazole	Renal	3-7	6-12	1-2 g q6h	Usual	1 g q8-12h	1 g q12-24h
Teicoplanin	Renal	6	41	—	Usual	One-half usual dose	One-third usual dose
Tetracycline	Renal	8	50-100	0.25-0.5 g q6h	Usual	Use doxycycline	Use doxycycline
Ticarcillin	Renal	1.0-1.5	16	—	Usual	2-3 g q6-8h	2 g q12h
Ticarcillin + clavulanic acid	Renal	1.0-1.5	16	—	Usual	2-3 g q6-8h	2 g q12h
Tobramycin	Renal	2.5	56	1.7 mg/kg q8h	0.03 × CCr mg/Kg/8h	0.03 × CCr mg/Kg/8h	0.03 × CCr mg/Kg/8h
Trimethoprim	Renal	8-15	24	100 mg q12h	Usual	100 mg q24h	Avoid
Trimethoprim-sulfamethoxazole (TMP-SMX)	Renal	TMP:8-15 SMX: 7-12	24 SMX: 22-50	1-2 tablets q12h or 1-2 double-strength tablets q12h	Usual	One-half dose	Avoid
Trimetrexate	Metabolized	11	No data	45 mg/m² q24h	Usual	3-5 mg/kg q12-24h	Avoid
Valacyclovir	Renal	2.5-3.3	14	1,000 mg tid	Usual	1 g q 12-24h	500 mg q 24h
				500 mg bid	Usual	500 mg q 12-24h	500 mg q 24h
Vancomycin	Renal	6-8	200-250	0.125-0.5 g q6h	Usual	Usual	0.125 g PO q6h
					1 g q24h	1 g q3-10d	1 g q5-10d
Zidovudine	Hepatic and renal metabolism	1	3	200 mg tid	Usual	Usual	100 mg q6-8h

Abbreviations: GI, gastrointestinal; CCr, creatinine clearance
Source: Adapted, in part, from American Hospital Formulary Service. *Drug information*. 1996:37-612.

Drugs and Vaccines

Table 3. Antimicrobial Dosing Regimens in Severe Liver Disease

Dose Unchanged	Dose Reduced	Avoid
Aminoglycosides	Cephalosporins[a,b]	Ketoconazole
Amphotericin B	Chloramphenicol	Pyrazinamide
Capreomycin	Clindamycin	Sulfonamides
Cephalosporins	Clofazimine	Tetracycline
Cycloserine	Dapsone	
Doxycycline	Erythromycin,[c] other macrolides	
Ethambutol	Isoniazid	
Penicillin	Metronidazole	
Pentamidine	Nitrofurantoin	
Polymyxin	Penicillins (antistaphylococcal)	
Quinolones[d]	Penicillins (antipseudomonal)	
Spectinomycin	Ribavirin	
Trimethoprim	Rifampicin	
Vancomycin	Zidovudine	

Data are not as accurate as in kidney failure.

[a] Cephalothin, cefotaxime, cefoperazone, ceftriaxone, and cefotetan

[b] Dose reduced particularly for coexisting kidney and liver failure

[c] Avoid using estolate salt.

[d] Except pefloxacin

Drugs and Vaccines

Table 4. Guidelines for Adult Immunizations

Category/Vaccine	Dose	Comments
Age 18–24 years		
Td[a]	0.5 mL i.m.	Booster every 10 years at mid-decades (ages 25, 35, 45, etc.) or single dose at midlife (age 50) for those who completed primary series
Measles[b]	MMR, 0.5 mL s.c. × 1 or 2	Post–high school institutions should require 2 doses of live measles vaccine (separated by 1 month), the first dose preferably given before entry.
Rubella[c]	MMR, 0.5 mL s.c. one time	Especially susceptible females; pregnancy now or within 3 months postvaccination is contraindication to vaccination; avoid pregnancy for at least 3 months postvaccination.
Influenza		Advocated for young adults at increased risk of exposure (military recruits, students in dorms, sports teams, etc.)
Age 25–64 years		
Td[a]		As for 18–24 years
Mumps[c]		As for 18–24 years
Measles[b]	MMR, 0.5 mL s.c. one time	Persons vaccinated between 1963 and 1967 may have received inactivated vaccine and should be revaccinated.
Rubella[c]	MMR, 0.5 mL s.c. one time	Principally, females age ≤45 years with childbearing potential
Age >65 years		
Td[a]		As for 18–24 years
Influenza	0.5 mL i.m. annual	Annually, usually in November
Pneumococcal	23 valent, 0.5 mL i.m. or s.c.	Single dose; effectiveness for the elderly is not established, but case control and epidemiology studies suggest 60% to 70% effectiveness in preventing pneumococcal bacteremia.
Pregnancy		
		All pregnant women should be screened for hepatitis B surface antigen (HBsAg) and rubella antibody.
		Live virus vaccines[d] should be avoided unless specifically indicated; it is preferable to delay vaccines and toxoids until the second or third trimester; immunoglobulins are safe; most vaccines are a theoretical risk only.
Td[a]	0.5 mL i.m.	If not previously vaccinated, dose at 0, 4 weeks (preferably second and third trimesters) and at 6–12 months; protection to the infant is conferred by placental transfer of maternal antibody.
Measles		Risk for premature labor and spontaneous abortion; exposed pregnant women who are susceptible[b] should receive immunoglobulin within 6 days and then MMR postdelivery at least 3 months after immunoglobulin (MMR is contraindicated during pregnancy).
Mumps		No sequelae are noted, immunoglobulin is of no value, and MMR is contraindicated.
Rubella		Rubella during the first 16 weeks carries great risk, for example, 15% to 20% rate of neonatal death and 20% to 50% incidence of congenital rubella syndrome; history of rubella is an unreliable indicator of immunity; women exposed during the first 20 weeks should have rubella serology and, if not immune, should be offered abortion. Inadvertent vaccine administration to 300 pregnant women showed no vaccine-associated malformations.
Hepatitis A		Immunoglobulin, preferably within 1 week of exposure
Hepatitis B		All pregnant women should have prenatal screening for HBsAg; newborn infants of HBsAg carriers should receive HBIG and HBV vaccine; pregnant women who are HBsAg-negative and at high risk should receive HBV vaccine.
Inactivated polio	0.5 mL PO	Advised if exposure is imminent in women who completed the primary series over 10 years ago; unimmunized women should receive 2 doses separated by 1–2 months; unimmunized women at high risk who need immediate protection should receive oral live polio vaccine.
Influenza and pneumococcal		Not routinely recommended but can be given if there are other indications.
Varicella	VZIG 125 U/10 kg i.m. Maximum, 625 U	Varicella zoster immunoglobulin (VZIG) may prevent or modify maternal infection.
Family member exposure		
H. influenzae type B		H. influenzae meningitis; rifampin prophylaxis for all household contacts in households with another child <age 4 years; contraindicated in pregnant women
Hepatitis A		Immunoglobulin within 2 weeks of exposure
Hepatitis B		HBV vaccine (3 doses) plus HBV immunoglobulin for those with intimate contact and no serologic evidence of prior infection

(Continued)

Drugs and Vaccines

Table 4. Guidelines for Adult Immunizations (*Continued*)

Category/Vaccine	Dose	Comments
Influenza A		Influenza case should be treated with amantadine or rimantadine to prevent spread; unimmunized high-risk family members should receive amantadine or rimantadine (×14 days) and vaccine.
Meningococcal infection		Rifampin, ciprofloxacin, or ceftriaxone for close contacts of meningococcal meningitis
Varicella zoster		No treatment unless immunocompromised or pregnant; consider VZIG
Residents of nursing homes		
Influenza	0.5 mL i.m.	Annually for staff and residents; vaccination rates of 80% required to prevent outbreaks; for influenza A outbreaks, consider prophylaxis with amantadine or rimantadine
Pneumococcal	23 valent 0.5 mL i.m.	Single dose; effectiveness not clearly established in this population
Td[a]	0.5 mL i.m.	Booster dose at mid-decades
Residents of institutions for mentally retarded		
Hepatitis B		Screen all new admissions and long-term residents; HBV vaccine for susceptible individuals (seroprevalence rates are 30% to 80%)
Prison inmates		
Hepatitis B		As for residents of institutions for mentally retarded
Homeless		
Td[a]		Most need primary series or booster.
Measles, rubella, mumps	MMR 0.5 mL s.c.	Young adults
Influenza	Annual	
Pneumococcal	0.5 mL i.m. one time	
Health care workers		
Hepatitis B	1.0 mL i.m. ×3	Personnel in contact with blood or blood products; serologic screening with vaccination only of seronegatives is optional; serologic studies show 5% are nonresponders (negative for anti-HBs), even with repeat vaccinations.
Influenza	0.5 mL i.m. annual	
Rubella	MMR 0.5 mL s.c.	Personnel who might transmit rubella to pregnant patients or other health care workers should have documented immunity or vaccination.
Mumps	MMR 0.5 mL s.c.	Personnel with no documented history of mumps or vaccine should be vaccinated.
Measles	MMR 0.5 mL s.c.	Personnel who do not have immunity[b] should be vaccinated; those vaccinated in or after 1957 should receive an additional dose, and those who are unvaccinated should receive 2 doses separated by at least 1 month; during an outbreak in a medical setting, vaccinate (or revaccinate) all health care workers who have direct patient contact.
Polio		Persons with incomplete primary series should receive inactivated polio vaccine.
Varicella		Personnel with a negative history of chickenpox and/or negative serology (5% to 10% of adults have negative serology)
Immigrants and refugees		
Td[a]		Immunize if not previously done.
Rubella, measles, mumps	MMR 0.5 mL s.c.	Most have been vaccinated or had these conditions, although MMR is advocated, except for pregnant women.
Polio		Adults are usually immune.
Hepatitis B		Screen for HBsAg and vaccinate susceptible family members and sexual partners of carriers; screening is especially important for pregnant women.
Homosexual men		
Hepatitis B		Prevaccination serologic screening is advocated, because 30% to 80% have serologic evidence of HBV markers.
Hepatitis A		
Intravenous drug abusers		
Hepatitis B		As for homosexual men, seroprevalence rates of HBV markers are 50% to 80%.
Hepatitis A		
Immunodeficiency		

Drugs and Vaccines

Table 4. Guidelines for Adult Immunizations (*Continued*)

Category/Vaccine	Dose	Comments
HIV Infection		
Measles		Vaccine is contraindicated; postexposure prophylaxis with immunoglobulin for AIDS patients with CD4 counts <200/mm^3: immunoglobulin 0.5 mL/kg i.m. (15 mL maximum).
Pneumococcal	0.5 mL s.c.	Recommended as high priority
Influenza	0.5 mL i.m. annual	Consider amantadine during epidemics (vaccine may promote HIV replication)
Asplenia		
Pneumococcal	0.5 mL i.m.	Recommended, preferably given 2 weeks before elective splenectomy; revaccinate those who received the 14 valent vaccine and those vaccinated >6 years previously.
Meningococcal	0.5 mL s.c.	Indicated
H. influenzae b conjugate	0.5 mL i.m.	Consider
Renal failure		
Hepatitis B	1.0 mL i.m. ×3	For patients whose renal disease is likely to result in dialysis or transplantation, double-dose and periodic boosters are advocated.
Pneumococcal	0.5 mL s.c.	
Influenza	0.5 mL i.m. annual	
Alcoholics		
Pneumococcal	0.5 mL s.c. one time	
Diabetes and other high-risk diseases		
Influenza	0.5 mL i.m.	
Pneumococcal	0.5 mL s.c. one time	

[a] Td diphtheria and tetanus toxoids absorbed (for adult use). Primary series is 0.5 mL i.m. at 0, 4 weeks, and 6–12 months; booster doses at 10-year intervals are single doses of 0.5 mL i.m. Adults who have not received at least 3 doses of Td should complete the primary series. Persons with unknown histories should receive the series.

[b] Persons are considered immune to measles if there is documentation of receipt of 2 doses of live measles vaccine after the first birthday, prior physician diagnosis of measles, laboratory evidence of measles immunity, or birth before 1957.

[c] Persons are considered immune to mumps if they have a record of adequate vaccination, documented physician-diagnosed disease, or laboratory evidence of immunity. Persons are considered immune to rubella if they have a record of vaccination after their first birthday or laboratory evidence of immunity. (A physician diagnosis of rubella is considered nonspecific.)

[d] Live virus vaccines include measles, rubella, yellow fever, oral polio vaccine. The preferred vaccine for persons susceptible to measles, mumps, or rubella is MMR given as 0.5 mL s.c. for measles (1 or 2 doses), mumps (1 dose), or rubella (1 dose). Pregnant women should not be vaccinated until after delivery, and persons with HIV infection should not receive this vaccine.

Source: Adapted from *Guide for Adult Immunization*, 3rd ed. Philadelphia: American College of Physicians, 1994: 1–218; *MMWR Morb mortal Wkly Rep* 1991;12(RR-40):1–94; *MMWR Morb mortal Wkly Rep* 1994;(RR-43):1–38.

Drugs and Vaccines

Table 5. Guidelines for Childhood Immunizations

Vaccines[a] are listed under the routinely recommended ages. *Bars* indicate the range of acceptable ages for immunization. Catch-up immunization should be done during any visit when feasible. *Ovals* indicate vaccines to be assessed and given, if necessary during the early adolescent visit. More details for specific vaccine information (age ranges, dose, missed vaccinations, etc.) follow the table.

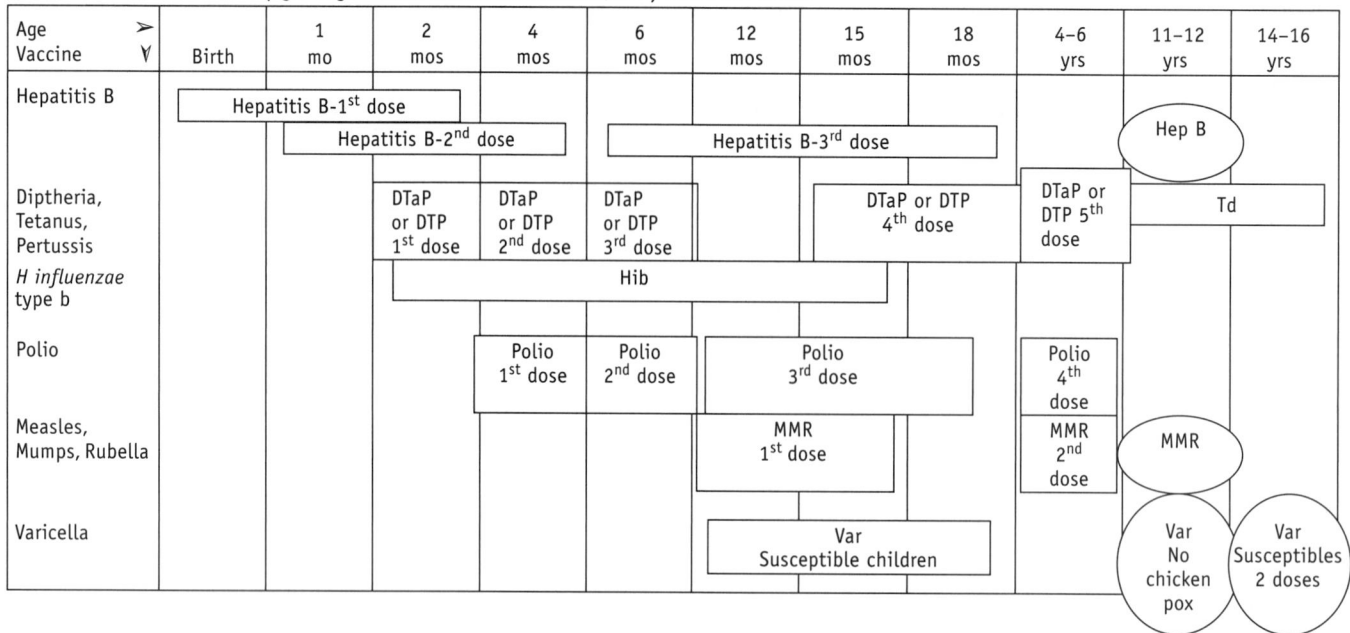

Age → Vaccine ↓	Birth	1 mo	2 mos	4 mos	6 mos	12 mos	15 mos	18 mos	4–6 yrs	11–12 yrs	14–16 yrs
Hepatitis B		Hepatitis B-1st dose								Hep B	
			Hepatitis B-2nd dose		Hepatitis B-3rd dose						
Diptheria, Tetanus, Pertussis			DTaP or DTP 1st dose	DTaP or DTP 2nd dose	DTaP or DTP 3rd dose		DTaP or DTP 4th dose		DTaP or DTP 5th dose	Td	
H influenzae type b			Hib								
Polio				Polio 1st dose	Polio 2nd dose	Polio 3rd dose			Polio 4th dose		
Measles, Mumps, Rubella						MMR 1st dose			MMR 2nd dose	MMR	
Varicella						Var Susceptible children				Var No chicken pox	Var Susceptibles 2 doses

[a] Recommended age for routine administration of currently licensed childhood vaccines; vaccines are listed under the ages for which they are routinely recommended. Catch-up immunization should be done during any visit when feasible. Some combination vaccines are available and may be used whenever administration of all components of the vaccine is indicated.

Drugs and Vaccines

Table 5. Guidelines for Childhood Immunizations (*Continued*)

HEPATITIS B

Infants born to *HBsAg-negative mothers* should receive 2.5 μg of Merck vaccine (Recombivax HB) or 10 μg of SmithKline Beecham (SB) vaccine (Energix-B). The *second dose* should be administered at least 1 month after the first dose. The *third dose* should be given at least 2 months after the second, but not before the age of 6 months.

Infants born to *HBsAg-positive mothers* should receive 0.5 mL of hepatitis B immunoglobulin (HBIG) within 12 hours of birth and either 5 μg Merck vaccine (Recombivax HB) or 10 μg SB vaccine (Energix-B) at a separate site. *Second dose* is recommended at the age of 1–2 months and the *third dose* at 6 months.

Infants born to *mothers whose HBsAg status is unknown* should receive either 5 μg Merck vaccine (Recombivax HB) or 10 μg SB vaccine (Engerix-B) within 12 hours of birth. The second dose of vaccine is recommended at the age of 1 month, and the third dose at 6 months. Blood should be drawn at the time of delivery to determine the mother's HBsAg status; if it is positive, the infant should receive HBIG as soon as possible (no later than the age of 1 week). Dosage and timing of subsequent vaccine doses should be based on the mother's HBsAg status.

Children and adolescents who have not been vaccinated against hepatitis B in infancy may begin the series with the first opportunity. *Those who have not previously received three doses* of hepatitis B vaccine should initiate or complete the series during the 11- to 12-year-old visit, and unvaccinated older adolescents should be vaccinated whenever possible. The *second dose* should be administered at least 1 month after the first dose, and the *third dose* should be administered at least 4 months after the first dose and at least 2 months after the second dose.

DIPTHERIA, TETANUS, PERTUSSIS

Diphtheria and tetanus toxoids and acellular pertussis vaccine (DTaP) is the preferred vaccine for all doses in the vaccination series, including completion of the series in children who have received one or more doses of whole-cell DTP vaccine. Whole-cell DTP is an acceptable alternative to DTaP. The fourth dose (DTP or DTaP) may be administered as early as age 12 months, provided 6 months have elapsed since the third dose and if the child is unlikely to return at 15 to 18 months. Tetanus and diphtheria toxoids vaccine (Td) is recommended at the age of 11 to 12 years if at least 5 years have elapsed since the last dose of DTP, DTaP, or DT. Subsequent routine Td boosters are recommended every 10 years.

HAEMOPHILUS INFLUENZAE

Three *H. influenzae* type b (Hib) conjugate vaccines are licensed for infant use. If PRP- OMP (PedvaxHIB [Merck]) is administered at ages 2 and 4 months, a dose at 6 months is not required.

POLIO

Two poliovirus vaccines are currently licensed in the United States: inactivated poliovirus vaccine (IPV) and oral poliovirus vaccine (OPV). The following schedules are all acceptable. Parents and providers may choose among these options:

- 2 doses of IPV, followed by 2 doses of OPV
- 4 doses of IPV
- 4 doses of OPV

Some authorities recommend two doses of IPV at 2 and 4 months of age, followed by two doses of OPV at 12 to 18 months and 4 to 6 years of age. IPV is the only poliovirus vaccine recommended for immunocompromised persons and their household contacts.

MEASLES, MUMPS, RUBELLA

A second dose of MMR is recommended routinely at 4 to 6 years of age but may be administered during any visit, provided at least 1 month has elapsed since receipt of the first dose and that both doses are administered beginning at or after 12 months of age. Those who have not previously received the second dose should complete the schedule no later than the visit at the ages of 11 to 12 years.

VARICELLA

Children who are susceptible to chickenpox may receive varicella vaccine at any visit after the first birthday, and those who lack a reliable history of chickenpox should be immunized during the visit at ages 11 to 12 years. Susceptible children age 13 years or older should receive two doses, at least 1 month apart.

Drugs and Vaccines

Table 6. Vaccines Available in the United States by Type and Recommended Routes of Administration

Vaccine	Type Indications (Adults)	Route and Usual Regimen[a]
Bacillus of Calmette and Guerin	Live bacteria; no longer advocated	Intradermal (0.2–0.3 mL)
Cholera	Inactivated bacteria; not recommended by the World Health Organization, but sometimes required for international travel	0.5 mL s.c. 2 times >1 week apart, or intradermal 0.2 mL 2 times
Diphtheria, tetanus, pertussis	Toxoids and inactivated bacteria Td or DT preferred for adults	0.5 mL i.m.
Hepatitis B	Inactived viral antigen (surface antigen); increased risk	1.0 mL i.m. 3 times at 0, 1, and 6 months
Hepatitis A	Inactivated virus	1.0 mL i.m. (deltoid muscle) + booster dose at ≥6 months
	Travel to endemic areas, homosexual men, injection drug users, persons with chronic liver disease, persons with occupational risk (laboratory workers who handle HAV)	
Haemophilus influenzae b conjugate	Polysaccharide conjugated to protein; adult at risk (splenectomy)	0.5 mL i.m. one time
Influenza	Inactivated virus or viral components; high risk, age >65 years, etc.	0.5 mL i.m. one time annually
Japanese B encephalitis	Inactivated JE virus; travel >1 month in epidemic area	1 mL s.c. at days 0, 7, and 30
Inactivated polio-viruses	Enhanced inactivated viruses of all 3 serotypes; travel to epidemic areas and immunocompromised patient or household contact. Note: Polio has been eradicated in the Western hemisphere.	0.5 mL s.c. one time
Measles	Live virus; unvaccinated adults born after 1956 without history of measles	0.5 mL s.c. one time or two, with second >1 month after first
Measles, mumps, rubella	Live viruses, usual form for persons susceptible to two of these viruses	0.5 mL s.c. one time or two, with second >1 month after the first
Meningococcal	Bacterial polysaccharides of serotypes A/C/Y/W-135; travel to epidemic area	0.5 mL s.c. one time
Mumps	Live virus; unvaccinated adults born after 1956 without history of mumps	0.5 mL s.c. one time
Oral poliovirus	Live viruses of all three serotypes; standard pediatric polio in U.S.	Oral

Drugs and Vaccines

Table 6. Vaccines Available in the United States by Type and Recommended Routes of Administration (*Continued*)

Vaccine	Type Indications (Adults)	Route and Usual Regimen[a]
Pertussis	Inactivated whole bacteria	Intramscular—distributed by Biologic Products Program, Michigan Department of Public Health (Phone: 517–335–8120)
Plague	Inactivated bacteria; selected travelers to epidemic areas	1.0 mL i.m., then 0.2 mL at 1 month and 4–7 months
Pneumococcal	Bacterial polysaccharides of 23 pneumococcal types; adults at risk or age >65 years	0.5 mL i.m. or s.c.
Rabies	Inactivated virus, HDCV and RVA postexposure	1.0 mL i.m. days 0, 3, 7, 14, and 28 postexposure
Rubella	Live virus; unvaccinated adults without history of rubella	0.5 mL s.c. one time
Tetanus	Inactivated toxin (toxoid); Td preferred	0.5 mL i.m. one time
Tetanus, diphtheria[b]	Inactivated toxins booster every 10 years or at midlife	0.5 mL i.m. one time
Typhoid	Inactivated bacteria	0.5 mL s.c. 2 times, separated by 1 month
	Live attenuated strain (Ty21a); travelers to epidemic area	Oral x 4 (dose every other day)
	Vi capsular polysaccharide vaccine; travelers to epidemic areas	0.5 mL i.m. one time
Varicella	Live attenuated virus	Adults: 0.5 mL s.c. 2 times, separated by 4–8 weeks
	Susceptible adults (negative history of chickenpox or negative serology). Also, health care workers, household contacts of immunosuppressed patient, persons living or working in high-risk area (schools, daycare centers), nonpregnant women of childbearing age, or international travelers	
Yellow fever (17 D strain)	Live virus; travel to epidemic areas	0.5 mL s.c. one time

[a] Assumes childhood immunizations have been completed.

[b] DT, tetanus and diphtheria toxoids for use in children age ≤7 years. Td, tetanus and diphtheria toxoids for use in persons age ≥7 years. Td contains the same amount of tetanus toxoid as DPT or DT but a reduced dose of diptheria toxoid.

Source: From MMWR Morb Mortal WKLY Rep 1994;43(RR-1); and *Ann Intern Med* 1996;124:35.

Drugs and Vaccines

Table 7a. Vaccines in the Immunocompromised Host

Vaccine	Routine (Not Immunocompromised)	HIV Infection or AIDS	Organ Transplantation, Chronic Immunosuppressive Therapy, Severly Immunocompromised (Non-HIV-related)[a]	Asplenia	Renal failure[b], Alcoholism, Alcoholic Cirrhosis, Diabetes
Td	Recommended	Recommended	Recommended	Recommended	Recommended
MMR (MR/M/R)	Use if indicated	Contraindicated	Contraindicated	Use if indicated	Use if indicated
Hepatitis B	Use if indicated	Use if indicated	Use if indicated	Use if indicated	Use if indicated
Hib	Not recommended	Considered	Recommended	Recommended	Use if indicated
Pneumococcal	Recommended if age ≥65 years	Recommended	Recommended	Recommended	Recommended
Meningococcal	Use if indicated	Use if indicated	Use if indicated	Recommended	Use if indicated
Influenza	Recommended if age ≥65 years	Recommended	Recommended	Recommended	Recommended

[a] Severe immunosuppression can be the result of congenital immunodeficiency, HIV infection, leukemia, lymphoma, generalized malignancy, or therapy with alkylating agents, antimetabolites, radiation, or large doses of corticosteroids.

[b] Patients with renal failure on dialysis should have their anti-HBs response tested after vaccination, and those found not to respond should be revaccinated.

Source: Recommendation of Advisory Committee on Immunization Practices of the CDC. *MMWR Morb Mortal Wkly Rep* 1993;42(RR-4).

Drugs and Vaccines

Table 7b. Summary of Recommendations on Nonroutine Immunization of Immunocompromised Persons

Vaccine	Not Immunocompromised	Organ Transplantation, Chronic Immunosuppressive Therapy, Severe Immunosuppression[a], and HIV/AIDS	Asplenia, Renal Failure, Alcoholism, and Alcoholic Cirrhosis
Live vaccines			
BCG	Use if indicated	Contraindicated	Use if indicated
OPV	Use if indicated	Contraindicated	Use if indicated
Vaccinia	Use if indicated	Contraindicated	Use if indicated
Typhoid, Ty21a	Use if indicated	Contraindicated	Use if indicated
Yellow fever[b]	Use if indicated	Contraindicated	Use if indicated
Killed or inactivated vaccines			
IPV	Use if indicated	Use if indicated	Use if indicated
Cholera	Use if indicated	Use if indicated	Use if indicated
Plague	Use if indicated	Use if indicated	Use if indicated
Typhoid, inactivated	Use if indicated	Use if indicated	Use if indicated
Rabies	Use if indicated	Use if indicated	Use if indicated
Anthrax	Use if indicated	Use if indicated	Use if indicated

[a] Severe immunosuppression can be the result of congenital immunodeficiency, HIV infection, leukemia, lymphoma, aplastic anemia, generalized malignancy, or therapy with alkylating agents, antimetabolites, radiation, or large amounts of corticosteroids.

[b] Yellow fever vaccine should be considered for patients when exposure to yellow fever cannot be avoided.

Drugs and Vaccines

Table 8a. Characteristics, Activity, and Adverse Effects of Immunoglobulins

Pooled Human Immunoglobulin	Hyperimmune-Specific Human Immunoglobulin	Animal (Equine) Immunoglobulin or Antitoxin
Characteristics		
Obtained from pooled human plasma Contains IgG for several common infections in the population	Obtained from immune persons. High concentration of specific IgG Half-life = 25 days	Obtained from animals immunized with toxoids (inactivated diphtheria or botulinum toxoids)
Half-life = 25 days	**Activity**	Half-life = 7 days

Prevention of
  Hepatitis A
  Measles
  Poliomyelitis if given early after exposure
Little protection against
 	
  Hepatitis B
  Congenital rubella (when given to pregnant women with rubella)
	Prevention of
	  Hepatitis B
	  Varicella zoster virus (VZV)
	  Rabies, Tetanus
	Effectiveness unclear and *not* recommended for
	  Whooping cough
	  Mumps
		Treatment relatively effective for
		  Diphtheria
		  Botulism

	Adverse Effects	
Local symptoms	Local symptoms	May cause anaphylaxis (perform intradermic testing before administration)
May be used in pregnancy Use only i.m.; Intravenous injection may cause anaphylaxis because it contains IgG aggregates of high molecular weight[a]	May be used in pregnancy Rarely causes anaphylaxis	Fever Serum sickness

Intravenous immunoglobulin may cause headache, abdominal pain, lumbar pain, nausea and vomiting, chills, fever, and myalgias, which may be alleviated by decreasing the infusion rate and administering aspirin or corticosteroids. In patients with IgA deficiency, a severe anaphylactic reaction may be seen. A preparation with low IgA content should be used (Gammagard).

[a] Human immunoglobulin preparations without anticomplement activity are available and may be given at high doses intravenously. They are indicated in patients with hypogammaglobulinemia, prevention of VZV and cytomegalovirus infections, Kawasaki disease, idiopathic thrombocytopenic purpura, and treatment of chronic parvovirus B19 infection in patients with immunosuppression.

Drugs and Vaccines

Table 8b. Use of Vaccines and Immunoglobulins

Disease	Indication	Vaccine	Immunoglobulin
Botulism	Patient with botulism	Not available	Horse antitoxin
CMV disease	Transplant recipient, especially bone marrow and liver transplant; seronegative for CMV	Not available	CMV IG *Dose*: 0.15–1.0 g/kg/wk *Efficacy*: Decreases frequency and severity of disease
Cholera	Travel to area where vaccination is required	*Action*: Killed bacteria *Dose*: 2 doses of 0.5 mL s.c. or i.m. with 1-week to 1-month interval *Efficacy*: <50% after 3–6 months	Not available
Diphtheria	Unimmunized persons	*Action*: Toxoid *Dose*: 3 doses of 0.5 mL i.m. at 0, 2, and 12 months	—
	Immunized persons	*Dose Booster*: Every 10 years (95% efficacy) *Efficacy*: Prevents toxic effects but does not prevent infection	—
	Patient with diphtheria	N/A	Horse antitoxin
Japanese encephalitis	Travel to endemic area (Southeast Asia and China)	*Action*: Killed virus *Dose*: 3 doses s.c. at days 0, 7, and 30	Not available
Yellow fever	Travel to endemic area (equatorial Africa and South America)	*Action*: Attenuated virus *Dose*: Single dose 0.5 mL s.c. Contraindicated in patients with egg protein allergy *Efficacy*: 10-year protection	Not available
Typhoid fever	Travel to endemic area; natural disasters (floods, earthquakes)	*Dose*: 4 capsules administered on alternative days; avoid antibiotics for at least 1 week Typhim Vi vaccine single 0.5-mL (25-μg) dose i.m. Booster recommended every 2 years *Efficacy*: Effectiveness of all typhoid vaccines is approximately 65%	Not available
Haemophilus influenzae serotype b	Children, especially those with Asplenia Sickle cell disease Nephrotic syndrome CSF fistulas Immunosuppression Adults with asplenia	*Action*: Capsular polysaccharide conjugated with a carrier protein *Dose*: Administer i.m. following the schedule of DTP vaccination. *Efficacy*: Greater than 90%	Not available
Influenza	Adults >age 65 years Health care workers, especially those caring for high-risk persons High-risk persons: Military, police headquarters Patients with chronic lung, heart, liver, kidney disease, diabetes, immunosuppression, or HIV Children 6 months to 18 years on chronic aspirin therapy	*Action*: Killed whole or fractionated virus or surface antigens *Dose*: Administer annually in a single 0.5-mL dose i.m. in the deltoid muscle in fall; intramuscular; contraindicated in patients with egg protein allergy. In children younger than the age of 13 years, must use fractionated virus vaccine *Efficacy*: 75% for 6 months in the young, but less in the elderly	Not available

(Continued)

Drugs and Vaccines

Table 8b. Use of Vaccines and Immunoglobulins (*Continued*)

Disease	Indication	Vaccine	Immunoglobulin
Hepatitis A	Susceptible persons older than the age of 2 years traveling to, living in, or relocating to an area of high endemic risk	Two vaccines available: Havrix and VAQTA	Pooled human IG 0.02 mL/kg i.m. for stays <3 months; for longer stays, 0.06 mL/kg/5 months; concurrent administration with vaccine at a different site for late initiation
	Military personnel	*Havrix for Adults*:	Pooled human IG 0.02 mL/kg i.m. within first 14 days after exposure
	Ethnic and geographic populations that experience cyclic hepatitis A epidemics, such as native peoples of Alaska and the Americas	*Dose*: single dose i.m. of 1440 EL.U. in 1 mL. Booster dose is recommended any time between 6 and 12 months after initiation of the primary course.	
	Persons engaging in high-risk sexual activity	*Havrix for Children 2–18 yr*:	
	Users of illicit injectable drugs	*Dose*: 2 doses containing 360 EL.U. each in 0.5 mL i.m. one month apart	
	Residents of a community experiencing outbreak of hepatitis A	*VAQTA for Adults*:	
	Persons with possible occupational exposure to hepatitis A virus, such as primate handlers and laboratory workers	*Dose*: Single dose i.m. of 50 U of hepatitis A virus antigen in 1 mL. Booster dose of 1 mL is recommended 6 months after the initial vaccination.	
	Children and adults in contact with a person with hepatitis A	*VAQTA for Children 2–17 yr*:	
		Dose: Single dose i.m. of 25 U of hepatitis A virus antigen in 0.5 mL. Booster dose of 0.5 mL is recommended 6–18 months after the initial vaccination.	
Hepatitis B	Unimmunized persons	Action: HBsAg	—
		Dose, Adult: 3 doses of 1 mL (20µg) i.m. in the deltoid at 0, 1, and 6 months	
		Dose, Children: 0.5 mL (10 µg)	
		Dose, Elderly and Immunosuppressed: 2 mL, (40 µg)	
		Efficacy: 95%	
		Rapid schedule for travelers: 2 doses at 2-week interval has >80% protection.	
	Newborn of HBsAg-positive mother	First dose of 0.5 mL at birth (10 µg) i.m. at different site from IG, then at 1 and 6 months	Specific IG, 0.5 mL i.m. at birth
	Accidental exposure (percutaneous, mucosa, sexual)	Immunize the week after administration of IG	Specific IG, 0.06 mL/kg i.m. within 48 hours after exposure. Obtain serum for HBsAg. If negative, give a second dose of specific IG 1 month later.
Pneumococcal	Adults age >65 years	Action: Capsular polysaccharide, 23 serotypes	Not available
	Adults and children older than age of 2 years with chronic lung disease, chronic heart disease, chronic liver disease, chronic kidney disease, diabetes, nephrotic syndrome, and immunosuppression, including asplenia (anatomic or functional), myeloma, immunosuppressive treatment, transplant, CSF fistulas, HIV	*Dose, Routine*: single dose of 0.5 mL SC or i.m. *Dose, High-Risk*: Consider booster in 4–5 years after "routine" dose; may be administered with flu shot (different sites)	

Drugs and Vaccines

Table 8b. Use of Vaccines and Immunoglobulins (*Continued*)

Disease	Indication	Vaccine	Immunoglobulin
		Dose, Transplant: Administer 2 weeks prior to transplant. *Efficacy*: 70%; lower in patients with immunosuppression or under the age of 2 years	
Meningococcal	Outbreak Complement deficiency Asplenia (anatomic or functional) Travelers visiting endemic areas Contact with meningococcus caused by serogroups included in the vaccine	*Action*: Polysaccharide of serotypes A, C, Y, and W135 *Dose*: single dose 0.5 mL i.m. or s.c. *Efficacy*: 90%; confers no protection against serogroup B	Not available
Mumps	Unimmunized persons	*Action*: Attenuated virus *Dose*: 0.5 mL s.c.; contraindicated in persons with egg protein allergy *Efficacy*: 95%	—
Plague	Exposure in an endemic area	*Action*: Killed bacilli *Dose*: Three 1-mL doses s.c. at 0, 1, and 4 months *Booster Dose*: At 6 months if exposure continues	Not available
Poliomyelitis	Unimmunized persons under age 18 years Unimmunized persons over age 18 years traveling to endemic area Immunosuppressed person Immunized persons over age 18 years traveling to an endemic area	*Action*: Live attenuated virus (Sabin) *Dose*: Orally *Action*: Killed virus (Salk) *Dose*: 3 doses of 0.5 mL s.c. at 0, 1, and 12 months *Booster Dose*: Live attenuated vaccine (Sabin)	—
Rabies[a]	Exposure to animals in areas where disease is endemic	*Action*: Killed virus *Dose*: 3 doses of 1 mL i.m. in deltoid area at 0, 7, and 28 days	—
	Animal bite or contact of a wound or the mucosae with saliva of an animal suspected of being rabid in an endemic area[a] (Unimmunized persons)	*Day 0*: 2 doses of 1 mL *Day 7*: 1 dose of 1 mL *Day 28*: 1 dose of 1 mL *Booster Dose*: Every 2–3 years	HRIG (specific human IG) 20 IU/kg; half i.m. and half around wound
	Immunized persons	*Dose*: 2 doses of 1 mL each i.m. at 0 and 3 days	Not needed if Ab response is good

(*Continued*)

Drugs and Vaccines

Table 8b. Use of Vaccines and Immunoglobulins (*Continued*)

Disease	Indication	Vaccine	Immunoglobulin
Rubella	Unimmunized persons	*Action*: Attenuated virus *Dose*: 0.5 mL s.c. *Efficacy*: 95% *Adverse Effects*: may cause arthralgias, adenopathy, and fever	—
Measles	Unimmunized persons	*Action*: Attenuated virus *Dose*: 0.5 mL s.c.; second dose given >1 month later	0.25 mL/kg i.m. up to 15 mL (healthy host) 0.5 mL/kg up to 15 mL (immunocompromised host)
	Susceptible contacts, in particular, children, pregnant women, and immunocompromised patients	—	IG
Tetanus	Unimmunized persons	*Action*: Inactivated toxin *Dose*: 3 doses of 0.5 mL i.m. at 0, 1, and 12 months	—
	Immunized persons Wound (prophylaxis)	*Booster Dose*: every 10 years	
	Tetanus (treatment)	—	Specific IG 3,000 IU i.m.
Pertussis	Unimmunized, <age 7 years	*Action*: Acellular vaccine (aP) *Dose*: Eight formulations available	—

Varicella (chickenpox)	Children >age 12 months
	Susceptible, immunocompetent adults
	  Health care workers
	  Household contacts of immunosuppressed persons living or working in high-risk areas (schools and day care centers)
	  Young adults in military or colleges
	  Nonpregnant women and those of childbearing potential
	  International travelers
		Children >12 months and <12 years:
		Dose: Single dose 0.5 mL s.c.
		Adults and children age >13 years
		Dose: 0.5 mL s.c. initial dose; 0.5 mL s.c. 4–8 weeks later
			—

	Immunocompromised or newborn contact	—	VZIG (specific IG) 125 U/10 kg i.m. up to 625 U
Tuberculosis	PPD-negative patients exposed to known TB who cannot be followed (immigrants, the noncompliant) Persons living in an area of high prevalence of resistant tuberculosis *Avoid* in HIV-infected patients and, possibly, in all immunosuppressed hosts	*Action*: Bacillus Calmette-Guérin *Dose*: single dose s.c. *Efficacy*: 60%–80% *Adverse Effects*: May cause ulcer at vaccination site and local adenopathy	—

Abbreviations: CMV, cytomegalovirus; IG, immunoglobulin.

[a] If the animal is captured, treatment may be delayed until the disease is confirmed with immunofluorescence testing of brain tissue. Immunized animals that exhibit normal behavior may be kept under continued observation for 10 days before the decision is made to kill them.

Drugs and Vaccines

Table 9a. Prophylaxis of Endocarditis

	Prophylaxis Recommended	Prophylaxis Not Recommended

Host Factors	High-risk patients
	  Prosthetic cardiac valves (bioprosthetic and homograft valves)
	  Previous bacterial endocarditis
	  Complex cyanotic congenital heart disease (e.g., single ventricle states, transposition of the great arteries, tetralogy of Fallot)
	  Surgically constructed systemic pulmonary shunts or conduits
	Moderate-risk Patients
	  Most other congenital cardiac malformations (other than those listed above and in the negligible-risk category on the right)
	  Acquired valvular dysfunction (e.g., rheumatic heart disease)
	  Hypertrophic cardiomyopathy
	  Mitral valve prolapse with valvular regurgitation and/or thickened leaflets[a]
		Negligible-risk Patients
		  Isolated secundum atrial septal defect
		  Surgical repair of atrial septal defect
		  Ventricular septal defect
		  Patent ductus arteriosis (without residua beyond 6 months)
		  Previous coronary artery bypass graft surgery
		  Mitral valve prolapse without valvular regurgitation[a]
		  Physiological, functional, or innocent heart murmurs
		  Previous Kawasaki disease without valvular dysfunction
		  Previous rheumatic fever without valvular dysfunction
		  Cardiac pacemakers (intravascular and epicardial)
		  Implanted defibrillators

Dental Procedures	Dental extractions Periodontal procedures, including surgery, scaling, root planing, probing, recall maintenance Dental implant placement Reimplantation of avulsed teeth Endodontic(root canal instrumentation or surgery only beyond the apex) Subgingival placement of antibiotic fibers or strips Initial placement of orthodontic bands but not brackets Intraligamentary local anesthetic injections Prophylactic cleaning of teeth or implants where bleeding is anticipated	Restorative dentistry[b] (operative and prosthodontic) with or without retraction cord Local anesthetic injections (nonintraligamentary) Intracanal endodontic treatment (including postplacement and buildup) Placement of rubber dams Postoperative suture removal Placement of removable prosthodontic or orthodontic appliances Taking of oral impressions Fluoride treatments Taking of oral radiographs Orthodontic appliance adjustment Shedding of primary teeth

(Continued)

Drugs and Vaccines

Table 9a. Prophylaxis of Endocarditis (*Continued*)

	Prophylaxis Recommended	Prophylaxis Not Recommended

Medical Procedures	**Respiratory Tract**
	Tonsillectomy and/or adenoidectomy
	Surgical operations that involve respiratory mucosa
	Bronchoscopy with a rigid bronchoscope
	
	Gastrointestinal Tract[d]
	Sclerotherapy for esophageal varices
	Esophageal stricture dilation
	Endoscopic retrograde cholangiography with biliary obstruction
	Biliary tract surgery
	Surgical operations that involve intestinal mucosa
	
	Genitourinary Tract
	Prostate surgery
	Cytoscopy
	Urethral dilation
		Respiratory Tract
		Endotracheal intubation
		Bronchoscopy with a flexible bronchoscope with or without biopsy[c]
		Tympanostomy tube insertion
		
		Gastrointestinal Tract
		Transesophageal echocardiogarphy[c]
		Endoscopy with or without gastrointestinal biopsy[c]
		
		Genitourinary Tract
		Cesarean section
		Vaginal hysterectomy[c]
		Vaginal delivery[c]
		  If tissue is not infected
		  Urethral catheterization
		  Uterine dilatation and curettage
		  Therapeutic abortion
		  Sterilization procedures
		  Insertion or removal of intrauterine devices
		Other Procedures
		Cardiac catheterization, including balloon angioplasty
		Implanted cardiac pacemakers
		Implanted defibrillators
		Coronary stents
		Incision or biopsy of surgically scrubbed skin
		Circumcision

[a] Patients with prolapsing and leaking mitral valves who have audible clicks and murmurs of mitral regurgitation of Doppler-demonstrated mitral insufficiency should receive prophylactic antibiotics.
[b] This includes restoration of decayed teeth (filling cavities) and replacement of missing teeth.
[c] Prophylaxis is optional for high-risk patients.
[d] Prophylaxis is recommended for high-risk patients; it is optional for medium-risk patients.

Drugs and Vaccines

Table 9b. Prophylactic Regimens for Dental, Respiratory Tract, or Esophageal Procedures

Situation	Agent	Regimen[a]
Standard general prophylaxis	Amoxicillin	*Adults:* 2 g PO *Children:* 50 mg/kg PO 1 hour before procedure
Cannot take oral medication	Ampicillin	*Adults:* 2 g i.m or i.v *Children:* 50 mg/kg i.m. or i.v. Within 30 minutes before procedure
Allergic to penicillin	Clindamycin	*Adults:* 600 mg PO *Children:* 20 mg/kg PO 1 hour before procedure
	Cephalexin[b] or Cefadroxil[b]	*Adults:* 2 g PO *Children:* 50 mg/kg PO 1 hour before procedure
	Azithromycin or Clarithromycin	*Adults:* 500 mg PO *Children:* 15 mg/kg PO 1 hour before procedure
Allergic to penicillin and cannot take oral medications	Clindamycin	*Adults:* 600 mg i.v. *Children:* 20 mg/kg i.v. Within 30 minutes before procedure
	Cefazolin[b]	*Adults:* 1 g i.m. or i.v. *Children:* 25 mg/kg i.m. or i.v. Within 30 minutes before procedure

[a] The total children's dose should not exceed the adult dose.
[b] Cephalosporins should not be used in individuals with immediate-type hypersensitivity reactions (urticaria, angioedema, or anaphylaxis) to penicillins.

Drugs and Vaccines

Table 9c. Prophylactic Regimens for Genitourinary and Gastrointestinal (Excluding Esophageal) Procedures

Situation	Agents[a]	Regimen[b]
High-risk patients	Ampicillin + gentamicin	Adults: Within 30 minutes of starting the procedure: Ampicillin 2 g i.m. or i.v. plus Gentamicin 1.5 mg/kg (not to exceed 120 mg) Six hours later: Ampicillin 1 g i.m. or i.v. or Amoxicillin 1 g PO Children: Within 30 minutes of starting the procedure: Ampicillin 50 mg/kg i.m. or i.v. (not to exceed 2.0 g) plus Gentamicin 1.5 mg/kg i.m. or i.v. Six hours later: Ampicillin 25 mg/kg i.m. or i.v. or Amoxicillin 25 mg/kg PO
High-risk patients allergic to ampicillin or amoxicillin	Vancomycin + gentamicin	Adults Vancomycin 1 g i.v. over 1–2 hours plus Gentamicin 1.5 mg/kg i.v. or i.m. (not to exceed 120 mg) Complete injection or infusion within 30 minutes of starting the procedure Children: Vancomycin 20 mg/kg i.v. or 1–2 hours plus Gentamicin 1.5 mg/kg i.v. or i.m. Complete injection or infusion within 30 minutes of starting the procedure
Moderate-risk patients	Amoxicillin OR ampicillin	Adults: Amoxicillin 2 g PO 1 hour before procedure or Ampicillin 2 g i.m. or i.v. within 30 minutes of starting the procedure Children Amoxicillin 50/kg PO 1 hour before procedure or Ampicillin 50 mg/kg i.m. or i.v. within 30 minutes of starting the procedure
Moderate-risk patients allergic to ampicillin or amoxicillin	Vancomycin	Adults: Vancomycin 1 g i.v. over 1–2 hours Complete infusion within 30 minutes of starting the procedure Children: Vancomycin 20 mg/kg i.v. over 1–2 hours Complete infusion within 30 minutes of starting the procedure

[a] Total children's dose should not exceed the adult dose.
[b] No second dose of vancomycin or gentamicin is recommended.

Drugs and Vaccines

Table 10. Trade Names of Antimicrobial Agents

Trade Name	Generic Name	Trade Name	Generic Name	Trade Name	Generic Name
Abelcet	Amphotericin (B-lipid complex)	Cloxapen	Cloxacillin	Grisactin	Griseofulvin
A-cillin	Amoxicillin	Cofatrim	Trimethoprim-sulfamethoxazole	Gulfasin	Sulfisoxazole
A-K-chlor	Chloramphenicol	Coly-Mycin M	Colistimethate	Halfan	Halofantrine
Achromycin	Tetracycline	Cotrim	Trimethoprim-sulfamethoxazole	Herplex	Idoxuridine
Aerosporin	Polymyxin B			Hetrazan	Diethylcarbamazepine
Aftate	Tolnaftate	Crixivan	Indinavir	Hiprex	Methenamine hippurate
Ala-Tet	Tetracycline	Cytovene	Ganciclovir		
Albamycin	Novobiocin	D-Amp	Ampicillin	HIVID	Zalcitabine
Alferon N	Interferon alfa-n3	Daraprim	Pyrimethamine	Humatin	Paromomycin
Amcap	Ampicillin	Declomycin	Demeclocycline	Ilosone	Erythromycin estolate
Amficot	Ampicillin	Diflucan	Fluconazole		
Amikin	Amikacin	Doryx	Doxycycline	Ilotycin	Erythromycin
Amoxil	Amoxicillin	Doxy-caps	Doxycycline	Intron A	Interferon-alfa-2b
Ancef	Cefazolin	Doxy-D	Doxycycline	Invirase	Saquinavir
Ancobon	Flucytosine	Duricef	Cefadroxil	Jenamicin	Gentamicin
Anspor	Cephradine	Dycill	Dicloxacillin	Kantrex	Kanamycin
Antepar	Piperazine	DynaPak	Dirithromycin	Keflex	Cephalexin
Antiminth	Pyrantel pamoate	Dynapen	Dicloxacillin	Keflin	Cephalothin
Aoracillin B	Penicillin G	E-mycin	Erythromycin	Keftab	Cephalexin
Aralen	Chloroquine	EES	Erythromycin ethylsuccinate	Kefurox	Cefuroxime
Arsobal	Melarsoprol			Kefzol	Cefazolin
Atabrine	Quinacrine	Elimite	Permethrin	Kwell	Lindane
Augmentin	Clavulanic acid plus amoxicillin	Emtet-500	Tetracycline	Lamisil	Terbinafine
		Epivir	Lamivudine	Lampit	Nifurtimox
Azactam	Aztreonam	Erothricin	Erythromycin	Lamprene	Clofazimine
Azulfidine	Sulfasalazine	ERYC	Erythromycin	Lanacillin	Penicillin V
Bactrim	Trimethoprim-sulfamethoxazole	Ery-Tab	Erythromycin	Lariam	Mefloquine
		Erythrocot	Erythromycin	Ledercillin VK	Penicillin V
Bactroban	Mupirocin	Eryzole	Erythromycin sulfisoxazole	Levaquin	Levofloxacin
Beepen-VK	Penicillin V			Lice-Enz	Pyrethrins
Biaxin	Clarithromycin	Famvir	Famciclovir	Lincocin	Lincomycin
Bicillin	Benzathine penicillin G	Fansidar	Pyrimethamine plus sulfadoxine	Lincorex	Lincomycin
				Lorabid	Loracarbef
Biltricide	Praziquantel	Fasigyn	Tinidazole	Lotrimin	Clotrimazole
Bitin	Bithionol	Femstat	Metronidazole	Lyphocin	Vancomycin
C-Lexin	Cephalexin	Floxin	Ofloxacin	Macrobid	Nitrofurantoin
Capastat	Capreomycin	Flumadine	Rimantadine	Macrodantin	Nitrofurantoin
Caropen-VK	Penicillin V	Fortaz	Ceftazidime	Mandelamine	Methenamine mandelate
Ceclor	Cefaclor	Foscavir	Foscarnet		
Cedax	Ceftibutin	Fulvicin	Griseofulvin	Mandol	Cefamandole
Cefadyl	Cephapirin	Fungizone	Amphotericin B	Marcillin	Ampicillin
Cefanex	Cephalexin	Furacin	Nitrofurazone	Maxaquin	Lomefloxacin
Cefizox	Ceftizoxime	Furadantin	Nitrofurantoin	Maxipime	Cefixime
Cefobid	Cefoperazone	Furamide	Diloxanide furoate	Mectizan	Ivermectin
Cefotan	Cefotetan	Furantoin	Nitrofurantoin	Mefoxin	Cefoxitin
Ceftin	Cefuroxime axetil	Furoxone	Furazolidone	Mepron	Atovaquone
Cefzil	Cefprozil	G-Mycin	Gentamicin	Merrem	Meropenem
Ceptaz	Ceftazidime	Gantanol	Sulfamethoxazole	Metric	Metronidazole
Chero-Trisulfa V	Trisulfapyrimidine	Gantrisin	Sulfisoxazole	Metro-IV	Metronidazole
Chloromycetin	Chloramphenicol	Garamycin	Gentamicin	Mezlin	Mezlocillin
Cinobac	Cinoxacin	Geocillin	Carbenicillin indanyl sodium	Minocin	Minocycline
Cipro	Ciprofloxacin			Mintezol	Thiabendazole
Claforan	Cefotaxime	Germanin	Suramin	Monocid	Cefonicid
Cleocin	Clindamycin	Grifulvin	Griseofulvin	Monodox	Doxycycline

(Continued)

Drugs and Vaccines

Table 10. Trade Names of Antimicrobial Agents (*Continued*)

Trade Name	Generic Name	Trade Name	Generic Name	Trade Name	Generic Name
Monurol	Fosfomycin	Proloprim	Trimethoprim	Tobrex	Tobramycin
Monistat	Miconazole	Pronto	Pyrethrins	Trecator SC	Ethionamide
Myambutol	Ethambutol	Prostaphlin	Oxacillin	Triazole	Trimethoprim-sulfamethoxazole
Mycelex	Clotrimazole	Protostat	Metronidazole		
Mycobutin	Rifabutin	Pyopen	Carbenicillin	Trimox	Amoxicillin
Mycostatin	Nystatin	Retrovir	Zidovudine	Trimpex	Trimethoprim
MyE	Erythromycin	RID	Pyrethrins	Trisulfam	Trimethoprim-sulfamethoxazole
Nafcil	Nafcillin	Rifadin	Rifampin		
Nallpen	Nafcillin	Rifamate	Rifampin-INH	Trobicin	Spectinomycin
Natacyn	Natamycin	Rifater	Rifampin, INH, pyrazinamide	Truxcillin	Penicillin G
Nebcin	Tobramycin			Ultracef	Cefadroxil
NebuPent	Pentamidine aerosol	Rimactane	Rifampin	Unasyn	Ampicillin-sulbactam
		Robicillin VK	Penicillin V		
NegGram	Nalidixic acid	Robimycin	Erythromycin	Unipen	Nafcillin
Netromycin	Netilmicin	Robitet	Tetracycline	Urex	Methenamine hippurate
Neutrexin	Trimetrexate	Rocephin	Ceftriaxone		
Niclocide	Niclosamide	Rochagan	Benzimidazole	Uri-Tet	Oxytetracycline
Nilstat	Nystatin	Roferon-A	Interferon-alpha-2a	Uroplus	Trimethoprim-sulfamethoxazole
Nix	Permethrin	Rovamycine	Spiramycin		
Nizoral	Ketoconazole	Seromycin	Cycloserine	V-Cillin	Penicillin V
Noroxin	Norfloxacin	Silvadene	Silver sulfadiazine	Valtrex	Valacyclovir
Nor-Tet	Tetracycline	Soxa	Sulfisoxazole	Vancocin	Vancomycin
Norvir	Ritonavir	Spectrobid	Bacampicillin	Vancoled	Vancomycin
Nydrazid	INH	Sporanox	Itraconazole	Vansil	Oxamniquine
Nystex	Nystatin	Staphcillin	Methicillin	Vantin	Cefpodoxime proxetil
Omnipen	Ampicillin	Storz-G	Gentamicin		
Ornidyl	Eflornithine	Stoxil	Idoxuridine	Veetids	Penicillin V
Ovide	Malathion	Sulfamar	Trimethoprim-sulfamethoxazole	Velosef	Cephradine
Paludrine	Proguanil			Vermox	Mebendazole
Panmycin	Tetracycline	Sulfamethoprim	Trimethoprim-sulfamethoxazole	Vibramycin	Doxycycline
PAS	Aminosalicylic acid			Vibra-Tabs	Doxycycline
		Sulfamylon	Mefenide	Videx	Didanosine
Pathocil	Dicloxacillin	Sulfimycin	Erythromycin sulfisoxazole	Vira-A	Vidarabine
Pediamycin	Erythromycin ethylsuccinate			Viracept	Nevirapine
		Sumycin	Tetracycline	Viramune	Nelfinavir
Peflacine	Pefloxacin	Suprax	Cefixime	Virazole	Ribavirin
Pen-G	Penicillin G	Suspen	Penicillin V	Viroptic	Trifluridine
Pen-V	Penicillin V	Symadine	Amantadine	Vistide	Cidofovir
Pen-VK	Penicillin V	Symmetrel	Amantadine	Wesmycin	Tetracycline
Penetrex	Enoxacin	TAO	Troleandomycin	Win-cillin	Penicillin V
Pentam 300	Pentamidine isethionate	Tazicef	Ceftazidime	Wintrocin	Erythromycin
		Tazidime	Ceftazidime	Wyamycin S	Erythromycin
Pentids	Penicillin G	Teebactin	Aminosalicylic acid	Wycillin	Penicillin G
Pentostam	Sodium stibogluconate			Wymox	Amoxicillin
		Tegopen	Cloxacillin	Yodoxin	Iodoquinol
Permapen	Penicillin G benzathine	Teline	Tetracycline	Zagam	Sparfloxacin
		Terramycin	Oxytetracycline	Zartan	Cephalexin
Pipracil	Piperacillin	Tetracap	Tetracycline	Zefazone	Cefmetazole
Plaquenil	Hydroxychloroquine sulfate	Tetracon	Tetracycline	Zinacef	Cefuroxime
		Tetralan	Tetracycline	Zentel	Albendazole
Polycillin	Ampicillin	Tetram	Tetracycline	Zerit	Stavudine (d4T)
Polymox	Amoxicillin	Tiberal	Ornidazole	Zithromax	Azithromycin
Povan	Pyrvinium pamoate	Ticar	Ticarcillin	Zolicef	Cefazolin
Primaxin	Imipenem plus cilastatin	Timentin	Clavulanic acid plus ticarcillin	Zosyn	Piperacillin-tazobactam
Principen	Ampicillin	Tinactin	Tolnaftate	Zovirax	Acyclovir

Drugs and Vaccines

Table 11. Prevention of Travel-related Illness

PRETRAVEL ASSESSMENT

The following information should be obtained from travelers to assess their medical needs and potential risks, to provide itinerary-specific advice, immunizations, and prophylactic medications:
- Date of departure
- Itinerary
- Types of accommodations
- Medical history
- Vaccination history
- Current medications
- Allergies
- For women: Are they pregnant or planning to conceive within the next 3 months?

TRAVEL MEDICAL KIT

Following are suggestions for a traveler's personal medical kit. The contents should be tailored to the type of trip, duration of travel, and potential risk of travel-related illness.
- Summary of medical history and drug allergies
- ABO blood and Rh-factor types
- List of current medications (including both trade and generic names)
- Names and telephone numbers of the traveler's usual physician and emergency contacts
- Current immunization record (ideally, the International Certificate of Vaccination)
- Medical insurance information
- Prescription medications (should have enough to last the whole trip plus a week, in case of unexpected delays)
- Antibiotics and/or antimotility drugs (such as a fluoroquinolone and loperamide) for the self-treatment of traveler's diarrhea
- Malaria pills
- Epinephrine for injection and an antihistamine (if the traveler has a history of severe, life-threatening allergic reactions)
- An antibiotic such as erythromycin (if the individual is prone to frequent respiratory tract infections)
- Analgesics (acetaminophen, aspirin, or ibuprofen)
- Antifungal vaginal cream or suppository (for women who have frequent episodes of vaginitis or who may be taking antibiotics en route)
- Topical antibacterial cream for minor cuts or abrasions
- Band-Aids, 2×2 or 4×4 sterile gauze pads, adhesive tape
- Thermometer
- Elastic bandage (i.e., Ace wrap) for minor sprains
- Venom-extractor pump
- An extra pair of eyeglasses (if corrective lenses are used)
- Insect repellent
- Insecticide
- Menstrual supplies
- Sunscreen (with sun protective factor > 15)
- Spare toilet paper
- Water disinfection device or tablets for water treatment

NONINFECTIOUS HAZARDS OF TRAVEL

Jet Lag

Symptoms

- Daytime sleepiness
- Insomnia
- Difficulty concentrating
- Slowed reflexes
- Indigestion
- Hunger at odd hours
- Irritability

Tips to Prevent Jet Lag

- Avoid alcohol during flights (but drink plenty of water or juices to prevent dehydration).
- Three days before departure, attempt to maintain the time schedule you will experience during the trip.
- Adjust the sleep pattern at home for a few days before departure.

Drugs and Vaccines

Table 11. Prevention of Travel-Related Illness (*Continued*)

- Exercise daily in the new setting during sunlight hours.
- Consider using a short-acting benzodiazepine at bedtime.

Approaches That May Help Reduce Effects of Jet Lag

- Phototherapy (makes use of bright lights to reset the circadian clock)
- Argonne National Laboratory Jet Lag Diet (alternately feasting and fasting before departure)
- Melatonin (5 mg PO qd for 3 days before departure and 3 days after arrival at destination). This hormonal preparation may be available in pharmacies and health food stores, but quality may vary because it is not an FDA-regulated preparation.

Motion Sickness

- Motion sickness usually manifested by nausea, which may be accompanied by loss of color, sweating, and vomiting.
- Preventive treatments include oral antihistamines, such as dimenhydrinate, meclizine, or terfenadine, and scopolamine patches. All measures are most effective if started before the onset of motion sickness.

Road Safety

- Driving in many developing countries can be dangerous because of poor road and automobile conditions, a lack of traffic regulations, and unsafe driving practices of vehicle operators. If a traveler plans to drive, he or she should learn the local rules of the road and be sure to bring a car seat for any infants or toddlers.

Altitude Sickness

- Acute mountain sickness (AMS) can occur at any altitude above 5,000 ft (1,600 m) but is more likely to occur at altitudes above 12,000 ft (3,600 m).
- Risk factors for AMS include rapid ascent (more than 2,000 ft in a 24-hour period) and a history of AMS.
- Symptoms of AMS include headache, loss of appetite, nausea, vomiting, insomnia, fatigue, and shortness of breath, especially with exertion.
- More severe forms of disease include high-altitude pulmonary edema (characterized by severe dyspnea, cough productive of frothy sputum, and cyanosis) and high-altitude cerebral edema (manifested by severe headache, drowsiness, ataxia, impaired judgment, erratic behavior, and loss of consciousness that may progress to coma).

Altitude Sickness Prevention

- Gradually ascending to higher altitude (600 m/d)
- Resting 1 day for every 900-m increase in altitude
- Avoiding overexertion
- Drinking plenty of fluids
- Consuming multiple small meals instead of a few large meals
- Consuming a high-carbohydrate diet
- Avoiding alcoholic beverages and smoking

Drugs Used for Prevention of Acute Mountain Sickness

- Acetazolamide 125 to 250 mg PO bid or tid should be started on the day of ascent and continued until peak altitude is reached. It is also useful for the treatment of mild AMS.
- Dexamethasone 4 mg PO q6h: This is generally not recommended, due to its potential to cause side effects such as hyperglycemia and dpsychosis, which may be especially dangerous at higher altitudes.
- Nifedipine, 20 to 30 mg (slow-release) PO tid

Sexually Transmitted Diseases

- High-risk groups include migrant laborers, younger travelers, long-distance truckers, seafarers, military personnel, and expatriates.
- High-risk travelers should be educated about the risks of HIV and other sexually transmitted diseases, regardless of destination.
- High-risk travelers should be advised to carry condoms and to avoid having unprotected sex, especially with prostitutes or casual acquaintances.
- High-risk travelers should receive the hepatitis B vaccine.

PREVENTION OF MALARIA

- Avoid exposure to mosquitoes by wearing clothing that covers the arms and legs when outside.
- Stay indoors in a screened area during the hours between dusk and dawn.
- Sleep under mosquito netting (ideally, permethrin-impregnated) in a screened room or in a closed, air-conditioned room.
- Apply a nonaerosol mosquito repellent to exposed skin when outdoors. Repellents that contain DEET are best. DEET concentrations greater than 35% may be toxic and should be avoided.
- Consider impregnating clothes with permethrin.
- At dusk, spray the sleeping area with an insect repellent containing pyrethroids, after securing screens and closing windows and doors.
- Depending on the region of travel and time of year, prophylactic medications should be prescribed (Table 1A, on page 519).

Drugs and Vaccines

Table 11. Prevention of Travel-Related Illness (*Continued*)

- The choice of prophylaxis depends on the traveler's itinerary, previous tolerance of antimalarials, and concomitant medications.
- Chloroquine-sensitive strains of *Plasmodium falciparum* exist in Central America, Mexico, Haiti, the Dominican Republic, and the Middle East (Figure 1 on page 521).
- Consider impregnating clothes with permethrin.
- At dusk, spray the sleeping area with an insect repellent containing pyrethroids, after securing screens and closing windows and doors.
- Depending on the region of travel and time of year, prophylactic medications should be prescribed (Table A).
- The choice of prophylaxis depends on the traveler's itinerary, previous tolerance of antimalarials, and concomitant medications.
- Chloroquine-sensitive strains of *Plasmodium falciparum* exist in Central America, Mexico, Haiti, the Dominican Republic, and the Middle East (Figure 1 on page 521).
- Chloroquine-resistant strains have been reported in all other malarious regions.
- Mefloquine-resistant strains of *P. falciparum* have been reported in rural areas of Thailand along the Myanmar and Cambodian borders and in Papua New Guinea.
- Doxycycline is the prophylactic agent of choice for these areas.

IMMUNIZATIONS

Routine Childhood Vaccines

- Guidelines for immunizations in travelers are reviewed in Table B, on page 520.
- All travelers who have not completed a primary series or who have not had a booster during the past 10 years should receive a booster.
- Travelers who will be visiting countries where poliomyelitis remains endemic should receive a single booster of the polio vaccine. Because of the rare risk of vaccine-associated poliomyelitis, the enhanced inactivated polio vaccine (eIPV) should be used, unless the traveler can verify previous immunization with the live attenuated oral vaccine (OPV).
- All adult travelers born after 1956 should have received at least two doses of the live attenuated MMR vaccine.
- Hepatitis B vaccination should be considered for travelers who plan to spend prolonged periods abroad (i.e., 6 months), health care workers not previously vaccinated, and short-term travelers who may engage in high-risk sexual activity.
- Varicella immunization should be considered for nonimmune travelers, especially if they plan to have extensive contact with local populations.

Vector-borne Disease

- Yellow fever, a mosquito-borne viral infection, is found in certain parts of sub-Saharan Africa and South America (Figure 2 on page 521). Although yellow fever is rare in travelers, the deaths in 1996 of two unvaccinated travelers to the Amazon region of Brazil underline the importance of vaccination for this disease. Yellow fever vaccine is required for all travelers for entry into some countries (e.g., Liberia). Some countries require travelers who have recently been in a yellow fever zone to provide documentation of vaccination (International Certificate of Vaccination).
- Japanese encephalitis is a mosquito-borne viral encephalitis common in many parts of Asia. Peak transmission generally occurs during the summer and autumn in regions with temperate climates. The vaccine should be considered for expatriates and travelers who will be spending 30 days in rural areas during seasons of peak transmission. Personal protection measures, as described for malaria prevention, should be followed.
- Tick-borne encephalitis is a form of viral encephalitis transmitted by the tick, *Ixodes ricinus*, in Scandinavia, western and central Europe, and many former Soviet Union countries. Peak transmission occurs from April to August. A closely related disease, Russian spring–summer encephalitis, is transmitted by *Ixodes persulcatus* ticks in eastern Russia, Korea, and China. Travelers who visit forested areas or consume unpasteurized dairy products should be advised. Effective vaccines are available in Europe but not in the United States.

Food- And Water-Borne Disease

- Proof of cholera vaccination is no longer officially required for entry into any country. Saudi Arabia usually requires proof of vaccination for people entering the country during the hajj. Because cholera is rare in travelers and because the vaccine is not very effective (only about 50% protective for *Vibrio cholerae* 01), it is rarely recommended. Travelers who will be staying in highly endemic areas with poor access to clean water, sanitary facilities, and medical care or who have compromised gastric defenses (achlorhydria, antacid therapy, or status postgastrectomy) should be considered for vaccination.
- Hepatitis A is hyperendemic in all developing countries and is the most common vaccine-preventable disease in returning travelers in whom it is responsible for significant morbidity and productive time lost from work. Young children tend to have mild to asymptomatic infections. The risk of severe infection with jaundice increases with age. For travelers, the risk of hepatitis A acquisition increases with the length of stay. At highest risk are travelers who visit rural areas, hike in back country, and consume food and beverages or have close contact with locals in settings with poor sanitation. Immigrants from developing countries frequently are immune; if time permits, serologic testing for hepatitis A antibody should be performed, because vaccination may be unnecessary. Immunoglobulin provides short-term protection from hepatitis A (85% effective). It should be considered for short-term travelers and can be administered in combination with the hepatitis A vaccines if immediate travel to a developing country is planned. For individuals who travel frequently to endemic areas or who will be at high risk, there are two highly effective, inactivated-virus vaccines for hepatitis A licensed in the United States: Havrix and Vaqta. Both provide 95% to 100% protection. Vaccines will develop a protective immune response in 2 to 4 weeks.
- Travelers who will be spending several weeks in endemic areas, eating or drinking in the setting of poor sanitation, or visiting rural areas should be considered for typhoid vaccination. Countries with especially high rates of typhoid fever include India, Nepal, Pakistan, and Peru. Three vaccines are

(*Continued*)

Drugs and Vaccines

Table 11. Prevention of Travel-Related Illness *(Continued)*

available for the prevention of typhoid fever, and they vary in terms of side effects. Ty21a is a live, attenuated, oral typhoid vaccine administered as four capsules; is must be stored in a refrigerator and must be taken on an empty stomach. A newer, purified, capsular polysaccharide vaccine consists of a single infection and can be used in young children who cannot swallow capsules. the original typhoid vaccine (composed of phenol-inactivated *Salmonella typhi*) is rarely used because it has many side effects. All three vaccines have similar protective efficacy (ranging from 50% to 80%) but have never been evaluated prospectively in travelers or in comparative clinical trials.

Additional Immunization

- Influenza vaccine should be considered for travelers to tropical countries at any time of the year, or to the Southern Hemisphere from April to September. The most recently released, available vaccine should be used.
- Meningococcal vaccination should be considered for travelers to countries known to have epidemic meningococcal disease caused by a vaccine-preventable serogroup (A, C, W-135, Y). High-risk countries include sub-Saharan countries in savanna areas from Mali to Ethiopia, Kenya, Rwanda, Burundi, Tanzania, India, and Nepal. Travelers to Saudi Arabia during the hajj also should be immunized.
- Dogs are an important reservoir of rabies in less-developed areas of the world. Preexposure vaccination is recommended for persons who will be living in or spending prolonged periods (30 days) in areas of the world where rabies is endemic. In addition, vaccination should be considered for short-term travelers involved in activities that place them at high risk of exposure, such as spelunking, hunting, trekking, and veterinary work. Travelers should be advised that, if bitten or scratched by a potentially rabid animal, they must clean the wound with soap and water and receive postexposure prophylaxis.

SPECIAL SITUATIONS

Immunocompromised Travelers

- Because morbidity and, potentially, mortality from many enteric infections may be increased in immunocompromised travelers, they should be advised to adhere strictly to food and water precautions. Attention to personal protection measures also must be emphasized, because certain vector-borne diseases may be more severe or more difficult to treat in certain immunocompromised groups (e.g., patients with HIV and visceral leishmaniasis). Certain countries have imposed restrictions on the entry of HIV-seropositive travelers and may even require HIV testing for certain risk groups before entry.
- All live attenuated vaccines should be avoided in immunocompromised subjects (although HIV-seropositive persons may receive the MMR vaccine). HIV-seropositive or other immunocompromised travelers should be given a letter of waiver for the yellow fever vaccine if they are traveling to regions where yellow fever is endemic or proof of vaccination is required. (Vaccination can be considered for asymptomatic HIV-seropositive patients with CD4 cell counts of 200 if the risk of yellow fever exposure is high). Inactivated vaccines should be considered for immunocompromised travelers as indicated by itinerary. However, the response to immunization may be impaired, depending on the degree of immune impairment. If time permits, postvaccination serologic testing should be performed to verify a response to vaccination.

Pregnant Travelers

- The pregnant traveler should be sure that proper prenatal and obstetric medical care will be available at her destinations and that her health insurance will provide coverage there for her and her child. Vigorous exercise, high altitude (generally 1,500 m), and high-risk adventure travel should be avoided.
- Flying after week 35 of pregnancy is not advised, and may be prohibited by many airlines. During the flight, pregnant travelers should frequently move about the cabin to prevent deep venous thrombosis.
- Chloroquine and proguanil are considered safe for use during pregnancy. Mefloquine may be considered for use after the first trimester. Doxycycline should be avoided because it may lead to staining of fetal bones and teeth.
- Pregnant travelers should adhere strictly to food and water precautions. Prophylactic drug therapy should generally be avoided. The antimotility agents loperamide and diphenoxylate are not known to be teratogenic and have been used safely in pregnancy. Fluoroquinolones and doxycycline should be avoided. Trimethoprim–sulfamethoxazole may be used safely for the treatment of traveler's diarrhea in the second trimester only.
- Live attenuated vaccines are generally contraindicated in pregnancy and during the 3 months before conception. Yellow fever and oral polio vaccines may be administered if the risk of exposure is high. Inactivated vaccines are probably safe, although there are few data on newer vaccines, such as hepatitis A.

SCHISTOSOMIASIS

- This infection is endemic in many areas of Latin America, the Caribbean, Africa, and Asia. Wading or swimming in freshwater bodies in rural areas where the appropriates nail host exists places travelers at risk for the acquisition of schistosomiasis. Swimming and wading in freshwater bodies in rural areas of endemic countries, therefore, should be avoided. Swimming in adequately chlorinated swimming pools or in salt water is unlikely to lead to schistosomiasis.

Drugs and Vaccines

Table A. Malaria Chemoprophylaxis Regimes

Drug	Adults	Children	Adverse Effects	Contraindications and Warnings
Chloroquine[a]	300 mg base/wk	5 mg base/kg/wk (maximum 300 mg)	Nausea, headache, pruritus, dizziness, blurred vision	May exacerbate psoriasis; may impede antibody response to intradermal rabies vaccine
Mefloquine[a]	250 mg (1 tablet)/wk	<3 mo or 5 kg: no data 5–9 kg; 1/8 tablet/wk 10–19 kg: 1/4 tablet/wk 20–30 kg: 1/2 tablet/wk 31–34 kg: 3/4 tablet/wk >45 kg: 1 tablet/wk	Nausea, dizziness, insomnia, rash, nightmares; rarely, seizures, psychosis, hallucinations, mood changes	Known hypersensitivity to mefloquine, history of seizures or severe psychiatric disorders, cardiac conduction abnormalities, concomitant use of β-blockers for arrhythmias
Doxycycline[b]	100 mg daily	Contraindicated if age <8 yr ≥8 yr: 2 mg/kg/d up to adult dose	Photosensitivity, nausea, vomiting, vaginal yeast infections	Pregnancy, children <8 yr
Chloroquine + proguanil[c]	300 mg base/wk + 200 mg daily	5 mg base/kg/wk to maximum of 300 mg <2 yr: 1/4 adult dose 2–6 yr: 1/2 adult dose 7–10 yr: 3/4 adult dose >10 yr: 200 mg daily	Proguanil may cause nausea, vomiting, mouth ulcers, hair loss	

[a]Should be started 2 weeks before entering malarious area, then each week during travel, and for 4 weeks after exiting the malarious region.
[b]Should be started 2 days before entering malarious area, continued daily during travel, and for 4 weeks after exiting the malarious region.
[c]Proguanil is not licensed for use in the United States but is available in Canada and most West European countries.
Source: From Gorbach SL. 1999 *Guidelines for infectious diseases in primary care*.

Drugs and Vaccines

Table B. Immunizations for Travel

Vaccine	Primary Series[a]	Booster	Adverse Effects	Contraindications and Precautions
Routine vaccines				
Tetanus/diptheria	Adults and children >7 yr: three doses (0.5 mL i.m. or s.c.) at 0, 4–8 wk, 6–12 mo	Every 10 yr	Pain or erythema at injection site, fever; rarely, anaphylaxis	History of neurologic or severe hypersensitivity reaction to the vaccine
Polio[b]	Adults: eIPV preferable. Three doses (0.5 mL s.c.) at 0, 4–8 wk, 6–12 mo	Single dose once as an adult if traveling to endemic areas	Pain or erythema at injection site	Concurrent moderate-to-severe illness; history of anaphylactic reaction to the vaccine or to neomycin, polymyxin B, or streptomycin
Measles, mumps, rubella[b]	Adults born in or after 1957 should have received two doses (0.5 mL s.c.) of MMR 1+ mo apart		Injection site discomfort, fever, lymphadenopathy, arthralgias; rarely, transient arthritis (especially in women)	Concurrent moderate-to-severe illness; history of anaphylactic reaction to the vaccine or to eggs; pregnancy; should not be given to immunocompromised persons, except those with HIV
Hepatitis B	Adults ≥20 yr: three doses (1.0 mL i.m.) at 0, 4, and 24 wk Children 11–19 yr: three doses (0.5 mL i.m.) at 0, 4, and 24 wk	Need for boosters has not yet been determined; nonresponders should receive three additional doses	Injection site discomfort, fatigue, fever, headache, nausea	Concurrent moderate-to-severe illness; history of anaphylactic reaction to the vaccine, thimerosal, or yeast
Varicella	Adults and adolescents ≥13 yr: 2 doses (0.5 mL s.c.) at 0 and 4–8 wk	Not currently recommended	Redness, swelling, or pain at the injection site; fever, varicella-like rash (may be local or generalized)	Concurrent moderate-to-severe illness; adolescents undergoing aspirin therapy; history of anaphylactic reaction to the vaccine, gelatin, or neomycin; pregnancy; should not be given to immunocompromised individuals
Vector-borne diseases				
Yellow fever[b]	>9 mo of age: 0.5 mL s.c.	One dose every 10 yr	Injection site discomfort, headaches, low-grade fevers, myalgias; rarely, hypersensitivity reactions	History of anaphylactic reaction to the vaccine or to eggs; avoid in children <4 mo of age, pregnancy, immunocompromised individuals

Drugs and Vaccines

Table B. Immunizations for Travel (*Continued*)

Vaccine	Primary Series[a]	Booster	Adverse Effects	Contraindications and Precautions
Japanese B encephalitis	≥3 yr: three doses (1.0 mL s.c.), at 0,7, 14–28 d 1–3 yr: three doses (1.0 mL s.c.) at 0, 7, 14–28 d	Single dose of 1.0 mL s.c. for all age groups at ≥3 yr	Local reactions, fever, headaches, myalgias; less commonly, hypersensitivity reactions (may be delayed as long as 1 wk after immunization)[c]	History of anaphylactic reaction to the vaccine; pregnancy; increased risk of allergic reactions in persons with a history of urticaria
Food- and water-borne diseases				
Cholera	Given as two doses, i.m. or s.c. ≥1 wk apart 6 mo–4 yr: 0.2 mL 5–10 yr: 0.3 mL ≥10 yr: 0.5 mL	Single dose every 6 mo	Pain, swelling, and redness at injection site; fever, fatigue, headache	Concurrent moderate-to-severe illness; history of anaphylactic reaction to the vaccine; should be administered ≥3 wk apart from yellow fever vaccine
Hepatitis A	Immunoglobulin: 2–5 mL i.m. shortly before travel	Immunoglobulin: must be repeated every 4 mo	Immunoglobulin: injection site discomfort	Concurrent moderate-to-severe illness; history of anaphylactic reaction to the vaccine
	Havrix or Vaqta: >18 yr—1.0 mL i.m. 2–18 yr—0.5 mL i.m.; both given ≥2 wk before travel	Havrix or Vaqta: >18 yr—1.0 mL i.m. at 6–12 mo; 2–18 yr—0.5 mL i.m. at 6–12 mo	Harvix or Vaqta: injection site pain, fatigue, fever, headache	
Typhoid fever	Ty21a (oral vaccine) ≥6 yr: four capsules on days 1, 3, 5, and 7 Purified Vi polysaccharide vaccine ≥2 yr: one dose (0.5 mL i.m.)	Ty21a: repeat full series every 5 yr Vi: every 2 yr	Ty21a: nausea, abdominal cramps; rarely, vomiting, fever, rash, headache Vi: local pain, fever, headache	Concurrent moderate-to-severe illness, history of anaphylactic reaction to either vaccine; Ty21a: avoid in immunocompromised patients, pregnancy, children <6 yr, and during antibiotic use

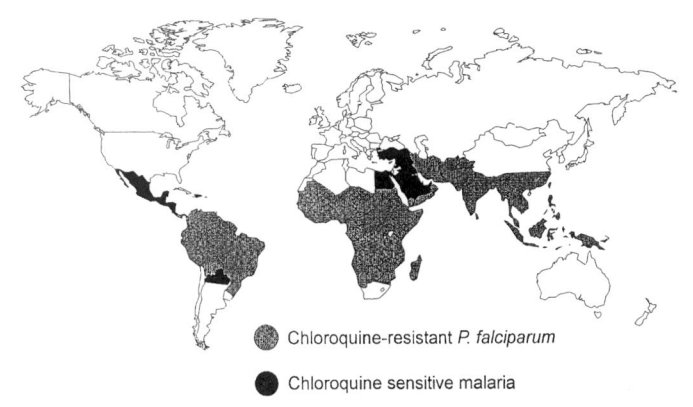

Figure 1. Distribution of malaria and chloroquine-resistant *Plasmodium falciparum*, 1995. From *Health Information for International Travel 1996*. U.S. Department of Health and Human Services. (Washington DC: U.S. Government Printing Office, 1996).

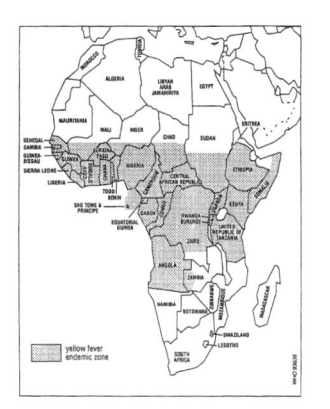

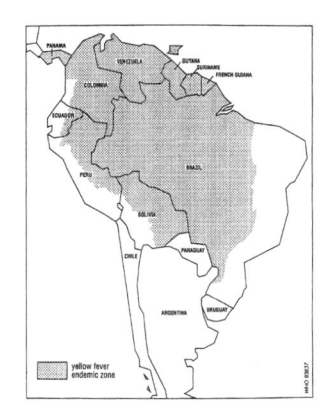

Figure 2. Yellow fever endemic zones. *Left*, Africa; *right*, South American and Panama. From *Health Information for International Travel 1996*. U.S. Department of Health and Human Service. (Washington, DC: U.S. Government Printing Office, 1996).

Index

Page numbers followed by f and t represent figures and tables respectively.

Abdominal pain and fever
  causes of, 2
  clinical manifestations of, 3
  diagnosis of, 3-4
  epidemiology of, 2-3
  treatment of, 5
Abscess
  cerebral, 104-105
  epidural, 176-177
  intraabdominal, 226-227
  lung, 250-251
  pilonidal, 322-323
Absidia corymbifera, 420
Acanthamoeba sp., 420
Acinetobacter sp., 420
Acne vulgaris (common acne), 64-65
Acquired immunodeficiency syndrome, HIV infection and, 218-221
Acremonium sp., 421
Actinobacillus sp., 421
Actinomadura sp., 421
Actinomycosis (*Actinomyces* sp.), 66-67
Acute inflammatory demyelinating polyneuritis, 290-291
Acute meningitis, 268-269. See also Meningococcal infection
Acute otitis externa, 304-305
Acute otitis media, 306-307
Acute sinusitis, 368-371
Acute suppurative thyroiditis, 388-389
Acute urethral syndrome, 16
Acute vasculitis, 230-231
Adenitis, mesenteric, 2, 272-273
Adenovirus infections, 68-69
Adults, immunization guidelines for, 495t-497t
Adverse reactions
  to antimicrobial agents, 482t-483t
    frequency of, 484t-485t
  to immunoglobulins, 504t
Aeromonas sp., 421
Afipia sp., 422
Africa, yellow fever endemic zones in, 521f
Age, immunization guidelines by
  for adults, 495t
  for children, 498t
Agrobacterium radiobacter, 422
AIDS (acquired immunodeficiency syndrome), HIV infection and, 218-221
Alcaligenes sp., 422
Alcoholics, immunization guidelines in, 497t
Allergic reactions, to antimicrobial agents, 482t
Alphavirus, 422-423
Alternaria sp., 423
Altitude sickness
  prevention of, 516t
  symptoms of, 516t
  treatment of, 516t
Amebiasis, 70-71, 441
Aminoglycosides, dosing regimens in renal failure, 487t-488t
Anaerobic infections, 72-73
Anaerobiospirillum, 423
Ancylostoma sp., 234-235, 354-355, 423
Anemia, aplastic, 36-37
Aneurysms, mycotic, 280-281
Angiomatosis, bacillary, 88-89
Angiostrongylus sp., 424
Animal bites, 6-7
Animal immunoglobulins, characteristics and adverse effects of, 504t
Anisakis sp., 424
Anorectal infections, 74-75
Anthrax, 76-77

vaccine for immunocompromised host, 503t
Antibiotic-associated diarrhea and colitis, 78-79
  frequency of, 484t-485t
Antimicrobial agents
  adverse reactions to, 482t-483t
    frequency of, 484t-485t
  dosing guidelines for, 489t-493t
    in renal failure, 487t-488t
    in severe liver disease, 494t
  drug-drug interactions involving, 486t
  trade names for, 513t-514t
Aplastic anemia, 36-37
Apophysomyces elegans, 424
Appendicitis, 80-81
Arcanobacterium sp., 424
Arenaviruses, 425
Argentine hemorrhagic fever, 425
Arthralgia, 30-31
Arthritis, 30-31
  septic, 364-365
Ascariasis (*Ascaris lumbricoides*), 354-355, 425
Aspergillosis (*Aspergillus* sp.), 82-83
Asplenia, immunization guidelines in, 497t
Assault, sexual, 52-53
Atypical lymphocytosis, 8-9
Atypical mycobacterial infections, 84-85
Aureobasidium pullulans, 425

Babesiosis (*Babesia* sp.), 86-87
Bacillary angiomatosis, 88-89
Bacillus sp., 426
Bacillus anthracis, 76-77
Bacillus of Calmette and Guerin
  availability and administration route, 500t
  in immunocompromised host, 503t
Back pain, with fever, 10-11
Bacteremia, 50-51
Bacterial vaginosis, 90-91
Bacteroides sp., 72-73, 426
Bacteroides fragilis, 72-73
Balanitis, 92-93
Balantidium coli, 427
Bartonella (Rochalimaea) henselae, 427
Bartonella (Rochalimaea) quintana, 427
Bartonellosis (*Bartonella bacilliformis*), 94-95
Basidiobolus ranarum, 427
Baylisascaris procyonis, 428
BCG. See Bacillus of Calmette and Guerin
Bell's palsy, 96-97
Bilophila wadsworthia, 428
Bipolaris sp., 428
Bite infections
  animal, 6-7
  human, 6-7
  insect, 26-27
Blastocystis hominis, 428
Blastomycosis (*Blastomyces dermatitidis*), 98-99
Blastoschizomyces capitatus, 429
Blepharitis, 100-101
Bolivian hemorrhagic fever, 454
Bone, infection of, 302-303
Bordetella sp., 316-317, 429
Bordetella bronchiseptica, 429
Bornholm disease, 172-173
Borrelia sp., 429
Borrelia burgdorferi (Lyme disease), 252-253
Botulism, 102-103
  vaccine and immunoglobulin use for, 505t
Brain
  abscess of, 104-105
  inflammation of. See Encephalitis
Breast infection, in nursing mothers, 260-261
Bronchiolitis, 106-107

Bronchitis, 108-109
Brucellosis (*Brucella* sp.), 110-111
Brugia sp., 430
Burkholderia (pseudomonas) sp., 336-337, 430
Burkholderia (pseudomonas) mallei, 336-337, 430
Burkholderia (pseudomonas) pseudomallei, 336-337, 430
Bursitis, 112-113

Calici-like viruses, 431
Calicivirus, 431
Calymmatobacterium granulomatis, 431
Campylobacter infections, 114-115
Candida vaginitis, 116-117
Candidiasis (*Candida* sp.), 118-119
CAP (community-acquired pneumonia), 328-329
Capillaria sp., 431
Capnocytophaga sp., 431
Cardiovascular symptoms, antimicrobial agents causing, 483t
Caries, 298-299
Cat-scratch disease, 120-121
Cephalosporins, adverse reactions to, frequency of, 484t
Cerebritis, 104-105
Cervicitis, 122-123
CFS (chronic fatigue syndrome), 134-135
Chalazion, 100-101
Chancroid, 22-23, 124-125
Chemoprophylaxis, for malaria, 519t
Chest pain, and fever, 40-41
Chickenpox, 126-127
  immunoglobulin for, 508t
  vaccine for, 508t
Chiggers (scabies), 274-275, 358-359
Children, immunization guidelines for, 498t-499t
Chlamydia sp., 432
Chlamydia psittaci, 338-339, 432
Chlamydia trachomatis, 74-75, 140-141, 394-395, 432
Cholangitis, 128-129
Cholecystitis, 128-129
Cholera, 130-131
  vaccine for, 500t
    in immunocompromised host, 503t
    travel and, 517t, 521t
    use of, 505t
Chorioretinitis, 132-133
Chromobacterium violaceum, 432
Chromomycosis agents, 432
Chronic bronchitis, 108-109
Chronic cough, defined, 12
Chronic fatigue syndrome, 134-135
Chronic meningitis, 34-35, 270-271. See also Meningococcal infection
Chronic otitis externa, 304-305
Chronic sinusitis, 368-371
Chronic suppurative otitis media, 306-307
Chryseomonas luteola, 432
Chrysosporium parvum, 433
Citrobacter sp., 433
CJD (Creutzfeldt-Jakob disease), 142-143
Clenched-fist injuries, 6-7
Clonorchis sinensis (*Opisthorchis sinensis*), 433
Clostridium sp., 72-73, 192-193, 433-434
Clostridium botulinum (botulism), 78-79
Clostridium difficile-associated diarrhea and colitis, 78-79
Clostridium tetani. See Tetanus
CMV. See Cytomegalovirus infections
Coccidioidomycosis (*Coccidioides immitis*), 136-137
Cold, common, 138-139

523

Index

Colitis
  antibiotic-associated, 78–79
  Clostridium difficile-associated, 78–79
Colorado tick fever virus, 434
Coma, 34–35
Comamonas sp., 434
Common acne (acne vulgaris), 64–65
Common cold, 138–139
Community-acquired pneumonia, 328–329
Condylomata acuminata, 22–23
Confusion, 34–35
Congenital toxoplasmosis, 392–393
Conidiobolus sp., 434
Conjunctivitis, 46–47, 140–141
  inclusion-type. *See* Inclusion conjunctivitis
Coronavirus, 435
Corynebacterium sp., 436
Corynebacterium diphtheriae. *See* Diphtheria
Corynebacterium jeikeium, 435
Corynebacterium minutissimum, 435
Corynebacterium pseudotuberculosis, 435
Corynebacterium urealyticum, 436
Cough
  in chronic bronchitis, 108–109
  and fever, 12–13
  whooping. *See* Pertussis
Coxiella burnetii (Q fever), 342–343
Coxsackievirus, 436
Crab lice (*Phthirus pubis*), 246–247, 463
Creutzfeldt-Jakob disease, 142–143
Crimean-Congo hemorrhagic fever virus, 436
Croup (laryngotracheobronchitis), 236–237
Cryptococcosis (*Cryptococcus neoformans*), 144–145
Cryptosporidiosis (*Cryptosporidium parvum*), 146–147
Cunninghamella bertholetiae, 437
Curvularia sp., 437
Cutaneous larvae migrans, 234–235
Cyclospora cayatanensis, 437
Cysticercosis, 148–149
Cystitis, 16–17, 150–151
Cytomegalovirus infections, 152–153
  atypical lymphocytosis and, 8–9
  infectious mononucleosis and, 222–223
  vaccine and immunoglobulin use for, 505t
Cytopenia, 36–37

de Quervain's thyroiditis, 388–389
Deep superficial incisional surgical site infection, 380–381
Demyelinating polyneuritis, acute inflammatory, 290–291
Dengue fever, 154–155
Dengue hemorrhagic fever-shock syndrome, 154–155
Dental infections, 298–299
Dental procedures
  endocarditis prophylaxis for, 510t
  prophylactic regimens for, 511t
Dermatobia hominis, 458
Devil's grip (epidemic pleurodynia), 172–173
Diabetes, immunization guidelines in, 497t
Diarrhea
  antibiotic-associated, 78–79
    frequency of, 484t–485t
  Clostridium difficile-associated, 78–79
  and fever, 14–15
  traveler's, 396–397
Dicrocoelium dendriticum, 438
Dientamoeba fragilis, 438
Diphtheria, 156–157
  immunization guidelines for
    in adults, 495t–497t
    in children, 498t, 499t
    in travelers, 520t
  immunoglobulin for, 505t
  vaccine for, 500t, 501t
    use of, 505t
Diphyllobothrium sp., 438
Dipylidium caninum, 439
Dirofilaria sp., 186, 439
Discharge
  urethral, 58–59
  vaginal, 60–61

Diverticular disease, 158–159
Diverticulitis, 158–159
Diverticulosis, 158–159
Donovanosis, 22–23, 200–201
Dosing guidelines, for antimicrobial agents, 489t–493t
  in renal failure, 487t–488t
  in severe liver disease, 494t
Dracunculus medinensis, 439
Drowsiness, 34–35
Drug therapy. *See* Antimicrobial agents; *individual classes of drugs*
DT vaccine
  availability and administration routes for, 501t
  in children, 498t, 499t
  for travelers, 520t
DTaP vaccine, in children, 498t, 499t
DTP vaccine, in children, 498t, 499t
Dysuria, 16–17
  with sterile pyuria syndrome, 58

Ear pain/earache, 18–19
Ebola virus, 439
EBV (Epstein-Barr virus). *See* Infectious mononucleosis
Echinococcosis (*Echinococcus* sp.), 160–161
Echinostoma ilocanum, 440
Echovirus, 440
Edwardsiella tarda, 440
Effusion
  otitis media with, 306–307
  pleural, and fever, 38–39
Ehrlichiosis (*Ehrlichia* sp.), 162–163
Eikenella corrodens, 440
Elderly, in nursing homes, immunization guidelines for, 496t
Emmonsia parva, 441
Emphysematous cholecystitis, 128–129
Empyema, 38–39
Encephalitis, 164–165
  flaviviruses causing, 441. *See also* Japanese B encephalitis
  tick-borne, vaccine for, 517t
Endemic zones
  for malaria, 521f
  for yellow fever, 521f
Endocarditis
  native valves, 166–167
  prophylaxis for, 509t–510t
  prosthetic valves, 168–169
Endolimax nana, 441
Endophthalmitis, 170–171
Entamoeba sp., 441
Entamoeba dispar. *See* Amebiasis
Entamoeba histolytica. *See* Amebiasis
Enteric fever, agents causing and conditions mimicking, 3t. *See also* Abdominal pain and fever
Enterobacter sp., 442
Enterobiasis (*Enterobius vermicularis*), 354–355, 442
Enterococcus sp., 442
Enterocytozoon bieneusi, 455
Enterohemorrhagic *Escherichia coli* infection, 2
  hemolytic-uremic syndrome and, 206–207
Enterovirus, 443
Eosinophilia, 2
Epidemic myalgia, 172–173
Epidemic pleurodynia, 172–173
Epidermophyton floccosum, 443
Epididymitis, 174–175
Epidural abscess, 176–177
Epiglottitis, 178–179
Epstein-Barr virus. *See* Infectious Mononucleosis
Equine immunoglobulins, characteristics and adverse effects of, 504t
Erysipelothrix rhusiopathiae, 443
Erythromycin, drug interactions with, 486t
Escherichia coli infections, 180–181
  enterohemorrhagic, 2, 206–207
Esophageal procedures, prophylactic regimens for, 511t
Esophagitis, infective, 182–183
Eubacterium sp., 443

Ewingella americana, 444
Exanthem subitum, 184–185
Exophiala sp., 444
Extrapulmonary tuberculosis, 404–405
Eye, redness of, 46–47

Family member exposure, immunization guidelines in, 495t–496t
Fasciola sp., 444
Fasciolopsis buski, 444
Fever
  abdominal. *See* Abdominal pain and fever
  back pain and, 10–11
  cough and, 12–13
  diarrhea and, 14–15
  hemorrhagic. *See* Hemorrhagic fevers
  hepatosplenomegaly and, 24–25
  jaundice and, 28–29
  joint disorders and, 30–31
  lymph node enlargement and, 32–33
  neurologic symptoms/signs and, 34–35
  pancytopenia and, 36–37
  pleural effusion and, 38–39
  pleuritic and chest pain and, 40–41
  postoperative, 42–43
  Q, 342–343
  rash and, 44–45
  rheumatic, 350–351
  Rocky Mountain spotted, 44–45, 352–353
  scarlet, 360–361
  splenomegaly and, 24–25
  typhoid, 408–409
  of unknown origin, 20–21
  yellow, 414–415
Filariasis, 186–187
Filovirus, 439
Flavimonas orzihabitans, 445
Flavivirus, 441
Flavobacterium sp., 445
Fluoroquinolones
  adverse reactions to, frequency of, 485t
  drug interactions with, 486t
Fonsecaea sp., as chromomycosis agent, 432
Food-borne diseases, 188–189
  immunization against, 517t, 521t
  and traveler's diarrhea, 396–397
Fournier's gangrene, 74–75
Francisella tularensis (tularemia), 406–407
Fulminant hepatitis, 208–209
Fungal infections
  of hair, nails, and skin, 190–191
  of sinuses, 368–371
Fungemia, 50–51
FUO (fever of unknown origin), 20–21
Fusarium sp., 445
Fusobacterium sp., 72–73, 445

Gangrene
  Fournier's, 74–75
  gas, 192–193
Gangrenous appendicitis, 80–81
Gardnerella vaginalis, 446
Gas gangrene, 192–193
Gaseous cholecystitis, 128–129
Gastrointestinal procedures
  endocarditis prophylaxis for, 510t
  prophylactic regimens for, 512t
Gastrointestinal symptoms, antimicrobial agents causing, 482t
Gemella sp., 446
Genital lesions, 22–23, 124–125
  herpes simplex virus, 194–195
  human papillomavirus, 413–413
Genitourinary procedures
  endocarditis prophylaxis for, 510t
  prophylactic regimens for, 512t
Geotrichum candidum, 446
German measles. *See* Rubella
Giant-cell thyroiditis, 388–389
Giardiasis (*Giardia lamblia*), 196–197, 446
Gingivitis, 198–199, 298–299
Glanders, 336–337
Gnathostoma spinigerum, 446

Index

Granuloma inguinale, 200-201
Guillain-Barré syndrome, 290-291

Haemophilus sp., 447
Haemophilus ducreyi, 447
Haemophilus influenzae, 447
  immunization guidelines for
    in adults, 495t, 497t
    in children, 498t, 499t
  vaccine for
    availability and administration route, 500t
    in immunocompromised patient, 502t
    use of, 505t
Hafnia alvei, 447
Hair, fungal infections of, 190-191
Hansenula sp., 448
Hantaan virus, 448
Hantavirus pulmonary syndrome, 202-203
Health care workers, immunization guidelines for, 496t
Heart valves, infection of. *See* Endocarditis
Helicobacter pylori infection, 204-205
Hematopoietic reactions, to antimicrobial agents, 482t
Hemolytic-uremic syndrome, and enterohemorrhagic *E. coli* infection, 206-207
Hemorrhagic fevers
  arenaviruses, 425
  Bolivian, 454
  dengue virus, 154-155
  Omsk virus and, 448
Hendersonula toruloidea, 448
Hepatic symptoms. *See* Liver disease
Hepatitis, 208-209
  serologic testing in, 28t
Hepatitis A virus, 208-209
  immunization guidelines, 500t
    in adults, 495t-497t
    for travel, 517t, 521t
  immunoglobulin for, 506t
  vaccine for, 506t
Hepatitis B virus, 208-209
  immunization guidelines, 500t
    in adults, 495t-497t
    in children, 498t, 499t
    in immunocompromised patient, 502t
    for travel, 517t, 520t
  immunoglobulin for, 506t
  vaccine for, 506t
Hepatitis C virus, 208-209
Hepatitis D virus, 208-209
Hepatitis E virus, 208-209, 431
Hepatitis G virus, 208-209
Hepatosplenomegaly, and fever, 24-25
Herpes simplex virus infections
  anorectal, 74-75
  genital, 22-23, 194-195
  types 1 and 2, 210-211
Herpes zoster, 212-213
Herpesvirus, human
  type 6, 448
  type 8, 449
Heterophyes heterophyes, 449
Hib conjugate vaccine
  in adults, 495t-497t
  availability and administration route, 500t
  in children, 498t, 499t
  in immunocompromised patient, 502t
High-risk patients
  endocarditis prophylaxis and, 510t
  immunization guidelines in, 497t
  prophylactic regimens for, 512t
Histoplasmosis (*Histoplasma* sp.), 214-217
HIV infection
  and AIDS, 218-221
  immunization guidelines in, 497t
Homeless, immunization guidelines for, 496t
Homosexual men, immunization guidelines for, 496t
Hookworm infection, 354-355
HPV (human papillomavirus), 412-413
HSV infections. *See* Herpes simplex virus infections
Human bites, 6-7

Human immunodeficiency virus infection. *See* HIV infection
Human immunoglobulins, characteristics and adverse effects of, 504t
Human papillomavirus, 412-413
Human pediculosis (*Pediculus humanus*), 246-247, 463
HUS (hemolytic-uremic syndrome), 206-207
Hymenolepsis sp., 449
Hyperbilirubinemia, 28-29
Hypersensitivity lung diseases, 82-83
Hypersensitivity reactions, to antimicrobial agents, 482t
Hypoderma sp., as myiasis agent, 458

Immigrants, immunization guidelines for, 496t
Immunization guidelines
  for adults, 495t-497t
  for children, 498t-499t
  for travel, 520t-521t
  for travelers, 517t-518t
Immunocompetent patients, toxoplasmosis in, 392-393
Immunocompromised patients
  immunization guidelines for, 496t-497t
  pneumonia in, 326-329
  toxoplasmosis in, 392-393
  vaccines in, 502t
  travel and, 518t
Immunoglobulins
  characteristics and adverse effects of, 504t
  use of, 505t-508t
Inactivated poliovirus vaccine
  in adults, 495t, 496t
  in children, 498t, 499t
  in immunocompromised host, 503t
Inclusion conjunctivitis, 140-141
  trachoma and, 394-395
Infectious mononucleosis, 222-223
  atypical lymphocytosis and, 8-9
Infectious thyroiditis, 388-389
Infective esophagitis, 182-183
Influenza, 224-225
  adult immunization guidelines for, 495t-497t
  vaccine for
    in immunocompromised patient, 502t
    travel and, 518t
    use of, 505t
Injuries, clenched-fist, 6-7
Insect bites, 26-27
Insect stings, 26-27
Institutional residents, immunization guidelines for, 496t
Intestines, roundworms infections in, 354-355
Intraabdominal abscess, 226-227
Intraperitoneal abscess, 226-227
Intravenous drug abusers, immunization guidelines for, 496t
Invasive aspergillosis, 82-83
Invasive otitis externa, 304-305
IPV. *See* Inactivated poliovirus vaccine
Isospora belli, 449

Japanese B encephalitis
  immunization guidelines for travelers, 521t
  vaccine and immunoglobulin use for, 505t
  vaccine for, 500t
  travel and, 517t
Jaundice, and fever, 28-29
JC virus, 332-333
Jet lag
  prevention of, 515t-516t
  symptoms of, 515t
Joint disorders, 30-31
Junin virus, 425

Kaposi's sarcoma, 228-229
Kawasaki syndrome, 230-231
Keratitis, 232-233
Kidney. *See* Renal *entries*
Kingella sp., 450
Klebsiella sp., 450
Kluyvera sp., 450

KS (Kaposi's sarcoma), 228-229
Kurthia sp., 450
Kyasanur forest disease virus, 451

Lactobacillus sp., 451
Larva migrans syndrome, 234-235
Laryngitis, 236-237
Laryngotracheobronchitis, 236-237
Lassa virus, 451
Leclercia adecarboxylata, 451
Legionnaire's disease (*Legionella* sp.), 238-239
Leishmaniasis (*Leishmania* sp.), 240-241
Leprosy, 242-243
Leptomyxid sp., 452
Leptospirosis (*Leptospira* sp.), 244-245
Leuconostoc sp., 452
Leukoencephalopathy, progressive multifocal, 332-333
LGV (lymphogranuloma venereum), 22-23, 256-257
Lice, 246-247
Lincosamide, adverse reactions to, frequency of, 485t
Linguatula serrata, 452
Listeriosis (*Listeria monocytogenes*), 248-249
Liver disease
  antimicrobial agents causing, 482t
  severe, antimicrobial dosing regimens in, 494t
Loa loa, 186-187, 452-453
Lung abscess, 250-251
Lyme disease, 252-253
Lymph node enlargement, and fever, 32-33
Lymphadenitis, 32-33
Lymphadenopathy, generalized, 32-33
Lymphangitis, 254-255
Lymphatic filariasis, 186-187
Lymphocytic choriomeningitis, 453
Lymphocytosis, atypical, 8-9
Lymphogranuloma venereum, 22-23, 256-257
Lymphotropic T-cell human virus, 453

MAC (*Mycobacterium avium* complex), 84-85
Machupo virus, 454
Macrolides, adverse reactions to, frequency of, 485t
Malaria, 258-259
  chemoprophylactic regimen, 519t
  distribution of, 521f
  prevention of, 516t-517t
Malassezia sp., 454
Malignant otitis externa, 304-305
Mansonella sp., 186, 454
Marburg virus, 439
Mastadenovirus, 68-69
Mastitis, 260-261
Mastoiditis, 262-263
Measles, 264-265
  immunization guidelines for
    in adults, 495t-497t
    in children, 498t, 499t
    in travelers, 520t
  immunoglobulin for, 508t
  vaccine for, 500t, 508t
    in immunocompromised patients, 502t
Measles virus. *See* Measles
Mediastinitis, 266-267
Medical kit, for traveling, 515t
Medical procedures, endocarditis prophylaxis for, 510t
Melioidosis, 336-337
Meningitis. *See also* Meningococcal infection
  acute, 268-269
  chronic, 34-35, 270-271
Meningococcal infection
  adult immunization guidelines for, 449t, 497t
  vaccine for, 500t, 507t
    in immunocompromised patient, 502t
    travel and, 518t
Mentally retarded, institutionalized, immunization guidelines for, 496t
Mesenteric adenitis, 2, 272-273
Mesenteric lymphadenitis, 32-33
Metabolic reactions, to antimicrobial agents, 483t
Metagonimus yokogawai, 455
Methylobacterium sp., 455

Index

Microsporidia, 455
Microsporum sp., 455
Mites (scabies), 274–275, 358–359
MMR vaccine
  availability and administration route, 500t
  in children, 498t, 499t
  in immunocompromised patients, 502t
  for travelers, 520t
Mobiluncus sp., 456
Moderate-risk patients
  endocarditis prophylaxis for, 510t
  prophylactic regimens for, 512t
Mold. *See* Fungal infections; *specific conditions and agents*
Molluscum contagiosum virus, 456
  genital lesions and, 22–23
Mononucleosis. *See* Infectious mononucleosis
Moraxella (Branhamella) sp., 456
Morganella morganii, 456
Motion sickness, 516t
Mouth, infections of, 298–299
Mucopurulent cervicitis, 122–123
Mucormycosis (*Mucor* sp.), 276–277
Muerto canyon virus, 448
Multiceps multiceps, 457
Mumps, 278–279
  immunization guidelines for
    in adults, 495t–496t
    in children, 498t, 499t
    in travelers, 520t
  vaccine for, 500t, 507t
  in immunocompromised patients, 502t
Mumps virus. *See* Mumps
Myalgia, epidemic, 172–173
Mycobacterial infections, atypical, 84–85
Mycobacterium avium infection, 84–85
Mycobacterium bovis, 457
Mycobacterium kansasii pneumonia, 84–85
Mycobacterium leprae (leprosy), 242–243
Mycobacterium marinum skin infections, 84–85
Mycobacterium tuberculosis. *See* Tuberculosis
Mycobacterium ulcerans, 84–85
Mycoplasma sp., 457
Mycotic aneurysms, 280–281
Myelitis, 282–283
Myiasis agents, 458
Myocarditis, 284–285
Myositis, 286–287

Naegleria fowleri, 458
Nails, fungal infections of, 190–191
Nanophyetus salmincola, 458
Nausea, from antibacterial drugs, frequency of, 484t–485t
Necator americanus, 354–355, 458
Necrotizing skin and soft-tissue infections, 288–289
Neisseria sp., 459
Neisseria gonorrhoeae, 58–59
Neisseria meningitidis, 268–269
Neuritis, 290–291
Neurologic signs/symptoms
  antimicrobial agents causing, 483t
  and fever, 34–35
"New variant CJD," 142–143
Nocardiosis (*Nocardia* sp.), 292–295
Nontyphoidal *Salmonella* infections, 296–297
Norwalk-like virus, 431
Norwalk virus, 431
Nosema sp. (Microsporidia), 455
Nosocomial pneumonia, 328–329
Nosocomial sinusitis, 368–371
Nursing home residents, immunization guidelines for, 496t

Obstructive appendicitis, 80–81
Ochrobactrum anthropi, 459
Ocular larvae migrans, 234–235
Odontogenic infections, 298–299
Oerskovia sp., 459
Oligella sp., 460
Omsk virus, 448
Onchocerciasis (*Onchocerca volvulus*), 186–187, 460
Ophthalmic symptoms, antimicrobial agents causing, 483t

Opisthorchis sp., 460
Opisthorchis sinensis (Clonorchis sinensis), 433
OPV. *See* Oral poliovirus vaccine
Oral poliovirus vaccine
  in children, 498t, 499t
  in immunocompromised host, 503t
Orchitis, 300–301
ORF virus, 460
Organ/space infection, postoperative, 380–381
Oroya fever, 94–95
Osteomyelitis, 302–303
Otalgia, 18–19
Otitis externa, 304–305
Otitis media, 306–307
Ototoxicity, antimicrobial agents causing, 483t

Paecilomyces sp., 461
Pain
  abdominal. *See* Abdominal pain and fever
  ear, 18–19
  joint, and fever, 30–31
  pleuritic and chest, and fever, 40–41
  spinal/paraspinal, and fever, 10–11
Pancytopenia, and fever, 36–37
Panophthalmitis, 17–171
Pantoea agglomerans, 461
Papillomavirus, human, 412–413
Paracoccidioides brasiliensis, 461
Paragonimus sp., 462
Parainfluenza virus, 462
Parapneumonic effusion, 38–39
Paraspinal pain, and fever, 10–11
Paratrachoma. *See* Inclusion conjunctivitis
Parvovirus infections (parvovirus B19), 308–309
Pasteurella sp., 463
Pediculosis, human (*Pediculus humanus*), 246–247, 463
Pediococcus sp., 464
Peliosis hepatica, 88–89
Pelvic inflammatory disease, 310–311
Penicillins, adverse reactions to, frequency of, 484t
Penicillium sp., 464
Peptococcus niger, 464
Peptostreptococcus sp., 72–73, 465
Perforated diverticulitis, 158–159
Perforating appendicitis, 80–81
Pericarditis, 312–313
Periodontitis, 298–299
Peritonitis, 314–315
Pertussis, 316–317
  childhood immunization guidelines for, 498t, 499t
  vaccine for, 500t, 501t, 508t
Pharyngitis, 318–321
Phialophora sp., 432
Phthirus sp. (lice), 246–247, 463
Piedraia hortae, 465
Pilonidal abscess, 322–323
Pinworm infection, 354–355
Plague, 324–325
  vaccine for, 501t, 507t
  in immunocompromised host, 503t
Plasmodium sp. *See* Malaria
Pleistophora sp. (Microsporidia), 455
Plesiomonas shigelloides, 466
Pleural effusion, and fever, 38–39
Pleuritic pain, and fever, 40–41
Pleurodynia, epidemic, 172–173
PML (progressive multifocal leukoencephalopathy), 332–333
Pneumococcal infection
  adult immunization guidelines for, 495t–497t
  vaccine for, 501t, 506t
  in immunocompromised patient, 502t
Pneumocystis carinii pneumonia, 326–327
Pneumonia, 328–329
  Mycobacterium kansasii, 84–85
  Pneumocystis carinii, 326–327
Poliomyelitis, 330–331
  immunization guidelines for
    in adults, 495t–496t
    in children, 498t, 499t
    in travelers, 520t
  vaccine for, 500t, 507t
Poliovirus infection. *See* Poliomyelitis

Polyneuritis, acute inflammatory demyelinating, 290–291
Polyomaviruses, 332–333
Porphyromonas sp., 72–73, 466
Postoperative fever, 42–43
Pregnancy
  immunization guidelines in, 495t
    travel and, 518t
  immunoglobulin use in, 504t
Prevotella sp., 72–73, 466
Prions, 467
Prison populations, immunization guidelines for, 496t
Progressive multifocal leukoencephalopathy, 332–333
Prophylaxis
  for endocarditis, 509t–510t
  for malaria, 519t
  regimens, 511t–512t
Propionibacterium sp., 467
Propionibacterium acnes, 64, 467
Propionibacterium propionica, 66–67
Prostatitis, 334–335
Prostatodynia, 334–335
Prosthetic valve endocarditis, 168–169
  prophylactic regimen for, 509t–510t
Proteus sp., 467
Protomonas sp., 455
Prototheca sp., 467
Providencia sp., 468
Pseudallescheria boydii, 468
Pseudomonas aeruginosa infections, 336–337
Psittacosis, 338–339
Psychrobacter immobilis, 468
Pubic lice (*Phthirus pubis*), 246–247, 463
Pulmonary symptoms, antimicrobial agents causing, 483t
Pulmonary tuberculosis, 404–405
PVE. *See* Prosthetic valve endocarditis
Pyelonephritis, 340–341

Q fever, 342–343

Rabies, 344–345
  immunoglobulin for, 507t
  vaccine for, 501t, 507t
    in immunocompromised host, 503t
    travel and, 518t
Rabies virus. *See* Rabies
Rape, 52–53
Rash
  from antibacterial drugs, frequency of, 484t–485t
  and fever, 44–45
Rectum, bacterial infections of, 74–75
Recurrent acute otitis media, 306–307
Recurrent sinusitis, 368–371
Red eye, 46–47
Refugees, immunization guidelines for, 496t
Relapsing fever, 346–347
Renal failure
  antimicrobial dosing regimens in, 487t–488t
    for maintenance, 489t–493t
  immunization guidelines in, 497t
Renal symptoms, antimicrobial agents causing, 483t
Respiratory syncytial virus infection, 348–349
Respiratory tract procedures
  endocarditis prophylaxis for, 510t
  prophylactic regimens for, 511t
Retinitis, 132–133
Retroperitoneal abscess, 226–227
Rheumatic fever, 350–351
Rhinocladiella aquaspera, 432
Rhinorrhea, 48–49
Rhinosporidium seeberi, 469
Rhinovirus, 469
Rhizomucor sp., 276–277
Rhizopus sp., 276–277
Rhodococcus sp., 470
Rhodotorula sp., 470
Rickettsia sp., 470–471
  typhus and, 410–411
Rickettsia rickettsii, 44–45, 352–353, 470–471
RMSF (Rocky Mountain spotted fever), 44–45, 352–353

Index

Road safety, 516t
Rocky Mountain spotted fever, 44–45, 352–353
Roseola, 184–185
Rotavirus, human, 471
Rothia dentocariosa, 471
Roundworms, intestinal, 354–355
RSV (respiratory syncytial virus) infection, 348–349
Rubella, 356–357
   immunization guidelines for
      in adults, 495t–496t
      in children, 498t, 499t
      in travelers, 520t
   vaccine for, 508t
      availability and administration route, 500t, 501t
      in immunocompromised patients, 502t
Rubella virus. *See* Rubella
Rubeola virus. *See* Measles

Saccharomyces cerevisiae, 472
Saksenaea vasiformis, 472
Salmonella sp.
   nontyphoidal infections and, 296–297
   typhoid fever and. *See* Typhoid fever
Sapporo-like virus, 431
Sarcocystis sp., 472
Sarcoma, Kaposi's, 228–229
Sarcoptes scabiei. *See* Scabies
Scabies, 274–275, 358–359
Scarlet fever, 360–361
Scedosporium prolificans, 472
Schistosomiasis (*Schistosoma* sp.), 362–363
   prevention of, 518t
Scleritis, 46–47
Scopulariopsis sp., 473
Sepsis syndrome, 50–51
Septata intestinalis, 455
Septic arthritis, 30–31, 364–365
Septic shock, 50–51
Septic thrombophlebitis, 386–387
Septicemia, 50–51
Serratia sp., 473
Severe sepsis, 50–51
Sexual assault, 52–53
Sexually transmitted diseases. *See also specific diseases and agents*
   genital lesions and, 22–23
   prevention of, 516t
Shigellosis (*Shigella* sp.), 366–367
Shingles, 212–213
Sinusitis, 368–371
SIRS (systemic inflammatory response syndrome), 50–51
Sixth disease, 184–185
Skin infections. *See also specific conditions and agents*
   fungal, 190–191
   necrotizing, 288–289
   superficial, 378–379
Smallpox virus, 473
Snow Mountain-like virus, 431
Soft-tissue infections
   necrotizing, 288–289
   superficial, 378–379
Solitary rectal ulcer syndrome, 74–75
Sore throat, 54–55. *See also specific conditions*
South America
   arenaviral hemorrhagic fevers in, 425
   yellow fever endemic zones in, 521f
Sphingobacterium sp., 474
Spinal pain, and fever, 10–11
Spirillum minus (minor), 474
Spirometra sp., 474
Splenomegaly, and fever, 24–25
Spongiform encephalopathies, 142–143
Sporobolomyces sp., 474
Sporotrichosis (*Sporothrix schenckii*), 372–373
Staphylococcus sp., 390–391, 475
Stenotrophomonas sp., 475
Sterile pyuria syndrome, dysuria with, 58
Stings, insect, 26–27
Stomatitis, 374–375
Stomatococcus mucilaginosus, 475

Streptobacillus moniliformis, 476
Streptococcus agalactiae (Group B), 476
Streptococcus pneumoniae. *See* Pneumonia
Streptococcus pyogenes (Group A β-Hemolytic *Streptococcus*), 360–361, 390–391, 476
Strongyloidiasis (*Strongyloides stercoralis*), 354–355, 376–377
Stupor, 34–35
Subacute granulomatous thyroiditis, 388–389
Subacute sinusitis, 368–371
Superficial incisional surgical site infection, 380–381
Superficial skin and soft-tissue infections, 378–379
Suppurative thrombophlebitis, 386–387
Suppurative thyroiditis, acute, 388–389
Surgery
   endocarditis prophylaxis prior to, 510t
   wound infections after, 380–381
Swimmer's ear, 304–305
Syphilis, 382–383
Systemic inflammatory response syndrome, 50–51

Taenia saginata, 476
Taenia solium (cysticercosis), 148–149
Tapeworm (*Taenia* sp.), 148–149, 476
TB (tuberculosis), 404–405
Td vaccine
   in adults, 495t–497t
   availability and administration routes for, 501t
   in immunocompromised patients, 502t
   for travelers, 520t
Testicles, infection of, 300–301
Tetanus, 384–385
   immunization guidelines for
      in adults, 495t–497t
      in children, 498t, 499t
      in travelers, 520t
   immunoglobulin for, 508t
   vaccine for, 508t
   vaccines for, 500t, 501t
      in immunocompromised patients, 502t
Tetracyclines, drug interactions with, 486t
Throat, sore, 54–55. *See also specific conditions*
Thrombophlebitis, suppurative, 386–387
Thyroiditis, infectious, 388–389
Tick-borne encephalitis, vaccine for, travel and, 517t
TMP-SMX. *See* Trimethoprim-sulfamethoxazole
Tonsillitis, 318–321
Toxic shock syndrome, 390–391
Toxocara sp., 234–235, 477
Toxoplasmosis (*Toxoplasma gondii*), 392–393
Trachoma, 140–141
   and inclusion conjunctivitis, 394–395
Trade names, for antimicrobial agents, 513t–514t
Trauma-related infections, 56–57
Travel
   immunization guidelines for, 520t–521t
   immunocompromised patient and, 518t
   noninfectious hazards of, 515t–516t
   pregnancy and, 518t
Travel medical kit, 515t
Travel-related illness, prevention of, 515t–518t
Traveler's diarrhea, 396–397
Treponema carateum, 477
Treponema pallidum, 382–383
Trichinosis (*Trichinella spiralis*), 398–399, 477
Trichomoniasis, 400–401
Trichomoniasis vaginitis (*Trichomonas vaginalis*), 400–401
Trichophyton sp., 378–379
Trichosporon beigelii, 478
Trichostrongylus sp., 478
Trichuriasis (*Trichuris trichiura*), 354–355, 478
Trimethoprim-sulfamethoxazole
   adverse reactions to, frequency of, 485t
   drug interactions with, 486t
Tropheryma whippelii, 478
Trypanosomiasis (*Trypanosoma* sp.), 402–403
TSLS (toxic shock-like syndrome), 390–391
TSS (toxic shock syndrome), 390–391
Tuberculosis, 404–405
   vaccine for, 508t
Tuberculous lesions, genital, 22–23
Tularemia, 406–407

Tunga penetrans, 479
Typhoid fever, 408–409
   vaccine for, 501t
      in immunocompromised host, 503t
      travel and, 517t–518t, 520t
      use of, 505t
Typhus, 410–411

Upper respiratory viral infection, 138–139
Upper urinary tract infection (pyelonephritis), 340–341
Ureaplasma urealyticum, 479
Urethral discharge, 58–59
Urethral syndrome, 58
   acute, 16
Urethritis, 58–59
Urinary tract infection, 16–17, 150–151
   upper (pyelonephritis), 340–341
URTI (upper respiratory viral infection), 138–139
UTI. *See* Urinary tract infection
Uveitis, 46–47, 132–133

Vaccines
   administration routes for, 500t–501t
   availability, 500t–501t
   in immunocompromised patients, 502t
   live, in immunocompromised host, 503t
   use of, 505t–508t
Vaccinia, in immunocompromised host, 503t
Vaginal discharge, 60–61
Vaginitis, 60–61
   Candida, 116–117
   trichomoniasis, 400–401
Vaginosis, bacterial, 90–91
Varicella zoster immunoglobulin
   in adults, 495t, 496t
   in children, 498t, 499t
   in travelers, 520t
   use of, 508t
Varicella zoster virus
   chickenpox and, 126–127
   immunization guidelines for
      in adults, 495t–496t
      in children, 498t, 499t
   reactivation of (herpes zoster), 212–213
   vaccine for, 501t
Vasculitis, acute, 230–231
Vector-borne disease
   differential diagnosis of, 3
   immunization for, 517t, 520t
   insect bites and stings and, 26
Veillonella parvula, 479
Verruga peruana, 94–95
Vibrio sp., 480
Vibrio cholerae. *See* Cholera
Visceral abscess, 226–227
Visceral larvae migrans, 234–235
Vomiting, from antibacterial drugs, frequency of, 484t–485t
VZIG. *See* Varicella zoster immunoglobulin
VZV. *See* Varicella zoster virus

Warts, 412–413
Water-borne diseases
   immunization for, 517t, 521t
   and traveler's diarrhea, 396–397
Weeksella sp., 480
Whipworm infection, 354–355
Whooping cough. *See* Pertussis
Wohlfahrtia magnifica, 458
Wound infections, surgical, 380–381
Wuchereria bancrofti (filariasis), 186–187

Yellow fever, 414–415
   in Africa and South America, 521f
   vaccine for, 501t
      in immunocompromised host, 503t
      travel and, 517t, 520t
      use of, 505t
Yellow fever virus. *See* Yellow fever
Yersinia sp. infections, 416–417. *See also* Plague

Zoonosis, defined, 26